# Neuroradiology
## The Core Requisites

# Neuroradiology
## The Core Requisites

**FIFTH EDITION**

**Rohini Nadgir, MD**
Associate Professor of Radiology
Division of Neuroradiology
Russell H. Morgan Department of Radiology and Radiological Sciences
Johns Hopkins University School of Medicine
Baltimore, Maryland

**Doris D.M. Lin, MD, PhD**
Professor of Radiology
Division of Neuroradiology
Russell H. Morgan Department of Radiology and Radiological Sciences
Johns Hopkins University School of Medicine
Baltimore, Maryland

**David M. Yousem, MD, MBA**
Professor of Radiology
Division of Neuroradiology
Russell H. Morgan Department of Radiology and Radiological Sciences
Johns Hopkins University School of Medicine
Baltimore, Maryland

ELSEVIER

**Elsevier**
1600 John F. Kennedy Blvd.
Ste 1800
Philadelphia, PA 19103-2899

**NEURORADIOLOGY**
**THE CORE REQUISITES**
**FIFTH EDITION**

ISBN: **978-0-323-75975-5**

Previous editions copyrighted 2017, 2010, 2003, and 1994.

*Senior Content Development Manager*: Somodatta Roy Choudhury
*Senior Content Strategist*: Melanie Tucker
*Publishing Services Manager*: Shereen Jameel
*Project Manager*: Vishnu T. Jiji
*Senior Designer*: Amy L. Buxton

Printed in India

Last digit is the print number: 9 8 7 6 5 4 3 2 1

# List of Contributors

**Chapter 1**
*Monica Watkins, MD*
Clinical Associate
Director of Neuroradiology
Johns Hopkins Hospital North Capital Region
Bethesda, Maryland

**Chapter 2**
*Margaret N. Chapman, MD*
Neuroradiologist
Virginia Mason Medical Center
Seattle, Washington

**Chapter 3**
*Oluwatoyin Idowu, MD*
Fairfax Radiology Centers
Fairfax, Virginia;
Adjunct Professor of Radiology
Russell H. Morgan Department of Radiology and
    Radiological Sciences
Johns Hopkins University School of Medicine
Baltimore, Maryland

**Chapter 4**
*Noushin Yahyavi-Firouz-Abadi, MD, MBA*
Associate Professor of Radiology and Nuclear Medicine
Vice Chair of Business Affairs
University of Maryland School of Medicine
Baltimore, Maryland

**Chapter 5**
*Karen Buch, MD*
Assistant Professor of Radiology
Harvard Medical School
Massachusetts General Hospital
Boston, Massachusetts

**Chapter 6**
*Doris D.M. Lin, MD, PhD*
Professor of Radiology
Division of Neuroradiology
Russell H. Morgan Department of Radiology and
    Radiological Sciences
Johns Hopkins University School of Medicine
Baltimore, Maryland

**Chapter 7**
*Memi Watanabe, MD*
Radiologist
Department of Radiology
Videbimus Toranomon Clinic
Tokyo, Japan

**Chapter 8**
*Melike Guryildirim, MD*
Assistant Professor
Section of Pediatric Neuroradiology
Russell H. Morgan Department of Radiology and
    Radiological Sciences
Johns Hopkins University School of Medicine
Baltimore, Maryland

*Aylin Tekes, MD*
Associate Professor
Section of Pediatric Neuroradiology
Russell H. Morgan Department of Radiology and
    Radiological Sciences
Johns Hopkins University School of Medicine
Baltimore, Maryland

**Chapter 9**
*Jarunee Intrapiromkul, MD*
Assistant Professor of Radiology
Russell H. Morgan Department of Radiology and
    Radiological Sciences
Johns Hopkins University School of Medicine
Baltimore, Maryland

**Chapter 10**
*Rohini Nadgir, MD*
Associate Professor of Radiology
Division of Neuroradiology
Russell H. Morgan Department of Radiology and
    Radiological Sciences
Johns Hopkins University School of Medicine
Baltimore, Maryland

**Chapter 11**
*Naoko Saito, MD, PhD*
Associate Professor of Radiology
Juntendo University
Tokyo, Japan

**Chapter 12**
*Karen Buch, MD*
Assistant Professor of Radiology
Harvard Medical School
Massachusetts General Hospital
Boston, Massachusetts

**Chapter 13**
*Elcin Zan, MD*
Assistant Professor
Department of Radiology
Weill Cornell Medicine
New York, New York

**Chapter 14**
*Karen Buch, MD*
Assistant Professor of Radiology
Harvard Medical School
Massachusetts General Hospital
Boston, Massachusetts

**Chapter 15**
*Rohini Nadgir, MD*
Associate Professor of Radiology
Division of Neuroradiology
Russell H. Morgan Department of Radiology and
    Radiological Sciences
Johns Hopkins University School of Medicine
Baltimore, Maryland

**Chapter 16**
*Margaret N. Chapman, MD*
Neuroradiologist
Virginia Mason Medical Center
Seattle, Washington

# Foreword

## Neuroradiology: Core Requisites, 5e

Congratulations to Drs. Rohini Nadgir, Doris D.M. Lin, and David M. Yousem for producing *Neuroradiology: Core Requisites*, Fifth Edition, the fourth edition to be published in the new format of the *Requisites in Radiology* series. Previous editions of *Neuroradiology: The Requisites* have been very well received for their concise and effective style in providing the key information radiologists need in their practices. The new outline format of the *Core Requisites* series is designed to further enhance ease of access to this key information. Drs. Nadgir, Lin, and Yousem have done a terrific job in pivoting their text to the new format to achieve this.

Although the format of *Neuroradiology: Core Requisites, 5e*, has changed, it builds on the outstanding tradition of the first four editions. The book is laid out logically in three sections covering the brain, head and neck, and spine. Within each major section, the text addresses both fundamentals and specific diseases and conditions. The reader is first given the tools to understand image content and is then presented with the most common and important conditions affecting the respective locations. Each chapter is written by an expert in the subject matter.

The invention of CT scanning for studies of the brain in the early 1970s put neuroradiology in the driver's seat to lead the entire field of radiology into the age of digital and cross-sectional imaging. CT was followed quickly by the invention and development of other methods based on magnetic resonance imaging, positron emission scanning, and ultrasound imaging to greatly expand the scope and importance of radiology. Each method has also continued to rapidly evolve. This has made it challenging for radiologists to stay current and up to date. The authors of *Neuroradiology: Core Requisites, 5e*, do an outstanding job in presenting the current state of the art to help close potential knowledge gaps.

Given the richness and diversity of imaging possibilities, a corollary challenge to the need to stay current about each method per se is to understand when to employ each one of them. To this end, the material in *Neuroradiology: Core Requisites, 5e*, is presented in the context of diseases and conditions with the discussion indicating the most useful and appropriate imaging methods rather than clustering the discussions based on modality as many texts do.

As noted, the format of the *Core Requisites* series is substantially different than the traditional series, but the philosophy remains the same—the production of books covering the core material required across the spectrum of what radiologists need to know from their first encounters as residents to studying for Board exams and later for reference in clinical practice. The books are not intended to be encyclopedic but to be practical and to still cover the vast majority of material encountered in daily practice. We hope that radiologists, whether in training or in practice, will find the books of the *Core Requisites* series useful, as will physicians in related fields, such as neurology and neurosurgery. The books in the *Core Requisites* series continue to be richly illustrated.

Congratulations again to Drs. Nadgir, Lin, and Yousem for adding this excellent text to the new *Core Requisites* series. I hope that this and the other new *Core Requisites* books will find the same excellent reception and be regarded with the same fondness as so many of the books that have come before.

*James H. Thrall, MD*
Chairman Emeritus
Department of Radiology
Massachusetts General Hospital
Distinguished Taveras Professor of Radiology
Harvard Medical School
Boston, Massachusetts

# *Preface*

Since the inception of this fifth edition of *Neuroradiology: The Core Requisites*, the world I thought I knew has changed a thousand-fold. I know that I am not alone in saying that it has been tough to stay afloat, maintain hope, and have the courage to take on a new day in a world fraught with human/women's rights violations, global health inadequacies, climate crises, international conflicts, economic anxiety, and feelings of isolation. In this context, the desire to bring friends and colleagues closer together and share in the joy of writing became the driving force in the making of this book.

Building on the foundation of core neuroradiology tenets set forth by the inimitable Drs. Grossman and Yousem in the first three editions of *Neuroradiology: The Requisites*, this latest edition carries with it the weighty knowledge and experience of 12 additional brilliant neuroradiologists, all women, many of color and from around the world, whom I have had the privilege of learning from and with over the past decade or so.

This edition includes the latest updates in neuroradiology, new figures, essential teaching points, and physics pearls, all in a much more streamlined bulleted format for ease of reading by the radiology trainee and radiologist in practice. In the spirit of brevity (your time is valuable, we know!), this version may be a little less funny than before, but there is still "fun" to be had in these 16 chapters covering all of neuroimaging from head to coccyx.

I am indebted to our contributing authors who have transformed this text into its current modernized form. I am immensely grateful to Drs. Yousem and Lin for their guidance, support, generosity, and kindness as we pieced this book together; I am blessed to call them my forever mentors and friends. I would like to extend gratitude to the staff at Elsevier for their patient encouragement. Last but not least, I want to thank trainees past, present, and future for keeping me honest and on my toes; I hope this fifth edition reveals to you the beauty and joy of neuroimaging, just as the prior editions by the esteemed Drs. Grossman and Yousem did for me many moons ago.

**Rohini Nadgir, MD**

# Contents

# PART I

# BRAIN

# 1 *Cranial Anatomy*

MONICA WATKINS

Neuroimaging gives us a finite representation of a brain that is infinitely complex in structure with functions we have yet to fully discover. Much of determining pathology begins with mastering normal anatomy. This chapter intends to provide an overview of intracranial structures with a focus on their location, nomenclature, and functional neurologic systems to serve as a baseline guide for interpretation at the workstation.

## Topographic Anatomy
## Supratentorial Brain

### CEREBRAL HEMISPHERES

■ The superior aspect of the brain is formed by the left and right cerebral hemispheres. The hemispheres are divided at midline by a large cerebrospinal fluid (CSF) cleft, the interhemispheric fissure, and a dural reflection, the falx cerebri. Each cerebral hemisphere contains a frontal, parietal, temporal, and occipital lobe. The inferior aspect of the brain consists of the cerebellum and brain stem separated from the superior brain by another dural reflection, the tentorium. The supratentorial brain containing the cerebral hemispheres and the infratentorial brain contains the brain stem and cerebellum.

■ Each cerebral hemisphere brain surface is a complex layered shell of gray matter cortex arranged in a pattern of gyri with CSF-filled clefts (sulci) in between. The surface gyral pattern varies from person to person. The pattern is variable within each individual person when compared left to right and anterior to posterior. However, there are key anatomic constants to identify to ensure consistency in radiology reports.

■ We aim to approach cortical anatomy the way one would interpret images at the workstation, in the axial, coronal, and sagittal planes. Beginning with an axial computed tomography (CT) image at the top of the head (Fig. 1.1), the frontal gyri from medial to lateral are the superior frontal gyrus and middle frontal gyrus. Between these two gyri is the superior frontal sulcus. Posterior to the middle frontal gyrus is the precentral sulcus, which joins the superior frontal gyrus in a T-shaped intersection.

■ The primary motor strip of the cerebral cortex lies posterior to the precentral sulcus. The primary motor strip contains a posterior lobulation (the "knob") that corresponds with the hand motor cortex. The appearance of the "knob" is also known as the "sigmoid hook sign" or the "upside down omega sign." The central (Rolandic) sulcus is posterior to the primary motor strip. Brain parenchyma anterior to the central sulcus is the frontal lobe with the parietal lobe posterior to the central sulcus.

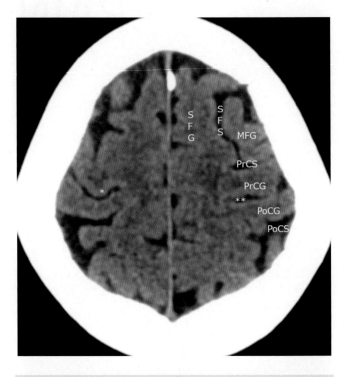

**Fig. 1.1 Axial computed tomography (CT) through the superior aspect of the brain shows the first gyrus to the left of midline, the superior frontal gyrus (SFG) followed by the middle frontal gyrus (MFG) with the superior frontal sulcus (SFS) between these two structures.** The SFS connects posteriorly with the precentral sulcus (PrCS). The precentral gyrus (PrCG) or motor strip is posterior to the PrCS, followed by the central sulcus (\*\*), postcentral gyrus (PoCG) or sensory strip, and the postcentral sulcus (PoCS). The asterisk (\*) on the right marks a knob-shaped region corresponding to the hand motor area in the precentral gyrus.

The central sulcus is a critical structure to reliably identify, particularly in surgical planning for a peri-Rolandic lesion to determine the expected location of primary motor cortex in an effort to preserve motor function.

■ The sagittal plane at midline provides additional ways to identify the central sulcus by magnetic resonance imaging (MRI) (Fig. 1.2A). The corpus callosum, the curvilinear band of white matter connecting the cerebral hemispheres, is easily discernable. The first gyrus draping over the corpus callosum is the cingulate gyrus, part of the limbic system to be described later in this chapter. The cingulate sulcus overlies and follows the course of the corpus callosum anteriorly but posteriorly makes an abrupt turn superiorly toward the brain surface and is known as the *pars marginalis*.

■ Proceeding anterior to the pars marginalis is the postcentral gyrus, the center for somatic sensation, followed

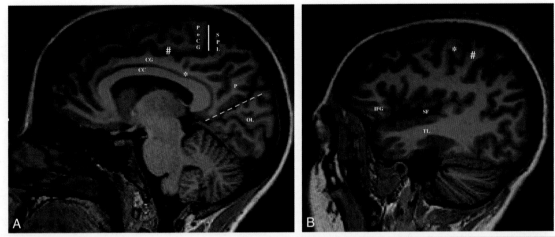

**Fig. 1.2 Important anatomic landmarks on sagittal imaging.** (A) Midline sagittal T1-weighted image (T1WI) with the corpus callosum *(CC)* easily identified. The asterisk marks the callosal sulcus at the superior margin of the CC followed by the cingulate gyrus *(CG)*. The cingulate sulcus (#) outlines the superior margin of the CG. The pars marginalis *(solid white line)* is a vertically oriented continuation of the cingulate sulcus and extends to the brain surface with the postcentral gyrus *(PoCG)* anterior to it. Posterior to the PoCG is the superior parietal lobule *(SPL)*. The parietal occipital sulcus (dashed line) demarcates parietal lobe *(P)* from occipital lobe *(OL)*. (B) Sagittal T1WI further lateral. The sylvian fissure demarcates the frontal and parietal lobes from the temporal lobes with the inferior frontal gyrus *(IFG)*, lying just above the sylvian fissure anteriorly *(SF)*. The curved "knob" of precentral sulcus *(\*)* sits anterior to the postcentral gyrus *(#)*.

by the central sulcus and the precentral gyrus. Together, these structures are known as the *paracentral lobule*. More lateral in the sagittal plane, the curved "knob" of the precentral gyrus can be seen laying within the postcentral gyrus (see Fig. 1.2B). Fig. 1.3 summarizes additional clues to identifying the central sulcus. In the sagittal plane, posterior to the postcentral gyrus of the parietal lobe lies the superior parietal lobule.

**TEACHING POINTS**

Helpful Tricks in Localizing the Central Sulcus

- The central sulcus enters the paracentral lobule anterior to the marginal ramus of the cingulate sulcus.
- The medial end of the postcentral sulcus is shaped like a bifid "y," and the bifid ends enclose the marginal ramus of the cingulate sulcus.
- The superior frontal sulcus terminates in the precentral sulcus, and the central sulcus is the next sulcus posterior to the precentral sulcus.
- The interparietal sulcus intersects the postcentral sulcus.
- The knob representing the hand motor area is in the precentral gyrus.
- The precentral gyrus's cortical gray matter thickness is greater than that of the postcentral gyrus thickness. Usually pre/post thickness ratio is about 1.5:1.
- The peri-Rolandic cortex is more hypointense than surrounding cortex on fluid-attenuated inversion recovery (FLAIR).

- In the coronal plane, if we begin anterior and inferior at the skull base, the gyrus rectus is positioned just lateral to the lowest portion of the interhemispheric fissure. Lateral to the gyrus rectus is the olfactory sulcus followed by the orbitofrontal gyrus directly overlying the orbits (Fig. 1.4).

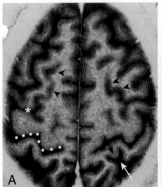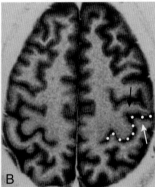

**Fig. 1.3 Central sulcus.** (A) Note the shape of the medial end of the postcentral sulcus, the bifid "y" (between *white* and *black arrows*) and how the superior frontal sulcus *(arrowheads)* terminates in the precentral sulcus *(asterisk)*. (B) The central sulcus is the next sulcus posterior to the precentral sulcus (between *white* and *black arrows*). Note that precentral gyrus's cortical gray matter *(black arrow)* thickness is greater than that of the postcentral gyrus *(white arrow)* cortical thickness. The central sulcus is indicated by dotted line in both images.

- Moving posterior in the coronal plane, we can divide the frontal lobes into the superior frontal gyrus, middle frontal gyrus, and inferior frontal gyrus (Fig. 1.5). The most posterior portion of the inferior frontal gyrus is the pars operculum, which essentially means the "lid" that covers the sylvian fissure and the insular cortex and contains portions of the Broca motor speech area. The insular cortex is a discrete region separate from the frontal, parietal, and temporal lobes with somatosensory function. Along the undersurface of the inferior frontal gyrus is the sylvian fissure demarcating the frontal lobe from the temporal lobe as well as the parietal lobe from the temporal lobe.
- The anatomy of the temporal lobe, whose primary functions include elements of speech, memory, emotion, and hearing, is well evaluated in the coronal plane (see

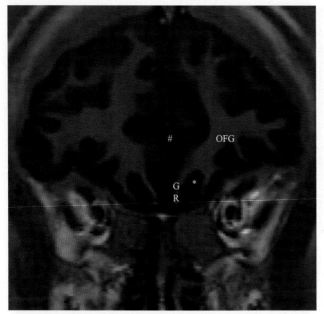

Fig. 1.4 **Coronal T1-weighted image (T1WI) demonstrating anatomy of the rostral brain over the orbits.** Lateral to the interhemispheric fissure (#) is the gyrus rectus (GR). The olfactory sulcus (*) separates the GR from the orbitofrontal gyrus (OFG) lying over the orbits.

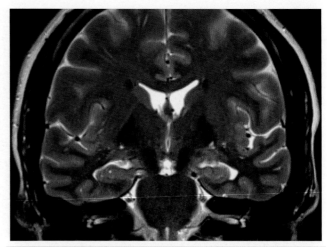

Fig. 1.6 **The characteristic curved shape of the hippocampus (*),** a part of the limbic system, is easy to identify in the mesial temporal lobe adjacent to the temporal horn of the lateral ventricles. The structure contains two layers of gray matter: dentate gyrus and Ammon horn (cornu ammonis). The hippocampus serves in memory function and is highly susceptible to anoxic injury.

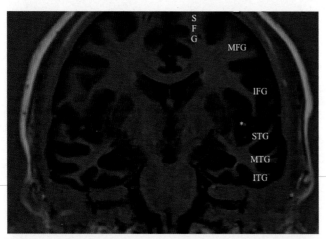

Fig. 1.5 **Coronal T1-weighted image (T1WI) through the temporal lobes region with lobes marked superior to inferior**: Superior frontal gyrus (SFG), middle frontal gyrus (MFG), inferior frontal gyrus (IFG), superior temporal gyrus (STG), middle temporal gyrus (MTG), and inferior temporal gyrus (ITG). The opercular (meaning lid) portion of the IFG covers the insular cortex (*).

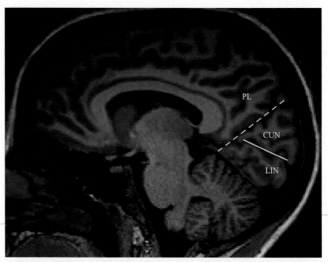

Fig. 1.7 **Sagittal T1-weighted image (T1WI).** The parieto-occipital sulcus (dashed line) demarcates the parietal lobe (PL) from the occipital lobe (OL). Within the occipital lobe, the calcarine sulcus (solid line) extends obliquely, with the cuneus (CUN) above and the lingual gyrus (LIN) below it.

Fig. 1.5). The temporal lobe lies just inferior to the sylvian fissure with three main gyri including the superior temporal gyrus, middle temporal gyrus, and the inferior temporal gyrus. The most recognizable portion of the medial aspect of the temporal lobe is the curved layered hippocampus, which is important in forming memories and highly susceptible to anoxic injury (Fig. 1.6). The almond-shaped amygdala lies just anterior to the hippocampus. Both the hippocampus and amygdala are part of the limbic system.

- The occipital lobe, whose primary function concerns vision, is well demonstrated in the sagittal plane at midline. The parieto-occipital sulcus demarcates the parietal lobe from the occipital lobe. The calcarine sulcus extends obliquely in the sagittal plane with the portion of the occipital lobe above the sulcus named the *cuneus* and the portion inferior to the sulcus named the *lingual gyrus* (Fig. 1.7).
- As a reminder, the central sulcus separates the frontal from the parietal lobe. The parieto-occipital sulcus separates the parietal lobe from the occipital lobe. The sylvian fissure separates the temporal lobe from the frontal and parietal lobes.

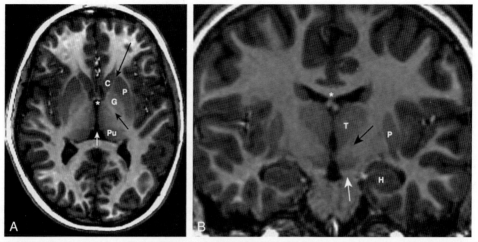

**Fig. 1.8 Deep gray matter anatomy.** (A) Axial T1-weighted image (T1WI) shows the caudate *(C)*, putamen *(P)*, and globus pallidus *(G)*, as well as the anterior limb *(long black arrow)* and posterior limb *(short black arrow)* of the internal capsule. White matter tracts pass between the basal ganglia. The thalamus and periaqueductal gray matter line the third ventricle. The tiny dots of the fornix anteriorly (just ventral to the *asterisk*) and the posterior commissure posteriorly *(white arrow)*, as well as pulvinar thalamic gray natter *(Pu)*, are also evident. (B) On this coronal T1WI, the subthalamic nucleus *(black arrow)* and substantia nigra *(white arrow)* can be seen under the thalami *(T)*. The hippocampus *(H)* is present further laterally. The thalami are joined in the midline at the massa intermedia, and one can also see the forniceal columns (just below the *asterisk*) projecting above the thalami.

## THALAMUS AND HYPOTHALAMUS

■ The thalamus is found on either side of the third ventricle and connects across the midline by the massa intermedia (Fig. 1.8). Its other functions include motor relays, limbic outputs, and coordination of movement. Portions of the thalamus also subserve pain, cognition, and emotions. The thalamus is subdivided into many different nuclei by white matter striae. The medial and lateral geniculate nuclei, located along the posterior aspect of the thalamus, serve as relay stations for auditory and visual function, respectively. The pulvinar is the posterior expansion of the thalamus. Behind the pulvinar are the wings of the ambient cistern.

■ The hypothalamus is located at the floor of the third ventricle, above the optic chiasm and suprasellar cistern. The hypothalamus is connected to the posterior pituitary via the infundibulum, or stalk, through which hormonal information to the pituitary gland is transmitted. The hypothalamus is critical to the autonomic functions of the body.

## BASAL GANGLIA

■ The basal ganglia are known by a number of names in the neuroanatomic literature. These gray matter structures lie between the insula and midline. The globus pallidus is the medial gray matter structure identified just lateral to the genu of the internal capsule (see Fig. 1.8). Lateral to it lies the putamen. The caudate nucleus head indents the frontal horns of the lateral ventricle and is anterior to the globus pallidus; however, the body of the caudate courses over the globus pallidus, paralleling the lateral ventricle and ending in a tail of tissue near the amygdala.

■ Additional terms used for the various portions of the basal ganglia include the corpus striatum, consisting of the caudate and the lentiform or lenticular nuclei. The lentiform is made up of the globus pallidus and putamen.

One can use the term "striatocapuslar region" to include the basal ganglia with the internal and external capsules. The basal ganglia receive fibers from the sensorimotor cortex, thalamus, and substantia nigra, as well as from each other. Efferents go to the same locations and to the hypothalamus. The main function of the basal ganglia appears to be coordination of smooth movement.

# Infratentorial Brain

## CEREBELLUM

■ The cerebellum is located in the infratentorial compartment posterior to the brain stem. The anatomy of the cerebellum is complex, with many named areas. For simplicity's sake, most people separate the cerebellum into the midline superior and inferior vermis and reserve the term "cerebellar hemispheres" for the rest of the lateral and central portions of the cerebellum.

■ The hemispheric portions of the cerebellum receive information from the pons and help control coordination of voluntary movements. Abnormalities within the cerebellar hemispheres result in dysmetria, dysdiadochokinesis (say THAT five times fast!), intention tremors, nystagmus, and ataxia. Ventrally, there is a bump called the *flocculus* on either side of the cerebellar hemisphere, which may extend toward the cerebellopontine angle cistern. This is a potential "pseudomass," often misidentified as a vestibular schwannoma. The tonsils are located inferiorly and are the structures that herniate downward through the foramen magnum in Chiari 1 malformations. The superior vermis has a central lobule and lingula visible anteriorly, and the inferior vermis has a nodulus, uvula, pyramid, and tuber on its inferior surface (Fig. 1.9). The superior surface provides a view of the culmen, declive, and folium of the superior vermis. The superior vermis and most of the inferior vermis receive spinocerebellar sensory information.

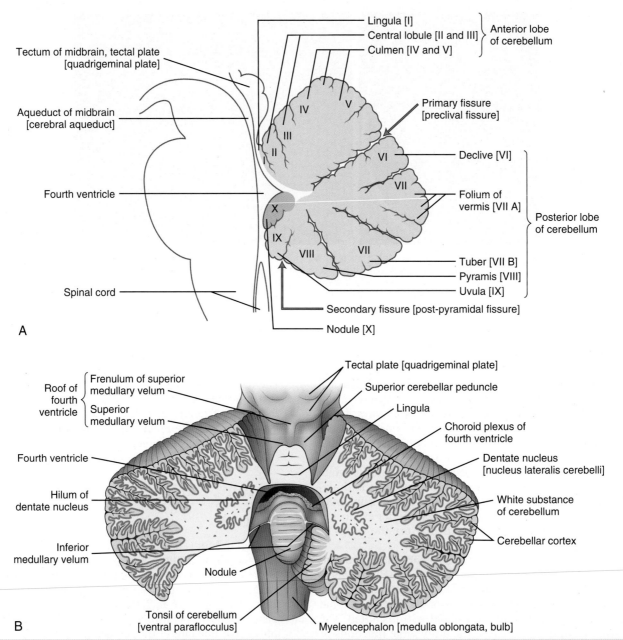

**Fig. 1.9  Cerebellar anatomy.** (A) Median and (B) coronal diagrams of the cerebellar lobes, lobules, and vermis. The cerebellar hemispheres and vermis are divided into 10 lobules (I–X). The primary fissure divides the cerebellum into anterior lobes (lobules I–V, including lingula, central lobule, and culmen) and posterior lobes (lobules VI–IX, including declive, folium, tuber, pyramid, and uvula). The secondary fissure separates the posterior lobe from the nodular lobe (lobule X). (From Putz R, Pabst R, eds. *Sobotta Atlas of Human Anatomy.* 13th ed. Philadelphia: Lippincott Williams & Wilkins; 1996:292, 293.)

- The cerebellum is made of cortex, white matter, and four paired of deep gray nuclei. Gray matter masses in the cerebellum include the fastigial, globose, emboliform, and dentate nuclei. The dentate nuclei are situated laterally in the white matter of the cerebellum and can be seen on CT because they may calcify in later life. The dentate nucleus, the largest deep gray matter structure, has connections to the red nuclei and to the thalami.
- Three major white matter tracts connect the cerebellum to the brain stem bilaterally (Fig. 1.10). The superior cerebellar peduncle (brachium conjunctivum) connects midbrain structures to the cerebellum, the middle cerebellar peduncle (brachium pontis) connects the pons to the cerebellum, and the inferior cerebellar

peduncle (restiform body) connects the medulla to the cerebellum.

## BRAIN STEM

- Starting superiorly, the brain stem consists of the midbrain, pons, and medulla.
- The midbrain is the site of origin of the third and fourth cranial nerves. Additionally, the midbrain contains the red nucleus, substantia nigra, and cerebral aqueduct, or aqueduct of Sylvius (Fig. 1.11). White matter tracts conducting the motor and sensory commands pass through the midbrain. The midbrain is also separated into the tegmentum and tectum, which refer to portions of the

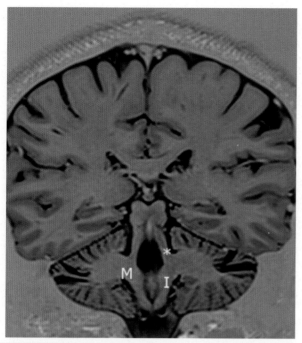

**Fig. 1.10 Cerebellar peduncles.** The paired cerebellar peduncles contain white matter tracts that connect the cerebellum to the brainstem. The inferior cerebellar peduncle (indicated on the left, I) aka restiform body contains spinocerebellar tracts from medulla. The middle cerebellar peduncle (indicated on the right, M) aka brachium pontis contains corticospinal fiber tracts from the pons, including corticopontine and pontocerebellar tracts terminating in the contralateral cerebellar hemisphere and vermis. The superior cerebellar peduncle (indicated on the left, *) aka brachium conjunctivum contains efferent fibers from the dentate nucleus, decussate at the inferior colliculus and extend to the contralateral red nucleus and thalamus.

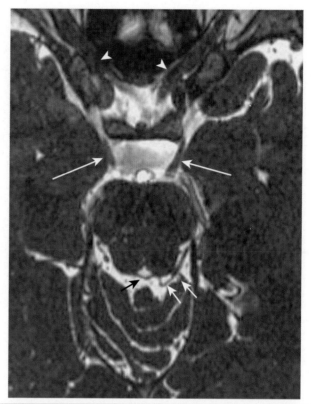

**Fig. 1.11 Midbrain anatomy.** This constructive interference steady state (CISS) image shows both oculomotor nerves *(long white arrows)* in their cisternal portions, leading to the cavernous sinus, the left trochlear nerve *(double arrows)* emanating from the posterior midbrain and coursing the ambient cistern, and the right trochlear nerve decussating posteriorly in the midline *(small black arrow)*. The optic nerves can be seen in the optic canals bilaterally *(arrowheads)*.

midbrain anterior and posterior to the cerebral aqueduct, respectively.

- The tectum, or roof, consists of the quadrigeminal plate (corpora quadrigemina), which houses the superior and inferior colliculi.
- The tegmentum contains the fiber tracts, red nuclei, third and fourth cranial nerve nuclei, and periaqueductal gray matter. The substantia nigra is within the anterior border of the tegmentum.
- Anterior to the tegmentum are the cerebral peduncles, which have somewhat of a "Mickey Mouse ears" configuration.

■ The pons contains the nuclei for cranial nerves (CN) V, VI, VII, and VIII (Figs. 1.12 and 1.13). Pontine white matter tracts transmit sensory and motor fibers to the face and body. The pons also houses major connections of the reticular activating system for vital functions. You can identify the pons on the sagittal scan by its "pregnant belly."

■ The medulla contains the nuclei for CN IX, X, XI, and XII. The sensory and motor tracts to and from the face and brain are transmitted through the medulla. Other named portions of the medulla include the pyramids, an anterior paramedian collection of fibers transmitting motor function, and the olivary nucleus in the mid medulla (Fig. 1.14A-B).

■ The Triangle of Guillain-Mollaret or the dentato-rubro-olivary pathway connects the brain stem and cerebellum

to coordinate motor activity (see Fig. 1.14C-D). The pathway consists of the red nucleus of the pons, the ipsilateral inferior olivary nucleus of the medulla, and the contralateral dentate nucleus of the cerebellum. Dysfunction along the pathway between the red nucleus and the ipsilateral inferior olivary nucleus (central tegmental tract) or between the red nucleus the contralateral dentate nucleus (dentato-rubral tract through the superior cerebellar peduncle) result in increased T2 signal and enlargement of the olive. For example, an acute hemorrhage in the left dorsal pons can result in hypertrophy of the left inferior olivary nucleus over several months. This entity is named *hypertrophic olivary degeneration* (HOD), with patients presenting with palatal myoclonus and limb ataxia.

## White Matter Tracts

There are three main categories of white matter tracts: commissural, association, and projection. Prominent commissural tracts connecting structures across midline are easily identified by conventional MRI sequences. Advances in diffusion tensor imaging (DTI) and three-dimensional (3D) fiber tracking help delineate axonal pathways of the association and projection tracts (Fig. 1.15).

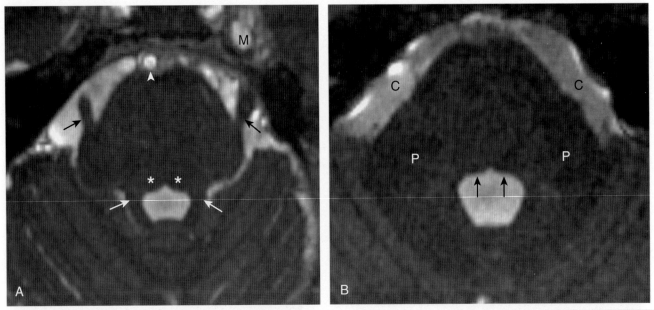

**Fig. 1.12 Pontine anatomy.** (A) Axial T2 constructive interference steady state (CISS) image shows cranial nerve V exiting the pons *(black arrows)*. Note the superior cerebellar peduncles *(white arrows)*, the Meckel's cave on the left *(M)*, medial longitudinal fasciculus *(asterisks)*, and basilar artery *(white arrowhead)*. (B) Facial colliculi *(arrows)* are clearly seen on this axial T2 CISS image. The middle cerebellar peduncle *(P)* is the dominant structure leading to the cerebellum. Also shown is the cerebellopontine angle cistern *(C)*.

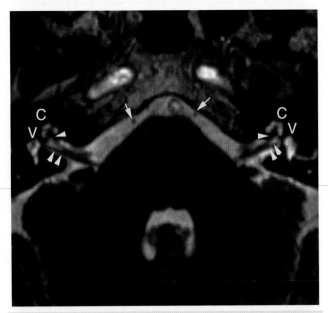

**Fig. 1.13 Lower pontine anatomy.** This constructive interference steady state (CISS) image shows the abducens nerve denoted by the white arrows, whereas the cochlear (more anterior) and inferior vestibular nerves (more posterior) are seen bilaterally in the cerebellopontine angle cistern *(single and double white arrowheads,* respectively). The fluid-filled cochlea *(C)* and vestibule *(V)* are hyperintense on T2.

Commissural: Bundles of fiber that extend across the midline

- Corpus callosum: Large midline white matter tract that spans the two cerebral hemispheres. Its named parts include the rostrum (its tapered anteroinferior portion just above the anterior commissure), the genu (the anterior sweep), the body or trunk (the most superior aspect),

and the splenium (the most posterior aspect) (Fig. 1.16). Often, there may be a focal narrowing within the posterior body, the so-called "isthmus," which is a normal anatomic variation and should not be confused with focal pathology.

- Anterior commissure: Located at the inferior aspect of the corpus callosum just above the lamina terminalis. The anterior commissure transmits tracts from the amygdala and temporal lobe to the contralateral side.
- Posterior commissure: Just anterior to the pineal gland near the habenula. The habenula and hippocampal commissures cross-connect the two hemispheres and thalami.

Association: Fibers can be long, connecting distant gyri, or short ("U" fibers), connecting gyri within the same lobe. Major tracts include the cingulum, uncinate fasciculus, superior longitudinal fasciculus, inferior longitudinal fasciculus, and inferior fronto-occipital fasciculus.

- The superior longitudinal fasciculus (SLF)/arcuate fasciculus complex connects the frontal lobe to the parietal and temporal cortex. The arcuate fasciculus has an arc-like trajectory linking the Wernicke (receptive) area in the temporal gyrus to the Broca (expressive) area in the inferior frontal gyrus, therefore playing a key role in language processing.
- The cingulum extends inferior to the cingulate gyrus along the medial aspect of each cerebral hemisphere connecting sections of the frontal, parietal, and temporal lobes. It allows communication between different components of the limbic system.

Projection: Include ascending and descending tracts connecting the cerebrum with the brain stem, cerebellum, and spinal cord. These tracts include the corona radiata, internal capsule, corticospinal tract, and corticobulbar tract.

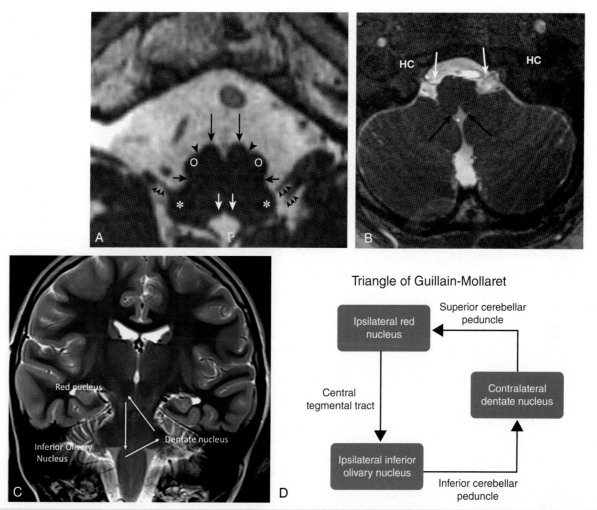

**Fig. 1.14 Medulla anatomy.** (A) Axial T2 constructive interference steady state (CISS) shows the postolivary sulcus *(short black arrows)*, the preolivary sulcus *(single arrowheads)*, pyramidal tract *(long black arrows)* and the inferior cerebellar peduncle *(asterisks)*, hypoglossal nuclei *(white arrows)*, and cranial nerves IX-X complex; *small triple arrowheads)*. The olive *(o)* can be seen anteriorly. (B) *White arrows* point out hypoglossal nerves coursing to hypoglossal canals *(HC)*. On either side of the midline posterior cleft are the gracile nuclei *(black arrows)*. Lateral to them will be the cuneate nuclei. (C–D) Triangle of Guillain-Mollaret or the dentato-rubro-olivary pathway: Anatomic feedback triangle connecting the red nucleus with the ipsi- lateral inferior olivary nucleus through the central tegmental tract. The dentate is connected to the contralateral red nucleus through the dentato-rubral tract and with the contralateral inferior olivary nucleus through the inferior cerebellar peduncle.

# Meninges and Associated Potential Spaces

- Exploring the intracranial compartment, outside to in, we first encounter the three layers of meninges protecting the brain: the dura, arachnoid, and pia (Fig. 5.1). The dura (pachymeninges) is the outermost thickest layer (1–2 mm in width) formed from an outer periosteal layer and an inner meningeal layer. The dura is adherent to the inner table of the skull at the sutures. Between the inner table of the skull and the dura is a potential space, the epidural space, which is only visible in pathologic conditions, such as an epidural hematoma. Pathology in the epidural space usually does not cross the sutures. Subjacent to the dura is the subdural space, another potential space visualized only in pathologic conditions.
- The next tissue layer, the arachnoid, is a thin sheet that aligns with the dura but is not tightly bound to it. The

subjacent CSF-filled subarachnoid space overlies the last tissue layer, the pia. The pia is closely approximated to the brain surface invaginating into the sulci. The pia and arachnoid cannot always be readily distinguished on imaging and are collectively referred to as the *leptomeninges*.
- The pial layer accompanies the cortical arteries as they course into the brain parenchyma. Nonpathologic prominent perivascular spaces or "Virchow-Robin spaces" occur when the potential space between the outer and inner pial layer becomes dilated with interstitial fluid. Typical locations include the striatocapsular region and midbrain (Fig. 1.17).

# Ventricular System, Cerebrospinal Fluid, and Cerebrospinal Fluid Spaces

- The normal volume of CSF in the entire central nervous system (CNS) is approximately 150 mL, with 75 mL distributed around the spinal cord, 25 mL within the

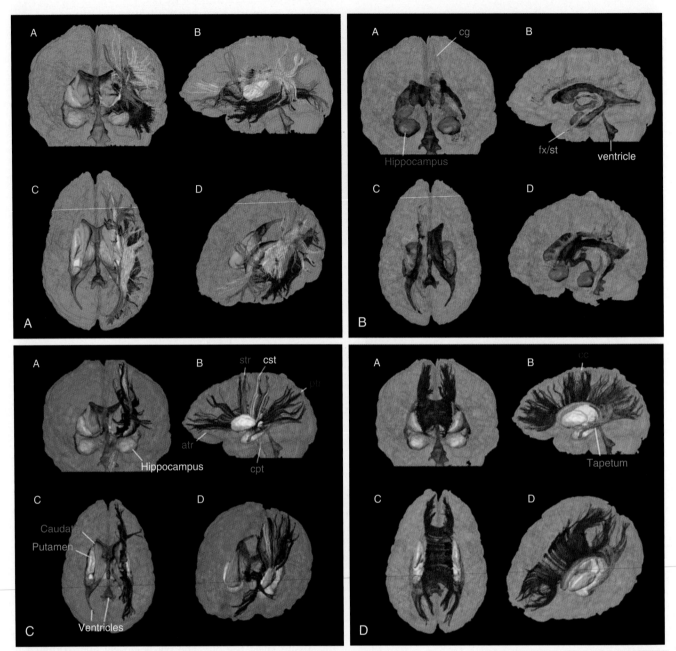

**Fig. 1.15 Diffusion tensor imaging (DTI) tractography.** Using DTI data, discrete fiber tracts in the brain can be isolated and color coded for your visual pleasure, demonstrating association fibers (those axon bundles connecting different parts of the brain in the same cerebral hemisphere), projection fibers (those axons connecting the cortex with lower parts of the brain and spinal cord), and commissural fibers (those axons connecting between the two cerebral hemispheres). (A) Three-dimensional (3D) reconstructions of association fibers are depicted, including in the anterior (A), left (B), superior (C), and oblique (left-anterosuperior) (D) orientations. Note the color-coded projections of the superior longitudinal fasciculus (*yellow*), inferior fronto-orbital fasciculus (*orange*), uncinate fasciculus (*red*), and inferior longitudinal fasciculus (*brown*). Thalami are yellow, ventricles are gray, caudate nuclei are green, and lentiform nuclei are light green. (B) 3D reconstruction results of association fibers in the limbic system viewed from the anterior (A), left (B), superior (C), and oblique (left- anterior) (D) orientations. The hippocampi are depicted in purple. (C) 3D reconstruction results of projection fibers viewed from the anterior (A), left (B), superior (C), and oblique (left-superior-anterior) (D) orientations. Depicted are anterior thalamic radiation (*atr*), corticopontine tract (*cpt*), corticospinal tract (*cst*), posterior thalamic radiation (*ptr*), and superior thalamic radiation (*str*). (D) 3D reconstructions of commissural fibers viewed from the anterior (A), left (B), superior (C), and oblique (left-anterior-superior) (D) orientations. The corpus callosum (*cc*) is color coded magenta and the tapetum (commissural fibers extending to temporal lobes) is color coded peach. *cg,* Cingulum; *fx,* fornix; *st,* stria terminalis. (From Oishi K, Faria AV, van Zijl PCM, Mori S. *MRI Atlas of Human White Matter.* 2nd ed. Philadelphia: Elsevier; 2011:18–21.)

ventricular system, and 50 mL surrounding the cortical sulci and in the cisterns at the base of the brain. In elderly persons, the intracranial CSF volume increases from 75 mL to a mean of approximately 150 mL in females and 190 mL in males. The normal production of CSF has been estimated to be approximately 450 mL/day, thereby replenishing the amount of CSF two to three times a day.

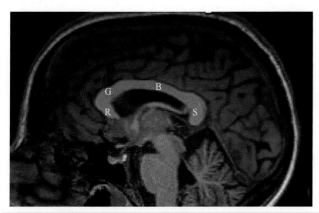

**Fig. 1.16 Midline sagittal T1 magnetic resonance (MR) of the corpus callosum.** The large white matter tract connects the cerebral hemispheres and consists of four parts: rostrum *(R)*, genu *(G)*, body *(B)*, and splenium *(S)*.

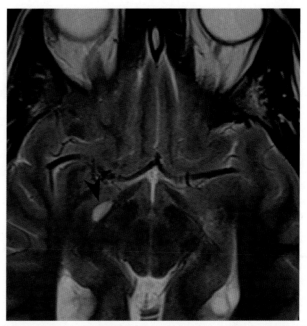

**Fig. 1.17 Virchow-Robin space.** Axial T2-weighted image shows prominent fluid-filled structure at the inferior aspect of the right basal ganglia *(arrowhead)*, typical appearance of Virchow-Robin space.

■ Each ventricle's choroid plexus contributes to CSF production, whereas the reabsorption of CSF occurs at the level of the arachnoid villi into the intravascular system from the extracellular fluid. Arachnoid villi reside on the surface of the brain and can project into the adjacent venous sinuses, appearing as fluid density/signal nonocclusive filling defects within the major venous sinuses.

■ The flow of CSF runs from the lateral ventricles via the foramina of Monro to the third ventricle, out the cerebral aqueduct of Sylvius, and into the fourth ventricle, finally exiting through the foramina of Luschka (bilaterally) and Magendie (in the midline; Fig. 1.18). CSF then flows into the cisterns of the brain and the cervical subarachnoid space and then down the intrathecal spinal compartments. The CSF ultimately percolates back up over the convexities of the hemispheres, where it is resorbed by the arachnoid villi into the intravascular space.

■ There are several named cisterns around the brain stem and midline structures (Fig. 1.19). The contents of these spaces can be compromised depending on the pathology at play, and critical structures coursing through these spaces may be affected and be the source of the patient's presenting complaint. Therefore, awareness of these cisterns and contents is critical in descriptions of different herniation syndromes and other pathologies that can be identified on imaging.

**TEACHING POINTS**

Cisterns of the Brain

| Name | Location | Structures Traversing Cistern |
|---|---|---|
| Cisterna magna | Posteroinferior to fourth ventricle | Vertebral arteries |
| Circum-medullary cistern | Around medulla | Posterior inferior cerebral artery |
| Superior cerebellar cistern | Above cerebellum | Basal vein of Rosenthal, vein of Galen |
| Prepontine cistern | Anterior to pons | Basilar artery, cranial nerves (CN) V and VI |
| Cerebellopontine angle cistern | Between pons and porus acusticus | Anterior inferior cerebellar artery, CN VII and VIII |
| Interpeduncular cistern | Between cerebral peduncles | CN III |
| Ambient (crural) cistern | Around midbrain | CN IV |
| Quadrigeminal plate cistern | Behind midbrain | Distal branches of posterior cerebral artery, superior cerebellar artery, CN IV, posterior choroidal artery |
| Suprasellar cistern | Above pituitary | Optic chiasm, CN III and IV, carotid arteries, pituitary stalk |
| Retropulvinar cistern (wings of ambient cistern) | Behind thalamus | Posterolateral choroidal artery |
| Cistern of lamina terminalis | Anterior to lamina terminalis, anterior commissure | Anterior cerebral artery (ACA) |
| Cistern of velum interpositum | Above third ventricle | Internal cerebral vein, vein of Galen |
| Cistern of the ACA | Above the corpus callosum | ACA |

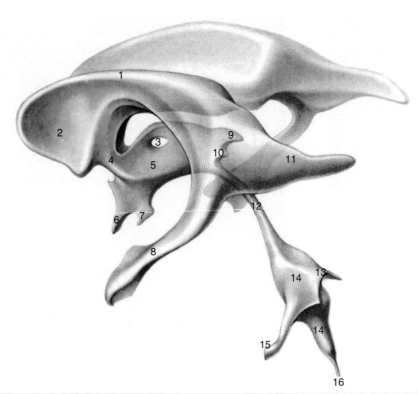

1 Lateral ventricle, body
2 Lateral ventricle, frontal horn
3 Massa intermedia
4 Foramen of Monro
5 Third ventricle
6 Optic recess, third ventricle
7 Infundibular recess, third ventricle
8 Temporal horn, lateral ventricle
9 Suprapineal recess, third ventricle
10 Pineal recess, third ventricle
11 Occipital horn, lateral ventricle
12 Aqueduct of Sylvius
13 Fastigium
14 Fourth ventricle
15 Lateral recess, foramen
   Luschka, fourth ventricle
16 Central canal

**Fig. 1.18  Ventricular system of the brain.** Three-dimensional diagram of the ventricular system of the brain is labeled. (From Nieuwenhuys R, Voogd J, van Huijen C. *The Human Central Nervous System: A Synopsis and Atlas.* Rev 3rd ed. Berlin: Springer-Verlag; 1988.)

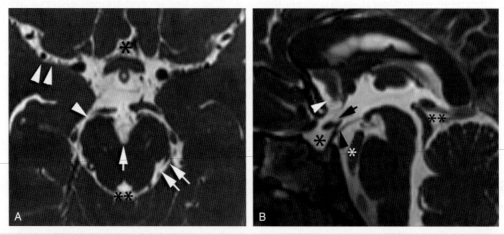

**Fig. 1.19  Cisterns of the brain.** (A) Axial constructive interference steady state (CISS) image shows the interpeduncular cistern *(single arrow)*, ambient cistern *(single arrowhead)*, perimesencephalic cistern *(double arrows)*, sylvian fissure *(double arrowheads)*, and quadrigeminal plate cistern *(double asterisk)*. The cistern of the lamina terminalis is indicated by a *single asterisk*. (B) Sagittal CISS image shows the cistern of the lamina terminalis *(arrowhead)*, suprasellar cistern *(single black asterisk)*, and quadrigeminal plate cistern *(double black asterisk)*. The basilar artery *(white asterisk)* is seen coursing the prepontine cistern. The chiasmatic recess *(black arrow)* and infundibular recess *(black arrowhead)* are also indicated.

## Physiologic Calcifications

- The pineal gland calcifies with age. A small percentage (2% of children younger than 8 years old and 10% of adolescents) of children show calcification of the pineal gland. By 30 years of age, most people have calcified pineal glands. Anterior to the pineal gland, one often sees the habenular commissure as a calcified curvilinear structure. The choroid plexus is calcified in about 5% of children by age 15, and most adults by age 40. Such calcifications may be seen in the lateral, third, and fourth ventricles, as well as the foramina of Luschka, Magendie, and choroid fissures.

- The dura of the falx and/or tentorium is virtually never calcified in children and should be viewed as suspicious for basal cell nevus syndrome in that setting. However, in adults, foci of calcification and even ossification of the dura, tentorium, and falx are not uncommon. The dura shows higher rates of calcification in patients who have had shunts placed or have been irradiated.

- Basal ganglia calcification is also rarely observed in individuals younger than 30 years of age and should provoke a search for metabolic disorders or a past history of perinatal infections if seen in youngsters. Over the age of 30, however, basal ganglia calcifications are very common to the point that these do not necessarily need to be mentioned in routine reporting unless true pathology is suspected. Such benign basal ganglia mineralization is typically bilateral, although in some cases it may be more conspicuous on one side compared with the other. Care must be made not to confuse these physiologic calcifications, which are hyperdense on CT, with hemorrhage, which is also hyperdense on CT. Dual-energy CT imaging can be useful in making the distinction in difficult cases. The choroid plexus also calcifies with increasing age, and the same caveats apply.

## Cranial Nerves

- How many medical students over the years have recited one of the classic mnemonics for the cranial nerves: On old Olympus' towering tops, a Finn and German viewed some hops (olfactory, optic, oculomotor, trochlear, trigeminal, abducens, facial, acoustic [vestibulocochlear], glossopharyngeal, vagus, spinal accessory, and hypoglossal nerves)? The phrase remains imprinted forever, but here is a refresher on the anatomy. We have already reviewed the site of CN nuclei within the brain stem. Each CN has a varied path through the intracranial compartment to traverse skull base foramina to reach extracranial structures. We will describe the function of each of their nuclei, intracranial pathways, and structures they innervate in more detail in a later section, but in brief summary:
- CN I, the olfactory nerve, provides information for smell.
- CN II, the optic nerve, provides a sense of vision.
- CN III, the oculomotor nerve, provides motor innervation to the extraocular muscles, except the lateral rectus and superior oblique with parasympathetic fibers to ciliary body controlling pupillary dilatation.
- CN IV, the trochlear nerve, provides motor innervation to the superior oblique muscles.
- CN V, the trigeminal nerve, provides sensory information from the head and face and motor innervation to the muscles of mastication.
- CN VI, the abducens nerve, provides motor innervation to the lateral rectus.
- CN VII, the facial nerve, provides motor innervation to the facial expression muscles; taste from the anterior two thirds of the tongue; and innervation to the lacrimal, submandibular, and sublingual glands.
- CN VIII, the vestibulocochlear nerve, serves our sense of hearing and balance.
- CN IX, the glossopharyngeal nerve, has functions that include taste for the posterior third of the tongue, sensation for the posterior third of the tongue, and the internal aspect of the tympanic membrane and parasympathetic innervation to the parotid gland. CN IX also supplies the stylopharyngeus muscles.
- CN X, the vagus nerve, provides motor to and transmits sensory and parasympathetic information from the pharynx and larynx and thoracic and abdominal viscera.
- CN XI, the accessory nerve, provides motor innervation to the sternocleidomastoid and trapezius muscles.
- CN XII, the hypoglossal nerve, provides motor supply to the intrinsic and extrinsic tongue muscles.
- MRI, particularly with thin section images, is typically performed when CN pathology is suspected. It is important to examine the entire course of the nerve, including the extracranial portion. For example, if pathology involving CN VII is suspected, the field of view should include the cerebellopontine angle, the temporal bone, and the parotid region. To evaluate the entire trigeminal nerve system, images would include the brain stem and the entire face. CN II, III, IV, and VI are well evaluated with dedicated images of the brain stem, cavernous sinuses, and the orbits.

**TEACHING POINTS CN I SUMMARY**

| Cranial Nerve (CN) I | Olfactory Nerve |
|---|---|
| Function | Provide afferent sensory information for smell to the central nervous system |
| Origin | Primary afferent neurosensory cells in the roof of both nasal cavities |
| Foramina | Efferent axons travel through numerous perforations within the cribriform plate of the ethmoid bone. |
| Destination | Secondary sensory neurons within the olfactory bulbs, which lie in the olfactory groove |
| Pathways in brain | Olfactory bulb becomes the olfactory tract, which divides into the lateral, intermediate, and medial striae. Largest amount of fibers travel within the lateral striae to the inferior medial temporal lobe amygdala |
| Important pathology | 1. Dysfunction results in anosmia with traumatic injury as leading etiology<br>2. Esthesioneuroblatoma: A tumor arising from the olfactory epithelium |

**TEACHING POINTS CN II SUMMARY**

| Cranial Nerve (CN) II | Optic Nerve |
|---|---|
| Function | Vision |
| Origin | Photoreceptors in the retina |
| Foramina | Optic canal |
| Destination | Optic chiasm |
| Pathways in brain | Extending posterior to the optic chiasm is the optic tract, which then divides into the lateral branch with fibers traversing to the lateral geniculate body of the thalamus and the medial branch with fibers traversing to the medial geniculate body of the thalamus. Efferent axons lead from the lateral geniculate body form the optic radiation terminating within the calcarine cortex |
| Important pathology | Visual deficits depending on portion of optic nerve affected, including demyelinating, ischemic, infectious/inflammatory, toxic/metabolic, neoplastic, and congenital processes, as well as glaucoma |

## TEACHING POINTS CRANIAL NERVE III SUMMARY

| Cranial Nerve (CN) III | Oculomotor |
|---|---|
| Function | Eye movement |
| Origin | 1. Oculomotor nuclei in the ventral midbrain just posterior to the red nucleus and anterior to the superior aspect of the cerebral aqueduct<br>2. Edinger-Westphal parasympathetic nuclei: Dorsal to the oculomotor nuclei |
| Intracranial pathway | Exits the midbrain in the interpeduncular cistern, travels between the posterior cerebral artery and superior cerebellar artery, and inferior to the posterior communicating artery. Travels along the superolateral wall of the cavernous sinus |
| Foramina | Superior orbital fissure |
| Destination/Extracranial branches | 1. Superior branch to the levator palpebrae superioris and superior rectus muscles<br>2. Inferior branch to the inferior rectus, medial rectus<br>3. Parasympathetic fibers to ciliary body controlling pupillary dilatation |
| Important pathology | 1. Compression by aneurysm of the posterior communicating artery (most common), posterior cerebral artery, and superior cerebellar artery can cause a third nerve palsy<br>2. Leptomeningeal disease including infectious, inflammatory, and neoplastic processes can affect CN III function<br>3. Horner's syndrome: Ptosis (because of sympathetic supply to superior tarsus portion of the levator palpebrae), anhidrosis, miosis, and enophthalmos |

## TEACHING POINTS CN IV SUMMARY

| Cranial Nerve (CN) IV | Trochlear |
|---|---|
| Function | Eye movement |
| Origin | Nucleus in the midbrain just below the nucleus of the CN III, anterior to the aqueduct |
| Intracranial pathway | The only nerve to exit from the dorsal aspect of the brain stem and the only nerve that crosses in entirety to the other side. Fibers of the trochlear nerve decussate just below the inferior colliculi posterior to the cerebral aqueduct. The nerve travels anteroinferiorly within the ambient cistern around the ambient cistern below the tentorium to enter the cavernous sinus |
| Foramina | Superior orbital fissure |
| Destination/Extracranial branches | Superior oblique muscle: Each muscle is supplied by the contralateral trochlear nucleus |
| Important pathology | Isolated palsy results in outward rotation of the eye usually from trauma of the cisternal segment or aneurysm from the superior cerebellar or posterior cerebral arteries |

## TEACHING POINTS CN V SUMMARY

| Cranial Nerve (CN) V | Trigeminal Nerve |
|---|---|
| Function | Sensory information from the face<br>Motor innervation to the muscles of mastication |
| Origin | Motor and sensory nuclei posterior aspect of the midpons just ventral to the superior cerebellar peduncle |
| Preganglionic pathway | Motor and sensory roots exit the lateral pons, pass through the prepontine cistern (cisternal portion of the nerve) to arrive at the trigeminal ganglion (Gasserian ganglion) within Meckel's cave |
| Postganglionic divisions | V1: Ophthalmic nerve travels in the inferior portion of the cavernous sinus. Provides sensory afferents to the upper portion of the face, the eye, the lacrimal gland, and the nose<br>V2: Maxillary nerve travels in the cavernous sinus, enters the foramen rotundum, and then courses anteriorly to the pterygopalatine fossa giving greater and lesser palatine nerves for sensation to the hard and soft palate. Continues along the inferior aspect of the orbits as the infraorbital nerve and exits through the infraorbital foramen where it supplies sensory innervation throughout the maxillofacial region below the orbits<br>V3: Mandibular nerve does not enter the cavernous sinus. From Meckel's cave, the mandibular nerve passes directly through the foramen ovale<br><br>a. Sensory branches<br>  i. Inferior alveolar: Enters the mandible through the mandibular (inferior alveolar) canal with fibers supplying the gingiva and teeth of the mandible<br>  ii. Lingual: Contains general sensory fibers and taste fibers with the chorda tympani (facial nerve) from the anterior two thirds of the tongue<br>  iii. Auriculotemporal nerve provides sensory information to skin of the lower face and temporal regions, external auditory canal and tympanic membrane, auricle, and temporomandibular joint. Several branches join the facial nerve<br>  iv. A meningeal branch returns through the foramen spinosum with the middle meningeal artery<br><br>b. Motor innervation to the muscles of mastication through the masticator nerve division and the mylohyoid and anterior belly of digastric muscles through the mylohyoid nerve, which are divisions of the inferior alveolar nerve |
| Foramina | V1: Superior orbital fissure<br>V2: Foramen rotundum<br>V3: Foramen ovale |
| Important pathology | Intimate relationship of branches of V and VII becomes very important when assessing for perineural tumor spread from head and neck cancers<br>Trigeminal neuralgia: "Tic douloureux" pain in the V2-V3 distributions, which can result from vascular compression of the cisternal portion of the trigeminal nerve |

## TEACHING POINTS CN VI SUMMARY

| Cranial Nerve (CN) VI | Abducens Nerve |
|---|---|
| Function | Eye movement |
| Origin | Nucleus at the dorsal pons at the level of the fourth ventricle |
| Intracranial pathway | Exits anterior brain stem at the junction of the pons and the pyramids of the medulla. The nerve courses through Dorello's canal before entering the cavernous sinus, where it lies lateral to the carotid artery |
| Foramina | Superior orbital fissure |
| Destination | Lateral rectus muscle |
| Important pathology | CN VI is the nerve closest to the internal carotid artery within the cavernous sinus and therefore most sensitive to cavernous sinus carotid artery diseases |

## TEACHING POINTS CN VII SUMMARY

| Cranial Nerve (CN) VII | Facial Nerve |
|---|---|
| Function | Motor innervations to facial muscles and stapedius. Taste from the anterior two thirds of the tongue. Innervation of the lacrimal and salivary glands (except the parotid) |
| Origin | Three nuclei:<br><br>1. Motor nucleus: Midpons anterolateral to abducens nucleus. Facial nerve encircles the nucleus of CN VI forming the facial colliculus, a nub on the anterior margin of the fourth ventricle<br>2. Superior salivatory nucleus: Efferent parasympathetic fibers to submandibular, sublingual, and lacrimal glands<br>3. Soltarius tract nucleus: Receives task afferents from VII (anterior tongue), IX (posterior tongue), and X(epiglottis) |
| Intracranial pathway | Exits the pons lateral to the abducens nerve and crosses the cerebellopontine angle cistern to enter the anterior superior margin of the internal auditory canal |
| Foramina | Internal auditory canal<br><br>Stylomastoid foramen |
| Destination/ Extracranial segment | 1. Greater superficial petrosal nerve arises at the geniculate ganglion to provide parasympathetic fibers to the lacrimal gland<br>2. Stapedius nerve arises from the mastoid segment of the facial nerve and provides motor innervation for the stapedius muscle<br>3. Chorda tympani arises from the mastoid segment of the facial nerve and provides taste fibers from the anterior two thirds of the tongue along with lingual branch of the V3 division of CN V<br>4. The distal mastoid portion of CN VII exits through the stylomastoid foramen to provide motor branches to supply muscles of facial expression |
| Important pathology | Facial nerve paralysis<br><br>Central: Supranuclear lesion (such as cortical stroke) results in paralysis of contralateral muscles of face with sparing of the forehead<br><br>Peripheral: Postnuclear injury (such as inflammatory process of CN VII within the internal auditory canal) results in paralysis of all ipsilateral muscles of facial expression |

## TEACHING POINTS CN VIII SUMMARY

| Cranial Nerve (CN) VIII | Vestibulocochlear Nerve |
|---|---|
| Function | Hearing and balance |
| Origin | The cochlear and vestibular nuclei are adjacent to each other, with the vestibular nuclei more medially. They are located in superior aspect of the medulla along the base of the inferior cerebellar peduncle |
| Intracranial pathway | The nerves exit the pontomedullary junction posterior to the inferior olivary nucleus |
| Foramina | Cochlear division: Travels in the anterior and inferior portion of the internal auditory canal.<br><br>Superior and inferior vestibular divisions: Travel in the posterior superior and posterior inferior portion of the internal auditory canal, respectively |
| Destination | Cochlear division: Enters the cochlea through the cochlear aperture, hair cells of the organ of Corti<br><br>Vestibular division: Enters the semicircular canals, hair cells of the vestibular labyrinth. |
| Important pathology | Vestibular schwannoma is the most common lesion to affect this nerve, interestingly most commonly presenting with hearing loss because of the mass effect on the cochlear division more so than vestibular symptoms |

## TEACHING POINTS CN IX SUMMARY

| Cranial Nerve (CN) IX | Glossopharyngeal Nerve |
|---|---|
| Function | Motor to stylopharyngeus muscle<br><br>Taste to posterior third of tongue<br><br>Parasympathetic to parotid gland<br><br>Viscerosensory to carotid body and sinus |

(Contiuned)

| Cranial Nerve (CN) IX | Glossopharyngeal Nerve |
|---|---|
| Origin | Glossopharyngeal nuclei are in the medulla posterior to the inferior olivary nucleus:<br><br>1. Nucleus ambiguous give rise to motor fibers to the pharynx-stylopharyngeus muscle.<br>2. Inferior salivary nucleus gives parasympathetic fibers to parotid gland for salivation<br>3. Nucleus of the solitary tracts: Receives taste fibers from the taste buds of the posterior third of the tongue |
| Intracranial pathway | The nerve fibers pass through the postolivary sulcus |
| Foramina | Pars nervosa of the jugular foramen |
| Extracranial Branches/ Destinations | 1. Jacobson nerve (tympanic branch): Middle ear sensory and parasympathetic fibers to parotid gland<br>2. Stylopharyngeus branch: Motor innervation to the stylopharyngeus muscles<br>3. Lingual branch: Posterior third of the tongue sensory and taste<br>4. Sinus nerve: Carotid sinus and carotid body |
| Important pathology | 1. Jacobson nerve: Glomus tympanicum paragangliomas arise from glomus bodies associated with this nerve<br>2. Isolated CN IX palsy is rare, usually in combination with CN X and XI palsies |

## TEACHING POINTS CRANIAL NEVE X SUMMARY

| Cranial Nerve (CN) X | Vagus Nerve |
|---|---|
| Function | Motor to muscles of the pharynx and larynx<br>Sensory from the larynx, trachea, esophagus, and abdominal viscera<br>Taste from the epiglottis and vallecula<br>Sensory to external tympanic membrane and external auditory canal |
| Central nervous system origin/Termination | Three parent nuclei within the medulla<br><br>1. Nucleus ambiguous gives rise to motor fibers to the larynx and pharynx<br>2. Dorsal nucleus receives sensory information and transmits motor information to and from the cardiovascular, pulmonary, and gastrointestinal tracts<br>3. Nucleus of the solitary tract receives taste afferents from the epiglottis and vallecula |
| Intracranial pathway | The vagus nerve exits the medulla through the postolivary sulcus. |
| Foramina | Pars vascularis of the jugular foramen |
| Extracranial branches/ Destination | 1. Recurrent laryngeal nerve loops under the aorta on the left side and subclavian artery on the right and travels in the tracheoesophageal grooves and provides motor to all laryngeal muscles except the cricothyroid muscle<br>2. Superior laryngeal nerve: Motor to the cricothyroid muscle<br>3. Arnold nerve: Sensation of the tympanic membrane and external auditory canal |
| Important pathology | Vocal cord paralysis from recurrent laryngeal nerve dysfunction:<br>If causative lesion between the medulla and hyoid bone: CN IX–XII involved with oropharyngeal and laryngeal dysfunction<br>If causative lesion below the hyoid bone: Isolated CN X with only laryngeal dysfunction |

## TEACHING POINTS CRANIAL NEVE XI SUMMARY

| Cranial Nerve (CN) XI | Spinal Accessory Nerve |
|---|---|
| Function | Motor supply to the sternocleidomastoid and trapezius muscles |
| Origin | Nucleus ambiguous: Gives bulbar motor fibers |
| | Spinal nucleus: Cells from the ventral horn of C1-C5 of the spinal cord give fibers that arise from the lateral aspect of the spinal cord and extend as a bundle called the *ansa cervicalis* along the carotid sheath to the foramen magnum |
| Intracranial pathway | Bulbar and spinal fibers combine and travel through the basal cistern |
| Foramina | Bulbar and spinal portions remain together in the posterior pars vascularis of the jugular foramen |
| Extracranial Branches/Destinations | 1. Bulbar portion travels with CN X to innervate muscles of pharynx and larynx<br>2. Spinal portion innervates the sternocleidomastoid and trapezius muscles |
| Important pathology | CN XI injury most commonly caused by radical neck dissection resulting in "frozen shoulder" with downward and lateral rotation of the scapula and shoulder drop |

## TEACHING POINTS CRANIAL NERVE XII SUMMARY

| Cranial Nerve (CN) XII | Hypoglossal Nerve |
|---|---|
| Function | Motor to the intrinsic and extrinsic muscles of the tongue |
| Origin | Nucleus along the paramedian area of the anterior wall of the fourth ventricle in the medulla |
| Intracranial pathway | Exits the medulla in the preolivary sulcus |
| Foramina | Hypoglossal canal |
| Destination | 1. Supplies the intrinsic muscles of the tongue and the genioglossus, styloglossus, and hyoglossus muscles<br>2. Ansa cervicalis branches run with the hypoglossal nerve to supply the anterior strap muscles |
| Important pathology | Tongue deviates to the side of hypoglossal nerve injury |

# Functional Anatomy

Understanding the functional anatomy requires a little bit of the cartographer in each of us (or a GPS-enabled smartphone). After having assimilated the destinations and points of departure, one should talk about the entire routes of neuronal travel. For functional anatomy, we can now use fMRI to identify the sites of cortical activation (the points of departure and destinations; Fig. 1.20).

## BRODMANN AREAS

- The functional units of the cerebral hemispheres have been separated into what are called *Brodmann areas* and include areas 1 through 47 (Fig. 1.21). These numbered areas correspond to different gyri that subserve various functions. The Brodmann areas are the currency with

which fMRI scientists transact business and are therefore important to be aware of. In addition, knowing which gyri are responsible for which properties can be critical to localizing lesions based on symptomatology and predicting deficits in patients with strokes.

- For example, Brodmann area 1 (i.e., S1) subserves primary somatosensory and position sense, and sits within the postcentral gyrus, in the paracentral lobule of the parietal lobe.
- Brodmann areas 2 and 3 subserve similar functions and are slightly posterior (2) and slightly anterior (3) to Brodmann area 1. Brodmann area 4 (M1) subserves primary motor function and resides within the precentral gyrus of the frontal lobe. Brodmann area 6 assists in planning and initiating movements.
- Wernicke areas are made up of Brodmann areas 21 and 22 (middle and superior temporal gyri, respectively) and serve functions of higher order audition and speech

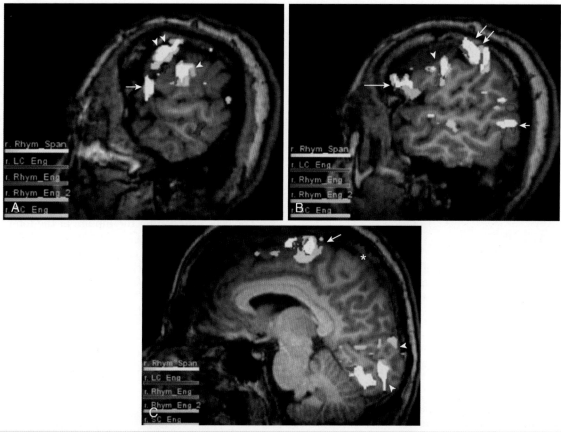

**Fig. 1.20 Functional magnetic resonance imaging (fMRI) with language task.** (A) fMRI blood-oxygen-level dependent (BOLD) activations overlayed onto anatomic T1-weighted images in sagittal plane. The left side of the brain is shown. Convergent activation is seen in the Broca region *(arrow)*. The Broca region typically corresponds to the pars opercularis/pars triangularis of the inferior frontal gyrus (Brodmann area 44-45), and in right-handed patients is typically lateralized to the left cerebral hemisphere. Even without overt movement, language-related motor areas can show concurrent activation, as is seen in the area of convergent activation in the subcentral gyrus *(single arrowhead)*, which represents the tongue/facial motor regions. The third convergent area of activation is seen in the ventral premotor cortex, also commonly activated during language tasks *(double arrowheads)*. (B) Convergent activation is seen in the left inferior frontal gyrus along the pars triangularis and pars opercularis corresponding to Brodmann areas 44 and 45, compatible with Broca activation *(large single arrow)*. Activation is also seen in the left ventral premotor cortex *(arrowhead)*, as well as language-related motor and sensory areas at the banks of the precentral and postcentral gyri *(double arrows)*. Posterior temporal lobe convergent activation represents Wernicke activation *(small single arrow)*. There are also smaller foci of language-related convergent activation seen just cranial to this in the supramarginal gyrus. (C) Convergent activation is seen in the presupplemental motor area *(arrow)*, which is activated during language tasks. This is anterior to the supplementary motor area, which is, in turn, anterior to the precentral gyrus. The central sulcus *(asterisk)* is seen as the sulcus immediately anterior to the marginal segment of the cingulate sulcus. Visual areas also demonstrate activation *(arrowheads)* as most of the language tasks used for this patient employed visual language task paradigms. (Courtesy Haris Sair, MD)

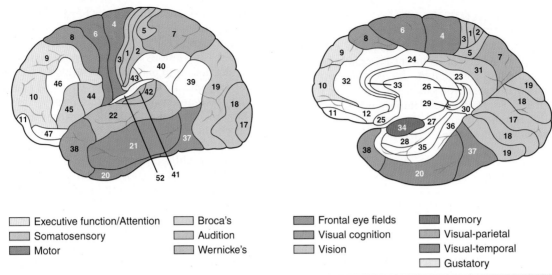

Executive function/Attention    Broca's    Frontal eye fields    Memory

Somatosensory    Audition    Visual cognition    Visual-parietal

Motor    Wernicke's    Vision    Visual-temporal

Gustatory

**Fig. 1.21 Brodmann areas.** Wernicke areas in Brodmann areas 21 and 22 (middle and superior temporal gyri) for higher order audition and speech reception, and areas 41 and 42 (A1-Wernicke and A2-Wernicke) in the superior temporal gyrus for primary audition and auditory association/speech recognition, respectively. Broca areas, Brodmann 44 and 45, are located within the inferior frontal gyrus laterally for speech expression and motor speech/tongue movement. (Source: Adapted by Gage NM and Baars BJ, *Fundamentals of Congitive Neuroscience: A Beginner's Guide*, 2nd Ed. 2019, Elsevier, Inc.)

reception, respectively (Can you hear me now?). Also, within the superior temporal gyrus are areas 41 and 42 (i.e., A1-Wernicke and A2-Wernicke), which subserve functions of primary audition and auditory association/speech recognition, respectively.

- Broca areas (Brodmann 44 and 45) located within the inferior frontal gyrus laterally subserve functions of speech expression and motor speech/tongue movement, respectively.

## Neural Systems

Knowing the anatomic locations of the flow of information for major neural pathways is essential for determining the site of pathology. To this end, we will review key pathways to be familiar with.

- The motor neurons of the precentral gyrus, the motor cortex, are arranged in an order that forms a map of the human body (the homunculus). However, the map is distorted with the face (especially the tongue and mouth) having an inordinately large area of motor representation along the inferiormost aspect of the precentral motor strip on the surface of the brain, just above the sylvian fissure.
- Motor neurons for the lower extremity are located superomedially along the paracentral lobule in the midline, whereas the upper extremity is located inferolaterally. The cells innervating the hip are at the top of the precentral sulcus; the leg is draped over medially along the interhemispheric fissure. Stimulation of the motor area of one precentral gyrus causes contraction of muscles on the opposite side of the body.
- After receiving input from multiple sensory areas, the motor neurons of the precentral gyrus send signals

## MOTOR SYSTEM

**TEACHING POINTS**

Motor Tracts

| Pathway | Course | Function |
|---|---|---|
| Lateral corticospinal tract | Primary motor cortex to corona radiata to posterior limb of internal capsule to cerebral peduncle to central pontine region to medulla through pyramidal decussation to posterolateral white matter of cord | Motor to contralateral extremities |
| Anterior corticospinal tract | Primary motor cortex to corona radiata to posterior limb of internal capsule to cerebral peduncle to central pontine region to medulla to anterior funiculus and anterior column of spinal cord | Motor to ipsilateral muscles |
| Rubrospinal tract | Red nucleus to decussation in ventral tegmentum of the midbrain through the lateral funiculus of the spinal cord to the posterolateral white matter of cord (with lateral corticospinal tract) | Motor control of contralateral limbs |
| Reticulospinal tract | Pons and medulla to ipsilateral anterior column of cord | Automatic movement of axial and limb muscles (walking, stretching, orienting behaviors) |
| Vestibulospinal tract | Vestibular nuclei to ipsilateral anterior columns in cord | Balance, postural adjustments, and head and neck coordination |

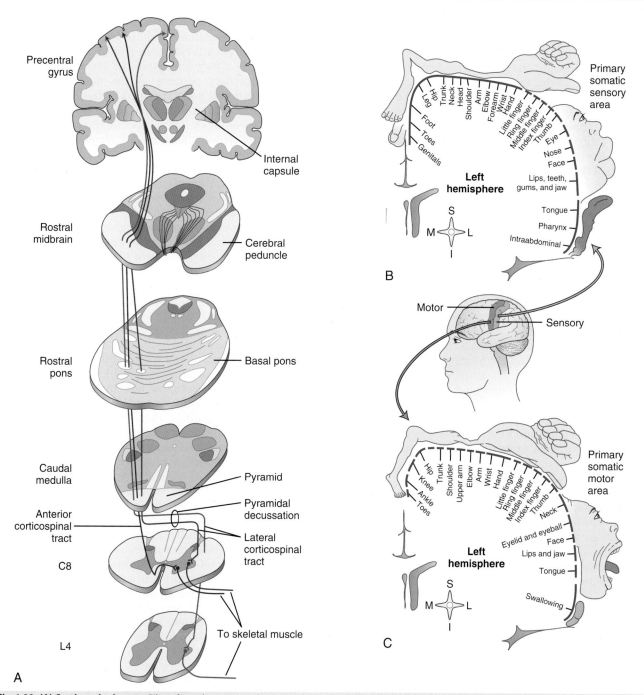

**Fig. 1.22 (A) Corticospinal tracts.** Fibers from the precentral gyrus and other nearby cortical areas descend through the cerebral peduncles, pons, and medullary pyramids; most cross in the pyramidal decussation to form the lateral corticospinal tract. Those that do not cross in the pyramidal decussation form the anterior corticospinal tract; most of these fibers cross in the anterior white commissure before ending in the spinal gray matter. Most corticospinal fibers do not synapse directly on the motor neurons. They are drawn that way here for simplicity. Primary somatic sensory (B) and motor (C) areas of the cortex, coronal view. The body parts illustrated here show which parts of the body are "mapped" to correlates in each cortical area. The exaggerated face indicates that more cortical area is devoted to processing information to/from the many receptors and motor units than for the leg or arm, for example. (A, From Nolte J. *The Human Brain: An Introduction to Its Functional Anatomy*. 4th ed. St. Louis: Mosby; 1999:249. B and C, From Thibodeau GA, Patton KT. *Anatomy and Physiology*. 4th ed. St. Louis: Mosby; 1999:394.)

through their axons through the white matter corticospinal tract. The signal extends through the white matter of the centrum semiovale and corona radiata to the posterior limb of the internal capsule (Fig. 1.22).

■ From the posterior portion of the posterior limb of the internal capsule, the corticospinal tract continues through the central portion of the cerebral peduncle in the anterior portion of the midbrain. These fibers continue in the anterior portion of the pons to the

pyramids of the medulla. At the medulla, tracts can proceed in one of two ways:

■ Lateral cortical spinal tract: Most fibers will cross to the other side in the medulla (the pyramidal decussation) and proceed inferiorly in the lateral corticospinal tract of the spinal cord.

■ Anterior corticospinal tract: 15% of fibers do not decussate in the medulla and will pass into the anterior funiculus along the anterior median fissure of the spinal cord as the anterior corticospinal tract. At the level of the spinal cord, these fibers cross the midline.

■ Axons in both tracts will synapse with the second order neuron anterior horn cell spinal cord nuclei whose axons innervate skeletal muscles. The lateral cortical spinal tract controls movement of the limbs. The anterior cortical spinal tract controls the central body musculature.

■ Motor supply to the face travels through a separate pathway called the corticobulbar tract. This tract extends from the cortex through the corona radiata and into the genu of the internal capsule. The corticobulbar fibers are located more anteromedially in the cerebral peduncles and have connections to the brain stem nuclei as they descend. Most of the connections to the various CN nuclei are contralateral to the cortical bulbar tract; however, some ipsilateral fibers are present as well.

■ The pyramidal system (referring to the pyramids of the medulla) is responsible for voluntary movement and is made up of corticospinal and corticobulbar fibers. Abnormalities of the pyramidal system mainly produce weakness, paralysis, or spasticity of voluntary motor function.

■ The extrapyramidal system includes the rubrospinal, reticulospinal, and vestibulospinal tracts, which course from the brain stem, pons, and medulla to the anterior columns of the spinal cord. Extrapyramidal system abnormalities often produce involuntary movement disorders, including tremors, choreiform (jerking) movements, athetoid (slow sinuous) movements, hemiballismic (flailing) motions, and muscular rigidity (think: pyramid, paralysis; extrapyramidal, extremity excesses).

## SENSORY SYSTEM

■ The sensory system of the CNS is separated into fibers that transmit the sensations of pain and temperature, position, vibration, and general fine touch. The three main tracts carrying sensation from the body include the spinothalamic, posterior column-medial lemniscus, and the spinocerebellar.

**TEACHING POINTS**

Sensory Tracts

| Tract | Course |
|---|---|
| Medial lemniscus | From posterior white matter of cord to dorsal nuclei of medulla, through decussation, to medial lemniscus to thalamus to anterior limb of internal capsule to primary sensory cortex |
| Spinothalamic tract | Dorsal horn of cord to spinal decussation to anterolateral spinal tract to reticular formation of pons, medulla, thalamus |
| Lateral lemniscus | From auditory fibers in caudal pons, crossed and uncrossed, to inferior colliculus, to medial geniculate of thalamus to primary auditory cortex |

■ The spinothalamic tracts (Fig. 1.23A) can be divided into the lateral, which carries pain and temperature, and the anterior tracts, which carry body crude touch and pressure sensation.

■ The first order neurons are in the dorsal root ganglia whose fibers may ascend or descend for one or two spinal segments before terminating in the region of the substantia gelatinosa of the dorsal horn. From the secondary neurons of the nucleus proprius of the dorsal horn, the fibers cross the midline in the anterior white commissures of the spinal cord and ascend in the lateral spinothalamic tract. The lateral spinothalamic tract is identified in the lateral midportion of the medulla and centrally in the pons where it is renamed the *spinal lemniscus*.

■ The spinal lemniscus proceeds through the anterolateral portion of the dorsal pons and along the lateral aspect of the midbrain. From there, the fibers synapse with tertiary neurons in the ventral posterolateral thalamic nucleus and then terminate in the somesthetic area of the parietal lobe in the postcentral sulcus region.

■ The posterior column-medial lemniscus tract (see Fig. 1.23B) transmits proprioception, fine touch, and pressure. First order sensory neurons are located within the dorsal root ganglia of the spinal cord. They send afferent fibers to the dorsal columns (either the fasciculus gracilis for spinal levels inferior to T6 or the fasciculus cuneatus for spinal levels superior to T6). The first axons synapse with the second order nuclei at the nucleus gracilis and nucleus cuneatus within the lower medulla. From the nucleus gracilis and nucleus cuneatus, the axons cross the midline of the medulla and continue superiorly as the medial lemniscus found in the posterior portion of the medulla and pons before synapsing with third order neurons in the ventral posterolateral (VPL) nucleus of the thalamus. From the VPL, the path is through the internal capsule to get to the primary somatosensory cortex.

■ Two spinocerebellar tracts carry information about the torso and lower extremities to the cerebellum.
  ▪ The dorsal spinocerebellar tract carries proprioception information from the torso to the cerebellum and remains ipsilateral along its entire course.
  ▪ The ventral spinocerebellar tract carries proprioception information from the lower extremities and joins to the cerebellum.

■ Sensations from the face are carried through the trigeminal nerve with the nuclei identified within the trigeminal ganglion. One usually separates the V1 sensation as from the lateral canthus of the eye upward, V2 from lateral canthus to junction of the lips, and V3 from the lower lip downward to the undersurface of the chin. Pain and temperature information travels along the axons from the trigeminal ganglion descending within the spinal trigeminal tract. The fibers terminate in the secondary neuron nucleus of the trigeminal spinal tract, which extends from the lower medulla to the C3 level of the spinal cord. At this point, the pain and temperature fibers cross the midline to the contralateral side and ascend as the trigeminothalamic tract, which passes medial to the lateral spinothalamic tract but terminates also in the ventral posterior (lateral) thalamic nucleus. Tertiary neuron fibers then pass to the somesthetic area of the cerebral cortex.

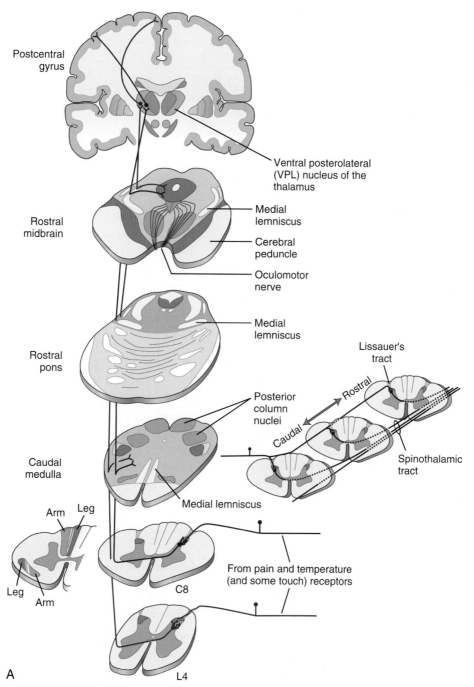

Postcentral gyrus

Ventral posterolateral (VPL) nucleus of the thalamus

Rostral midbrain

Medial lemniscus

Cerebral peduncle

Oculomotor nerve

Rostral pons

Medial lemniscus

Lissauer's tract

Rostral

Posterior column nuclei

Caudal

Spinothalamic tract

Caudal medulla

Arm    Leg

Medial lemniscus

From pain and temperature (and some touch) receptors

Leg
Arm

C8

A                    L4

**Fig. 1.23  The sensory pathways of the body.** (A) Spinothalamic tract. Pain, temperature, and some touch and pressure afferents end in the posterior horn. Second- or higher-order fibers cross the midline, form the spinothalamic tract, and ascend to the ventral posterolateral *(VPL)* nucleus of the thalamus (and also to other thalamic nuclei not indicated in this figure). Thalamic cells then project to the somatosensory cortex of the postcentral gyrus and to other cortical areas. Along their course through the brain stem, spinothalamic fibers give off many collaterals to the reticular formation. The inset to the *left* shows the lamination of fibers in the posterior columns and the spinothalamic tract, in a leg-lower trunk-upper trunk-arm sequence. The inset to the *right* shows the longitudinal formation of the spinothalamic tract. Primary afferents ascend several segments in Lissauer's tract before all their branches terminate; fibers crossing to join the spinothalamic tract do so with a rostral inclination. As a result, a cordotomy incision at any given level will spare most of the information entering the contralateral side of the spinal cord at that level, and to be effective the incision must be made several segments rostral to the highest dermatomal level of pain.

■ The pathway for light touch of the face is identical to that of pain and temperature. However, termination of these CN V fibers occurs in a more superior portion of the nucleus of the trigeminal spinal tract. In addition, these fibers may bifurcate on entering the pons and synapse with the chief sensory nucleus of V within the pons.

## VISUAL PATHWAY

■ The image received by the rods and cones of the retina is passed to secondary sensory ganglion cells of the retina and is then transmitted along the second CN—the optic nerve. The optic nerve ascends obliquely through the optic canal to join fibers from the contralateral optic nerve at the optic chiasm (Fig. 1.24A).

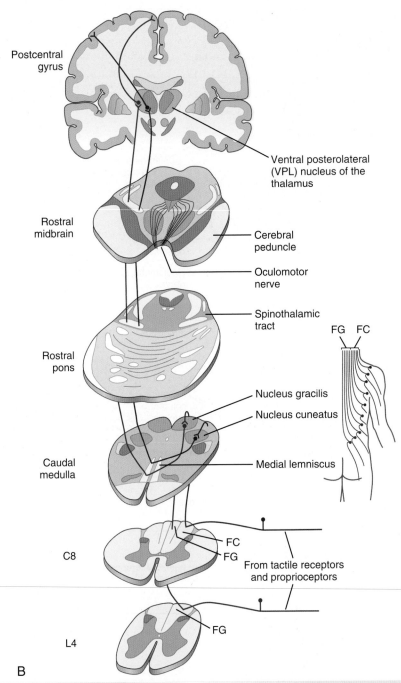

**(B) Posterior column-medial lemniscus pathway.** Primary afferents carrying tactile and proprioceptive information synapse in the posterior column nuclei of the ipsilateral medulla. The axons of second-order cells then cross the midline, form the medial lemniscus, and ascend to the ventral postero-lateral nucleus of the thalamus. Third-order fibers then project to the somatosensory cortex of the postcentral gyrus. A somatotopic arrangement of fibers is present at all levels. The beginning of this somatotopic arrangement, as a lamination of fibers in the posterior columns, is indicated in the inset to the *right*. *FC*, Fasciculus cuneatus; *FG*, fasciculus gracilis. (From Nolte J. *The Human Brain: An Introduction to Its Functional Anatomy*. 4th ed. St. Louis: Mosby; 1999:244, 245.)

- The temporal retina fibers (nasal field) remain uncrossed and pass to the ipsilateral optic tract.
- The fibers from the nasal retina (temporal fields) decussate to join the nondecussating nasal field fibers from the opposite optic nerve continuing in the postchiasmal optic tract.
  - However, before they cross, some of the inferonasal retinal fibers loop for a short distance up into the contralateral optic nerve in what is termed *Wilbrand knee*.

This accounts for the signs of the "junctional syndrome" found in a lesion that compresses one optic nerve and the looping contralateral Wilbrand fibers. This results in a central scotoma in the ipsilateral eye and a superotemporal visual defect in the contralateral eye.

- Ninety percent of the fibers in the chiasm are from the macula of the retina; the crossing fibers lie superiorly

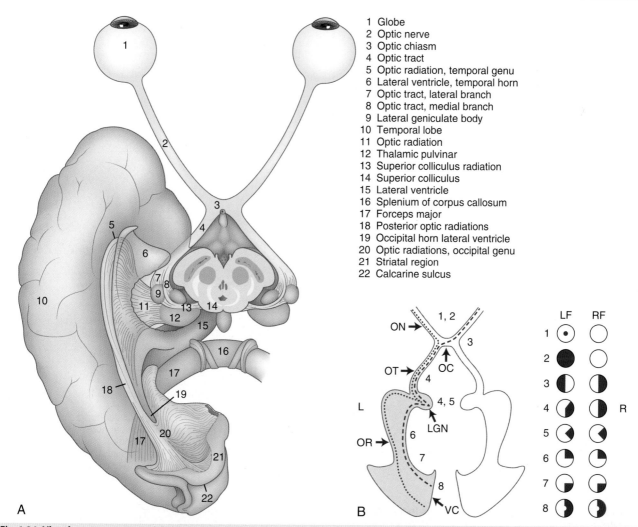

1 Globe
2 Optic nerve
3 Optic chiasm
4 Optic tract
5 Optic radiation, temporal genu
6 Lateral ventricle, temporal horn
7 Optic tract, lateral branch
8 Optic tract, medial branch
9 Lateral geniculate body
10 Temporal lobe
11 Optic radiation
12 Thalamic pulvinar
13 Superior colliculus radiation
14 Superior colliculus
15 Lateral ventricle
16 Splenium of corpus callosum
17 Forceps major
18 Posterior optic radiations
19 Occipital horn lateral ventricle
20 Optic radiations, occipital genu
21 Striatal region
22 Calcarine sulcus

**Fig. 1.24 Visual system anatomy.** (A) The anatomy of the optic nerves, tracts, and radiations is diagrammed. (B) Optic chiasm: Correlation of lesion site and field defect. Note the most ventral nasal fibers (mostly from inferior nasal retina) temporarily travel within the fellow optic nerve in Wilbrand knee. *LGN,* Lateral geniculate nucleus; *OC,* optic chiasm; *ON,* optic nerve; *OR,* optic radiations; *OT,* optic tract; *VC,* visual cortex. (A, From Nieuwenhuys R, Voogd J, van Huijen C. *The Human Central Nervous System: A Synopsis and Atlas.* Rev 3rd ed. Berlin: Springer-Verlag; 1988.)

and posteriorly in the chiasm. The optic tract encircles the anterior portion of the midbrain before terminating in the lateral geniculate body of the thalamus.

■ The lateral geniculate body is located in the posterolateral portion of the thalamus within the pulvinar nucleus. A few fibers ascend to the Edinger-Westphal nucleus (CN III) in the pretectal portion of the midbrain as part of the pupillary reflex, and some connect to the superior colliculus for tracking ability.

■ From the lateral geniculate nucleus, tertiary neuronal fibers pass in the geniculocalcarine tract (optic radiations), course through portions of the posterior limb of the internal capsule and around the lateral ventricle, and terminate in the visual calcarine cortex in the medial occipital lobe.

■ The superior optic radiations (inferior visual fields) pass through the parietal lobe on their way to the superior visual cortex of the occipital lobe. The inferior optic radiations (superior visual fields) are called Meyer's loop fibers. They pass over the anteroinferior aspect of the lateral ventricle (around the temporal horn) into the

temporal lobe to terminate in the inferior visual cortex just below the calcarine sulcus. An optic radiation lesion is localized depending on whether there are signs of neglect or sensory loss (superior radiation: parietal lobe lesion) or dysphasia and memory loss (Meyer's loop: temporal lobe lesions).

■ Thus, lesions in the optic nerve cause blindness of the ipsilateral eye. Lesions in the midline at the level of the optic chiasm will cause bitemporal defects. Lesions compressing the lateral edge of the optic chiasm cause a nasal hemianopsia of the ipsilateral eye. Lesions of the optic tract extending to the lateral geniculate and primary lesions of the lateral geniculate nucleus cause a contralateral homonymous hemianopsia. Lesions of the geniculocalcarine tract or visual cortex cause a contralateral homonymous hemianopsia (see Fig. 1.24B).

■ Sparing of macular vision with cortical strokes is common, and one of four explanations is possible: (1) localization of macular fibers to the watershed area of middle and posterior cerebral artery (PCA) supply, allowing for

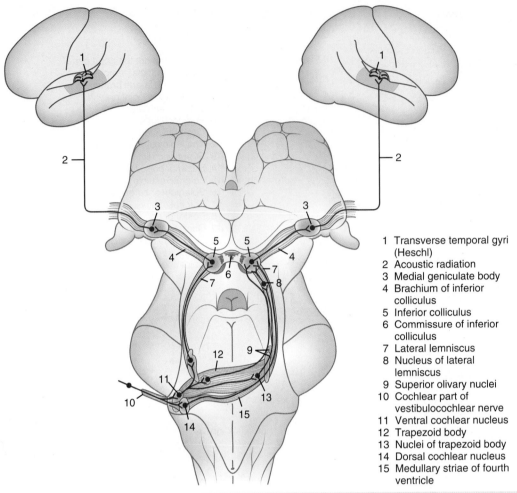

1  Transverse temporal gyri
   (Heschl)
2  Acoustic radiation
3  Medial geniculate body
4  Brachium of inferior
   colliculus
5  Inferior colliculus
6  Commissure of inferior
   colliculus
7  Lateral lemniscus
8  Nucleus of lateral
   lemniscus
9  Superior olivary nuclei
10 Cochlear part of
   vestibulocochlear nerve
11 Ventral cochlear nucleus
12 Trapezoid body
13 Nuclei of trapezoid body
14 Dorsal cochlear nucleus
15 Medullary striae of fourth
   ventricle

**Fig. 1.25 The auditory system in the brain stem (dorsal view) and in the cerebrum (lateral view).** (From Kretschmann H-J, Weinrich W. *Cranial Neuroimaging and Clinical Neuroanatomy: Magnetic Resonance Imaging and Computed Tomography*. Rev 2nd ed. New York: Thieme; 1993:284.)

dual vascular supply to be present; (2) a very large cortical area devoted to central vision, meaning that small strokes will not affect all fibers; (3) some decussation of macular fibers, so that they are bilaterally represented; and (4) testing artifact because of poor central fixation by the subject.

- The optic nerve is unique among the CNs in that it consists of an extension of the CNS white matter surrounded by dural sheath and is therefore not a peripheral nerve like the other CNs. The optic nerve is subject to the pathologies intrinsic to white matter in the brain (such as multiple sclerosis), and its sheath is subject to dural-based processes.

## AUDITORY SYSTEM

- What goes on in your head when your cell phone chirps? Sound is transmitted through the external ear via vibrations of the tympanic membrane to the middle ear ossicles. It is then transmitted to the hair cells of the organ of Corti in the cochlea. The cochlear division of the eighth CN runs in the anterior inferior portion of the internal auditory canal.

- From the canal, the nerve enters the brain stem at the junction between the pons and the medulla. The fibers end in the dorsal and ventral cochlear nuclei, which are identified in the upper part of the medulla along its dorsal surface (Fig. 1.25). After this primary synapse, the secondary nerves for hearing may cross the midline at the level of the pons and ascend in the lateral lemniscus in what is termed the *trapezoid body*. A synapse may occur in the trapezoid body, but other fibers may synapse in the superior olivary nucleus. Some fibers may remain on the ipsilateral side and synapse in the ipsilateral superior olivary nucleus to ascend in the ipsilateral lateral lemniscus.

- The tertiary neurons of the lateral lemniscus pass through the ventral portion of the pons and midportion of the midbrain before synapsing at the inferior colliculus (thought to be instrumental in frequency discrimination).

- From the inferior colliculus, the fourth-order fibers pass to the medial geniculate nucleus of the thalamus. It should be noted, however, that fibers may bypass each of these nuclei to get to the next level in the auditory pathway.

- Fibers from the medial geniculate course in the posterior limb of the internal capsule as the auditory radiations and terminate in the anterosuperior transverse temporal gyri (also called *Heschl's gyri*) and superior temporal gyrus.

- The auditory association cortex is also located in the temporal lobe. Unilateral lesions in the auditory cortex do not induce complete deafness in the contralateral ear, but there is a decrease in auditory acuity because of crossing fibers in the lateral lemniscus and crossed connections between the nuclei of the lateral lemniscus and the inferior colliculi. Most causes of unilateral hearing loss (speak up, please!) are at the level of the inner and middle ear.

## LIMBIC SYSTEM

- The main components of the limbic system include the fornix, the mammillary bodies, the hippocampus, the amygdala, and the anterior nucleus of the thalamus. The limbic system controls the emotional responses to visceral and other stimuli. In addition, portions of memory function are contained within the limbic system.
- The olfactory and gustatory systems tie into the limbic system. The olfactory bulb receives nerve fibers located in the upper nasal cavity, the ciliary nerves. The olfactory bulbs feed into the olfactory tracts lying just under the gyrus rectus region in the olfactory sulcus of the frontal lobes. The olfactory tracts penetrate the brain just under the lamina terminalis and send nerve fibers to the septal nuclei, the parahippocampus, the uncus, and the amygdala via medial and lateral striae.
- The amygdala is a primary workstation for emotions. In addition to input from the olfactory system, it receives fibers from the thalami and the hypothalamus. Efferent fibers are sent from the amygdala to the temporal and frontal lobes, the thalamus, the hypothalamus, and the reticular formation in the brain stem. Lesions of the amygdala and other portions of the limbic system may cause anhedonia with a lack of emotional response to what are normally pleasurable stimuli.
- The fornices are white matter tracts lying medially beneath the corpus callosum and are the major white matter relays from one hippocampus to the other and on to the hypothalamus. The forniceal columns invaginate into the lateral and third ventricles as they sweep anteroinferiorly to end in the mammillary bodies. The anterior portions of the fornices parallel the corpus callosum but are more inferiorly and centrally located.
- The hippocampal formation includes the hippocampus (located in the temporal lobe above the parahippocampus), the indusium griseum (a fine gray matter tract situated between the corpus callosum and cingulate gyrus connecting septal nuclei to parahippocampal gyri; don't misinterpret this as ectopic gray matter in imaging of seizure patients!), and the dentate gyrus (just above the parahippocampal gyrus). The hippocampus is found along the medial temporal lobe adjacent to the inferior temporal horn of the lateral ventricle and the choroidal fissure. The hippocampus is involved primarily with visceral responses to emotions (with the hypothalamus) and memory, with less input into olfaction.

## TASTE

- Taste from the anterior two thirds of the tongue is transmitted by the chorda tympani, a branch of CN VII that runs with fibers from the third division of CN V as the lingual nerve. From the chorda tympani, the fibers run through the otic and geniculate ganglia to end at the cell bodies in the nucleus solitarius.
- The taste papillae of the posterior third of the tongue are supplied by CN IX. These fibers course through the petrosal ganglion of CN IX to reach the cell bodies in the nucleus solitarius (Fig. 1.26).
- Some bitter taste fibers may be supplied via the vagus nerve's nodose ganglion from the epiglottis.
- From the nucleus solitarius, projections are made to the pons, both ventromedial nuclei of the thalamus, hypothalamus, and amygdala. These limbic structures monitor the visceral (nausea, vomiting, sweating, flushing, salivation) and emotional responses (elation, disgust, satiation) to certain foods, like jalapeños. From the thalamus, fibers track up to both sides of the sensory cortex, where the tongue occupies a huge proportion of the homunculus projection of the body on the brain surface.

## SPEECH

- Obviously, speech ties into the motor and auditory pathways described previously. Nonetheless, a brief description of the speech pathway is warranted because of its critical role in humans.
- Speech requires coordination between the left hemisphere's temporoparietal areas assigned to the sensation of speech and the inferior frontal gyrus (Broca area) assigned to motor function. Portions of the arcuate fasciculus connect these two areas. In a few persons (usually left-handed people), speech may be localized to the right hemisphere. Portions of the superior and middle temporal gyri and the inferior parietal lobule control ideational language.
- The auditory association cortex of the superior temporal gyrus (Wernicke area) handles receptive understanding of speech and is deficient in most politicians. If the inferior frontal gyrus is injured, coordination of intelligible expressive speech is lost (motor aphasia). Receptive aphasia develops with lesions in the Wernicke area, and conductive aphasia (disturbance in speech in response to verbal command but not spontaneously [ideomotor dyspraxia]) occurs with arcuate fasciculus lesions.

# Vascular Anatomy

- Advancements in noninvasive cross-sectional imaging modalities, CT, and magnetic resonance (MR) angiography have greatly improved accuracy in displaying vascular system anatomy and its pathology. Conventional angiography continues to have role in delineating vascular disease, including aneurysms, vasculitis, and arteriovenous malformations, and serves as a prerequisite for therapeutic interventions.

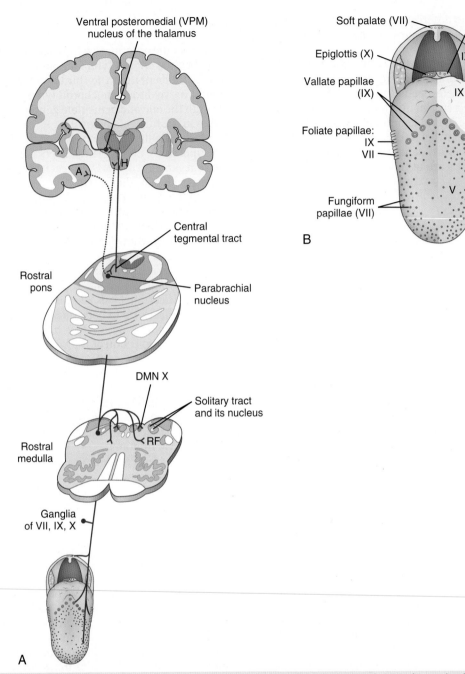

**Fig. 1.26 Taste pathways.** (A) Second-order neurons feed into reflexes both by direct projections (e.g., to the nearby dorsal motor nucleus of the vagus) and by connections with the reticular formation. The projection from the parabrachial nucleus to the hypothalamus and amygdala is dashed because its existence in primates has not been demonstrated conclusively. (B) Distribution and innervation of taste buds and innervation of the lingual epithelium. The trigeminal nerve *(V)* subserves general sensation from the anterior two thirds of the tongue, and the glossopharyngeal nerve *(IX)* has a similar function with taste for the posterior third of the tongue. Taste is controlled anteriorly by the chorda tympani of the facial nerve *(VII)*. *DMN,* Dorsal motor nucleus. (A and B, From Nolte J. *The Human Brain: An Introduction to Its Functional Anatomy.* 4th ed. St. Louis: Mosby; 1999:324, 320, respectively.)

## CERVICAL ARTERIAL VASCULATURE

- The great vessels arising from the aortic arch provide vascular supply to the neck and brain. Approximately 80% of the time, there is a "classic branching pattern" with the brachiocephalic artery arising first followed by the left common carotid artery followed by the left sub-clavian artery. The most common variant is a common origin of the brachiocephalic artery and the left common carotid artery. Occasionally, the left vertebral artery can be observed arising directly from the arch. Another anomaly, the aberrant right subclavian artery arises beyond the left subclavian artery, courses behind the esophagus, and travels in the right neck.

- The common carotid artery bifurcates into an external and internal carotid artery approximately at the level of the third or fourth cervical vertebral body in most persons. The angle of the mandible is another good marker for the carotid bifurcation. The external carotid artery typically courses anteromedially to the internal carotid artery from the bifurcation. However, the internal

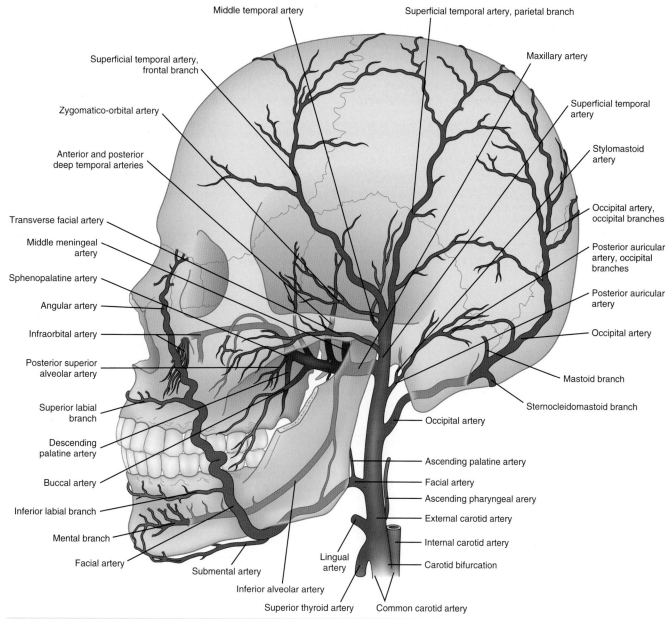

**Fig. 1.27 External carotid artery (ECA) anatomy.** The ECA and its branches, lateral aspect.

carotid artery typically crosses medial to the external carotid artery at approximately the C1 to C2 level as it turns to enter the skull.

- Both vertebral arteries arise most typically from the subclavian arteries on either side and ascend the neck within transverse foramina of the cervical spine, entering the foramina at variable levels, to supply the posterior fossa intracranially. In the neck the vertebral arteries give off muscular branches to the neck as well as spinal branches that supply the cervical spinal cord and vertebral bodies. Vertebral arteries can be codominant in terms of caliber, but not infrequently, one may be larger (dominant) compared to the other.

## EXTERNAL CAROTID BRANCHES

- The branches of the external carotid artery can be remembered by presented this way: "She Always Likes Friends Over Pop, Mom, and Sis." With this memory aid, you can remember the eight external carotid artery branches of superior thyroidal, ascending pharyngeal, lingual, facial, occipital, posterior auricular, (internal) maxillary, and superficial temporal arteries (Fig. 1.27).

- Knowing the branches of the external carotid artery is important for understanding the vascular supply to head and neck and skull base tumors. Anterior and middle cranial fossa meningiomas by and large are supplied by the anterior and posterior divisions of the middle meningeal artery, a branch of the internal maxillary artery. The ascending pharyngeal artery is the artery that is typically implicated in supply of glomus jugulare, glomus tympanicum, and carotid body tumors, whereas the internal maxillary artery is typically implicated in the supply of juvenile nasopharyngeal angiofibromas.

- The branches of the external carotid arteries have multiple anastomoses with the internal carotid artery and vertebral arteries, which can serve as an important source of collateral blood in cases of arterial stenosis. For example, branches of the internal maxillary artery are significant for supplying collateral circulation to the distal internal carotid artery when internal carotid artery occlusion occurs. The middle meningeal artery may anastomose with ethmoidal branches of the ophthalmic artery, or collateral circulation may be achieved by way of the meningolacrimal artery to the ophthalmic artery. The ophthalmic artery, an important branch of the intracranial internal cerebral artery (ICA) that supplies the orbit, the globe, the frontal scalp region, the frontal and ethmoidal sinuses, and the upper part of the nose has anastomoses with facial and internal maxillary artery branches.

## TEACHING POINTS

### External Carotid Artery Branches

| Branches | Origin | Supplies | Anastomotic Channels |
|---|---|---|---|
| Superior thyroidal artery | Arises from the anterior aspect of the external carotid artery branches (ECA) | Superior thyroid and larynx | Nasal and orbital branches anastomose with ophthalmic artery branches of the internal carotid artery (ICA)<br><br>Anastomoses with the vertebral artery |
| Ascending pharyngeal artery | Arises from the posterior ECA or central carotid artery (CCA) bifurcation | 1. Anterior (pharyngeal branch)-posterolateral pharyngeal wall and palatine tonsil<br>2. Middle (neuromeningeal)<br>3. Posterior branches supply the vasa nervorum of cranial nerves IX, X, and XI | |
| Lingual artery | Second branch to arise anteriorly from the ECA with characteristic hook appearance of its course | Floor of the mouth, hyoid muscles, tongue, and submandibular and sublingual glands | |
| Facial artery | May arise independently or common trunk with the lingual artery | Face from the inferior aspect of the mandible to the medial corner of the eye, the palate, and submandibular gland | |
| Occipital artery | Arises posteriorly from the ECA | Sternocleidomastoid muscle, meninges of the posterior fossa. Could supply skull base mass such as glomus tumors through the stylomastoid branch | Anastomoses to the vertebral artery |
| Posterior auricular | Arises from the posterior ECA | Scalp posterior to auricle | Meningeal anastomoses to the posterior fossa<br><br>Anastomoses to the vertebral artery |
| Superficial temporal artery | Smaller of the terminal branches of the ECA | Parotid gland, masseter, buccinators muscles, lateral part of the scalp, then anterior scalp and cheek | Anterior branches anastomose with ophthalmic artery branches, whereas posterior branches join the posterior auricular and occipital artery supply |
| Internal maxillary artery | Large terminal branch of the ECA | Deep structures of the face with numerous branches traveling within several skull base foramina and fissures | Branches of the internal maxillary artery are significant for supplying collateral flow to distal ICA when there is proximal ICA occlusion |

■ Several anastomotic channels that are present in fetal life and connect carotid and vertebral circulations usually regress in utero but can remain patent in rare instances. The persistent trigeminal artery is the most common persistent anastomosis, which connects the cavernous carotid artery to the upper basilar artery in 0.1% to 0.2% of people (Fig. 1.28). This normal variant may be associated with hypoplasia of the vertebrobasilar system below the anastomosis. There is a Saltzman classification of persistent trigeminal arteries that specifies type I as ending on the basilar artery (BA) and supplying the PCA and superior cerebellar artery (SCA), and type II terminating on the BA, supplying the SCA with a persistent fetal posterior communicating artery supplying the PCA. Other persistent trigeminal artery variants have it terminating on the SCA, the anterior ICA, and the posterior ICA.

## TEACHING POINTS

### Persistent Vascular Connections

| Persistent Artery | Origin | Feeds | Location | Coexistent Findings |
|---|---|---|---|---|
| Trigeminal | Cavernous carotid | Top of basilar | Suprasellar cistern | Aneurysms, hypoplastic vertebrobasilar system |
| Otic (real or imagined?) | Petrous carotid | Mid basilar | Internal auditory canal | Hypoplastic vertebrobasilar system |
| Hypoglossal | High cervical internal carotid at skull base | Intracranial vertebrobasilar circulation | Hypoglossal canal | Hypoplastic vertebrobasilar system |
| Proatlantal type 1 | Low internal carotid | Cranial and cervical vertebrobasilar circulation | C2 level | Hypoplastic vertebrobasilar system |
| Proatlantal type 2 | External carotid | Cranial and cervical vertebrobasilar circulation | C2 level | Hypoplastic vertebral arteries |

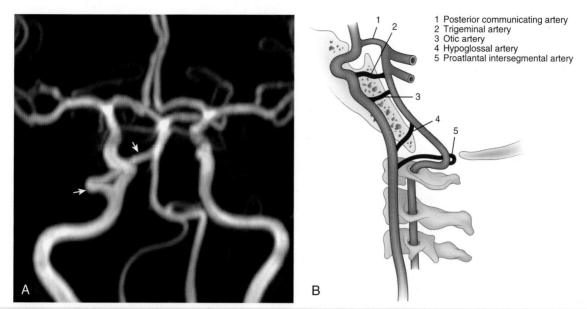

Fig. 1.28 **Persistent fetal connections.** (A) Magnetic resonance angiogram shows the persistent trigeminal artery *(arrows)* connecting the cavernous internal carotid and basilar arteries. The hypoplastic basilar artery below the trigeminal contribution is also evident. (B) Anatomic diagram depicts the embryonic carotid-basilar and carotid-vertebral anastomoses. The posterior communicating artery is the only vessel that normally persists; the other four, shown in black, usually regress completely. (B, From Osborne AG. *Diagnostic Cerebral Angiography.* 2nd ed. Philadelphia: Lippincott, Williams & Wilkins; 1998:69, Fig. 3.14.)

- The persistent otic and hypoglossal arteries are found more inferiorly (and much more rarely) connecting the petrous (otic) and cervical (hypoglossal) internal carotid artery to the lower basilar artery. Persistent otic arteries are so incredibly rare that some feel they don't actually exist. A persistent proatlantal artery can arise from the cervical carotid (type I) or the external carotid artery (type II) to anastamose with the vertebral artery at the foramen magnum.

## INTRACRANIAL CIRCULATION

- The intracranial circulation is supplied by paired internal carotid arteries giving rise to the anterior circulation (Fig. 1.29) and paired vertebral arteries, the latter of which join to form the basilar artery forming the posterior circulation (Fig. 1.30). Because of the collateral network inherent in the circle of Willis, where the left and right carotid and vertebrobasilar systems are interconnected via anterior and posterior communicating arteries, the brain possesses a redundant defense against major-vessel occlusive disease (Fig. 1.31). Such is not the case wsith the branches distal to the circle of Willis, where collateral circulation is less easily supplied.

- The course of the internal carotid arteries can be divided into seven segments. The first segment, C1, extends from the internal carotid artery origin through the cervical portion and has no branches. The six intracranial nerve segments include petrous (i.e., horizontal) (C2), lacerum (C3), cavernous (C4), clinoid (C5), ophthalmic (i.e., supraclinoid) (C6), and communicating (i.e., terminal) (C7).

**TEACHING POINTS**

Intracranial Internal Carotid Artery Segments

| Segment | Location | Major Branches |
|---|---|---|
| C2: Petrous | Carotid canal within the petrous temporal bone | Vidian: Within the pterygoid canal |
| | | Caroticotympanic: Supplies the middle ear |
| C3: Lacerum | Above the petrous apex | None |
| C4: Cavernous | Within the cavernous sinus | 1. Inferolateral trunk: Supplies cavernous sinus<br>2. Meningohyophyseal trunk: Supplies pituitary. Tentorial artery branch (Bernasconi-Cassinari can supply tentorial bases lesions such as meningioma and arteriovenous malformation |
| C5: Clinoid | Above the cavernous sinus to the distal dural ring | None |
| C6: Ophthalmic | Distal dural ring to the PCOM | Ophthalmic artery: 80%–90% arises intradural just below the anterior clinoid process. |
| C7: Communicating | From the PCOM to the ICA terminus | 1. Posterior communicating artery (PCOM): Connects anterior and posterior circulation. Supplies parts of thalamus, hypothalamus, optic chiasm, and mammillary bodies. Variant anatomy "fetal origin of the PCA" when the PCOM is larger than the first segment of the posterior cerebral artery<br>2. Anterior choroidal artery: Supplies the optic tract, medial temporal lobe, uncus, amygdala, hippocampus, anterior limb of the internal capsule, choroid plexus of the lateral ventricle, inferior globus pallidus, caudate, cerebral peduncles and midbrain |

Legend (from figure):
1 Posterior communicating artery
2 Trigeminal artery
3 Otic artery
4 Hypoglossal artery
5 Proatlantal intersegmental artery

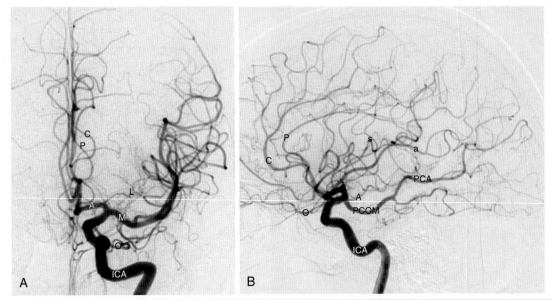

**Fig. 1.29  Internal carotid artery anatomy.** (A) Anteroposterior view of an internal carotid artery (ICA) injection shows filling of anterior cerebral artery and middle cerebral artery (MCA) branches. The M-1 *(M)* and A-1 *(A)* segments are labeled. Note that the pericallosal artery *(P)* remains closer to the midline than callosal-marginal *(C)* branches. Lenticulostriate branches *(L)* and the ophthalmic artery *(O)* can also be made out. (B) Lateral view in a different patient with persistent fetal origin of the posterior cerebral artery *(PCA)* demonstrates filling of the posterior communicating artery *(PCOM)* and PCA. There is opacification of the pericallosal *(P)* and callosal-marginal *(C)* branches. The ophthalmic artery *(O)*, anterior choroidal artery *(A)*, sylvian loops *of* the insula *(s)*, and angular branch *(a)* of the MCA can be identified.

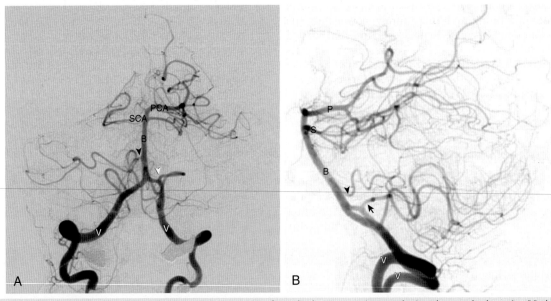

**Fig. 1.30  Vertebrobasilar artery circulation.** (A) Anteroposterior view of vertebral artery arteriogram depicts the vertebral arteries *(V)*, the posterior inferior cerebellar arteries (PICAs; *white arrowhead*), the basilar artery *(B)*, the anterior inferior cerebellar arteries (AICAs; *black arrowhead*), the superior cerebellar arteries *(SCAs)*, and the posterior cerebral arteries *(PCAs)*. Only the *left* PCA opacifies here because of persistent origin of the PCA on the *right*. (B) Lateral view shows the same vascular anatomy. Vertebral arteries *(V)*, basilar artery *(B)*, PICA *(black arrow)*, AICA *(black arrowhead)*, SCA *(S)*, and PCA *(P)* are shown.

- The ICA terminates into the anterior cerebral artery (ACA) and the middle cerebral artery (MCA) after giving off the posterior communicating artery in its supraclinoid segment.

## Anterior Circulation

### Anterior Cerebral Artery System.

- The ACA supplies medial aspects of the frontal and parietal lobes, olfactory cortex, and the corpus callosum

(Fig. 1.32). Therefore ACA infarctions affect olfaction, thought processes (the medial inferior frontal lobe), motor function of the leg (precentral gyrus medially), sensation to the leg (postcentral gyrus medially), memory, and emotion (the cingulate gyrus). The ACA has three segments as follows:

- A1: The first, horizontal portion gives rise to two main segments:
  a. Medial lenticulostriates: Extending superiorly through the perforating substance and suppling the

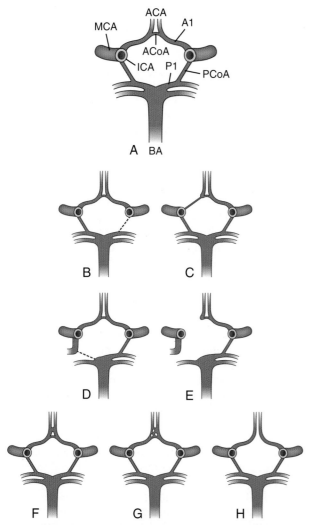

Fig. 1.31 **Circle of Willis.** Anatomic diagrams depict the circle of Willis (A) and its common variations (B-H). (A) A "complete" circle of Willis is present. Here all components are present, and none are hypoplastic. This configuration is seen in less than half of all cases. (B) Hypoplasia of one or both posterior communicating arteries (PCoAs) is the most common circle of Willis variant, seen in 25% to 33% of cases. (C) Hypoplasia, or absence of the horizontal *(A1)* anterior cerebral artery segment, is seen in approximately 10% to 20% of cases. Here the right A1 segment is hypoplastic. (D) Fetal type origin of the right posterior cerebral artery (PCA) with hypoplasia *(dotted line)* of the precommunicating *(P1)* PCA segment, seen in 15% to 25% of cases. (E) If both a fetal origin PCA and an absent A1 occur together, the internal carotid artery *(ICA)* is anatomically isolated with severely restricted potential collateral blood flow. (F) Multichannel (two or more) anterior communicating artery segments, seen in 10% to 15% of cases. Here the duplicated anterior communicating arteries *(AcoAs)* are complete, and both extend across the entire AcoA. (G) In a fenestrated AcoA, the AcoA has a more plexiform appearance. (H) Absence of an AcoA is shown. *ACA*, Anterior cerebral artery; *BA*, basilar artery; *MCA*, middle cerebral artery. (From Osborne AG. *Diagnostic Cerebral Angiography.* 2nd ed. Philadelphia: Lippincott Williams & Wilkins; 1999:113.)

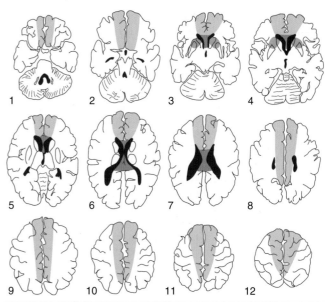

Fig. 1.32 **Anterior cerebral artery (ACA) distribution.** Shaded areas of these axial diagrams, arranged in sequence from base to vertex, outline the territory of the ACA, including the medial lenticulostriate *(orange)*, callosal *(blue)*, and hemispheric branches *(green)*. (From Latchaw RE. *MR and CT Imaging of the Head, Neck, and Spine.* 2nd ed. St. Louis: Mosby; 1991.)

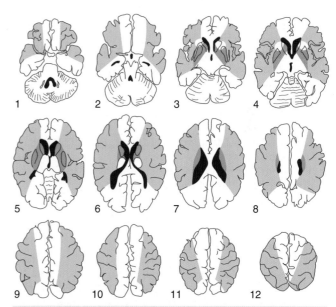

Fig. 1.33 **Middle cerebral artery (MCA) distribution.** This diagram of the axial sections, arranged in sequence from base to vertex, outlines the MCA distribution with the lateral lenticulostriate *(orange)* and hemispheric branches *(green)*. (From Latchaw RE. *MR and CT Imaging of the Head, Neck, and Spine.* 2nd ed. St. Louis: Mosby; 1991.)

basal ganglia and anterior limb of the internal capsule. Infarcts in this region affect motor function of the face and arm.
  b. Recurrent artery of Heubner: Supplies the head of the caudate and anteroinferior internal capsule.
- A2: Vertical segment extending superiorly along the genu of the corpus callosum, which bifurcates into the following branches:
  a. Orbitofrontal artery
  b. Frontopolar artery

- A3: Wraps around the corpus callosum genu, dividing into the following branches:
  a. Pericallosal artery
  b. Callosomarginal artery

**Middle Cerebral Artery System.**

- The MCA has a large vascular distribution with cortical branches supplying most of the lateral surface of the cerebral hemispheres and anterior temporal lobe (Fig. 1.33).

MCA infarcts may affect motor and sensory function of the face, arm, and trunk (lateral precentral and postcentral gyri), speech (inferior lateral frontotemporal gyri), thought processes (anteroinferolateral frontal lobes), hearing (superior temporal gyri), memory and naming of objects (temporal lobe), and taste (insular cortex). Perforating branches supply most of the putamen, globus pallidus, and caudate and the superior aspect of the internal capsule. The MCA has four segments as follows:

- M1: Horizontal segment extending to the sylvian fissure giving rise to the lenticulostriate vessels and typically the anterior temporal artery.
- M2: Sylvian segment after the MCA bifurcates into superior and inferior divisions, or less commonly trifurcates.
- M3: Loops around the frontal operculum to form the "candelabra" effect on the lateral surface of the cortex.
- M4: The most distal MCA branches course over the lateral convexities.

## Posterior Circulation

### Vertebral Arteries

- The vertebral arteries typically arise from the subclavian arteries. The left vertebral artery arises directly from the aortic arch before the left subclavian artery in 1% of the population. The left is larger (dominant) compared with the right in 75% of people. The vertebral arteries can be divided into four segments:
- V1: Extending from their origin, coursing superiorly between the longus colli and scalene muscles to the foramen transversarium. Branches include the occipital, segmental cervical, muscular, and spinal branches.
- V2: From the entrance within the spinal canal (beginning at C6 in 95% of the people), coursing within the foramen transversarium to the exit from the spinal canal at the C1 to C2 transverse foramen. Branch: Anterior meningeal artery.
- V3: From the exit of the spinal canal at C1 to C2 to the dura. Branch: Posterior meningeal artery.
- V4: Piercing the dura entering the intracranial compartment via the foramen magnum. Branches:
  - Anterior and posterior spinal arteries supplying the spinal cord artery.
  - Posterior inferior cerebellar artery(PICA) usually arises from the V4 segment but can arise from the V3 segment. This vessel loops around the medulla and tonsil while supplying the posterolateral medulla, the inferior vermis, the choroid plexus of the fourth ventricle, and the inferior aspect of the cerebellum.
    - The size of the PICA is inversely proportional to the size of the anterior inferior cerebellar artery (AICA), which arises from the basilar artery. Occasionally, one vertebral artery may terminate in PICA, without contributing to the basilar system. Also, common trunk origins of AICA and PICA (AICA-PICA complex) may be seen.
    - PICA infarcts can induce the lateral medullary (Wallenberg) syndrome. This causes loss of pain and temperature of the body on the contralateral side (lateral spinothalamic tract) and face on the ipsilateral side (descending trigeminothalamic tract), ataxia (cerebellar connections), ipsilateral swallowing and taste disorders (ninth cranial nerve), hoarseness

(tenth cranial nerve), vertigo and nystagmus (eighth nerve), and ipsilateral Horner syndrome.

### Basilar Artery Branches

- The two vertebral arteries join to form the basilar artery at the pontomedullary level. The basilar artery has many tiny branches to the pons and medulla that are never seen at angiography. The major branches and the structures they supply are as follows:
  - AICA arises as the first branch of the basilar artery and often loops into the internal auditory canal. It supplies the labyrinthine branches of the inner ear and anterior inferior cerebellum.
  - The superior cerebellar artery (SCA) is the last infratentorial branch and supplies the superior vermis, superior cerebellar peduncle, and the brachium pontis.
  - The posterior cerebral artery (PCA) is the termination of the basilar artery feeding the occipital, posterior inferior frontal, and inferior temporal lobes.
  - Artery of Percheron with additional small perforating vessels arise from the basilar dome. They serve paramedian thalamus and midbrain. Infarctions can affect CN III and IV, causing oculomotor deficits; the cerebral peduncles, affecting motor strength; the medial lemniscus, altering sensation; the red nucleus and substantia nigra, affecting coordination and motor control; and the reticular activating system, affecting level of consciousness.
- The PCAs wrap around the midbrain and can be divided into four segments:
- P1 segment: From the terminus of the basilar artery to its junction with the posterior communicating artery, traveling above the cisternal segment of CN III. Main branch: Posterior thalamoperforating arteries, which supply the medial thalami and wall of the third ventricle.
- P2 segment: From the posterior communicating artery (PCOM) junction through the ambient cistern. Branches include:
  - Thalamogeniculate arteries: Supply medial and lateral geniculate nucleus and the pulvinar of the thalamus
  - Medial posterior choroidal arteries: Supply the tectum, the choroid plexus of the third ventricle, and the thalami
  - Lateral posterior choroidal arteries, which run behind the pulvinar into the choroidal fissure and supply the choroid of the lateral and third ventricles, the posterior thalamus, and the fornix
  - Anterior temporal artery: Supplies the anterior aspect of the inferior temporal lobe including hippocampus
  - Posterior temporal artery: Supplies the posterior parahippocampal gyrus
- P3 segment: Within the quadrigeminal plate cistern. Anterior and posterior inferior temporal arteries arise from the P3 segment.
- P4 segment: Within the calcarine fissure dividing into the medial and lateral branches.
- PCA infarctions affect vision most commonly (occipital lobes) but also affect memory (posteroinferior temporal lobe), smell (hippocampal region), and emotion (posterior fornix) (Fig. 1.34). Disease of the perforating branches, such as the posterior thalamoperforating arteries and the thalamogeniculate arteries that form the P1 and P2 segments, may affect memory and emotion (anterior

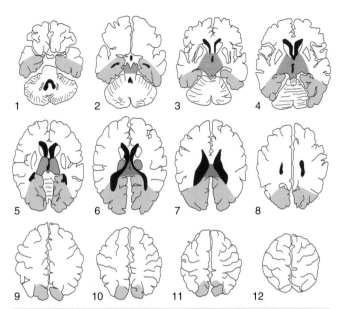

**Fig. 1.34 Posterior cerebral artery (PCA) distribution.** Axial diagrams arranged in sequence from base to vertex outline supply from the PCA, the thalamic and midbrain perforators *(orange),* callosal *(blue),* and hemispheric branches *(green).* (From Latchaw RE. *MR and CT Imaging of the Head, Neck, and Spine.* 2nd ed. St. Louis: Mosby; 1991.)

thalamus), endocrine function (hypothalamus), language (pulvinar), pain sensation (thalami), sight (lateral geniculate), and motor control (subthalamic nuclei).

## VENOUS ANATOMY

- The intracranial venous system consists of dural sinuses, large venous channels within the dural reflections, and cerebral veins that drain to the sinuses (Fig. 1.35).

### Superficial Drainage

- Superficial drainage patterns are highly variable from person to person. However, the superficial drainage of the brain is notable for the superficial vein of Labbé (draining from the sylvian fissure laterally into the transverse sinus) and the superior superficial vein of Trolard (draining from the sylvian fissure into the superior sagittal sinus).
- Superior cerebral veins also empty directly into the superior sagittal sinus (see Fig. 1.35). The superficial middle cerebral vein drains from the sylvian fissure into the cavernous sinus, which drains into the petrosal sinuses. The vein of Labbé may arise from the posterior extent of the superficial middle cerebral vein.

### Deep Supratentorial Drainage

- The deep venous drainage of the supratentorial space centers on the internal cerebral vein and the vein of Galen. Medullary veins radiate downward from the superficial white matter to drain to the subependymal veins, which include the septal veins extending along the septum pellucidum and the thalamostriate veins, which course over the caudate. The septal veins and the thalamostriate veins join to form the internal cerebral veins.
- The septal veins course around the anteromedial aspect of the lateral ventricle before passing behind the foramen of Monro to join the internal cerebral vein at the "true venous angle." If the septal vein joins the internal

cerebral vein further posteriorly than the demarcation of the foramen of Monro, the junction is called the "false venous angle." Thus, the internal cerebral veins usually begin at the foramina of Monro and run on either side of the roof of the third ventricle (velum interpositum).

- The internal cerebral veins unite to form the great vein of Galen, which curves under the splenium of the corpus callosum. The vein of Galen drains into the straight sinus. The internal cerebral veins are a marker for midline shift, behind the foramen of Monro. They should not deviate more than 2 mm from the midline.

### Deep Infratentorial Drainage

- The anatomy of posterior fossa venous drainage is more complex and can be divided into three main drainage systems (Fig. 1.36).
  - The superior group includes a drain into the vein of Galen and includes the superior vermian vein traveling over the vermis, the precentral cerebellar vein midline terminating adjacent to the inferior colliculi, and the anterior pontomesencephalic vein, which drains a venous plexus over the ventral pons and cerebral peduncles. The vein of Galen and the inferior sagittal sinus drain to the straight sinus, which, in turn, drains into the torcular Herophili (torcula). The torcula is the common dumping ground (toilet) of the venous system. It also receives the drainage from the superior sagittal sinus.
    - From the torcula, blood flows to the transverse sinus, which receives drainage from the superior petrosal sinus, diploic veins, and lateral cerebellar veins. It courses laterally in the leaves of the tentorium and continues as the sigmoid sinus, which also drains the occipital sinus. Transverse sinus size asymmetry is very common and often one side may be hypoplastic with diminished caliber throughout its course. In addition, arachnoid granulations (often seen as focal rounded hyperintense CSF spaces on T2-weighted imaging [T2WI]) often invaginate the transverse sinus and lead to focal narrowings. These two factors (frequent sinus hypoplasia and focal narrowings from extrinsic arachnoid granulation indentations) make the evaluation for transverse sinus stenosis in idiopathic intracranial hypertension (pseudotumor cerebri) problematic. These granulations may also result in bony excavations in the adjacent skull, most commonly at the occipital skull but also along the frontal calvarium and sphenoid bone.
    - The sigmoid sinus terminates as the internal jugular vein.
  - The second infratentorial group is the anterior or petrosal group with its dominant vein, the petrosal vein, taking drainage from the cerebellum, pons, and medulla. The petrosal vein then drains into the superior petrosal sinus.
  - The third division, the posterior group, drains the inferior vermis and tentorium consisting mainly of the inferior vermian veins. The inferior vermian veins drain into the straight sinus.

## BLOOD-BRAIN BARRIER

- It is probably appropriate after a vascular anatomy section to emphasize the role of the blood-brain barrier

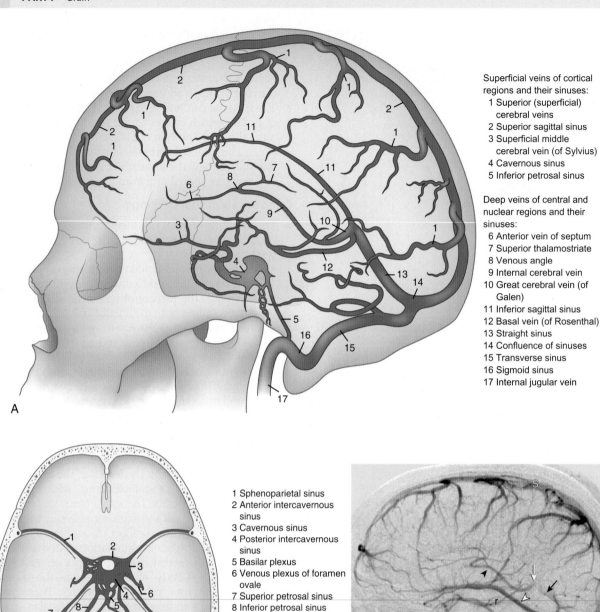

Superficial veins of cortical
regions and their sinuses:
  1 Superior (superficial)
    cerebral veins
  2 Superior sagittal sinus
  3 Superficial middle
    cerebral vein (of Sylvius)
  4 Cavernous sinus
  5 Inferior petrosal sinus

Deep veins of central and
nuclear regions and their
sinuses:
  6 Anterior vein of septum
  7 Superior thalamostriate
  8 Venous angle
  9 Internal cerebral vein
  10 Great cerebral vein (of
     Galen)
  11 Inferior sagittal sinus
  12 Basal vein (of Rosenthal)
  13 Straight sinus
  14 Confluence of sinuses
  15 Transverse sinus
  16 Sigmoid sinus
  17 Internal jugular vein

1 Sphenoparietal sinus
2 Anterior intercavernous
  sinus
3 Cavernous sinus
4 Posterior intercavernous
  sinus
5 Basilar plexus
6 Venous plexus of foramen
  ovale
7 Superior petrosal sinus
8 Inferior petrosal sinus
9 Internal jugular vein
  (running caudally)
10 Sigmoid sinus
11 Transverse sinus
12 Occipital sinus
13 Superior sagittal sinus
14 Confluence of sinuses

**Fig. 1.35 Venous anatomy.** (A) Lateral view of the head illustrating the cerebral veins and sinuses. The sequence of the numbers takes into account both the areas drained by the veins and the direction of blood flow. (B) Top-down view of the skull base depicts the basal sinuses. (C) Venous anatomy on angiography. This lateral view shows the internal cerebral vein *(black arrowhead),* vein of Galen *(white arrow),* straight sinus *(black arrow),* torcular (T), and superior sagittal sinus (S). The vein of Labbé *(white arrowhead)* drains into the transverse sinus (t). Sigmoid sinus *(sig)* and jugular vein (J) are also readily appreciable. Faintly seen are the basal vein of Rosenthal (r) and blush of the cavernous sinus (c). (A and B, Modified with permission from Kretschmann H-J, Weinrich W. *Cranial Neuroimaging and Clinical Neuroanatomy: Magnetic Resonance Imaging and Computed Tomography.* Rev 2nd ed. New York: Thieme; 1993:214, 215.)

(BBB) in neuroimaging and in CNS pathology. The anatomy of the BBB is based on the microanatomy of the capillary endothelial cells. There are tight junctions between normal endothelial cells without gaps or channels. The basement membrane maintains the tubular conformation of the capillary and holds the endothelial cells together.

- In only a few regions in the brain do channels exist so that direct communication is present between the capillary and extracellular fluid or neurons. Such sites play a role in the feedback mechanism for hormonal homeostasis and as a port of entry into the brain for certain disease processes. They include the choroid plexus of the ventricles, the pineal gland, pituitary gland, median eminence,

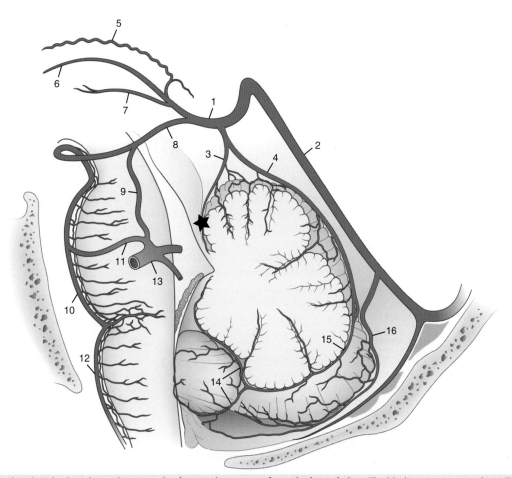

**Fig. 1.36 Anatomic drawing depicts the major posterior fossa veins as seen from the lateral view.** The black star represents the colliculocentral point, an angiographic landmark that should be about halfway between the tuberculum sellae and the torcular herophili. 1, Vein of Galen; 2, straight sinus; 3, precentral cerebellar vein; 4, superior vermian vein; 5, superior choroid vein (in lateral ventricle); 6, internal cerebral vein; 7, thalamic vein; 8, posterior mesencephalic vein; 9, lateral mesencephalic vein; 10, anterior pontomesencephalic venous plexus; 11, transverse pontine vein; 12, anterior medullary venous plexus; 13, petrosal vein; 14, tonsillar veins; 15, inferior vermian veins; and 16, hemispheric vein. (From Osborne AG. *Diagnostic Cerebral Angiography*. 2nd ed. Philadelphia: Lippincott William & Wilkins; 1998:234.)

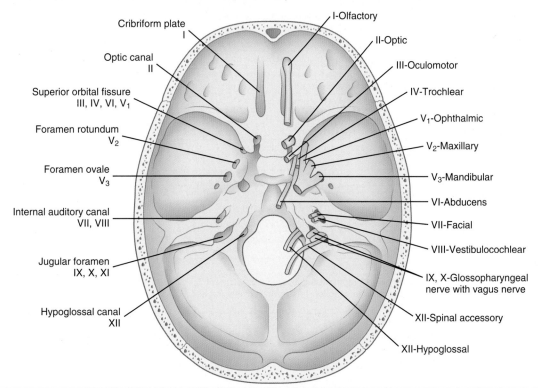

**Fig. 1.37 Skull base foramina.** This diagram illustrates the exits of the cranial nerve through the skull base foramina.

subcommissural organ, subfornical organ, area postrema, and organum vasculosum of the lamina terminalis.

- After injection of contrast, enhancement on CT or MRI is noted in the vessels of the brain and structures without a BBB. Slightly increased density on CT is also demonstrated in the cerebral parenchyma (gray matter denser than white matter) because of the cerebral blood volume (4%–5% of total brain volume). The normal cerebral parenchymal enhancement is minimal.
- Any alteration of the BBB from factors such as inflammation, infection, neoplasm, infarct, and trauma can produce intraparenchymal enhancement. The alteration is usually in the form of unlocking of the tight junctions, increased pinocytosis of contrast agents, vascular endothelial fenestration (formation of transendothelial channels), or increased permeability of the endothelial membrane.
- In many neoplastic conditions, the BBB is not competent and contrast material is distributed into the

extravascular spaces. A minority of enhancement is caused by increased blood volume in certain neoplastic lesions. This has recently been demonstrated by perfusion-weighted MR studies of high-grade neoplasms. Lack of angiographic vascularity has little bearing on contrast enhancement. Angiogenesis at a microvascular level may also be an important factor in enhancement.

## Skull Base Foramina

- The skull base contains numerous canals, fissures, and foramina which house important structures including arteries, veins and nerves. It is important to have a working knowledge of these structures and their contents, depicted in Figs. 1.37 and 1.38. These are discussed in further detail in dedicated orbit, skull base, temporal bone and sinonasal chapters (Chapters 9-12) coming up ahead!

**TEACHING POINTS**

Skull Base Foramina and Their Contents

| Skull Base Foramen | Contents | Noteworthy Pathology |
|---|---|---|
| Cribriform plate | Olfactory nerves, anterior ethmoidal artery | Anterior skull base tumors, trauma |
| Optic canal | Optic nerve, ophthalmic artery | Optic neuritis, gliomas, meningiomas |
| Superior orbital fissure | Oculomotor, trochlear, abducens, and ophthalmic (V–1) nerves, ophthalmic veins, sympathetic nerve plexus, orbital branch of middle meningeal artery, recurrent branch of lacrimal artery | Schwannomas, meningiomas, perineural spread of cancer (PNS) |
| Foramen rotundum | Maxillary (V–2) nerve | Schwannomas, meningiomas, PNS |
| Foramen ovale | Mandibular (V–3) nerve, accessory meningeal artery, emissary veins | Schwannomas, meningiomas, PNS |
| Stylomastoid foramen | Facial nerve, stylomastoid artery | PNS, Bell palsy, schwannoma |
| Internal auditory canal | Facial and vestibulocochlear nerves, labyrinthine artery (branch of anterior inferior cerebellar artery [AICA]) | Schwannomas, meningiomas, epidermoids, arachnoid cysts |
| Jugular foramen, pars nervosa | Glossopharyngeal nerve, inferior petrosal sinus | Schwannomas, meningiomas, PNS |
| Jugular foramen, pars vascularis | Vagus, spinal accessory nerves, internal jugular vein, ascending pharyngeal and occipital artery branches | Glomus tumors, schwannomas, meningiomas, PNS |
| Hypoglossal canal | Hypoglossal nerve, meningeal branch of ascending pharyngeal artery, emissary vein | Schwannomas |
| Foramen magnum | Spinal cord, vertebral arteries, spinal arteries, and nerves | Meningiomas, chordomas, schwannomas |
| Foramen spinosum | Middle meningeal artery, meningeal branch of V–3 | Supplies meningiomas, PNS |
| Foramen lacerum | Carotid artery lies on top of it, greater petrosal nerve, vidian nerve pass above it | PNS |
| Incisive canal/nasopalatine canal | Nasopalatine nerve, palatine arteries | Cysts |
| Greater palatine canal | Greater palatine nerve, palatine vessels | PNS |
| Lesser palatine canal | Lesser palatine nerve and artery | PNS |
| Carotid canal | Internal carotid artery, sympathetic plexus | Aneurysms |
| Foramen of Vesalius | Emissary veins | Spread of cavernous sinus disease |
| Foramen cecum | Emissary vein | Nasal glioma, encephalocele |
| Vestibular aqueduct | Endolymphatic duct, meningeal branch of occipital artery | Ménière disease, congenital stenosis, or enlargement |
| Condylar canal | Emissary vein, meningeal branch of occipital artery | — |
| Mastoid foramen | Emissary vein, meningeal branch of occipital artery | — |
| Palatovaginal canal | Pharyngeal branches of pterygopalatine ganglion and maxillary artery | PNS |
| Cochlear aqueduct | Perilymphatic duct, emissary vein | Congenital stenosis or patulousness |
| Inferior orbital fissure | Maxillary nerve, zygomatic nerve, orbital branches of pterygopalatine ganglion, infraorbital vessels, inferior ophthalmic veins | PNS, schwannomas |
| Infraorbital foramen | Infraorbital nerve and vessels | Blow-out fractures |
| Mental foramen | Mental nerves and vessels | PNS |
| Mandibular foramen | Inferior alveolar nerve and vessels | PNS |
| Pterygomaxillary fissure | Maxillary artery, maxillary nerve, sphenopalatine veins | Juvenile angiofibromas |
| Vidian canal | Vidian nerve and artery | PNS |

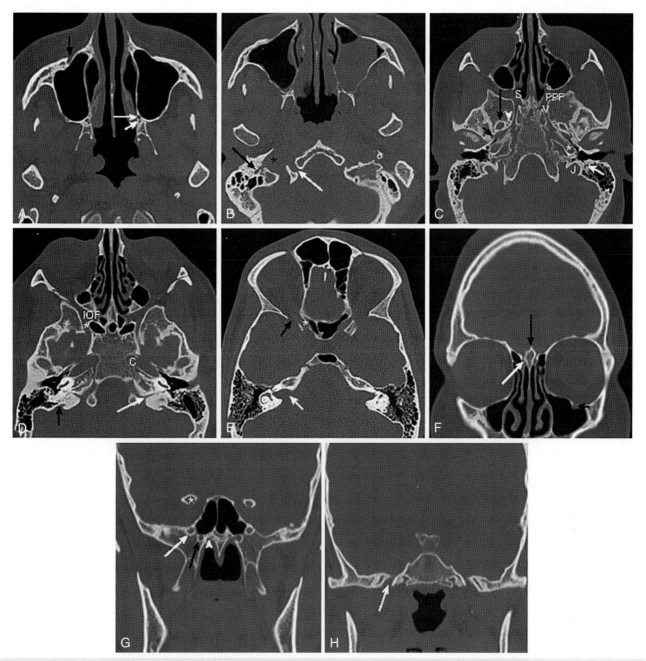

**Fig. 1.38 Skull base foramina on computed tomography (CT).** From inferior to superior on axial CT images and anterior to posterior on coronal CT images, skull base foramina are depicted. (A) At the level of the pterygoid plates, the greater *(long white arrow)* and lesser *(short white arrow)* palatine foramina are clearly seen. The canal of the infraorbital nerve *(black arrow)* can also be seen on this image. (B) At the posterior cranial fossa, the hypoglossal canal *(white arrow)*, stylomastoid foramen *(black arrow)*, and jugular foramen *(asterisk)* are shown. (C) More superiorly, the pterygopalatine fossa *(PPF)*, sphenopalatine foramen *(S)*, vidian canal *(V)*, and jugular foramen *(J)* are depicted. The foramen ovale *(large black arrow)* is adjacent to foramen of Vesalius *(white arrowhead)* along its anteromedial margin and the foramen spinosum *(small black arrow)* along its posteromedial margin. The carotid canal is depicted with an *asterisk*. The stylomastoid foramen is shown *(white arrow)*. (D) Slightly more superiorly, the inferior orbital fissure *(IOF)*, foramen rotundum *(asterisk)*, and carotid canal *(C)* are seen. At the same level within the temporal bone, the vestibular aqueduct *(black arrow)* and cochlear aqueduct *(white arrow)* are indicated. (E) At the level of the mid orbit, the optic canal is seen *(asterisk)* along with the superior orbital fissure *(black arrow)*. At the same level in the temporal bone, the internal auditory canal is depicted *(white arrow)*. (F) On this coronal CT, the crista galli is shown at the midline *(long black arrow)*, and the olfactory groove at the cribriform plate is seen as well *(white arrow)*. The canal of the inferior orbital nerve is again demonstrated *(short black arrow)* coursing the floor of the orbit. (G) More posteriorly, the anterior clinoid process is depicted *(asterisk)*, and the foramen rotundum *(white arrow)* and vidian canal *(black arrow)* are seen adjacent to the floor of the sphenoid sinus. The palatovaginal canal *(white arrowhead)* is also seen medial to vidian canal. (H) Even more posteriorly, foramen ovale can be seen *(white arrow)*.

Congratulations! You've made it through Chapter 1 and a not-so-brief overview of anatomy and functional neurologic systems. Now onto some more good stuff …

# 2  *Intracranial Neoplasms*

MARGARET N. CHAPMAN

In this chapter, we will review the more common neoplastic processes that occur in the intracranial compartment. Regional specific neoplasms, including those occurring in the orbit, sella, temporal bone, and sinonasal cavity, are discussed in detail in Chapters 9 to 12, respectively.

## Relevant Anatomy

### INTRA-AXIAL VERSUS EXTRA-AXIAL TUMORS

- Determining whether a lesion is intra-axial or extra-axial is essential in formulating a differential diagnosis when one encounters an intracranial lesion.
- It may be difficult to determine whether a lesion is intra-axial or extra-axial because some extra-axial lesions may invade the brain parenchyma and some parenchymal lesions can invade the meninges. This distinction has been made easier by the multiplanar capabilities of magnetic resonance imaging (MRI) and three-dimensional computed tomography (3D-CT)
- Intra-axial lesions are defined by their location within the brain parenchyma.

#### TEACHING POINTS

Characteristics of Intra-axial Lesions

- Expansion of brain cortex
- No expansion of the subarachnoid space
- The dura and pial blood vessels are peripheral to the mass.

- Extra-axial lesions are centered outside of the brain substance and include meningeal, dural, subarachnoid, or intraventricular locations (Fig. 2.1).

#### TEACHING POINTS

Characteristics of Extra-axial Lesions

- Buckling of the adjacent gray-white interface
- Expansion of the ipsilateral subarachnoid space
- Adjacent reactive bony changes (in some cases)
- Visualization of a thin rim of cerebrospinal fluid (CSF) between the lesion and adjacent parenchyma (*CSF cleft sign*)

- Once this distinction is made, secondary features of the lesion, such as shape/margination, internal architecture (solid, hemorrhagic, calcified, fatty, cystic), diffusivity, and enhancement characteristics will help lead to a specific diagnosis. The parenchymal location of a tumor may also assist in arriving at a specific diagnosis because some tumors have a predilection for certain lobes.

## Imaging Techniques/Protocols

### COMPUTED TOMOGRAPHY

- An unenhanced computed tomography (CT) scan of the brain is often the first imaging modality obtained in previously undiagnosed brain tumors in the setting of new and/or progressing neurologic symptoms. The tumor, associated mass effect, and other features, including hemorrhage or calcifications, can often be readily identified.
- The addition of iodinated intravenous (IV) contrast may help to better define the margins of a tumor and may improve sensitivity and the detection of smaller masses that may not have a significant amount of mass effect or adjacent edema and/or may be isodense to brain on unenhanced scanning.

### MAGNETIC RESONANCE IMAGING

- Multiplanar imaging of the brain before and after the administration of IV gadolinium is the preferred modality to characterize intracranial lesions. The following sequences are often obtained: sagittal T1, axial diffusion-weighted imaging (DWI), T1, T2, fluid-attenuated inversion recovery (FLAIR), gradient-recalled echo (GRE)/susceptibility-weighted imaging (SWI), postcontrast T1-weighted images (often in axial, coronal, and sagittal planes).
- If imaging is performed for presurgical planning, thin section T1- and T2-weighted images may help aid neurosurgical navigation in the operative field, following placement of fiducial markers.
- Perfusion imaging helps to predict tumor grade.
- Diffusion tensor imaging (DTI) and functional MRI may be helpful for surgical guidance.
- Postoperative imaging after resection of intracranial tumors is preferred within 24–48 hours of craniotomy to help distinguish a residual tumor from developing granulation tissue adjacent to the resection cavity and to serve as a baseline for follow-up imaging.

### ADVANCED IMAGING TECHNIQUES

- *Magnetic resonance (MR) perfusion* techniques may serve as a noninvasive method of measuring tissue perfusion, most often using the dynamic susceptibility contrast (DSC) enhanced method following intravenous administration of a gadolinium-based contrast agent.

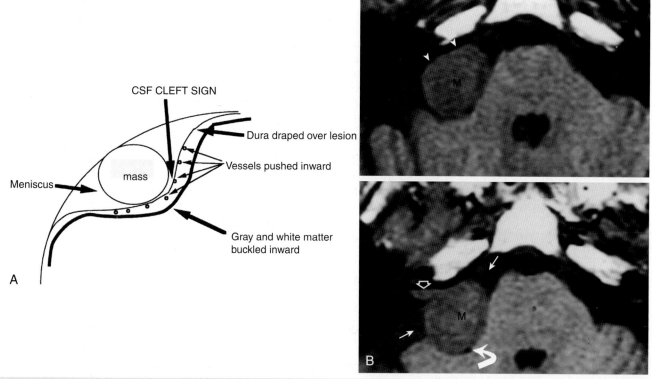

**Fig. 2.1 Extra-axial lesion signs.** (A) A skull-based extradural mass is depicted diagrammatically, producing a meniscus sign, displacement of the subarachnoid veins inward, and buckling of the gray-white interface. The dura may be draped over the lesion. (B) Extra-axial mass *(M)* abuts the petrous ridge *(arrowheads* in upper image), displaces blood vessels *(curved arrow* in lower image), and widens the subarachnoid space *(small arrows)*. The clincher here is the soft-tissue component extending into the internal auditory canal *(open arrow)*, nailing the diagnosis of vestibular schwannoma. *CSF,* Cerebrospinal fluid.

### PHYSICS PEARLS

Magnetic Resonance (MR) Perfusion

- This technique provides hemodynamic measurements, including cerebral blood volume (CBV), cerebral blood flow (CBF) and mean transit time (MTT).
- Perfusion maps can be used to evaluate vascularity in tumors and may correlate with tumor grade and malignant histology. The designation "corrected normalized" CBV maps means that data provided on these maps accounts for contrast leakage through the disrupted blood-brain barrier at the tumor site. These corrected maps are more accurate in determining tumor grade than noncorrected maps, which artificially lower CBV.
- Perfusion imaging techniques are often used in the posttreatment setting to differentiate recurrent tumor from posttreatment changes such as radiation necrosis.

### PHYSICS PEARLS

Magnetic Resonance (MR) Spectroscopy

- The relative concentrations and ratios of various metabolites can increase confidence in a suspected diagnosis.
- Generally speaking, NAA (N-acetyl aspartate) is a marker of neuronal viability and will be decreased in processes that decrease neurons such as high-grade tumors, metastases, and radiation necrosis.
- Cho (choline) is a component of cell membranes, and a marker of cellular membrane turnover, and will be elevated in processes that increase cellular turnover, such as neoplasms, gliosis, demyelination, and inflammation.
- Lactate is a marker of anaerobic metabolism and can be seen in the setting of necrotic tumors and abscesses.
- The ratios of the metabolites (for example, Cho/Cr, Cho/NAA, and NAA/Cr) in comparison to "normal" brain may also assist in differentiating processes such as recurrent tumor from posttreatment changes.

■ *MR spectroscopy* refers to an advanced imaging technique where a selected region of tissue is interrogated for the presence/concentration of various metabolites.

■ MR spectroscopy and perfusion are adjuncts to traditional anatomic MR imaging of the brain, and in combination, they can increase the sensitivity and specificity in differentiating tumors from nonneoplastic lesions, to suggest the best target for a biopsy, and to predict the grade of the tumor.

- *Functional MRI (fMRI)* refers to an advanced imaging technique that enables visualization of hemodynamic changes in the brain that occur while the patient performs specific tasks (task-based fMRI) or networks that are present even in the resting state (resting state fMRI). These techniques are often performed to further localize a lesion's relationship near or within centers in the brain responsible for controlling important functions, such as language, motor, or visual tasks.
- *DTI* is a useful technique to show white matter tracts. This is useful in surgical planning of tumor removal to determine the safest approach to a tumor that does not transect important functional white matter pathways.

# Pathology

- The World Health Organization (WHO) classification remains the worldwide standard for the classification of brain tumors and uses a combination of histologic, clinical, and imaging features to predict response to therapy and outcome. The 2016 WHO revision considers the molecular footprint of tumors as an important prognostic factor in classification, and this has been further expanded in the updated 2021 WHO classification.
- Specific molecular markers either present or absent in various tumor types will be described in their respective sections later in the chapter.
- Generally speaking, higher-grade tumors have higher malignant potential and a lower chance of long-term survival.

### EXTRA-AXIAL LESIONS

#### Meningiomas

- Meningiomas are a group of mostly benign, slow-growing, dural-based extra-axial neoplasms that arise from meningothelial cells of the arachnoid layer (arachnoid cap cells). They are the most common extra-axial neoplasm, accounting for approximately 36% of all brain tumors. Females are at a slightly greater risk for developing a meningioma than males.
- Most meningiomas are WHO grade I.

---

**TEACHING POINTS**

World Health Organization (WHO) Classification of Meningioma Variants

**Grade I**

Meningothelial, fibrous (fibroblastic), transitional (mixed), psammomatous, angiomatous, microcystic, secretory meningioma, lymphoplasmacyte-rich, metaplastic

**Grade II**

Chordoid meningioma, clear cell meningioma, atypical meningioma

**Grade III**

Papillary, rhabdoid, anaplastic

---

- 90% of meningiomas occur in the supratentorial compartment. Common locations (in descending order) are the parasagittal dura, convexities, sphenoid wing, cerebellopontine angle cistern, olfactory groove, and planum sphenoidale, although they can occur anywhere arachnoid exists.
- On unenhanced CT examinations, approximately 60% of meningiomas are slightly hyperdense compared with adjacent brain parenchyma (Fig. 2.2). Calcifications can be seen in approximately 20% of cases.
- MRI is superior to CT in detecting the full extent of meningiomas and for evaluation of associated or secondary findings, such as venous sinus invasion and/ or thrombosis, hypervascularity, adjacent edema, or intraosseous extension (Fig. 2.3). Classic meningiomas are isointense to gray matter on all pulse sequences and demonstrate avid enhancement, although variability often occurs depending on internal architecture.
- Meningiomas are characterized by high levels of alanine and absent N-acetyl aspartate on MR spectroscopy.
- A "dural tail"—dural enhancement adjacent to the lesion, often tapering in a crescentic fashion—is commonly encountered and may correspond to reactive fibrovascular tissue as opposed to neoplastic infiltration. This may serve as a useful feature in differentiating meningiomas from other extra-axial lesions, such as schwannoma.
- The "cleft sign" can be seen and refers to CSF, dura, and/ or marginal vessels interposed between the brain and meningioma.

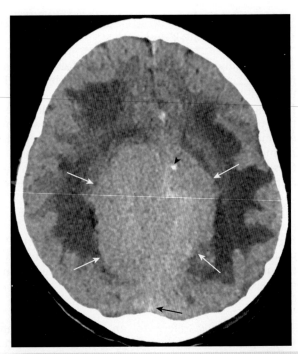

**Fig. 2.2 Meningioma.** A hyperdense extra-axial mass arising from the falx and extending into both cerebral hemispheres *(white arrows)*. Note calcification *(arrowhead)*. There is very likely invasion of the superior sagittal sinus *(black arrow)*. Note the extensive vasogenic edema within the surrounding brain tissue on the unenhanced computed tomography scan.

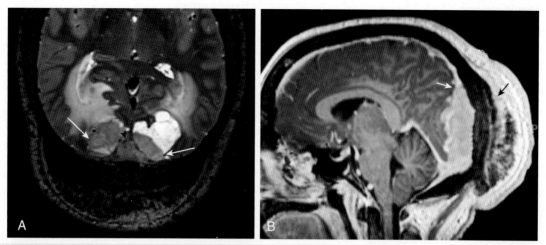

**Fig. 2.3 Parasagittal meningioma.** (A) This meningioma *(white arrows)* is isointense on T2-weighted imaging (T2WI), and demonstrates adjacent hyperintense intra-axial vasogenic edema. Because the lesion crosses midline outside a normal white matter tract and is invading the dura of the superior sagittal sinus *(black arrowhead)*, it is clearly extra-axial. (B) Other imaging features include a dural tail, tumor growth along the sagittal sinus *(white arrow)*, bone reaction *(black arrow)*, and strong enhancement, imaging features most consistent with a meningioma.

- Other imaging features that can be seen with meningiomas include:
  - Vascular encasement and narrowing
  - Vasogenic edema in adjacent brain parenchyma, more commonly seen with convexity and larger meningiomas. This may be secondary to compressive ischemia, venous stasis, aggressive growth, or parasitization of pial vessels. Venous sinus occlusion or venous thrombosis can also result in parenchymal edema.
  - Adjacent hyperostotic or osteolytic bone changes. Hyperostosis is particularly common when the tumor is located near the skull base or anterior cranial fossa.
  - Pneumosinus dilatans is the expansion of a paranasal sinus from an adjacent meningioma (usually anterior cranial fossa meningioma with an adjacent large frontal sinus).
- Less common meningiomas:
  - Intraosseous meningiomas appear as expansions of the calvarium and can extend into the scalp soft tissues. These are most commonly found along the sphenoid wing (Fig. 2.4). A blastic osseous metastasis is a differential consideration. That said, intraosseous meningiomas are much less common than dural origin meningiomas that grow into or through the bone.
  - Intraventricular meningiomas typically occur near the choroid plexus in the trigone of the lateral ventricle (80%), more often on the left, but may be seen in the third (15%) and fourth ventricles (5%) (Fig. 2.5). These commonly calcify.
  - Multiple meningiomas are associated with neurofibromatosis type 2.

## Atypical Meningiomas

- Atypical meningiomas are classified as WHO grade II, intermediate between benign and malignant types, with more aggressive-appearing histopathologic features. These recur more frequently.

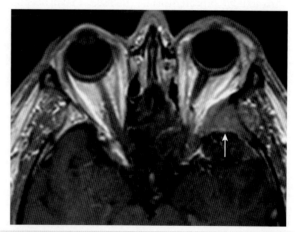

**Fig. 2.4 Intraosseous meningioma.** Contrast enhanced T1-weighted image *(T1WI)* demonstrates evidence of an intraosseous meningioma expanding the left sphenoid wing *(white arrow)*. The patient has mild asymmetric proptosis and a small amount of intraorbital soft tissue. A small amount of soft tissue extends extracranially into the left temporalis muscle.

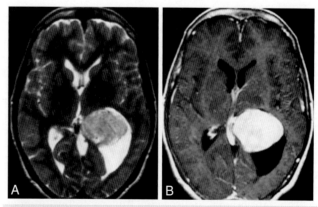

**Fig. 2.5 Intraventricular meningioma.** (A) Axial T2 WI shows a well-defined large intraventricular mass isointense to gray matter in a dilated left lateral ventricular trigone. (B) Note the avid homogeneous enhancement.

## Malignant Meningiomas

- Malignant meningiomas are classified as WHO grade III and demonstrate malignant cytology, very high mitotic rate, anaplasia, or sarcomatous degeneration. Rapid growth, intraparenchymal infiltration, and recurrence are more common with more aggressive grades.

## Mesenchymal, Nonmeningothelial Tumors

- There are a number of relatively rare benign and malignant mesenchymal tumors that can affect the meninges.
- Solitary fibrous tumor (SFT) has now replaced the term "hemangiopericytoma" and represents mesenchymal tumors of a fibroblastic type, derived from smooth muscle pericyte cells of Zimmerman around the capillaries of the meninges. Most tumors are located supratentorially.
- These are more aggressive than most meningiomas, have a higher rate of recurrence, and can metastasize. Hence some consider them malignant and distinct from meningiomas.
- They tend to be large (over 4 cm in size), lobular, extra-axial supratentorial masses. Hydrocephalus, edema, and mass effect are common.
- The "mushroom sign" refers to a narrow dural attachment despite parenchymal invasion (opposite of what is expected from meningiomas) in some cases.
- They are often dural-based and more frequently seen in the skull base and in parasagittal/parafalcine locations.
- In the CNS, there is a three-tiered grading system based on mitotic counts and necrosis.
  - Grade I tumors are considered benign and resectable. These demonstrate a classic SFT phenotype histologically.
  - Grade II and III tumors are malignant and are treated with adjuvant therapy, usually radiation.
- CT shows solitary, irregularly contoured, heterogeneous masses that enhance. Calcification and/or hyperostosis are rare. These tumors are isointense with variable enhancement on T1-weighted imaging (T1WI) and demonstrate high or mixed signal on T2-weighted imaging (T2WI).

## Melanocytic Lesions

- These processes include diffuse melanocytosis, melanocytoma, neurocutaneous melanosis, and malignant melanoma. These diagnoses are difficult to distinguish from metastatic melanoma to the dura.
- Hyperintensity on T1WI is often seen but varies with melanin content.
- Malignant melanoma of the meninges may bleed or spread from the dura to the adjacent nerves, brain, or skull. Prognosis is poor, as is malignant melanoma of the meninges with distant metastases.

## TUMORS OF NEUROGENIC ORIGIN

- The intracranial neurogenic tumors (schwannomas, neurofibromas) are similar in imaging appearance.

## Schwannomas

- Schwannomas are benign (WHO grade I), typically encapsulated nerve sheath tumors composed of well-differentiated Schwann cells.
- Histologically, schwannomas arise from the perineural Schwann cells. Two types of tissue may be seen with schwannomas: Antoni A and Antoni B tissue. The Antoni A tissue typically has a darker signal on T2WI because of the compactness of the fibrils. Antoni B tissue is a looser, myxomatous tissue that is typically brighter on T2WI.
- The distinction between meningiomas and schwannomas is a common one that radiologists must make at the skull base, although it is sometimes difficult to distinguish between the two.

---

**TEACHING POINTS**

Differential Diagnosis of Meningioma versus Schwannoma

| Feature | Meningioma | Schwannoma |
| --- | --- | --- |
| Dural tail | Frequent | Extremely rare |
| Bony reaction | Osteolysis or hyperostosis | Rare |
| Angle made with dura | Obtuse | Acute |
| Calcification | 20% | Rare |
| Cyst/necrosis formation | Rare | Up to 10% |
| Enhancement | Uniform | Inhomogeneous in 1/3 |
| Extension into IAC | Rare | 80% |
| Precontrast CT attenuation | Hyperdense | Isodense |

CT, Computed tomography; GABA, gamma-aminobutyric acid; IAC, internal auditory canal.

---

- Schwannomas of cranial nerve VIII (vestibular schwannoma) are the most common. One of the distinguishing features of vestibular schwannomas from meningiomas is the expansion of and growth into the internal auditory canal (IAC) seen in schwannomas. The porus acusticus (the bony opening of the IAC to the cerebellopontine angle cistern) is typically flared and enlarged with vestibular schwannomas, whereas the amount of tissue seen in the IAC with meningiomas is usually small or absent.
- Vestibular schwannomas account for more than 90% of purely intracanalicular lesions, but only 20% of them are solely intracanalicular (Fig. 2.6A). Approximately 20% of vestibular schwannomas present only in the cerebellopontine angle cistern without an IAC stem. About 60% of vestibular schwannomas have both a canalicular and cisternal portion (see Fig. 2.6B).

---

**TEACHING POINTS**

Cerebellopontine Angle Masses

Vestibular schwannoma (75%)
Meningioma (10%)
Epidermoid (5%)
Facial nerve schwannoma (4%)

(Continued)

Aneurysm (vertebral, basilar, posterior inferior cerebellar artery)
Exophytic brain stem glioma
Arachnoid cyst
Paraganglioma (from temporal bone)
Hematogenous metastasis
Subarachnoid spread of tumors
Lipoma
Exophytic desmoplastic medulloblastoma

- Multiple schwannomas are associated with neurofibromatosis type 2. Malignant schwannomas (and peripheral nerve sheath tumors) may be seen in patients with neurofibromatosis type 1 but are usually *not* intracranial.
- On MRI, schwannomas are usually well-circumscribed and isointense to slightly hypointense compared with white matter tissue on all pulse sequences, although they may be heterogeneous and/or cystic. Enhancement is nearly always evident and is homogeneous in around 70% of cases. Peritumoral edema may be seen in one third of cases, usually in the larger schwannomas.
- After lesions of cranial nerve VIII, schwannomas of cranial nerves VII (Fig. 2.7) and V are the most common

sites of intracranial neurogenic tumors, although any cranial nerve (excluding CN I and II) may be involved. Trigeminal schwannomas may arise anywhere along the pathway from the pons to the Meckel cave, to the cavernous sinus, and to and beyond the exit foramina (ovale, rotundum, and superior orbital fissure).
- Postoperatively, it is not unusual to see linear gadolinium enhancement in the internal auditory canal after vestibular schwannoma resection as a dural reaction.
- Acoustic neuroma is a term commonly misused for vestibular schwannoma. Since the cochlear (acoustic) nerve is not the one typically involved (as opposed to the superior and inferior **vestibular** nerves) and the lesion is not a "neuroma" (defined as a posttraumatic nonneoplastic enlargement of the nerve), this term should not be used by *REQUISITES* readers.

## METASTASES

### Dural Metastases

- Dural metastases usually result from hematogenous dissemination from extracranial primary tumors (Fig. 2.8) or from extension from adjacent bone metastases.

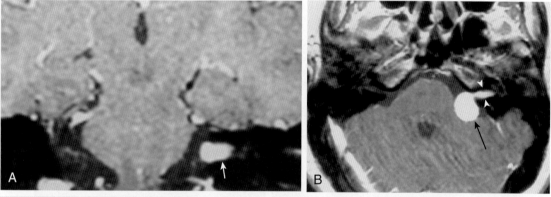

**Fig. 2.6 Intracanalicular vestibular schwannoma.** (A) Left intracanalicular vestibular schwannoma: Postgadolinium enhanced T1-weighted coronal image show an intracanalicular mass *(arrow)* on the *left* side. Fat saturation techniques can be performed to ensure that this does not represent fat. (B) Cerebellopontine angle and intracanalicular vestibular schwannoma. A brightly enhancing mass with both cisternal *(black arrow)* and intracanalicular *(arrowheads)* components is seen. The ipsilateral prepontine cistern is enlarged.

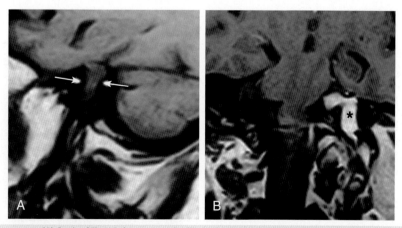

**Fig. 2.7 Facial nerve schwannoma.** (A) Sagittal T1-WI shows a markedly thickened descending portion of the facial nerve *(arrows)*. (B) The course of this enhancing mass suggests a facial nerve schwannoma by virtue of its tympanic segment and descending portion on this coronal postcontrast T1-WI *(asterisk)*.

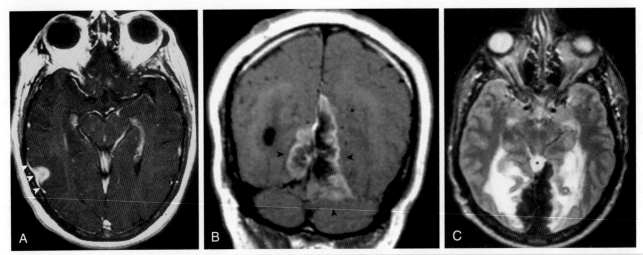

**Fig. 2.8 Metastases with dural tails.** (A) Postgadolinium enhanced T1WI in a patient with adenocarcinoma of the lung demonstrates a dural metastasis in the right temporal region. Although a dural tail *(arrowheads)* is suggestive of a meningioma, it is not pathognomonic for it. (B) Another patient with mucinous adenocarcinoma metastatic to the dura on coronal unenhanced T1WI shows a dural-based mass with low signal centrally and peripheral high-signal intensity *(arrowheads)*. The lesion was calcified on computed tomography. (C) On axial *(T2WI)* of the same patient as in (B), the lesion has low intensity but incites high-signal intensity edema. The low signal could be from the mucinous content and/or calcification.

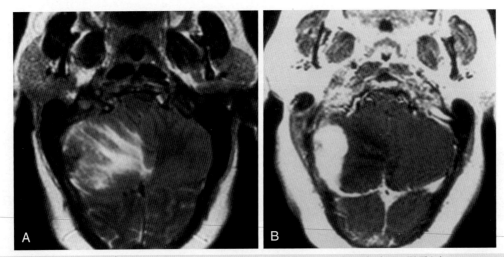

**Fig. 2.9 Dural lymphoma.** (A) A low-signal dural mass on the T2WI with associated intraparenchymal edema. (B) This becomes more apparent on the postcontrast T1WI. Lymphoma will nearly always enhance. Include meningioma, sarcoidosis, plasmacytoma, and other dural metastases in the differential diagnosis.

- Lung, breast, prostate, and melanoma cancers produce most dural metastases. Breast carcinoma is the most common neoplasm to be associated with purely dural metastases. Lymphoma is the next most common but is unique in that the dural lymphoma may sometimes be the primary focus of the neoplasm (Fig. 2.9). Dural plasmacytomas will look identical to dural lymphoma.
- In children, dural metastases are most commonly associated with neuroblastomas (typically centered on sutures) and leukemia.
- Occasionally, one can identify an adjacent parenchymal metastasis with dural spread (Fig. 2.10), and, alternatively, an osseous-dural metastasis (breast, prostate primaries) occasionally invades the parenchyma (Fig. 2.11).

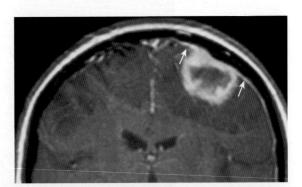

**Fig. 2.10 Leiomyosarcoma with dural-based metastasis.** Postgadolinium coronal T1WI shows a high left frontal intraparenchymal metastasis, which demonstrates dural invasion *(arrows)* along its superomedial margin.

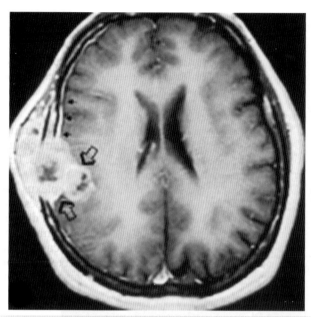

**Fig. 2.11 Intraparenchymal growth of renal cell carcinoma metastasis.** Postcontrast T1WI show a lesion centered on the calvarium with extracalvarial, dural, and intraparenchymal invasion *(open arrows)*. Dural enhancement located more peripherally *(small black arrows)*.

**Table 2.1**  Sources of Subarachnoid Seeding

| CNS Primary | Non-CNS Primary |
| --- | --- |
| **CHILDREN** | |
| Medulloblastoma | Leukemia/Lymphoma |
| Ependymoma | Neuroblastoma |
| Pineal region tumors | |
| Malignant astrocytomas | |
| Retinoblastoma | |
| Choroid plexus papilloma | |
| **ADULTS** | |
| Glioblastoma | Leukemia/Lymphoma |
| Primary CNS lymphoma | Breast |
| Oligodendroglioma | Lung |
| | Melanoma |
| | Gastrointestinal |
| | Genitourinary |

*CNS,* Central nervous system.

- On MRI, the T1WI and T2WI characteristics are variable depending on the cellular content (see Fig. 2.8). On CT, these lesions are identified as isodense thickening of the meninges. Contrast enhancement is prominent. Contrast-enhanced T1WI or enhanced FLAIR scans can readily demonstrate the abnormality.
- Inflammatory lesions that may simulate dural metastases include granulomatous processes, including infections (mycobacterial, syphilitic, and fungal), as well as sarcoidosis and Langerhans cell histiocytosis.

### Leptomeningeal Metastases

- Subarachnoid seeding (SAS) refers to leptomeningeal spread of tumor. The other terms you will see for subarachnoid seeding from cancers outside the CNS include *meningeal carcinomatosis* or *carcinomatous meningitis.*
- Clinically, patients present with multiple cranial neuropathies, radiculopathies, and/or mental status changes secondary to hydrocephalus or meningeal irritation. The cranial neuropathies may be irreversible. Although an initial CSF sample is positive in only 50% to 60% of cases, by performing multiple taps, the positive cytology rate approaches 95%. Patient survival is usually less than 6 months.
- SAS may occur with primary CNS tumors or non-CNS primary tumors (Table 2.1). Lymphoma and leukemia are the most common tumors to seed the CSF. However, because they only rarely invade the meninges and do not incite reactions in the CNS, most leukemic and lymphomatous SAS is not perceptible on neuroimaging even with IV contrast administration; the diagnosis is usually made by multiple spinal taps for CSF sampling. Breast, lung, and melanoma are the most common non-CNS primaries to seed the CSF.

- Primary CNS tumors may also seed the subarachnoid space. Although medulloblastomas have the highest rate of seeding (35%), glioblastomas, because of their higher prevalence, are the most common primary CNS tumor to have subarachnoid seeding. However, a wide variety of intracranial tumors may grow/shed cells in the subarachnoid space (including those of ependymal or choroid plexus origin).
- The malignant cells in the CSF and/or the associated elevated protein in the CSF will cause the usually low signal of CSF to be bright on an unenhanced FLAIR scan. Although this may be a difficult diagnosis to make in the basal cisterns because of artifact, the presence of such high signal over the convexities implies subarachnoid seeding, subarachnoid hemorrhage, or meningeal inflammation. Diffusion-restricting material within cerebral sulci can also raise alarm for SAS in the context of metastatic disease workup. Enhancement will be seen on postcontrast T1 and FLAIR images. You may see tiny nodules of leptomeningeal enhancement, or if diffuse, the whole pial surface may be studded with disease.
- The typical locations where one identifies SAS are at basal cisterns, in the interpeduncular cistern, at the cerebellopontine angle cistern, along the course of cranial nerves, and over the convexities (Fig. 2.12). Secondary communicating hydrocephalus may be present.

## INTRAVENTRICULAR MASSES (EXCLUDING MENINGIOMAS)

### Choroid Plexus Masses

#### Choroid Plexus Papillomas.

- Choroid plexus papillomas (WHO grade I) make up 3% of intracranial tumors in children. Eighty-six percent of these tumors are seen in patients younger than 5 years old. In children, 80% occur at the trigone/atria of the lateral ventricles; in adults, they may also be seen in the fourth ventricle. If you also include adults, 43% are located in the lateral ventricle, 39% in the fourth

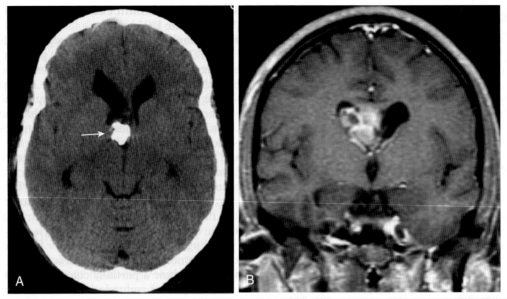

**Fig. 2.22 Grade I benign subependymal giant cell astrocytoma.** (A) Note the calcified mass *(arrow)* near the right foramen of Monro on unenhanced CT. (B) On the coronal T1WI, one is more impressed with the component of the tumor that extends intraventricularly. The septum also seems to be involved.

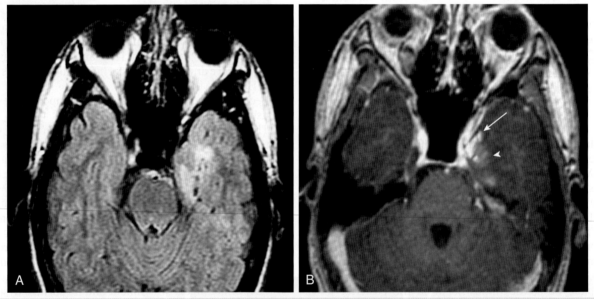

**Fig. 2.23 Pleomorphic xanthoastrocytoma of the temporal lobe.** (A) A FLAIR image shows an ill-defined mass in the left medial temporal lobe. (B) There is nodular enhancement at the periphery adjacent to the left cavernous sinus *(arrow)* and less well-defined enhancement in the area of FLAIR signal abnormality *(arrowhead)*.

- On CT, a poorly defined hypodense mass with no enhancement may be seen. Calcifications and/or cystic change may rarely occur. On MRI, diffuse astrocytomas are expansile lesions that are hypointense on T1WI and hyperintense on T2WI. There is usually no enhancement, although this may appear as the tumor progresses.
- The "T2-FLAIR mismatch" sign, evidenced by solid mass with high signal on T2WI but decreased signal on FLAIR, has been shown to be highly specific for an IDH-mutant, non- 1p/19q codeleted molecular genetic marker for lower grade infiltrating astrocytoma.

### Anaplastic Astrocytomas (WHO Grade III).

- Anaplastic Astrocytomas (AAs) are also diffusely infiltrating astrocytomas that occur in young adults with median survival of 3 to 5 years. These may also have mutations in the *IDH1* or *IDH2* genes and as with diffuse astrocytoma, the IDH mutant type is more common and has a more favorable course than the IDH wild-type variant.
- These may evolve from lower-grade astrocytomas but can be diagnosed without a precursor lesion. They have ill-defined borders with prolific vasogenic edema (Fig. 2.25). They can occur anywhere but are most commonly seen in the frontal lobes.

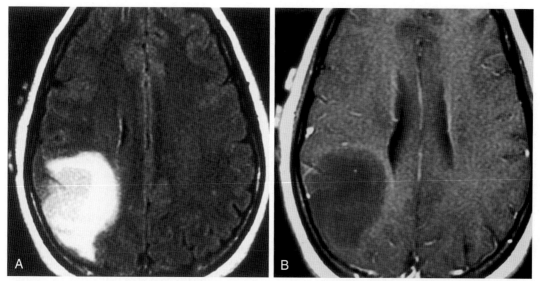

**Fig. 2.24 Grade II astrocytoma.** (A) The mass is somewhat well-defined on a FLAIR image but is still bulky. (B) It does not enhance.

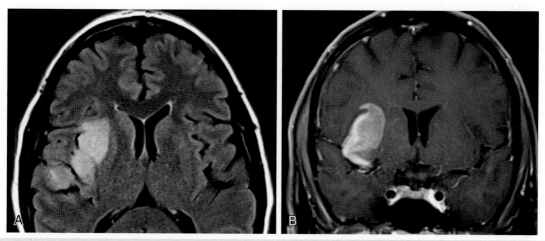

**Fig. 2.25 Grade III astrocytoma.** (A) An axial FLAIR image shows peri-insular high signal extending from right temporal lobe to right frontal opercular zone. (B) After contrast, administration enhancement is seen along the perisylvian region on coronal T1WI.

- Compared with diffuse astrocytoma, AAs are much more likely to show contrast enhancement. If necrosis is seen, grade IV astrocytoma should be considered. These tend to progress to grade IV astrocytoma. Restricted diffusion is often seen in AAs, and their cerebral blood flow is intermediate between lower-grade astrocytomas and grade IV astrocytoma.

### Glioblastoma (WHO Grade IV).

- GBs are the most common malignant brain tumor in adults, accounting for 15% of intracranial neoplasms and approximately 50% to 60% of primary malignant brain tumors. These are the most lethal of the gliomas, having a 10% to 15% 2-year survival rate.
- In the 2016 update, GBs were characterized by the presence or absence of the IDH mutation (IDH mutant or IDH wild-type). However, recent 2020 updates have moved to classify all GBs as IDH wild-type tumors.
- The IDH wild-type is the more common type, accounting for 90% of all GBs. These typically arise de novo without

a precursor lesion in older patients and are associated with poorer prognosis.

- The IDH mutant astrocytomas can be malignant and demonstrate necrosis, formerly considered as "glioblastoma, IDH-mutant, WHO grade IV." However, since they are clinically and genetically distinct, based on the 2021 updated classification they are now simply denoted as grade IV astrocytoma, or "astrocytoma, IDH mutant, WHO grade IV." These usually develop from lower-grade lesions such as diffuse astrocytoma or AA, may occur in slightly younger patients, and may be associated with a better prognosis. These are almost always O-6-methylguanine-DNA methyltransferase (MGMT) methylated. The MGMT methylation portends a favorable response to temozolamide but may also put the patient at risk for "pseudoprogression."
- GBs are typically supratentorial and diffusely infiltrate the subcortical white matter and deep gray matter. These tumors can appear anywhere in the cerebrum but are seen most commonly in the temporal lobes, followed by the parietal, frontal, and occipital lobes.

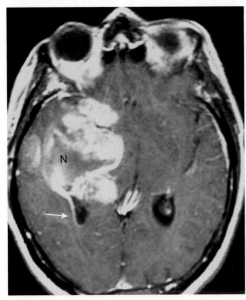

**Fig. 2.26 Glioblastoma.** This glioblastoma demonstrates irregular enhancement, necrosis *(N)*, and mass effect with displacement of midline structures to the *left* side. Note the ependymal spread of tumor *(arrow)*, which also is a bad prognostic sign.

- GBs are characterized on imaging by the presence of necrosis within the tumor (Fig. 2.26). Ring enhancement, enhancement in general, marked mass effect, intratumoral necrosis and hemorrhage, and restricted diffusion may be seen.
- Daughter/satellite lesions around the periphery of the mass may look like a cluster of grapes. The tumor frequently crosses the corpus callosum, anterior commissure, or posterior commissure to reach the contralateral hemisphere.
- Of the adult astrocytomas, a GB is the most common to have intratumoral hemorrhage and subarachnoid seeding (2%–5% of cases). Occasionally, it coats the ventricles. When you see a lesion involving the corpus callosum, GB and lymphoma are top differential considerations for etiology (Fig. 2.27).
- The extent of a neoplasm is not defined by its enhancing rim. In fact, radiation oncologists treat the entire area of abnormal T2WI/FLAIR high intensity with radiation, followed by a coned-down portal encompassing the enhancing portion with a 2-cm rim around the enhancing edge. Microscopic infiltration clearly extends beyond the confines of enhancement, however the high-signal intensity on T2WI may not represent tumor in all instances.
- The presence of high choline/NAA ratios or lactic acid peak on MR spectroscopy have been linked to a higher grade (Fig. 2.28). Most people are using a Cho/NAA ratio of greater than 2.2 to denote a high-grade astrocytoma and the presence of myoinositol to suggest lower-grade lesions.
- For lesions adjacent to eloquent cortex (e.g., near speech, memory, or motor areas), it is helpful to the neurosurgeons to know the involvement and/or proximity of the lesion to these critical areas so that they can reduce the operative morbidity associated with the resection.
- fMRI can be used preoperatively to define the speech areas (and other eloquent areas) in relation to the tumor or even intraoperatively to direct the surgical resection to include the maximum amount of tumor and minimal

amount of eloquent cortex (Fig. 2.29). A word of caution, the blood oxygenation level–dependent (BOLD) fMRI contrast effect may be reduced near an astrocytoma secondary to (1) compression of vessels and neurovascular uncoupling, (2) vasoreactive substances (nitric oxide), (3) neurotransmitter substances expressed by tumors, (4) reduced neuronal function, and (5) invasion of vascular structures by the tumor.

- The lower the ADC in an astrocytoma, the higher the grade. The higher the perfusion, the higher the grade. These adages show exceptions for tumors like JPAs (where the nodule may show hyperperfusion) and some GBs that have intermediate ADC values.

### "Gliomatosis Cerebri" Redefined.

- Gliomatosis cerebri was previously recognized as a defined tumor entity with a pattern of disease, which involves "at least 3 lobes and is usually bilateral, extending from the cerebral white matter, including the deep and subcortical portions, and often infiltrating the brain stem and the spinal cord" (Fig. 2.30).
- In the 2016 WHO revision, it has been redefined as a pattern of widespread tumor (rather than tumor type) that can be seen with any of the infiltrating gliomas including astrocytoma, AA, and GB.
- A CT scan may be interpreted as normal in appearance, but loss of the gray-white differentiation and subtle mass effect may be seen. The more sensitive T2W1/FLAIR MRI shows diffuse increased signal intensity throughout. Both gray and white matter may be involved, and the lesion may spread bilaterally. Enhancement, if present at all, is minimal.

### Diffuse Midline Glioma (WHO Grade IV).

- Diffuse midline gliomas are infiltrative, high-grade gliomas previously referred to as *brain stem glioma* and *diffuse intrinsic pontine glioma* (DIPG). In addition to the pons, these tumors may also be seen in the thalami, cerebellum, and other midline structures, such as hypothalamus and pineal region.
- Diffuse midline glioma tumors are characterized by mutations in the histone *H3F3A* gene (K27M mutations) or, less frequently, *HIST1H3B* and *HIST2H3C* genes.
- Three attributes have to be fulfilled to call it diffuse midline glioma: (1) the tumor shows diffuse infiltrative growth in the parenchyma; (2) it affects "midline" structures (e.g., brain stem, thalamus, spinal cord); and (3) glioma histology and the presence of an H3 K27M mutation.
- Most of these lesions occur in the pediatric population. They make up 20% of posterior fossa masses in children, less common than cerebellar astrocytomas and medulloblastomas. Symptoms occur late during the disease and are often related to brain stem dysfunction or from increased intracranial pressure (ICP) and include cranial neuropathies, ataxia, motor weakness/hemiparesis, and gait disturbances. The prognosis for diffuse midline H3 K27M-mutant gliomas is a 10% 2-year survival.
- Pontine brain stem gliomas are most common. The masses may be isolated to one part of the brain stem and may grow exophytically (20% of cases). Pontine and exophytic brain stem gliomas have a better prognosis than midbrain or medullary ones, and exophytic ones may benefit from surgical resection.

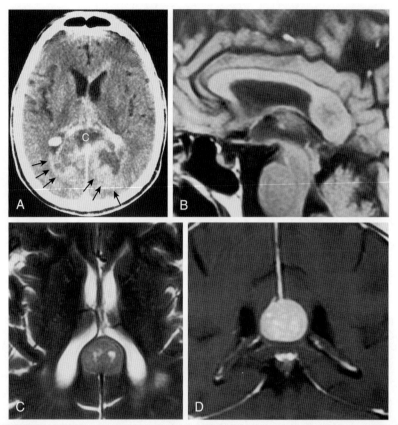

**Fig. 2.27 Lesions invading the corpus callosum.** (A) Glioblastoma crossing the corpus callosum. Enhanced CT reveals an irregularly enhancing tumor in a garland wreath pattern *(arrows)* crossing the splenium of the corpus callosum. Note that the genu of the corpus callosum also shows subtle enhancement denoting tumor infiltration. (C) marks the splenium of the corpus callosum, which appears to be somewhat necrotic. (B) Lymphoma of the splenium: Sagittal T1WI shows expansion of the splenium with abnormal signal intensity. (C) The T2WI shows a focal mass in the splenium without significant edema. (D) The lesion enhances strongly on coronal T1WI. Would this favor lymphoma over an intermediate-grade astrocytoma? Try diffusion. (Courtesy Stuart Bobman.)

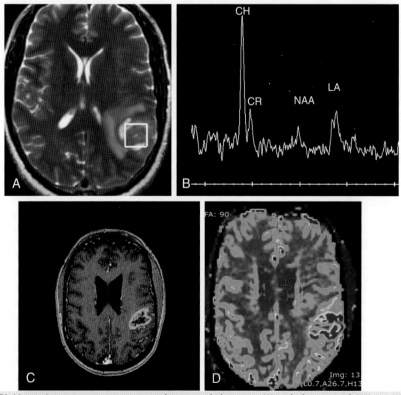

**Fig. 2.28 Glioblastoma (GB).** Magnetic resonance spectroscopy shows voxel placement (A) and a lactate peak *(LA)* at 1.3 PPM and a very high choline *(CH)* to N-acetyl aspartate *(NAA)* ratio of peak heights (B). Creatine peak *(CR)* is also indicated. GB in a different patient shows heterogeneously enhancing left posterior frontal lobe mass on postcontrast T1WI (C) with corresponding dramatic increased perfusion on cerebral blood volume map (D), indicating viable tumor.

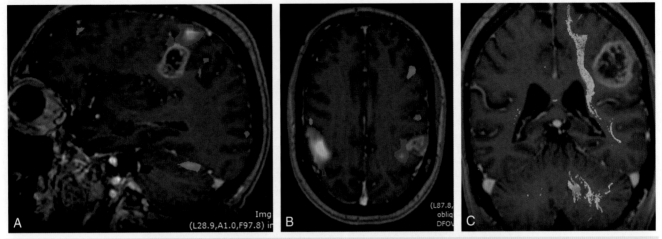

**Fig. 2.29 Functional magnetic resonance imaging (fMRI) in action.** In this patient with a heterogeneously enhancing mass in the left posterior frontal lobe (same patient as in Fig. 2.28 C–D), advanced imaging using blood oxygenation level–dependent (BOLD) fMRI and with a finger tapping paradigm showed close motor activation, with right finger tapping abutting the superior and medial aspects of the mass on sagittal (A) and axial (B) images. Multidimensional diffusing imaging with fiber tracking also shows the relationship of the corticospinal tracts to the mass (C). Surgeons beware!

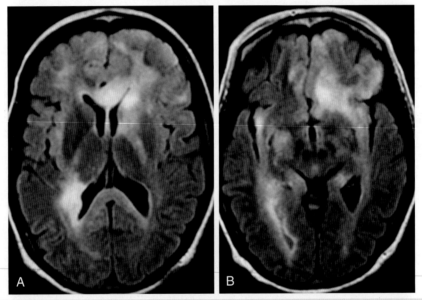

**Fig. 2.30 Infiltrating glioma.** (A and B) This FLAIR image shows multiple lobes, bilateral involvement, and relatively low mass effect for the size of the abnormality, characteristic of infiltrating pattern of tumor involvement. Do not expect avid enhancement.

- On MRI, the lesions are high in intensity on T2WI/FLAIR amid the normal decreased signal intensity of the white matter tracts of the brain stem (Fig. 2.31). They may (33%) or may not (67%) enhance. Cystic degeneration may occur. Subtle enhancement that cannot be seen with CT may be apparent on MRI. As they enlarge, they often appear to encircle the basilar artery.
- Other lesions that expand the brain stem in a child include tuberculosis (most common brain stem lesion worldwide), lymphoma, rhomben-cephalitis (caused by *Listeria*), and demyelinating disorders (acute disseminated encephalomyelitis and multiple sclerosis).

## Oligodendroglial Tumors

The WHO 2016 revision defines these tumors as possessing both the IDH mutant and 1p/19q codeletion molecular markers (Table 2.6). This is in contradistinction to astrocytomas, which may have the IDH mutation but never contain the 1p/q19 codeletion. The term *oligoastrocytoma* has been eliminated in the WHO classification—they either are oligodendrogliomas based on 1p/19q codeletion or not.

### Oligodendrogliomas (WHO Grade II).

- Oligodendrogliomas are diffusely infiltrating, slow-growing gliomas, making up just 4% to 8% of intracranial gliomas but typified by their high rate of calcification (40%–80%; Fig. 2.32).
- These tumors involve the white matter and cortex of the cerebral hemispheres with the frontal lobe the most common location (>50%), followed by the temporal, parietal, and occipital lobes.
- On CT, the lesions are hypodense or isodense on unenhanced scans (unless hemorrhage or calcification is present). On MRI the tumor is hypointense on T1WI and hyperintense on T2WI/FLAIR except in the areas of calcification (Fig. 2.33). Edema associated with the mass is typically minimal, a distinguishing point from other more aggressive tumors. Enhancement, when present

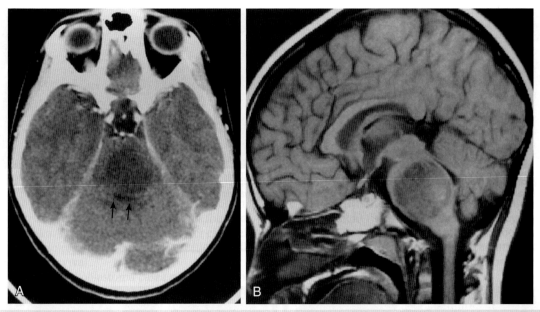

**Fig. 2.31 Diffuse midline glioma.** (A) Pontine brain stem glioma on this enhanced CT scan compresses the fourth ventricle *(arrows)*. Note the lack of enhancement of the tumor. (B) Sagittal T1WI better defines the extent of the tumor on this midline scan.

**Table 2.6** World Health Organization Classification of Oligodendroglial Tumors

| Tumor | Grade | Peak Age (years) |
|---|---|---|
| Oligodendroglioma | II | 30–55 |
| Anaplastic oligodendroglioma | III | 45–60 |

in oligodendrogliomas, is variable occurring in less than 20% of grade II tumors. Hemorrhage occurs in 20% of cases, as does cyst formation.

### Anaplastic Oligodendrogliomas (WHO Grade III).
- Anaplastic oligodendrogliomas (WHO grade III) have a worse prognosis than the WHO grade II oligodendrogliomas, although they have a better prognosis than AAs.
- These may arise either de novo or by progression from a WHO grade II oligodendroglioma.
- They account for one fourth to one half of all oligodendrogliomas, with a mean age of 49 years old. Over 90% are found in either the frontal lobe or temporal lobe. Hemorrhage, necrosis, calcification, cystic degeneration, and avid enhancement alone or in combination may occur in these tumors. Five-year survival is approximately 30%.

## Embryonal Tumors

### Medulloblastoma (WHO Grade IV).
- Medulloblastomas are the most common embryonal neuroepithelial tumors and the most common solid tumors in children. They arise in the cerebellum or dorsal brain stem and account for more than one third of posterior fossa neoplasms and 50% of cerebellar tumors in children. These tumors are usually seen in the midline arising from the vermis and then growing into the inferior

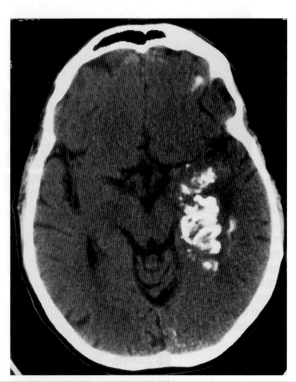

**Fig. 2.32 Calcification in an oligodendroglioma.** This lesion shows typical calcification of this low-grade tumor on unenhanced CT image. The serpentine nature of the calcification should raise additional differential considerations of an arteriovenous malformation or even Sturge-Weber.

or superior velum of the fourth ventricle (Fig. 2.34). Medulloblastomas typically occur in the 5- to 12-year age range, with boys twice as commonly affected as girls. Patients usually present with hydrocephalus. Brain stem dysfunction may also be present.

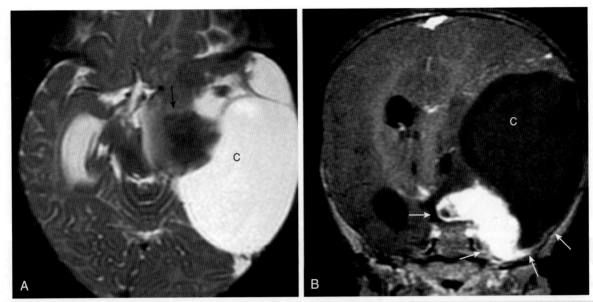

**Fig. 2.40 Desmoplastic infantile ganglioglioma.** (A) This large cystic mass *(C)* in the temporal region has a solid component *(arrow)* more medially seen as intermediate signal on the T2WI. (B) Typical of a desmoplastic infantile ganglioglioma, a peripherally located mass with a solidly enhancing component, which has a dural attachment *(arrows)* and a huge cyst, is demonstrated on this post contrast fat-suppressed T1WI. The differential diagnosis of desmoplastic infantile ganglioglioma (DIG) is dysembryoplastic neuroectodermal tumor (DNET) or pleomorphic xanthoastrocytoma (PXA).

and parietal lobes, are large in size, and have a meningeal base. Cyst formation is the rule, and peripheral rim or nodular enhancement usually is present as well. Some may show a calcified rim. Although this lesion may look like a huge necrotic GB in an infant, it has a good prognosis with a benign histology (Fig. 2.40).

■ Desmoplastic infantile astrocytoma probably represents a variant of DIG and has features of glial and mesenchymal histology. It has been grouped together with DIG in the 2016 WHO classification of CNS tumor because of clinicoradiological and pathologic similarities. Absence of neuronal components histologically distinguishes this tumor from a DIG. It is a benign tumor found in early life. In general, there is a dural-based mass with cystic change. Although the dural-based mass will enhance, the cyst does not, not even on the periphery. Mass effect and vasogenic edema are rare. It also presents in the first 18 months of life and is usually seen supratentorially.

### Other Gliomas

#### Angiocentric Gliomas (WHO Grade I).
■ These tumors are slow-growing cerebral tumors with an angiocentric pattern of growth, most commonly affecting children and young adults. Seizure is a common presenting symptom. Surgical resection is often curative.
■ On MRI, a circumscribed, superficial, cortically-based lesion with hyperintense signal on FLAIR images will be seen. There is no associated enhancement.

#### Chordoid Gliomas (WHO Grade II).
■ These are slow-growing, solid, well-circumscribed, and avidly enhancing tumors of the hypothalamus and anterior third ventricle. They are hyperdense to gray matter on a CT scan and reasonably isointense on standard T1WI and T2WI but may have central necrosis or cystic regions. They occur in adults over age 30 and can cause acute hydrocephalus because of their obstructive nature.

### Astroblastomas

■ Astroblastomas are rare tumors of variable aggressiveness and of unknown origin with no definite grade. They are tumors of young adulthood affecting the cerebral hemispheres. They are well-circumscribed tumors with peripheral enhancement, central necrosis, and usually a large size. Prognosis is good as long as the surgeon does a complete resection.

### Hemangioblastomas (WHO Grade I)

■ These are mesenchymal, nonmeningothelial tumors arising in the CNS parenchyma and are the most common primary intraparenchymal tumor in the infratentorial space in adults.
■ Hemangioblastoma (HBs) are benign, slow-growing tumors of adults, typically occurring in the cerebellum, although they may also involve the brain stem and spinal cord. Approximately 30% are associated with von Hippel Lindau (VHL) disease, although they may arise sporadically. HBs associated with VHL syndrome generally present at an earlier age.

---

**TEACHING POINTS**

Lesions Associated With von Hippel-Lindau Syndrome

**Central Nervous System**

Cerebellar HB (66%–80%)
Spinal HB (28%–40%)
Medullary HB (14%–20%)
Extra-axial HB (<5%)
Retinal HB (50%–67%)

**Renal**

Cysts (50%–75%)
Hypernephroma, or renal cell carcinoma (25%–50%)
Hemangioblastoma
Adenoma

(Continued)

**Pancreatic**

Cysts (30%)
Adenoma
Adenocarcinoma
Islet cell tumor

**Liver**

Hemangioma
Cyst
Adenoma

**Spleen**

Angioma

**Adrenal**

Pheochromocytoma (10%)
Cyst

**Lung**

Cyst

**Bone**

Endolymphatic sac tumor of temporal bone (10%)
Hemangioma

**Cardiac**

Rhabdomyoma

**Epididymis**

Cyst
Cystadenoma

**Hematologic**

Polycythemia (25%–40%)

*HB,* Hemangioblastoma.

- Symptoms usually arise from increased ICP and hydrocephalus related to impaired CSF flow.
- MRI will show a cystic mass with a solid mural nodule in 60% of cases. There is no associated calcification. The solid component is usually peripherally located. Flow voids may be seen (Fig. 2.41). Solid HBs (40%) and, less commonly, purely cystic HBs occur as well.
- On angiographic examination, a vascular nodule amid an avascular mass, usually with serpentine vessels, may be identified with or without draining veins.
- It may be difficult to distinguish an HB from a pilocytic astrocytoma. The age of presentation (pilocytic astrocytomas are seen in the 5–15 age range versus 30–40 for HBs), pial attachment, a tiny nodule with a huge cyst, and multiplicity and association with other findings of VHL syndrome suggests HB.
- VHL is associated with the *VHL* gene, which provides instructions for making a protein that functions as part of the VCB-CUL2 complex, which cleans up degraded proteins in the cell. It is found on the short arm of chromosome 3.

## Metastases

- The most common infratentorial and supratentorial malignant neoplasm to occur in the adult population is a metastasis (Fig. 2.42). They are usually seen as well-defined, round masses, which are identified near the gray-white junction. Metastases lodge at the gray-white interface in 80% of cases, basal ganglia in 3%, and cerebellum in 15%. These lesions show contrast enhancement and are one of the lesions of the brain that often causes nodular or ring enhancement.
- The most common primary extracranial tumors in adults to metastasize to the brain are lung and breast carcinomas. Other neoplasms that have a propensity for metastatic spread to the brain include melanoma (third most common, after lung and breast), renal cell carcinoma, colorectal carcinoma, and thyroid carcinoma. Virtually all metastases evoke some vasogenic edema, however, the amount is variable.
- Fifty percent of metastases are solitary. The other 50% are multiple; of these, 20% have two lesions only (Fig. 2.43).
- Unless the metastatic deposit is hemorrhagic, calcified, hyperproteinaceous, or highly cellular, where it would be hyperdense (Fig. 2.44), most metastases are low density on unenhanced CT. Rarely, one may identify calcification in metastatic deposits.
- Metastatic deposits may have variable intensity on T2WI. Some lesions are isointense to gray matter on T2WI (probably from hypercellularity) and can be readily distinguished from the high intensity of the edema they elicit. Other metastatic deposits, however, are hyperintense to gray matter on T2WI.
- Hemorrhagic metastases are usually seen as areas of high-signal intensity on T1WI and T2WI with a relative absence of hemosiderin deposition. Primary neoplasms that have a propensity to hemorrhage include melanoma (Fig. 2.45), renal cell, choriocarcinoma, and thyroid carcinomas; however, because lung and breast cancers are more common than these other primary tumors, a hemorrhagic metastasis is most often from breast or lung. Hemorrhagic metastases must be differentiated from occult cerebrovascular malformations, such as cavernomas or nonneoplastic hematomas (Table 2.9).

**TEACHING POINTS**

Hemorrhagic Metastases

Melanoma
Renal cell carcinoma
Breast cancer
Lung cancer
Thyroid cancer
Retinoblastoma
Choriocarcinoma

- Although virtually all metastases enhance to a variable degree, the pattern may be solid, ring-like, regular, irregular, homogeneous, or heterogeneous (Fig. 2.46).
- The vasogenic edema is often out of proportion to the size of the metastasis, except in cortical metastases, where edema may be minimal or absent and the enhanced studies are essential to their detection.

## Lymphomas

- Primary CNS lymphoma is often referred to as PCNSL. These account for approximately 2% to 3% of all brain

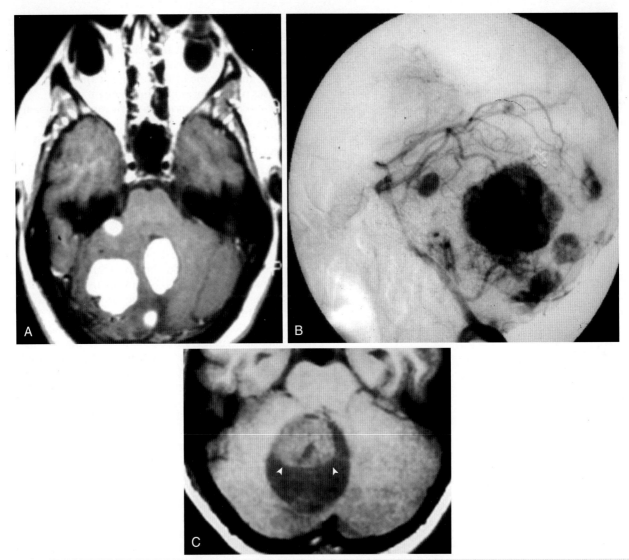

**Fig. 2.41 Hemangioblastomas of the cerebellum.** (A) Note the numerous enhancing masses in the posterior fossa. There may have been ocular lesions as well judging from the distorted appearance of the globes. (B) On angiography the hypervascular nature of the masses is evident as well as their multiplicity. The supply is from pial, not dural, branches. (C) A hemangioblastoma with both cystic and solid components *(arrowheads)* is seen on this unenhanced axial T1WI.

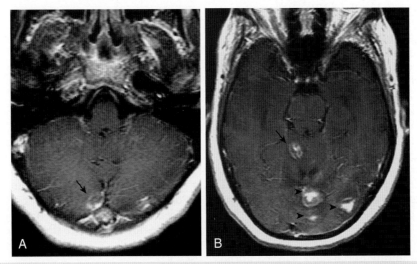

**Fig. 2.42 Multiple posterior fossa metastases.** (A) With contrast enhancement, a ring-enhancing metastasis *(arrow)* is well seen in the right cerebellum. (B) Additional metastases are seen in the superior vermis of the cerebellum *(arrow)* and in the left occipital lobe *(arrowheads)* at the gray matter-white matter junction.

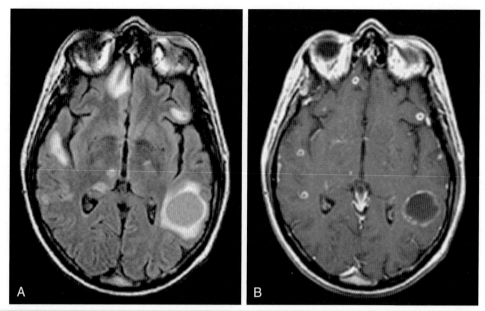

**Fig. 2.43 Multiple metastases.** (A) Cystic and solid metastases are present in this patient. The cystic lesion in the left temporal lobe does not have the same intensity as cerebrospinal fluid on FLAIR because of high protein. (B) The masses enhance along the periphery and the posterior right temporal lesion reveals its nature on this post contrast T1WI. The differential diagnosis would include a brain abscess, and a diffusion-weighted scan could be useful if bright (suggesting an abscess and differentiating the two).

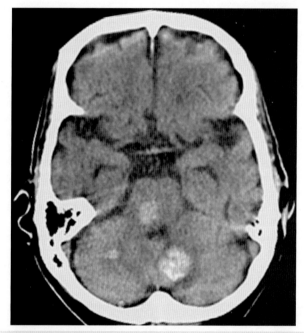

**Fig. 2.44 Hemorrhagic metastases.** Hyperdense masses are seen in the brain stem and cerebellum on noncontrast CT image. Although one might consider cavernomas in the differential diagnosis, this patient had renal cell carcinoma. There is edema around the mass in the left cerebellar hemisphere.

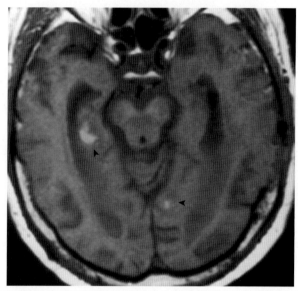

**Fig. 2.45** Paramagnetic high signal in metastases *(arrowheads)*. This was a case of metastatic melanoma where the high signal was a result of melanin (or hemorrhage) on noncontrast T1WI.

- About 60% of CNS lymphomas involve the supratentorial compartment, most often seen in the frontal lobe, followed by the temporal, parietal, and occipital lobes, the basal ganglia and periventricular regions, and corpus callosum (Fig. 2.47). The posterior fossa and spinal cord are less commonly involved. More than half present with a single intracranial tumor.
- CNS lymphoma is often associated with an immunodeficient state, including that resulting from acquired immunodeficiency syndrome (AIDS), organ transplantation, Wiskott-Aldrich syndrome, Sjögren syndrome, and prolonged immunosuppressive therapy. Care must be taken to distinguish CNS toxoplasmosis from lymphoma in the AIDS population.

tumors and 4% to 6% of extranodal lymphomas. This is a non-Hodgkin, large B-cell lymphoma.
- PCNSL can affect patients of any age with a peak incidence in the fifth through seventh decades of life. Symptoms include cognitive dysfunction, focal neurologic signs, and, less frequently, headache, seizures, and cranial neuropathies. There is often rapid improvement with steroids.

**Table 2.9** Features of Recently Bled Cavernomas versus Hemorrhagic Metastases

| Feature | Hemorrhagic Cavernomas | Hemorrhagic Metastases |
|---|---|---|
| Edema | Only with acute episode, resolves by 8 weeks | Persistent |
| Mass | Variable but resolves | Moderate to large, persistent |
| Hemosiderin ring | Complete | Incomplete or absent |
| Nonhemorrhagic tissue | Absent | Present |
| Enhancement | Minimal and central | Nodular, ring, or eccentric |
| Progression of hemorrhagic stages | Orderly | Delayed |
| Follow-up | Decreases in size with time | Increases in size with time |
| Calcification | Approximately 20% | Rare |

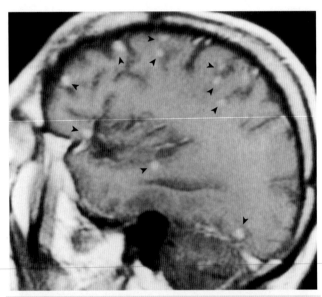

**Fig. 2.46 Multiple small cell carcinoma lung metastases.** The preponderance of small enhancing lesions *(arrowheads)* at the gray-white junction on this sagittal postcontrast T1WI suggests a diagnosis of metastatic disease.

**TEACHING POINTS**

Lymphoma versus Toxoplasmosis in Acquired Immunodeficiency Syndrome

| Feature | Lymphoma | Toxoplasmosis |
|---|---|---|
| ADC value | Low | High |
| Calcification | Rare | Common especially after treatment |
| Perfusion | Intermediate | Low |
| Density on NCCT | Hyperdense | Hypodense (unless calcified) |
| Size of lesions | Can be quite large; >3 cm | Rare over 3 cm |
| Thallium avidity | Yes | No |
| FDG PET avidity | Yes | Less |
| T2 dark | Common | Unusual unless calcified |
| Subependymal spread | Characteristic | Rare |
| Response to steroids/XRT | Rapid | Laughable |
| Hemorrhagic | Rare | More common |
| MRS | Choline high | Lactate possible |

*ADC,* Apparent diffusion coefficient; *FDG,* fluorodeoxyglucose; *MRS,* magnetic resonance spectroscopy; *NCCT,* noncontrast computed tomography; *PET,* positron emission tomography; *XRT,* radiation therapy.

- MRI findings in CNS lymphoma are varied. Periventricular (40%), subcortical, and deep gray matter abnormalities (27%) and mixed patterns (20%) are most common, with masses less than 2 cm in size in patients with AIDS and greater than 2 cm in size in non-AIDS patients. Close to 50% touch along the ventricular surface from a white matter origin.
- PCNSL does not calcify and is most commonly seen in the frontal lobes and basal ganglia.
- Multiple lesions occur more commonly in patients with AIDS. The signal intensity is variable on T2WI scans, with approximately 50% of cases isointense to slightly

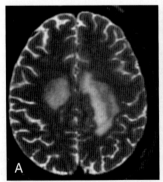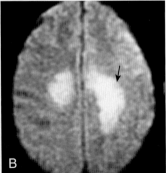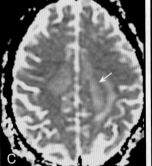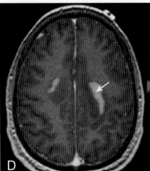

**Fig. 2.47 Low apparent diffusion coefficient (ADC) value in lymphoma.** Despite the bright edema on the T2WI (A) and diffusion-weighted imaging (B), one can make out on the ADC map (C) a lower ADC value area *(arrows)* indicating restricted diffusion amid higher ADC values indicating vasogenic edema. Hypercellular/small cell tumors can show reduced ADC. (D) This area also shows enhancement and should be the target for biopsying.

hypointense. Gadolinium enhancement is marked and homogeneous in over 90% of non-AIDS cases, but beware when steroids are given as treatment because these drugs may suppress the enhancement. Ring enhancement is often seen in immunodeficient (AIDS) patients but is rarely seen in the immunocompetent PCNSL population (Fig. 2.48).

■ Because lymphoma and GB may often appear similar by conventional imaging, it is useful to note that the ADC values of lymphoma are significantly lower than those of GB because of its dense cellularity and high nucleus to cytoplasm ratio (see Fig. 2.47C). The choline/creatine ratio is elevated in CNS lymphoma,

and cerebral blood volume is lower compared with high-grade astrocytomas (although higher than toxoplasmosis).

■ The classic teaching used to be that lymphoma is typically hyperdense on a noncontrast CT scan and enhances to a moderate degree (Fig. 2.49). Hemorrhage is distinctly uncommon in lymphomas (<8%).

## PINEAL REGION MASSES

■ The pineal gland grows steadily until age 2, and then the size stabilizes into early adulthood. No difference in size exists between males and females.

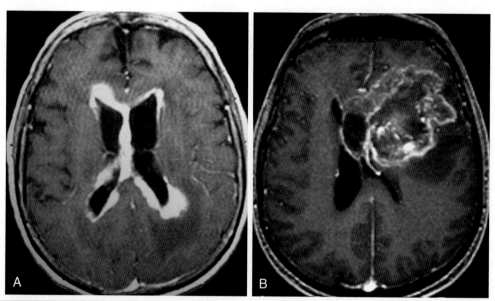

**Fig. 2.48  Lymphoma.** Periventricular ependymal enhancement (A) is present in this patient on post contrast T1WI, whereas parenchymal necrotic enhancement is seen in another patient on post contrast T1WI, abutting the ventricle (B). Lymphoma typically shows solid enhancement, but in the immunocompromised can show regions of necrosis, as seen here.

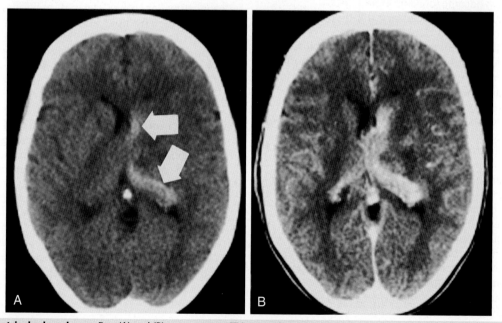

**Fig. 2.49  Periventricular lymphoma.** Pre- (A) and (B) post contrast CT images demonstrate the classic findings of lymphoma—a hyperdense mass on an unenhanced scan *(arrows),* which shows enhancement after iodinated contrast a dministration (B) and infiltrates the ependymal surface of the ventricular system.

- The normal pineal gland is calcified in 7% to 10% of patients before 10 years of age, in 30% of patients in their midteens, and peaks by age 20 to 40 in 33% to 40% of individuals.
- A calcified pineal gland before the age of 6 should be viewed with suspicion for adjacent tumor.
- Pineal region masses constitute 1% of all CNS tumors. They are generally separated into two categories: those of germ cell origin (60%) and those of pineal cell origin (40%).
- The manifestations of pineal region masses are based on their site near many critical structures: the aqueduct, the tectal plate, the midbrain, and the vein of Galen. Pineal region masses may cause (1) hydrocephalus through obstruction of the aqueduct of Sylvius, (2) precocious puberty, (3) headache, or (4) paresis of upward gaze (Parinaud syndrome).
- Because the signal intensity characteristics of pineal parenchymal tumors, malignant germ cell tumors, germinomas, and gliomas may overlap, some investigators have suggested that serum markers may be more specific than imaging features for histology.

### TEACHING POINTS

Syndromes Associated With Brain Tumors

Basal cell nevus syndrome (chromosome 9q31)/Gorlin syndrome
    Basal cell nevi and carcinomas, odontogenic keratocysts, ribbon ribs, phalangeal deformity and pitting, falcine calcification, craniofacial deformities, scoliosis, and medulloblastomas
Cowden syndrome (chromosome 10q23)
    Multiple hamartomas, mucocutaneous tumors, fibrocystic breast disease, polyps, thyroid adenoma, and Lhermitte-Duclos syndrome
von Hippel-Lindau (see Chapter 8)
Li-Fraumeni syndrome (chromosome 17p13)
    Increased rate of breast cancers, soft-tissue sarcomas, osteosarcomas, and leukemia
    Autosomal dominant with astrocytomas, primitive neuroectodermal tumors, and choroid plexus tumors
    Central nervous system tumors
Maffucci syndrome
    Enchondromas, soft-tissue cavernomas, and CNS neoplasms including astrocytoma and chondrosarcoma
Neurofibromatosis 1 and 2 (see Chapter 8)
Ollier syndrome
    Multiple enchondromas
Retinoblastoma
    Pineoblastoma (trilateral retinoblastoma)
Sturge-Weber
    Choroid plexus hemangioma
Tuberous sclerosis (see Chapter 8)
Turcot syndrome (chromosomes 5q21, 3p21, 7p22)
    Colonic familial polyposis, glioblastoma, rare medulloblastoma

## Tumors of Germ Cell Origin

### Germinomas.

- The most common pineal tumor of the germ cell line is the germinoma, accounting for 60% of pineal germ cell tumors and 36% of pineal region masses. It has also been termed *seminoma* and *dysgerminoma* in the medical literature.
- This tumor has a male predominance when seen in the pineal region (in some series as high as 33:1) and a slight female predilection when seen in suprasellar location. The tumor may be multifocal in suprasellar and pineal locations. It is a tumor of adolescence and young adulthood, rarely seen in patients older than 30 years.
- The characteristic appearance of the germinoma is that of a hyperdense mass on unenhanced CT scans, which enhances markedly (Fig. 2.50). The tumor engulfs the pineal gland.
- On MRI, the germinoma has intermediate signal intensity on T1WI, slightly hypointense signal (similar to gray matter) on T2WI because of the tumor cells' high nucleus/cytoplasm ratio, and enhancement. Germinomas show higher ADC values than the pineal cell tumors, and the patients are younger.
- Germinomas are extremely radiosensitive and also respond well to chemotherapy. CSF seeding is not uncommon. The best imaging study to evaluate for CSF seeding is contrast-enhanced MRI of the entire neuroaxis; nonetheless, repeated CSF cytologic studies are still more sensitive than imaging.
- Most of the remaining CNS germinomas occur in the suprasellar cistern (Fig. 2.51), but some have been reported to occur in the basal ganglia and thalami as well.

### Teratomas.

- Teratomas are the second most common pineal region germ cell neoplasm, but they also abound in the suprasellar cistern.
- Teratomas may have fat, bone, calcification, cysts, sebaceum, or other dermal appendages associated with them. The lipid and calcification or bone have distinctive CT and MRI densities or intensities. A chemical shift artifact may signal the presence of fat rather than blood on the T2WI. Enhancement is irregular because of the nonenhancing fatty or calcified component.

### Choriocarcinomas and Other Germ Cell Line Tumors.

- Choriocarcinoma is commonly hemorrhagic, human chorionic gonadotropin (HCG) and human placental lactogen positive on immunohistochemistry. The others are not.
- Yolk sac tumors often show more cystic change than other germ cell line lesions. Alpha-fetoprotein titers are positive in yolk sac tumors.
- Embryonal carcinoma is most commonly solid. Teratomas and choriocarcinomas, as well as embryonal cell carcinoma and endodermal sinus tumors, are more common in male patients and have a worse prognosis. Placental alkaline phosphatase characterizes the embryonal tumor.

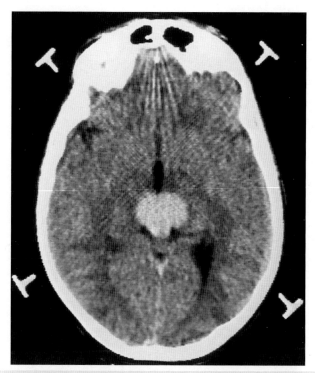

**Fig. 2.50 Germinoma in stereotactic biopsy frame.** A hyperdense mass in the pineal region is seen on this axial CT image.

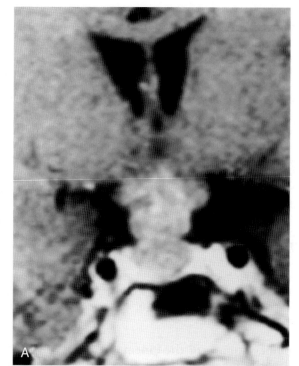

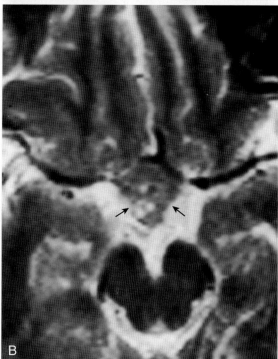

**Fig. 2.51 Suprasellar germinoma.** (A) An enhancing suprasellar mass is seen infiltrating the optic chiasm on the coronal scan. The patient had precipitous diabetes insipidus and a germinoma. (B) Axial T2WI shows the low signal you would expect for this tumor *(arrows)*.

## Others.

- The pineal gland is often referred to as the "third testes" because of the prevalence of the germ cell line of tumors in males.
- It is also the "third eye"; retinoblastomas occur here as part of the retinoblastoma oncogene complex. The occurrence of bilateral retinoblastomas in association with pineoblastomas (see the following section) has been termed *trilateral retinoblastoma* (although the third primitive neuroectodermal tumor may also occur in a suprasellar location). This occurs in 3% of patients with bilateral retinoblastomas. There is a high rate of subarachnoid seeding.

## Tumors of Pineal Cell Origin
### Pineocytomas (WHO Grade I).

- Pineocytomas are slower-growing, well-differentiated pineal parenchymal neoplasms and can occur in any age group, with the mean age in the thirties. These tumors are smaller than the pineoblastomas, often less than 3 cm in size, and they may demonstrate a higher rate of calcification or cyst formation than the pineoblastoma. The 5-year prognosis is 86%.
- Expansile growth may cause symptoms of increased ICP, Parinaud syndrome, and brain stem and cerebellar dysfunction. Hydrocephalus is a common feature.
- On CT, a globular, well-defined hypodense mass, usually less than 3 cm in diameter with possible peripheral or central calcification, is seen.
- Pineocytomas are hypointense to isointense on T1WI, hyperintense on T2WI, and demonstrate avid homogeneous enhancement.

### Pineoblastomas (WHO Grade IV).

- Pineoblastomas are highly cellular malignant neoplasms arising from the pineal gland.
- The pineoblastoma occurs in a younger age group (peak in first decade of life) than the pineocytoma. The 5-year survival is 50% to 60%. Pineoblastomas may occur in association with retinoblastomas.

- Their appearance at imaging is nearly identical, but pineoblastomas may be slightly more invasive and larger than pineocytomas and have a higher rate of subarachnoid seeding (SAS).
- Because these tumors are of the round cell variety with high nucleus/cytoplasm ratios, they often will be dense on unenhanced CT and intermediate in signal intensity on T2WI with low ADC values (Fig. 2.52). They enhance avidly.
- Calcification is not common, yet may be intrinsic to the tumor rather than within the pineal gland itself. Alternatively, the pineal gland calcification may appear exploded because it is displaced peripherally by the pineal tumor. We say germinomas "engulf" the pineal gland, but pineoblastomas "explode" the gland.

### Pineal Parenchymal Tumors of Intermediate Differentiation.

- These lesions appear similar by imaging to pineocytomas and pineoblastomas and are of intermediate malignancy. On imaging, they appear as bulky pineal region masses with local invasion. "Exploded" calcifications may also be seen.

### Papillary Tumors of the Pineal Region (PTPR).

- Papillary tumors of the pineal region (PTPR) are a very rare, recently described entity that occurs in the pineal region but felt to arise from the posterior commissure rather than the pineal gland itself (WHO II and III). On imaging, these lesions are difficult to distinguish from pineocytomas but can be distinguished histopathologically based on immunohistochemistry including vimentin positivity.

## NONNEOPLASTIC MASSES

### Cysts

#### Pineal Cysts.

- Pineal cysts are particularly common, found in 40% of autopsy series, and because some pineal masses (pineocytomas) may be cystic, it is important to attempt to identify a solid portion to the lesion to distinguish the two (Fig. 2.53).
- Despite their CSF content, pineal cysts do not have the same intensity as CSF on FLAIR, T1WI, or proton density weighted sequence. This may be because of hemorrhage, hemorrhagic debris, or high protein seen histologically in these cysts.
- Pineal cysts may compress or occlude the aqueduct and may be calcified. They may be round or oblong and can be equal to or greater than 2 cm in size. The key to distinguishing a pineal cyst from a cystic astrocytoma is the lack of growth during long-term follow-up. Nonetheless, it is not necessary to follow every pineal cyst because more than 99% are developmental and nonprogressive; allow the clinicians to use patient symptoms to determine appropriate follow-up.
- Because pineal cysts are often surrounded by the two limbs of the internal cerebral veins, one must be careful not to misread vascular enhancement as solid mass enhancement.

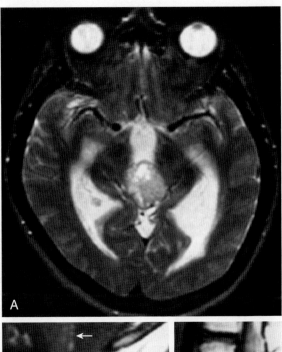

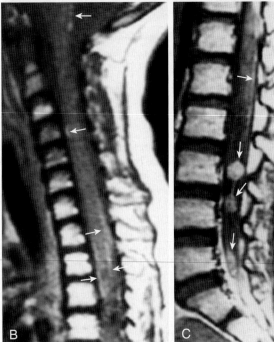

**Fig. 2.52 Pineoblastoma.** (A) Axial T2WI shows a pineal mass that is intermediate in signal intensity with some heterogeneity to the lesion. Low signal is characteristic of the highly cellular primitive neuroectodermal tumors. Note the dilatation of the third ventricle and occipital horns of the lateral ventricles caused by the compression of the aqueduct, signifying hydrocephalus. Subarachnoid seeding *(arrows)* in the form of sugarcoating (B) or gumdrops on the cauda equina (C) is not unusual in pineoblastomas.

#### Colloid Cysts.

- Colloid cysts (neuroendodermal or paraphyseal cysts) arise in the anterior portion of the third ventricle near the foramen of Monro. They occur with an incidence of three cases per one million individuals per year, usually presenting with positional headaches and/or hydrocephalus in the fourth decade of life. Sudden death because of acute hydrocephalus is one scenario. Usually the lesion is hyperdense on a CT scan because of high-protein concentration; the same factor may account for its high signal seen 50% of the time on T1WI (Fig. 2.54). The rim of the cyst may faintly enhance.

■ Treatment may include biventricular shunting, craniotomy for cyst resection, endoscopic excision or fenestration of cyst, or stereotactic aspiration.

■ Rarely, colloid cysts may occur within the body of the lateral ventricles, fourth ventricle, or outside the ventricular system. When one sees an intraventricular cyst, the differential diagnosis should include a choroid plexus cyst, an ependymal cyst, a colloid cyst, and a cysticercal cyst. Ependymal cysts occur in the frontal horns of the lateral ventricles and are asymptomatic unless they obstruct the foramen of Monro.

### Neuroepithelial Cysts.

■ Neuroepithelial cysts are most commonly seen as a curiosity in the brain parenchyma (Fig. 2.55) that leads to angst about whether it represents a pilocytic tumor. The fluid in these cysts simulates CSF on CT scans and T2WI MRI but may be bright on T1WI or FLAIR owing to cholesterol debris or high-protein concentration. These cysts are lined by epithelium. Differential considerations include epidermoid cysts and traumatized arachnoid cysts.

### Paraneoplastic Syndromes

■ Paraneoplastic conditions of the brain may occur in association with non-CNS primary tumors.

■ Among these, limbic encephalitis, an abnormality affecting the temporal lobes causing memory and mental status changes, has been described extensively. The appearance simulates a herpes simplex encephalitis, usually bilateral (although it may be unilateral in 40%) with extensive disease in the temporal lobes, bright on T2WI with possible enhancement (Fig. 2.56). Atrophy of the temporal lobe may coexist, but hemorrhage is exceedingly uncommon.

■ Abnormal signal intensity in the brain stem and/or hypothalamus may be seen in about 10% to 20% of cases of limbic encephalitis.

■ Many different primary tumors have been associated with limbic encephalitis: small cell carcinoma of the lung is classic; testicular germ cell, thymic, ovarian, breast, hematologic, and gastrointestinal malignancies have also been reported. Another paraneoplastic syndrome is that of cerebellar atrophy with clinical manifestations of ataxia. Ovarian carcinoma and lymphoma may cause this finding.

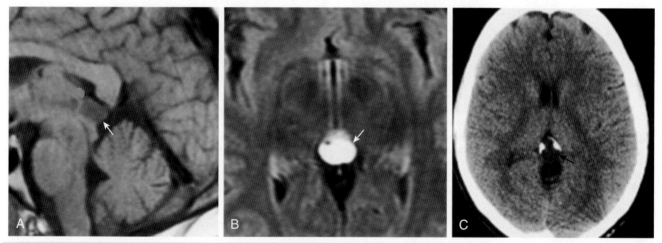

**Fig. 2.53 Cyst or cystic tumor?** Although the signal intensity *(arrow)* on the sagittal T1WI (A) and FLAIR image (B) is dissimilar to cerebrospinal fluid, this may still represent a benign pineal cyst. (C) This cystic lesion in the pineal gland displaces the pineal calcification apart. Is it a benign cyst or a neoplasm? In the absence of an enhancing mass or hydrocephalus, one could probably follow this based on patient symptoms only to assess for growth.

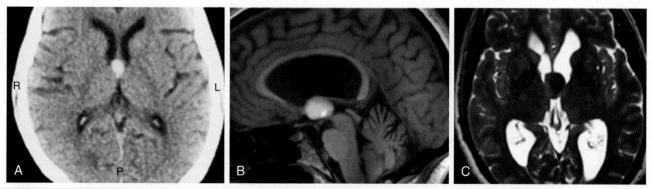

**Fig. 2.54 Colloid cyst.** (A) On computed tomography the colloid cyst is hyperdense from high protein. (B) On T1WI the colloid cyst is hyperintense because of proteinaceous contents. (C) Axial T2WI shows the low signal intensity mass in the midline at the foramen of Monro.

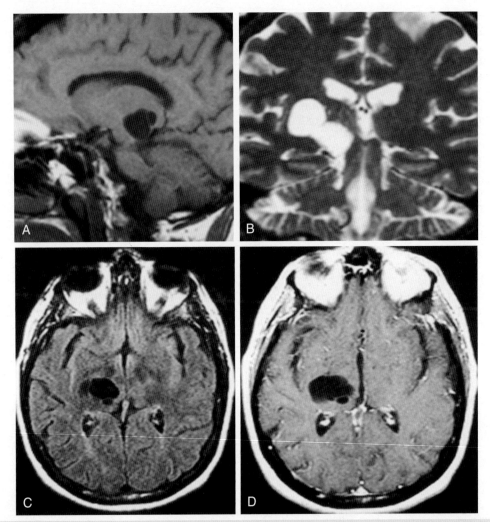

**Fig. 2.55 Neuroepithelial cyst.** (A) Unenhanced T1 sagittal scan shows a multiloculated cystic lesion in the right thalamus. (B) Coronal T2-weighted scan shows no significant mass effect and high signal similar to cerebrospinal fluid. (C) The FLAIR image scan also shows intensity identical to cerebro-spinal fluid. (D) There is no contrast enhancement. This may represent a neuroepithelial cyst, which is a benign lesion that does not require surgical intervention. Differential point: Arachnoid cysts are usually not intraparenchymal but can exist along perivascular spaces. This could be a huge Virchow-Robin space in fact.

- There are a series of antibodies that indicate paraneo-plastic syndromes. (see Chapter 5)
- Treatment of the primary tumor usually results in improvement of the paraneoplastic syndrome.

## Posttreatment Evaluation

### POSTOPERATIVE IMAGING

- Determining whether residual neoplasm is present in the postsurgical tumor bed is one of the most daunting tasks facing a neuroradiologist. Prognostic considerations for the patient (see Table 2.10), potential repeated surger-ies, and nonsurgical therapeutic decision-making often depend on the imaging interpretation.
- Surgical margin contrast enhancement almost always presents after the second postoperative day and is usu-ally thin and linear. The margin may become thicker or more nodular after a week. It thus becomes difficult to tell whether enhancing tissue in a surgical bed is because of granulation tissue or marginal tumor enhancement (provided that the tumor enhanced preoperatively). A

**Table 2.10    Five-Year Survival Rates by Tumor Type**

| Neoplasms | Survival (%) at 5 Years |
| --- | --- |
| Pilocytic astrocytoma (WHO I) | 90% |
| Ependymoma | 64% |
| Oligodendroglioma | 62% |
| Mixed glioma | 59% |
| Embryonal type | 51% |
| Diffuse astrocytoma (WHO II) | 49% |
| Anaplastic astrocytoma (WHO III) | 30% |
| Glioblastoma (WHO IV) | 3% |

*WHO*, World Health Organization.

scan within 48 hours showing nodular enhancement in or along the margins of the surgical bed should lead one to suggest residual neoplasm. The precontrast and post-contrast images must be carefully scrutinized to detect the extra thickness of enhancement along a hematoma cavity—do not confuse T1 hyperintense blood products with residual tumor!

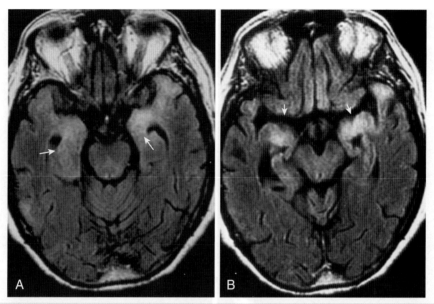

**Fig. 2.56 Limbic encephalitis.** (A) Bilateral mesial temporal lobe hyperintensity is present on the FLAIR scan *(arrows)* in this patient with ovarian cancer. (B) Atrophy argues against acute herpes encephalitis. Note prominence of sylvian fissures bilaterally *(arrows)*. In this case FLAIR hyperintensity is likely from anti-Hu antibodies from a paraneoplastic syndrome.

- Elevated cerebral blood volume on perfusion mapping at the site of nodular enhancement can increase your confidence in calling residual or recurrent tumor (Fig. 2.57).
- Granulation tissue enhancement may persist for months postoperatively, but intraparenchymal enhancement and mass effect after 1 year should be viewed with suspicion. Dural enhancement is nearly always seen even at 1 year and can persist as long as decades after surgery. Enhancement appears sooner and persists longer on MRI than on CT scans. Table 2.11 describes imaging features that can help differentiate residual tumor from granulation tissue.

## POSTRADIATION

- The radiologist's challenge in the postradiotherapy evaluation is to differentiate residual or recurrent tumor from radionecrosis.
- Several factors influence the development of radiation necrosis. These include total dose, overall duration of administration, size of each fraction of irradiation, number of fractions per irradiation, patient age, and survival time of patients. Because patients survive longer with more effective treatment, the incidence of radiation necrosis will rise, because it is usually a late effect of treatment. The signs and symptoms of radiation necrosis are nonspecific and do not differentiate it from recurrent tumor.
- The effects of irradiation have been separated into those occurring early (within weeks) and late (4 months to many years later; Table 2.12). The former is transient, may actually occur during radiotherapy, and is usually manifested by high-signal intensity in the white matter caused by increased edema (beyond that associated with the tumor).
- The delayed effects are separated into early delayed injury (within months after therapy) or late injury (months to years after therapy).

**Table 2.11    Granulation Tissue versus Residual Tumor**

| Feature | Scar | Residual Tumor |
|---|---|---|
| Enhancement within 1–2 days | No | Yes |
| Enhancement after 3–4 days | Yes | Yes |
| Change in size with time | Decreases | Increases |
| Type of enhancement | Linear, outside preoperative tumor bed | Nodular, solid |
| Mass effect | Decreases | Increases |
| Perfusion | Low | High (with higher-grade tumor) |

- Early delayed injury is also a transient effect and is of little consequence other than recognizing it as such (as opposed to tumor growth) directly after therapy.
- The late effects are usually irreversible, affect white matter to a much greater extent than gray matter, and histologically involve vascular changes that include coagulative necrosis and hyalinization. The late injury to the brain may be focal or diffuse and occurs in approximately 5% to 15% of irradiated patients. Seventy percent of focal late radiation injuries occur within 2 years after therapy. Diffuse late injury to the brain takes the form of severe demyelination, particularly in periventricular and posterior centrum semiovale regions. CT scans demonstrate decreased white matter density, but T2WI/FLAIR is more sensitive and shows high-signal intensity in the white matter. Usually the abnormality does not show enhancement.
- Disseminated necrotizing leukoencephalopathy is a severe form of radiation-related injury usually seen in conjunction with chemotherapy, whether intrathecal or

CBV, elevation in ADC, and low uptake on fluorodeoxy-glucose (FDG) PET, which would suggest tumor regression rather than progression.

- *MGMT*, a gene located on chromosome 10q26, encodes a DNA-repair enzyme that has been shown to contribute to the resistance of GB cells to alkylating agents like temozolomide. When the MGMT is methylated, pseudoprogression occurs in more than 90% of GBs (Fig. 2.59), and the overall survival is also improved, because the tumors are more responsive to chemotherapy.

- With respect to pseudoresponse, it makes sense that vascular endothelial growth factor (VEGF) receptor signaling pathway inhibitors like bevacizumab would be associated with diminished gadolinium enhancement of the tumor, thus suggesting tumor regression. Unfortunately, this may be a reversible treatment effect. It is a phenomenon seen beginning after 2 weeks of therapy and can last 2 to 3 months after therapy. The findings that suggest a treatment effect and not tumor

regression include the absence of reduction in FLAIR signal abnormality, progression/persistence of reduced diffusivity, and persistent perfusion increase.

## RESPONSE ASSESSMENT IN NEURO-ONCOLOGY

- These pseudoresponse and pseudoprogression phenomena have laid waste to the traditional Macdonald criteria for determining tumor response to therapy. These criteria have been used extensively in drug treatment trials. Response is based on the product of two-dimensional tumor measurements of the tumor on the image with the largest contrast-enhancing tumor area. A complete response is determined by resolution of all contrast-enhancing tumor. A partial response is defined by an at least 50% decrease in the product of two orthogonal diameters. Progressive disease is defined by at least a 25% increase in the product of orthogonal diameters.

- However, there is a misleading increase in enhanced lesion volume from treatment effect by temozolomide and decreased lesion enhancement volume with anti-VEGF drugs, which can cloud the assessment of treatment response or lack thereof.

- The response assessment in neuro-oncology (RANO) working group now has advocated new criteria, with the recognition that contrast enhancement is nonspecific during therapy and may not always be an accurate indicator of tumor response. The revision takes into account the increased importance of the nonenhancing component of the tumor, namely the T2/FLAIR signal changes.

- Specifically, the RANO response criteria indicate that complete responders (CR) must not be on steroids and be stable or improved clinically and must show no enhancing tissue and stable or decreasing T2/FLAIR signal change.

- Partial responders (PR) may be on stable or decreasing doses of steroids and be clinically stable or improving

**Table 2.13**  Distinction Between Tumor versus Radiation Necrosis

| Feature | Residual or Recurrent Tumor | Radiation Necrosis |
|---|---|---|
| Timing | Immediate or delayed | Months to years |
| Mass effect/edema | Present | Present |
| Enhancement | Yes | Yes, soap bubbles or Swiss cheese |
| PET (18-FDG) | Positive | Negative |
| SPECT (Thallium201, methionine-11C) | Positive | Negative |
| MRS | Elevated choline | Decreased choline |
| Perfusion-weighted MR | Elevated rCBV | Decreased rCBV |

*FDG*, Fluorodeoxyglucose; *MR*, magnetic resonance; *MRS*, magnetic resonance spectroscopy; *PET*, positron emission tomography; *rCBV*, relative cerebral blood volume; *SPECT*, single-photon emission computed tomography.

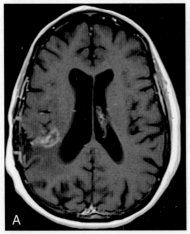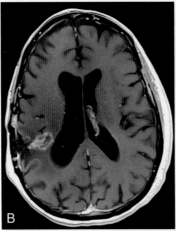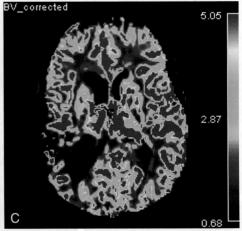

**Fig. 2.59 Pseudoprogression.** In this patient with right parietal O-6-methylguanine-DNA methyltransferase (MGMT) methylated glioblastoma treated with radiation and temozolomide, an area of heterogeneous contrast enhancement is seen adjacent to the resection cavity on postcontrast T1WI (A), which could represent tumor progression or treatment-related change. On follow-up imaging a few months later, the enhancing lesion appears increased in size on postcontrast T1WI (B); however, there is no increased perfusion on corrected cerebral blood flow map (C), favoring this enhancing tissue to reflect treatment related change (pseudoprogression) rather than increased viable tumor burden.

and have greater than or equal to a 50% reduction in the volume of enhancing tissue and stable or decreasing T2/FLAIR signal change.

- Stable disease (SD) may be on stable or decreasing doses of steroids and shows less than 50% reduction or less than 25% increase in enhancing tumor with stable or decreasing T2/FLAIR signal change.
- Finally, progressive disease (PD) shows either greater than 25% increase in enhancing tissue or increasing T2/FLAIR signal intensity tissue or declining clinical status.

# 3 *Vascular Diseases of the Brain*

OLUWATOYIN IDOWU

## Relevant Anatomy

- Good news! Vascular anatomy in the head and neck has not changed much since Chapter 1. Please take a look back at that chapter to refresh your memory.

## Imaging Techniques/Protocols

### CAROTID ULTRASOUND/TRANSCRANIAL DOPPLER

- Ultrasound is a fast, convenient, noninvasive technique to assess vasculature, using sound waves to image structures or measure the velocity and directions of blood flow with two-dimensional (2D) gray scale and color Doppler techniques.
    - Less than 50% internal carotid artery (ICA) stenosis is suggested by a peak systolic velocity (PSV) of less than 125 cm/sec and no visible plaque or intimal thickening.
    - Fifty to sixty-nine percent ICA stenosis is suggested by PSV 125 to 230 cm/sec with visible plaque.
    - At least 70% ICA stenosis is suggested by PSV greater than 230 cm/sec with visible plaque and luminal narrowing. ICA to common carotid artery (CCA) peak systolic ratio greater than 4, and ICA end-diastolic velocity greater than 100 cm/sec are additional criteria to identify ICA stenosis of at least 70%.
    - With near occlusion of the ICA, velocity parameters may not apply because velocity may be high, low, or undetectable; however, significant luminal narrowing is visualized with some flow on color Doppler.
- Color-coded Doppler ultrasound can depict the residual lumen of the extracranial carotid artery more accurately than conventional duplex Doppler. However, the results from color-coded Doppler ultrasound can be confounded by artifacts related to plaque contents and limited by vessel tortuosity. Problems include distinguishing high-grade stenosis from occlusion, calcified plaques interfering with visualization of the vascular lumen, inability to show lesions of the carotid near the skull base, difficulty with tandem lesions, and inability to image the origins of the carotid or the vertebral arteries.
- Transcranial Doppler ultrasound is a noninvasive means to evaluate the basal cerebral arteries through the infratemporal fossa. It evaluates the flow velocity spectrum of the cerebral vessels and can provide information regarding the direction of flow, patency, vessel narrowing from atherosclerotic disease or spasm, and cerebrovascular reactivity. It can determine adequacy of middle cerebral artery (MCA) flow in patients with carotid stenosis and evaluate for embolus within the proximal MCA. It is very useful in the detection of cerebrovascular spasm after subarachnoid hemorrhage or after surgery in the intensive care setting bedside and can rapidly assess the result of intracranial angioplasty or intra-arterial vasodilators to treat vasospasm.

### COMPUTED TOMOGRAPHY ANGIOGRAM

- Advances with multidetector computed tomography (CT; increased detector rows of 256, 320, and up to 640 slice scanners, and increased gantry rotation speeds contributing to higher spatial and temporal resolution) allow for excellent visualization of the extracranial and intracranial vasculature.
- Dual-energy CT is an additional technique that can produce a data set at two x-ray photon energy spectra. Tissues that demonstrate varying attenuation based on K edge at higher (120–140 kVp) versus lower (50–80 kVp) energy values can be differentiated. This may be applicable, for example, in vascular imaging to help distinguish calcium in atherosclerotic plaque and to better evaluate vessels coursing in the skull by subtracting out bone and in distinguishing extravasated contrast from blood products.
- CT angiogram (CTA) requires administration of an iodinated contrast agent usually into an antecubital vein to opacify the vasculature. A timing technique (bolus tracking to threshold HU or initial injection of test bolus run before the formal CTA) is used to identify the start of arterial phase opacification of the vessels during imaging. Helical axial CT images through the head and/or neck are then acquired to produce angiographic images.
- Reconstructive techniques process the axial source data imaging set to provide additional angiographic views. These include multiplanar reformats (MPR) in sagittal and coronal planes, 2D maximum intensity projections (MIPs) that increase slice thickness and superimposition of the brightest density structures, 2D curved formats, and three-dimensional (3D) volume-rendering images (Fig. 3.1).
- At the cost of radiation and iodinated contrast dye, CTA allows for faster imaging acquisition and higher spatial resolution compared with magnetic resonance angiography (MRA) techniques. Extremely slow flow and tandem lesions are more reliably detected on CTA than MRA. Postimaging manipulations may be necessary to improve visualization and reduce artifacts at the skull base or related to significant vascular calcification.

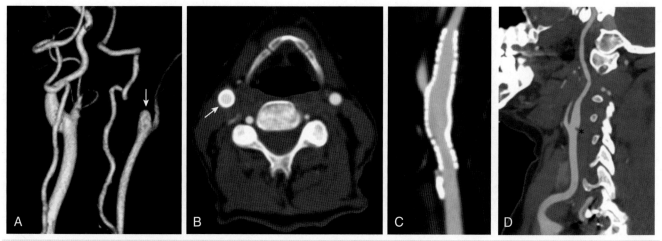

**Fig. 3.1 Computed tomography angiography (CTA) of the neck.** (A) Three-dimensional (3D), volume-rendered reconstructions of the cervical arterial vasculature with bone subtraction elegantly show abrupt occlusion of the internal carotid artery (ICA; *arrow*) indicating dissection, with remainder of vessels normal in appearance. (B) Axial CTA source image in a different patient to assess patency of a right ICA after stent placement shows the stent to be intact with normal enhancement in the vessel lumen *(arrow)*. (C) Sagittal maximum intensity projection reconstruction shows the same stent in the craniocaudal dimension to be widely patent. (D) Curved radial reconstructed CTA image shows shelf-like intraluminal projection at the origin of the ICA *(asterisk)*, consistent with carotid web.

- Four-dimensional (4D) CTA is a dynamic acquisition technique that combines the noninvasive nature of CTA with the dynamic acquisition of digital subtraction angiography (DSA) techniques by performing multiple or continuous CT acquisitions over a period of time. This is useful in evaluating flow dynamics. The high temporal resolution of this technique is particularly useful in characterizing arteriovenous malformations (AVMs) and arteriovenous fistulas (AVFs). However, a limitation can be the higher radiation dose compared with conventional CTA.

## MAGNETIC RESONANCE ANGIOGRAM

- This alternative angiographic imaging technique eliminates the use of ionizing radiation compared with CT but requires screening the patient for any ferromagnetic metal hardware or implants and takes more time than CTA imaging from start to finish.
- Time-of-flight (TOF) MRA does not require administering a contrast medium, which is helpful for those pesky contrast allergies or those individuals with compromised renal function given previously reported concerns for development of nephrogenic systemic sclerosis in patients with low glomerular filtration rates ($<30\,mL/min/1.73m^2$). That said, a recent 2020 consensus statement from the American College of Radiology and the National Kidney Foundation reported that the risk of nephrogenic systemic fibrosis (NSF) in patients with impaired renal function is extremely low using standard dosing (0.1 mmol/kg) of group II or III gadolinium-based contrast media and that the harm of delaying or withholding contrast may outweigh the risk of NSF.
- With this technique, the signal from flow-related spins within the moving water protons in blood are captured on 2D or 3D gradient echo (GRE) sequences, showing as a "bright" signal on the T1-weighted images (T1WI). To highlight arterial (cranially directed) signal, a venous

saturation band can be applied to remove flow-related signal from venous structures (caudally directed). TOF imaging is accomplished by first demagnetizing (i.e., saturating out the signal) water protons in a slice/volume of tissue by applying a radiofrequency (RF) magnetic pulse. Fresh blood entering that same volume of tissue will, in turn, have "high" signal relative to the surrounding demagnetized tissues, and the slice can be imaged. The technique is repeated to acquire multiple slices throughout the region of interest, and multiple volumes are combined to produce angiographic images.

- MIP images are reconstructed from the source images to obtain 3D views of the vessels. A presaturation band can be added ahead of the volume of tissue being imaged to prevent signal from vessels flowing in the opposite direction (i.e., venous flow) into the slab being imaged for arterial TOF. For venous TOF imaging, the direction of the saturation band is reversed.
- A 2D TOF technique is used for long vascular segments but is not great for detection of in-plane flow, and motion can contribute to misregistration of slices (step artifact). A 2D cervical TOF MRA also tends to overestimate stenosis. A 3D TOF technique offers higher spatial resolution and signal to noise compared with 2D but is not great in the case of slow-flow vessels. Saturation effects limit slab thickness with 3D TOF, and it is generally a longer acquisition. A 3D TOF is used for more compact vascular regions with various flow directions (circle of Willis and carotid bifurcation, for example).
- Phase-contrast (PC) MRA relies on the concept that a moving spin (proton) subject to a pair of bipolar flow-sensitizing gradient will experience a net phase shift or position change proportional to its velocity. The change in phase can be used to compute velocity. Spins flowing at the same speed but in the opposite direction will have equal but opposite shifts. The operator adjusts a parameter known as *velocity encoding* (VENC), which controls the amplitude, duration, and spacing of the bipolar gradients and contributes to the degree of flow sensitivity. VENC

ranges from about 30 cm/sec for arterial flow to 15 cm/sec for venous flow. Complex subtraction of data from the two acquisitions (one which inverts the polarity of the bipolar gradient) will cancel all phase shifts except those resulting from flow. The flow data obtained can be used to depict a magnitude image similar to a TOF MRA. This technique provides excellent background suppression to differentiate flow from other causes of T1 shortening, such a subacute thrombus, subacute hemorrhage, or fat because stationary spins experience no net phase shift.

- Contrast-enhanced (CE) MRA technique uses a gadolinium-based contrast agent to opacify the vasculature instead of the iodinated contrast used with CT. The contrast contributes to T1 shortening, which shows as increased signal on a T1WI sequence. The technique is less affected by flow-related artifacts compared with TOF and can be useful in confirming vessel patency when there is reversal of flow, such as in subclavian steal syndrome (Fig. 3.2).
  - Similar to CTA, timing of the contrast bolus and image acquisition during the arterial phase is essential for the arteriogram and to prevent venous contamination. Bolus tracking or a test bolus can be used for this. A precontrast "mask" image is acquired that can be subtracted from the postcontrast images to produce the vascular arteriogram images.
  - Time-resolved imaging is a dynamic CE MRA technique where cine images are obtained from the arterial through the venous phases of imaging, providing information on flow dynamics.
- With black-blood MRA, the signal from inflowing blood is suppressed, rendering it "black" compared with the enhanced bright signal seen with traditional "bright-blood" techniques, such as TOF or CE MRA. The loss of

intraluminal signal highlights the surrounding walls of vessels, making it a uniquely helpful technique for evaluating head and neck vasculature for pathologies such as atherosclerosis, dissection, vasculitis/arteritis, or aneurysm stability. This requires high magnet field strength (3 T preferred) and high spatial and contrast resolution imaging, most commonly obtained with precontrast and postcontrast T1W sequences.

## CONVENTIONAL CATHETER ANGIOGRAPHY

- Conventional angiography is a minimally invasive interventional procedure. The vasculature is accessed from a peripheral site with the use of dedicated catheters and wires and the intra-arterial injection of iodinated contrast. Selective catheter angiography is used to evaluate the intracranial vasculature. Dynamic fluoroscopic imaging is performed, often with a rotating imager such as a C-arm. DSA techniques allow for subtraction of the underlying tissues/bones to produce a vascular arteriogram. The images produced are high resolution and can be assessed in real time and in multiple imaging projections.
- Catheter angiography remains a gold standard for assessment of vessel stenoses and occlusions where serial images can show the presence, source, and extent of collateral supply. A 4D catheter angiography combines 3D spatial resolution with temporal-related information for assessment of AVMs and AVFs, where time-resolved arterial and venous phase imaging is essential for characterizing the lesion. Detection of ulcerated plaque on catheter angiography is more accurate than with noninvasive angiography. Minimally invasive interventions can also be performed with this technique, including

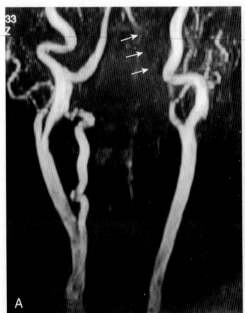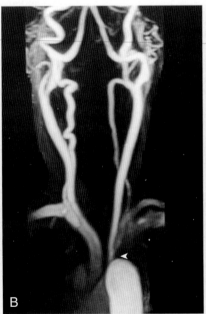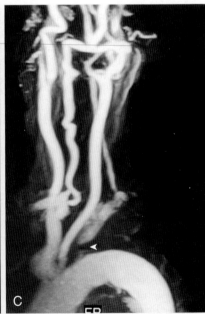

**Fig. 3.2 Subclavian steal.** (A) Anterograde flow in the left vertebral artery *(arrows)* is not appreciated on time-of-flight magnetic resonance angiography (MRA). This is because flow within this vessel is in the opposite direction and has been suppressed along with the venous structures by the intentionally applied saturation pulse. (B) Gadolinium-enhanced MRA now shows the left vertebral artery, which is opacifying in a retrograde fashion. The cause is a stenosis of the proximal left subclavian artery *(arrowhead)*, which is hard to believe on this projection but much more plausible *(arrowhead)* on the oblique view (C).

aneurysm treatment with embolization or coiling, vascular stenting, or thrombectomy/thrombolysis in the case of vascular occlusion.

## PERFUSION IMAGING

- Perfusion imaging represents an advanced form of vascular imaging that provides a map of the hemodynamic status of the brain at the capillary level. CT- and magnetic resonance (MR)-based imaging techniques can measure the amount of an exogenous (iodinated or paramagnetic contrast material) or endogenous tracer (magnetically labeled blood) within a volume of tissue during dynamic imaging. Perfusion parameters are calculated from the acquired data based on the central volume principle that cerebral blood flow (CBF) = cerebral blood volume (CBV) / mean transit time (MTT).
- The CBF of a normal brain ranges between 45 to 110 mL/min/100 g of tissue. Cerebral oligemia (about 20–30 mL/min/100 g) is defined as an underperfused asymptomatic region of the brain that will recover spontaneously, whereas ischemic hypoperfused brain is symptomatic and at risk to develop irreversible infarct without revascularization. This ischemic threshold where there is cessation of action potential generation occurs around 20 mL/min/100 g, and the infarction threshold associated with irreversible neuronal damage is at approximately 10 mL/min/100 g.
- Changes in MTT and CBV reflect the autoregulatory process that occurs in the setting of CBF and cerebral perfusion pressure (CPP) changes because of vessel occlusion or stenosis. The initial autoregulatory response of the brain is vasodilatation of the vascular bed distal to the occlusion or stenosis, which increases CBV and can initially maintain CBF. MTT is also prolonged so red blood cells have longer contact at the capillary level with increased time for oxygen extraction. With prolonged or further decreases in CBF, maximal vasodilation is reached and tissue oxygen extraction capabilities are overwhelmed. This can ultimately result in collapse of the vascular bed and a decrease in CBV.
- CT perfusion requires administration of iodinated contrast (e.g., 40–50 cc at 5–6 cc/sec injection followed by a 40 mL saline bolus), and after an initial (7–10 sec) delay, an axial dynamic imaging acquisition is performed (e.g., every 1.5–2 sec for a 40–50 sec acquisition). Partial volume (minimum 4 cm) or up to whole brain acquisitions are possible, dependent on scanner capabilities. The imaging slices should cover the main intracranial vessels of interest. Intravascular changes in density from the iodinated contrast are measured during passage of the contrast. From a dynamic perfusion scan, a time versus density curve can be established and is used to calculate perfusion parameters.
- Perfusion imaging in MR imaging (MRI) can be performed with or without contrast. The most commonly used contrast technique is dynamic susceptibility contrast-enhanced (DSC) imaging. This is most commonly a GRE-based technique that relies on the T2* effects of gadolinium contrast, which result in a drop in intravascular signal intensity.

- From a dynamic imaging scan, a time versus signal intensity curve can be established. The decrease in signal intensity is converted to contrast concentration and used to calculate perfusion parameters. Conversion formulas take into account the natural course of cerebral blood flow into the brain from arterial across capillary bed to venous, with the assumption that contrast remains intravascular (no leakage).
- Alternatively, the dynamic contrast-enhanced (DCE) technique relies on the intrinsic T1 shortening properties of gadolinium-based contrast on T1W images to measure increased signal within the vessels as a means of calculating the perfusion parameters. The DCE imaging can depict the wash-in, plateau, and washout contrast kinetics of the tissue, more useful in tumor imaging. The most commonly calculated parameter is k-trans, which mainly reflects vessel permeability and has been shown to be higher in tumor recurrence. Leakage-corrected CBV measurements from DSC exams take into account blood–brain barrier breakdown in the setting of tumor and can provide insight into viable tumor burden following treatment.
- The arterial spin–labeled (ASL) MR technique uses labeled water as an endogenous tracer, meaning it requires no contrast! The inflow of labeled blood into an imaging slab can be measured over a dynamic imaging sequence. Subtraction of a baseline image with unlabeled blood produces the signal changes that represent blood flow to the brain. However, ASL tends to be limited by low signal to noise and affected by motion and poor hemodynamic status.
- Both CT and DSC MR perfusion techniques produce time versus density/signal intensity curves where the area under the curve represents CBV. The time it takes from injection for contrast to reach max concentration in the brain (time to peak), the time it takes for contrast in the red blood cell to traverse the capillary bed (MTT), or the time it takes for contrast to reach the capillary bed from an index artery/arterial input function (Tmax) are all time-sensitive parameters that evaluate the transit characteristics of blood. CBF can be calculated from this data set based on the central volume theorem and with the application of a deconvolution algorithm that factors in the contrast agent travel within peripheral arteries and veins before reaching capillaries within the region of interest. Delay-insensitive algorithms are ideal because delay-sensitive methods may overestimate changes in CBF and CBV that correlate to core infarct volume. Differences in these deconvolution algorithms can also contribute to the variability in perfusion imaging postprocessing software outputs.

# Pathologies

## PARENCHYMAL HEMORRHAGE

- With hemorrhage, there is a linear relationship between CT attenuation (density) and hematocrit. The attenuation of whole blood with a hematocrit of 45% is approximately 56 Hounsfield units (HUs). Normal gray matter ranges from 37 to 41 HU, and normal white matter is from 30 to 34 HU. Thus freshly extravasated blood in a patient with a normal hematocrit can be readily demonstrated on CT. In severely anemic patients, there is a small possibility that the acute hemorrhage will be isodense to brain because of low hematocrit (<10%). Conversely, in infants with high hematocrit or patients with polycythemia, the dural sinuses, large veins, and proximal arteries may normally appear dense (mimicking thrombosis).

■ After initial hemorrhage, the CT density of blood products progressively increases for approximately 72 hours and then subsequently decreases to isodensity with the brain over the next 2 weeks (Fig. 3.3). This is caused by increasing hemoglobin concentration attributed to clot formation and retraction and eventual macrophage digestion and resorption of blood products. The presence of fluid levels within a hematoma suggests active bleeding, absence of coagulation (e.g., in patients on blood thinners), or coagulopathy, resulting in nonfunctioning or absent clotting factors.

■ The use of intravenous (IV) contrast is indicated for CTA or CTV to evaluate for associated vascular anomalies (aneurysm, arteriovenous malformations) and thrombosis (arterial or venous). Focal extravasation of contrast (the "dot sign") into the center of a hematoma on source images is a sign of active hemorrhage and is often associated with continued growth of the hematoma (Fig. 3.4). If contrast is given, intraparenchymal hemorrhage is often associated with a smooth peripheral rim of enhancement from approximately 6 days to 6 weeks, resulting from the breakdown of the blood–brain barrier at the margin of the hematoma.

■ The MR imaging features of hemorrhage are complex compared with CT secondary to key effects created by the hemoglobin (Hb) molecule within the red blood cell (RBC). Temporal changes in parenchymal attenuation and signal are summarized below.

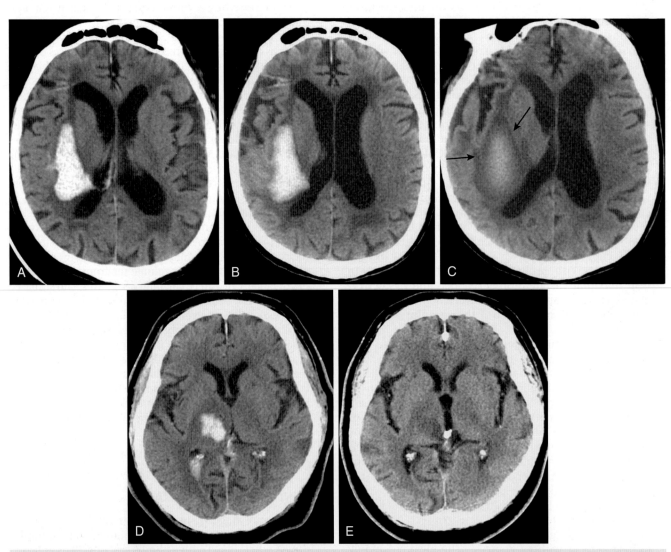

**Fig. 3.3 Computed tomography (CT) scan of hematoma evolution.** (A) CT scan 6 hours after onset of symptoms in a patient with chronic hypertension reveals a large lenticular nucleus homogeneous hyperdense hematoma with mild surrounding edema and relatively little mass effect. (B) Follow-up exam at 6 days reveals decreased density at the margin of the hematoma. There is increased mass effect on the right lateral ventricle. (C) Examination at 3 weeks reveals decreased central hyperdensity that fades gradually at the periphery of the hematoma *(arrows)*, where hematoma is now hypodense. (D) A CT scan in a different hypertensive patient at 18 hours reveals discrete hyperdense right thalamic hemorrhage with surrounding edema and mass effect on the third ventricle. (E) Follow-up exam at 2 weeks reveals complete resolution of hyperdensity. Hypodense hematoma still has mass effect on the third ventricle.

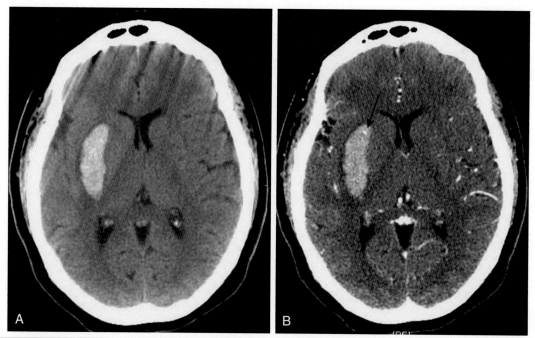

**Fig. 3.4 Hyperacute intracerebral hemorrhage.** (A) Hyperacute (3 hours) right lateral ganglionic hypertensive hemorrhage. Note the lack of surrounding edema and paucity of mass effect. (B) Computed tomography angiography source image reveals "dot sign" *(arrow)* within the anterior portion of the hematoma, indicative of acute extravasation and active hemorrhage.

### PHYSICS PEARLS

- With *hyperacute* hemorrhage (0–4 hours), early clot formation within mainly intracellular oxyhemoglobin (oxy-Hb) is seen as mildly T1W hyperintense/hypointense or isointense (because protein increases T1 and edema/water decreases T1) and T2 hyperintense. The periphery of the hematoma contains RBCs that have started to desaturate (deoxyhemoglobin, deoxy-Hb) producing peripheral hypointensity, particularly on susceptibility-weighted imaging (SWI) and at higher field strength (Fig. 3.5).

- During the *acute* hemorrhage period (4–72 hours), there is conversion of oxy-Hb to deoxy-Hb because of local hypoxia and acidosis. Clot formation and retraction leads to decreased water content. These effects produce profound T2 and T2* hypointensity from proton relaxation enhancement that begins at the periphery and extends to the center of the hematoma. The hematoma is mildly T1 hypointense because of the susceptibility effects. No T1 shortening is caused by proton-electron dipole-dipole interactions because water molecules are unable to bind the iron atom of deoxy-Hb at this stage. Peripheral vasogenic edema around the hematoma is increased (see Fig. 3.5).

- During the *early subacute* period (3–6 days), there is oxidation of the deoxy-Hb to methemoglobin (met-Hb) inside the RBC. Unlike deoxy-Hb, water molecules can approach the paramagnetic heme of met-Hb permitting proton-electron dipole-dipole interactions that shorten T1. This effect gives subacute hematomas their characteristic hyperintensity on T1WI, proceeding from the periphery to the center of the clot during the first week. Because the paramagnetic methemoglobin remains encapsulated within the RBC, marked hypointensity is present on T2-weighted imaging (T2WI) and T2* images because of the previously described proton relaxation enhancement susceptibility effects (Fig. 3.6). With cell lysis, these effects begin to decrease.

- The *late subacute* hemorrhage phase (6–14 days) is characterized by red cell and clot lysis. Met-Hb is less stable and can spontaneously lose the heme group from the protein molecule, promoting RBC lysis. Hyperintensity persists on T1WI because of the shortening effects of the residual intracellular and extracellular met-Hb. The hematoma progressively increases signal on T2WI because of loss of local field inhomogeneity and reduction in proton relaxation enhancement that results from RBC lysis and decreasing protein concentration. Paralleling this process is the accumulation of iron molecules, hemosiderin and ferritin, within macrophages at the periphery of the lesion, resulting in a hypointense rim variably visible on T1WI but increasingly prominent on T2WI and SWI (Fig. 3.7).

- In the *chronic* hemorrhage phase (>2 weeks), the hematoma becomes progressively smaller and, within months, the fluid and protein within the clot is broken down and resorbed. Peripheral edema and mass effect resolve. The iron atoms from the metabolized hemoglobin molecules are deposited in hemosiderin and ferritin molecules that are trapped permanently within the brain parenchyma because of restoration of the blood–brain barrier. Susceptibility effects of the iron cores of hemosiderin produce permanent hypointensity on all sequences, most prominent on the GRE and SWI sequences, where "blooming" is observed, particularly with larger hemorrhages (Fig. 3.8). Smaller petechial hemorrhages (microbleeds <5 mm) produce foci of T2* hypointensity on GRE or SWI sequences, which cannot be detected on CT.

**TEACHING POINTS**

Stages of Hemorrhage

| Stage | CT | T1WI | T2WI | Mass Effect | Time Course | Explanation |
|---|---|---|---|---|---|---|
| Hyperacute | High density | Mild hyper-intensity | High intensity with peripheral low intensity | +++ | 0–4 hrs | CT: High protein<br>T1WI, T2WI: Central oxyhemoglobin in with peripheral deoxyhemoglobin (deoxy-Hb) |
| Acute | High density | Isointense to low intensity | Low intensity | +++ | 4–72 hrs | CT: High protein<br>T1WI: High protein, susceptibility (deoxy-Hb)<br>T2WI: Susceptibility (deoxy-Hb) |
| Early subacute | High density | High intensity | Low intensity | +++/++ | 3–6 days | CT: High protein<br>T1WI: PEDDI (intracellular methemoglobin [met-Hb]), high protein<br>T2WI: Susceptibility (intracellular met-Hb), high protein |
| Late subacute | Isodense | High intensity | High intensity with rim of low intensity | ± | 6–14 days | CT: Absorption of high protein<br>T1WI: PEDDI (free met-Hb), absence of susceptibility effects (from intracellular met-Hb), dilution of high protein<br>T2WI: PEDDI (free met-Hb), absence of susceptibility effects, dilution of high protein, susceptibility effects from hemosiderin and ferritin in peripheral rim |
| Chronic | Low density | Low intensity | Low intensity | – | >2 weeks | CT: Atrophy<br>T1WI: Susceptibility effects from hemosiderin and ferritin (T2 effect on T1WI)<br>T2WI: Susceptibility effects from hemosiderin and ferritin |

*CT*, Computed tomography; *Hb*, hemoglobin; *PEDDI*, proton-electron dipole-dipole interaction; *T1WI*, T1-weighted image; *T2WI*, T2-weighted image.

■ The most common cause of nontraumatic parenchymal hemorrhage is hypertension, and these lesions are most often seen in the deep gray matter (basal ganglia and thalamus), brain stem, and cerebellum (see Fig. 3.3). Damage to small perforating arteries leads to fibrinoid necrosis and contributes to the deeper hemorrhages. Imaging often reveals evidence of underlying cerebrovascular disease, including lacunar infarcts, previous deep cerebral hemorrhages, or microvascular white matter disease. On SWI or GRE sequences, there is often evidence of prior occult microhemorrhages, situated primarily in central structures, including the basal ganglia, thalami, and brain stem, although deep white matter and cerebellar microbleeds can also be present.

■ Lobar hemorrhages may be seen with infarcts, hypertension, blood pressure swings that may be drug induced (cocaine), or from supratherapeutic anticoagulation. In patients over 50 years of age, lobar hemorrhages can be the result of cerebral amyloid angiopathy. Venous thrombosis can lead to parenchymal hemorrhages, typically in the white matter adjacent to the thrombosed dural sinus or cortical vein. Hemorrhage into underlying neoplastic lesions or from vascular abnormalities (AVMs, cavernous malformations, and aneurysms) can occur in any location at any age. Microbleeds typically occur in hypertensive cerebrovascular disease and amyloid angiopathy and as a result of head trauma with diffuse axonal injury (DAI). They may also be seen with multiple cavernous malformations and after radiation therapy.

## EXTRA-AXIAL HEMORRHAGE

■ Extra-axial hemorrhages, namely epidural, subdural, and subarachnoid bleeds, are most commonly seen in the trauma setting, and discussed in detail in Chapter 4 and are briefly revisited here in the context of vascular implications.

■ Epidural hemorrhages are most commonly seen in the trauma setting, most often secondary to laceration of the middle meningeal artery, less often because of venous injury. If small, they may resolve on their own, but if large, they require surgical decompression to avoid herniation syndromes. They are usually elliptical in shape, do not cross sutures, and, when related to venous sinus injury, may cross the midline and dissect between the dura and the subperiosteum.

■ Subdural hemorrhages (SDHs) in the acute trauma setting are most often because of rupture of veins bridging the subdural space. They may also be seen after surgical intervention. Elderly patients can present with SDHs, more often in a subacute context, wherein these patients come to medical attention after multiple rebleeding episodes. These hematomas tend to be anatomically complex, with blood products of variable age, multiple septations within the hematomas, and compartmentalized fluid levels. It is theorized that chronic inflammation from subdural bleeding results in angiogenesis centered about the middle meningeal artery, and it is, in fact, repeated bleeding events from this vessel that cause recurrent SDHs in this population. Recently it has been shown that rather than repeated subdural evacuation

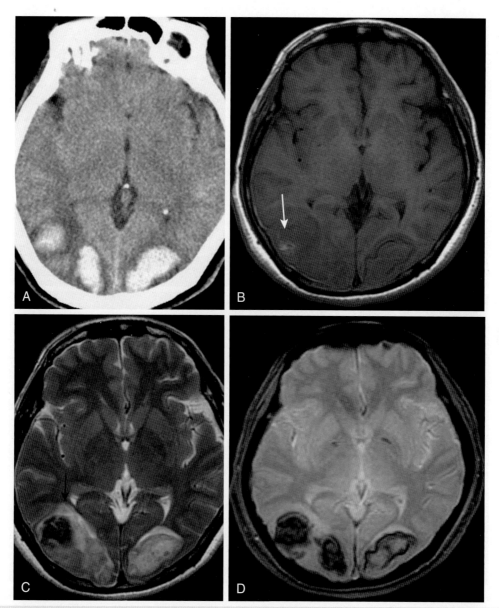

**Fig. 3.5 Imaging of hyperacute and acute intracranial hemorrhage.** Patient presented with left field cut 2 days before the examination. Approximately 4 hours before examination, the patient became blind. Both hyperacute left and acute right hematomas are present. (A) Computed tomography scan several hours after onset of new field cut reveals bilateral occipital hematomas. Right hematoma has more edema than left, suggesting slightly "older" bleed. (B) T1-weighted image (T1WI) reveals that the left hematoma is relatively isointense with a hypointense margin. The right hematoma has a focus of hyperintensity in its lateral margin *(arrow)* indicative of acute to subacute hematoma. (C) T2-weighted image (T2WI) reveals that left hematoma is hyperintense, whereas right hematoma has regions of marked hypointensity *(arrow)*. (D) Gradient-echo scan reveals that left hematoma has a hypointense margin and a relatively hyperintense center. Right hematoma is more diffusely hypointense.

procedures, these patients tend to do better after embolization of the middle meningeal artery (Fig. 3.9).

- Subarachnoid hemorrhage (SAH) may result from a variety of circumstances, including trauma, ruptured aneurysm, AVM, vasculopathy, venous thrombosis, and extension of parenchymal hemorrhage (e.g., hemorrhagic strokes or hypertensive bleeds) into the subarachnoid space.
  - On CT, acute SAH produces hyperdensity in the affected sulci, cisterns, and fissures. The hyperdensity rapidly evolves with complete resolution within 2 days for a small amount of isolated SAH and within 5 to 7 days for most aneurysmal SAH. Dissection of

hemorrhage into the adjacent parenchyma and ventricular system may occur.
- On routine T1WI, SAH produces only subtle T1 hyperintensity. Spinal fluid dilutes the blood and antifibrogenic elements in CSF, preventing or inhibiting clot formation. Rapid dilution and removal of blood, absence of clot formation, and presence of high $O_2$ concentration (which limits the amount of deoxy-Hb) prevent development of T2 and T2* hypointensity and subacute T1 hyperintensity via the mechanisms previously discussed.
- However, more notable changes are seen on fluid-attenuated inversion recovery (FLAIR) imaging,

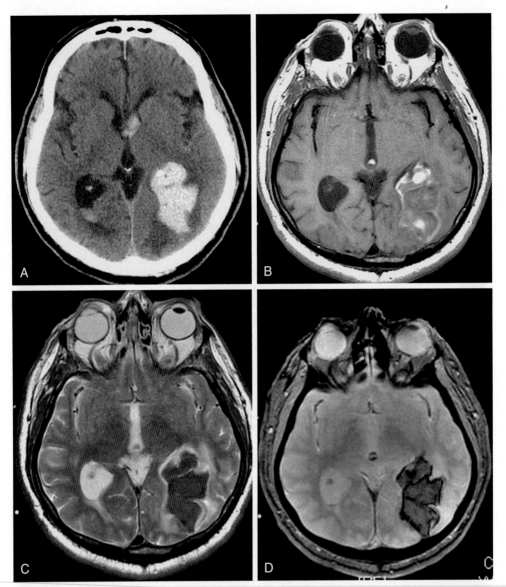

**Fig. 3.6  Imaging of subacute hematoma.** (A) Computed tomography scan at 1 day reveals a large irregular hyperdense left parieto-occipital hematoma with intraventricular hemorrhage. Magnetic resonance imaging performed at 3 days. (B) T1-weighted image (T1WI) reveals hyperintensity at the margin of the lesion and within the anterior and posterior portions of the hematoma. (C) T2-weighted image (T2WI) reveals homogeneous marked central hypointensity with mild surrounding T2 hyperintense edema. (D) Gradient-echo scan reveals diffuse hypointensity with a more hypointense rim.

where blood in the subarachnoid space changes the time inversion (TI) of the CSF and prevents CSF suppression. Because CSF is not suppressed, T2 effects are visible and the bloody CSF is bright on FLAIR (Fig. 3.10). Although sensitivity is high, specificity is low because nonsuppression of sulcal FLAIR signal can be seen with several pathologies, including inflammatory and neoplastic leptomeningeal disease, artifacts related to metal (shunt valves, dental devise), and when patients are breathing supplemental oxygen (e.g., anesthesia) during the exam ($O_2$ is paramagnetic, and its presence within the subarachnoid CSF shortens TI sufficiently to prevent suppression of signal). The most common CSF artifact on FLAIR sequences is a pulsation artifact at the skull base, which limits assessment for SAH in the basal cisterns.

■  When a subarachnoid space clot does form, the MR intensities are similar to those seen with parenchymal hemorrhage without hemosiderin. Acute clot is T2 and T2* hypointense and subacute clot is T1 hyperintense. Hemosiderin deposition on the surface of the brain (leptomeningeal and pial) and cranial nerves can occur as a result of chronic recurrent SAH (i.e., superficial (hemo)siderosis). Hemosiderin is neurotoxic, and when it involves the cranial nerves, patients may develop specific neuropathic symptoms. On MR, hypointense coating of the surface of the brain and cranial nerves is visible on T2WI and more extensively on SWI or T2*–weighted images (Fig. 3.11).

## CEREBRAL INFARCTION

The causes of cerebral infarction include large and small arterial vessel occlusions, vasculopathy, migraines, venous sinus thrombosis, and systemic/metabolic processes

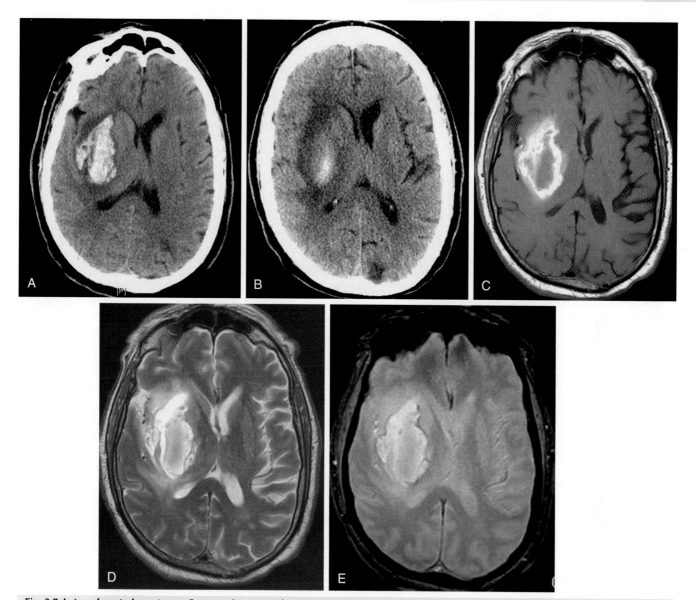

**Fig. 3.7 Late subacute hematoma.** Computed tomography scans at 24 hours (A) and 14 days (B) reveal evolution of right ganglionic hematoma. Magnetic resonance (MR) scan also performed at 14 days reveals peripheral hyperintensity and central isointensity on T1-weighted image (T1WI) (C); marked peripheral hyperintensity, central mild hyperintensity, and a subtle hypointense margin on T2-weighted image (T2WI) (D); and central hyperintensity with a peripheral hypointense margin on gradient-echo image (E). Note that size of hematoma is more easily appreciated on MR than computed tomography (CT) at this stage. Hematoma is approximately the same size on MR as it was at time of initial CT.

contributing to anoxic or hypoxic brain injury. Atherosclerotic disease contributing to thromboembolic phenomenon in large vessels, cardioembolic phenomenon, and lacunar infarcts affecting small vessels are by far the most prevalent causes of acute stroke, particularly in high-risk populations (i.e., hypertensives, diabetic, smokers, and hyperlipidemics).

Identifying the cause, location, and severity of the infarct has important implications for treatment, outcomes, and prevention of future events. For instance, acute large vessel occlusions may be eligible for thrombolytic therapy or vascular intervention for thrombectomy. Carotid endarterectomy may be the treatment of severe carotid atherosclerosis, and anticoagulation/antiplatelet drugs with medical management of risk

factors may be the pathway of choice for cardiac origin or lacunar strokes.

## ARTERIAL INFARCTS

- Effective acute stroke management relies on streamlined imaging and treatment algorithms that quickly identify patients that could benefit from anticoagulation or advanced therapies. In the acute stroke setting, patients present with acute localizing neurologic deficits based on the stenotic or occluded vessel that can be assessed clinically in the acute setting with the National Institutes of Health Stroke Scale (NIHSS). The Modified Rankin Scale (MRS) is also used for scoring the degree of neurologic disability after stroke.

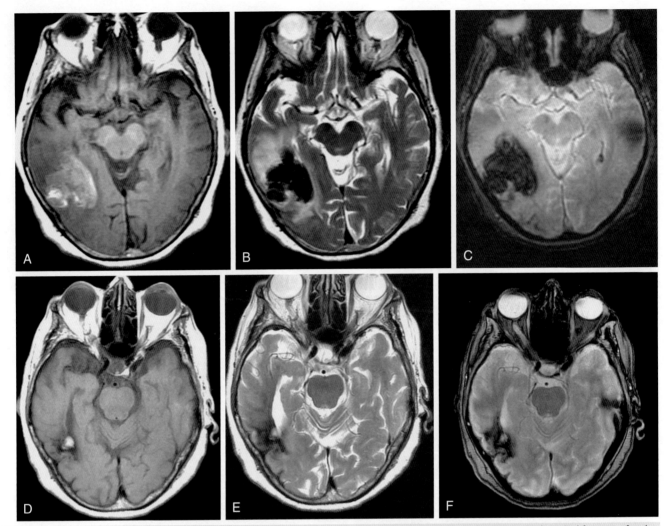

**Fig. 3.8 Magnetic resonance study of chronic hematoma.** Right temporal hematoma examined 4 days after ictus reveals typical features of early subacute hematoma with peripheral hyperintensity on T1-weighted image (T1WI) (A), diffuse hypointensity on T2WI with surrounding edema and mass effect (B), and marked hypointensity on gradient echo (C). (D–F) Repeat examination at 2 months reveals marked contraction of clot with focal volume loss and no edema. Residual central T1 (D) and T2 (E) hyperintensity is present. There is extensive T2 and susceptibility hypointensity in the adjacent tissue, and there is mild sulcal hemosiderin deposition in the leptomeninges (siderosis) adjacent on the gradient-echo scan (F).

## TEACHING POINTS

Hyperacute/Early Acute Stroke Management With Suspected Large Vessel Occlusion (LVO)

- Noncontrast computed tomography (CT) → check for bleed or large infarct
- CT angiography (CTA) → document LVO
- <4.5 hours → tissue plasminogen activator eligible
- <6 hours → intra-arterial thrombectomy eligible (up to 24 hours for posterior circulation infarcts)
- >6 hours up to 24 hours → advanced perfusion imaging to assess salvageable brain tissue based on: DAWN trial (clinical National Institutes of Health Stroke Scale mismatch to core infarct volume by Diffusion weighted imaging or cerebral blood flow [CBF]) or DEFUSE 3 trials (core infarct <70 cc based on relative 30% decrease in CBF, ischemic tissue based on Tmax >6 sec and core infarct:ischemic tissue volume mismatch of >1.8)
- "Malignant Profile" implies poorer outcomes after reperfusion (core >100 cc or >50% defect in collaterals on single or multiphase CTA)

## TEACHING POINTS

Clinical Stroke Assessment

- The National Institutes of Health Stroke Scale score of 0 indicates no stroke symptoms, and score less than 5 indicates a minor stroke increasing to severe stroke with a score of 21 to 42.
- Modified Rankin Scale ranges from 0 to 6 with increasing level of disability, where 0 to 2 represents functional independence, and a score of 4 to 5 indicates a more severe disability.

---

- Descriptive timing of infarct age can be variable. For the purposes of the chapter, we delineate hyperacute infarcts as less than 6 hours, early acute infarcts as 6 to 24 hours, late acute infarcts as 24 hours to 7 days, subacute infarcts as 1 to 2 weeks, and chronic infarcts as greater than 2 weeks.
- Arterial vessel occlusions can be secondary to thromboembolic phenomenon from vessel disease or from cardiac sources of which there are multiple risk factors.

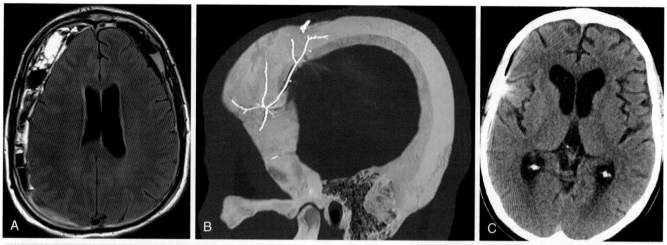

**Fig. 3.9 Middle meningeal artery embolization.** (A) Axial fluid-attenuated inversion recovery (FLAIR) image in an elderly patient shows right greater than left bilateral cerebral convexity complex appearing subdural hematomas with variably aged blood products, septations, and fluid levels suggesting ongoing hemorrhages. The patient had underdone bilateral subdural evacuation procedures in the past to no avail, so this time embolization of the right middle meningeal artery (MMA) was performed, with evidence of embolization material within the right MMA on subsequent computed tomography (CT) brain sagittal maximum intensity projection (MIP) reformat through the right skull (B). Axial CT brain image in soft-tissue windows (C) shows resolution of the right (and also incidentally left) subdural hematomas.

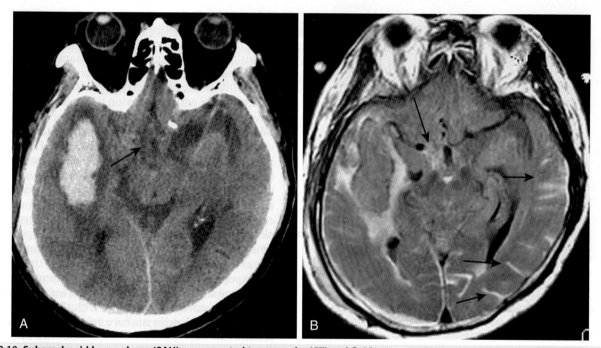

**Fig. 3.10 Subarachnoid hemorrhage (SAH) on computed tomography (CT) and fluid-attenuated inversion recovery (FLAIR) images.** (A) CT scan at the level of the suprasellar cistern reveals acute right sylvian fissure hematoma secondary to rupture of middle cerebral aneurysm. SAH in the suprasellar cistern (*arrow*) and interpeduncular cistern are also present, but less conspicuous compared to the dominant hematoma. (B) FLAIR image on same day reveals hyperintensity in the suprasellar cistern (*long arrow*) and superficial sulci (*short arrows*) indicative of SAH not as readily visible on CT. Hyperacute right sylvian fissure hematoma is isointense.

- Large vessel occlusions (LVOs) affect larger vascular territories reflected by greater neurologic deficits, particularly if the dominant hemisphere is involved. The MCA territory is most commonly involved. Unilateral weakness, aphasia, or gaze preference (toward side of cerebral infarct) are telltale signs of an MCA territory infarct. So hint, hint—get clinical history! Knowing the neurologic deficit can save you from overlooking subtle findings of acute infarct on imaging.

- Noncontrast CT head is often the initial imaging modality for suspected infarction. CT signs of acute infarct include hypodensity of the affected brain parenchyma and loss of gray-white matter differentiation, hyperdense thrombus within a vessel otherwise known as the "hyperdense

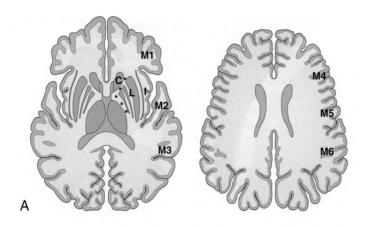

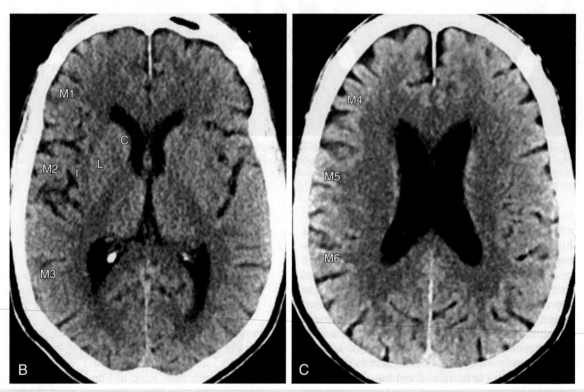

Fig. 3.13 **Alberta Stroke Program Early computed tomography (CT) Score (ASPECTS).** Schematic (A) and anatomic (B and C) axial noncontrast computed tomographic images at the level of the basal ganglia and corona radiata show the specific regions to be assessed for involvement by infarct to provide ASPECTS results. Starting with an initial score of 10, 1 point is deducted if infarct is observed in the following structures: caudate *(C)*, lentiform nucleus *(L)*, internal capsule*, insular cortex *(I)*, frontal operculum *(M1)*, anterior temporal lobe *(M2)*, posterior temporal lobe *(M3)*, anterior middle cerebral artery *(MCA)* territory superior to M1 *(M4)*, lateral MCA territory superior to M2 *(M5)*, posterior MCA territory superior to M3 *(M6)*. A score of less than 7 indicates that the patient is a less than ideal candidate for thrombolytic therapy.

## LACUNAR INFARCTS

- Small vessel occlusions often lead to lacunar infarcts. These tend to affect the centrum semiovale and corona radiata white matter, basal ganglia, internal and external capsules, and pons. Although originally thought to arise from small vessel atherosclerosis and lipohyalinosis associated with hypertension, many other causes have been proposed, including emboli, hypercoagulable states, vasospasm, and small intracerebral hemorrhages.

- By definition, a lacunar infarct measures less than 15 mm in size. Given the smaller nature of these infarcts, they tend to have less prominent neurologic symptoms and better outcomes, although this is also highly dependent on infarct location. Often times, these lesions are small enough to be invisible on conventional noncontrast CT. If visible, acute infarcts can be difficult to distinguish from chronic infarcts.

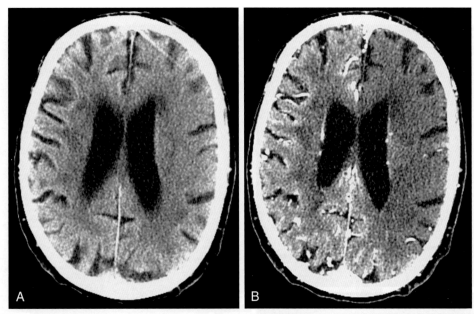

**Fig. 3.14 Computed tomography angiography (CTA) source images in the detection of hyperacute infarction.** (A) Unenhanced scan reveals subtle loss of normal gray matter density in the left middle cerebral artery (MCA) distribution. (B) Source image from CTA reveals obvious relative hypodensity in the left MCA and anterior cerebral artery distributions. Lesion is more conspicuous and extensive than on unenhanced scan because of the markedly diminished vascularity in the affected territory.

■ On MRI, lacunes demonstrate the typical signal characteristics of infarct with elevated diffusion signal, decreased ADC values, and mild edema in the acute phase. Diffusion and ADC appearances evolve in the subacute phase in a manner similar to large vessel occlusions, and enhancement may also be seen on post contrast T1WI in this phase. In the chronic phase, there is resolution of diffusion signal hyperintensity and signs of encephalomalacia (increased T2/FLAIR signal and volume loss).

## CARDIOEMBOLIC INFARCTS

■ Cardioembolic and thromboembolic infarcts from cardiac or vessel sources demonstrate distinct imaging features in that they tend to involve multiple vascular territories or multiple foci within a unilateral vascular distribution as dislodged clot showers the brain (Fig. 3.21). The extracranial carotids are often the source of thromboembolic disease, particularly at the carotid bifurcations. Build-up of atherosclerotic and especially ulcerated or exposed plaque can serve as a breeding ground for emboli (Fig. 3.22).

■ Carotid occlusions, often superimposed on pre-existent stenosis, can also lead to distal emboli. In the setting of systemic hypotension, high-grade carotid stenosis can lead to infarcts in distal watershed distributions (Fig. 3.23). Border zone infarcts occur in the posterior parietal region (between the middle and posterior cerebral artery zones), in the frontal lobes (between the anterior cerebral artery [ACA] and MCA zones), and in the basal ganglia. The major distinguishing feature is the presence of multiple infarcts at the interface between the different vascular territories and evidence of carotid occlusion, stenosis, or slow flow.

■ Interest in the detection and treatment of extracranial carotid artery disease has been heightened by the results of two large trials for the treatment of symptomatic and asymptomatic patients, the North American Symptomatic Carotid Endarterectomy Trial (NASCET) and Asymptomatic Carotid Atherosclerosis Study (ACAS). The NASCET trial demonstrated benefit of endarterectomy in patients with 70% or higher stenosis of the cervical ICA in symptomatic patients, and the ACAS study showed benefit of endarterectomy in patients with more than 60% cervical ICA stenosis in asymptomatic patients. The assessment of the degree of stenosis is complicated by the existence of various methods of measurement. NASCET uses the ratio of the tightest point of carotid stenosis to the "normal lumen" distal to the stenosis (Fig. 3.24), which may underestimate stenosis if the distal lumen narrows as a result of severe proximal stenosis as seen in the "string sign." ACAS and the European-based studies use the degree of stenosis relative to the estimated normal lumen at the same site, which means the observer must extrapolate what is thought to be the true lumen.

## TRANSIENT ISCHEMIC ATTACK

■ Transient ischemic attack (TIA) is a sudden functional neurologic disturbance caused by inadequate blood supply, limited to a vascular territory that usually persists for less than 15 minutes, with complete resolution of symptoms by 24 hours and no associated diffusion restriction on MRI. TIA may be a harbinger for thromboembolic stroke, and assessment for intracranial or extracranial vessel disease in this setting is often indicated, with the goal to treat the cause before the development of a completed cerebral infarct. The TIA work-up typically includes vascular imaging of the head and neck with one stop shop or combination of CTA, MRA, or ultrasound. Perfusion imaging can help confirm presence of at-risk brain tissue.

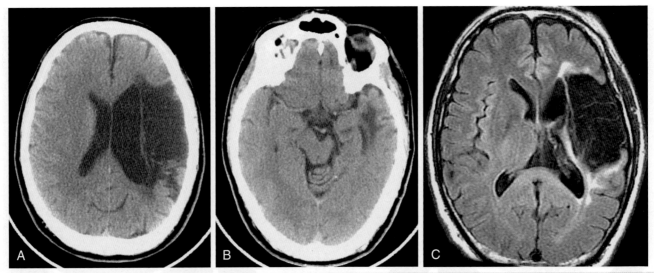

**Fig. 3.20 Chronic infarct computed tomography (CT) and magnetic resonance imaging.** (A) CT scan reveals a large discrete focus of hypodensity in the left frontal lobe. Lesion is more hypodense than acute infarct and it has irregular, somewhat concave margins. There is ex vacuo dilatation of the left lateral ventricle. (B) CT scan at lower level reveals atrophy of the ipsilateral cerebral peduncle (Wallerian degeneration). (C) Fluid-attenuated inversion recovery scan performed 1 day after CT reveals large fluid collection with T2 hyperintense margins indicative of cystic encephalomalacia.

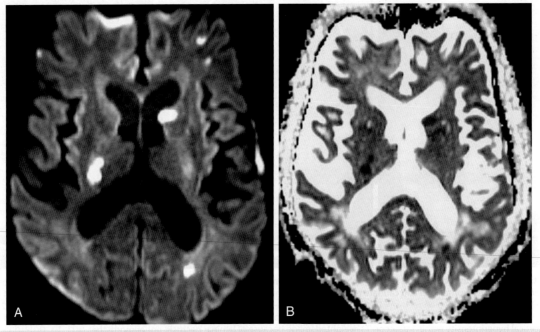

**Fig. 3.21 Embolic infarcts.** (A) Diffusion-weighted imaging shows numerous foci of hyperintensity within both cerebral hemispheres and in multiple vascular territories. Cortical, subcortical, and deep structures are affected. (B) Restriction is confirmed on apparent diffusion coefficient (ADC) maps, indicating that these represent acute infarcts. This distribution raises concern for central embolic (cardiac) source.

can sort out slow or turbulent flow areas that mimic sinus thrombosis and/or sinus stenosis.

■ Arachnoid granulations can also mimic a filling defect but fortunately have characteristic increased T2 signal on the conventional MR sequences that distinguish them from acute clots.

■ Chronically occluded sinuses tend to be smaller, often with partial recanalization and development of venous collaterals.

■ Concomitant findings can include subcortical hemorrhage near the thrombosed sinus, subarachnoid hemorrhage and subdural hemorrhage, and focal leptomeningeal enhancement that reflects venous congestion. Treatment

is primarily anticoagulation, although endovascular treatment to extract clot may also be considered.

## GLOBAL ANOXIC/HYPOXIC ISCHEMIC INJURY

■ Anoxic injuries occur when there is near complete absence of oxygen in the blood for more than 5 minutes, while hypoxia occurs when there is a partial but more prolonged decreased oxygenation. Anoxic injuries can be seen in the setting of cardiac arrest, prolonged seizure, strangulation/hanging, near drowning, and smoke/carbon monoxide inhalation. The metabolically active areas of the brain are most severely affected, including the basal ganglia and

Ammon's horns (dentate nucleus and hippocampus) in the adult population (Fig. 3.27).

- CT initially will be normal, but there is subsequent development of diffuse cerebral edema with generalized loss of definition of the gray-white interface within 12 hours.
- MRI can demonstrate abnormalities much earlier (3 hours) as cytotoxic edema and cell death set in, resulting in DWI hyperintensity and restriction on ADC maps. With prolonged hypoxia, the basal ganglia and

hippocampi are relatively spared. MRI reveals T2 and restricted diffusion at the gray-white junction bilaterally.

- In severe cases, anoxia and/or hypoxia progress to the point of diffuse edema with sulcal and cisternal effacement demonstrable on CT and MRI. The increased intracranial pressure produces transtentorial and tonsillar herniation with complete cessation of cerebral blood flow (brain death). On CT, the brain is diffusely hypodense with no gray-white matter differentiation, and the ventricles and cisterns are effaced. The surrounding vessels may actually seem hyperdense relative to the low-density brain parenchyma and may be mistaken for subarachnoid or subdural hemorrhage (pseudosubarachnoid

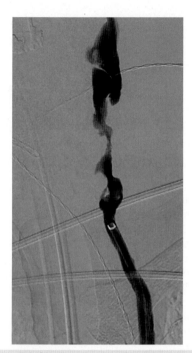

**Fig. 3.22 Ulcerated plaque.** Conventional common carotid angiogram in the lateral projection showing markedly ulcerated plaque within the distal left common carotid artery resulting in critical stenosis. The patient presented with embolic left middle cerebral artery (MCA) infarct, and it is very likely this nasty plaque was the source of the thrombus.

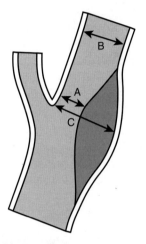

NASCET % stenosis = 100 [B–A] / B
ECST % stenosis = 100 [C–A] / C

**Fig. 3.24 Drawing of North American Symptomatic Carotid Endarterectomy Trial (NASCET) and European Carotid Surgery Trial (ECST) criteria for evaluation of carotid stenosis.** (A) The diameter of the residual lumen at the point of maximal stenosis. (B) The diameter of the normal artery distal to the stenosis. (C) The estimated "true" lumen at the point of stenosis. (Courtesy P. Kim Nelson, MD.)

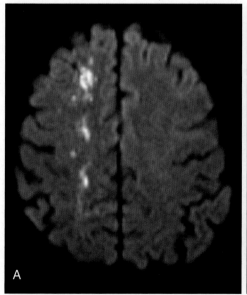
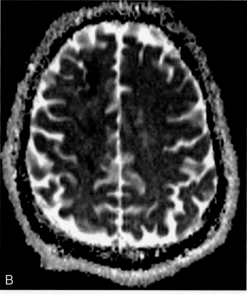

**Fig. 3.23 Border zone (watershed) infarcts.** (A) Diffusion-weighted image and (B) ADC map show diffusion restricting foci at the right middle cerebral artery–anterior cerebral artery border.

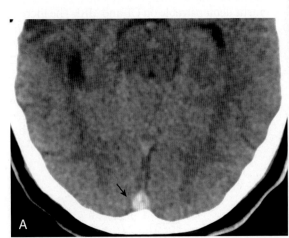
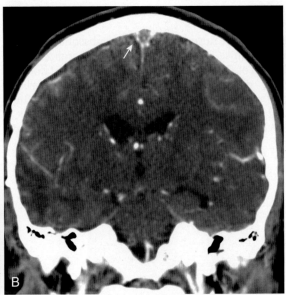

**Fig. 3.25 Venous sinus thrombosis on computed tomography (CT).** (A) Axial unenhanced CT showed hyperattenuation within the expanded sigmoid sinus *(arrow)*. (B) After contrast administration for venogram study, the same clot appears relatively hypodense *(arrow)* on coronal reformatted CT because of adjacent hyperattenuating contrast material and parenchymal contrast enhancement ("empty delta sign").

hemorrhage) (Fig. 3.28). The cerebellum in this setting can also be strikingly conspicuous because it is normal in density as opposed to the low-density remainder of the brain (i.e., the dense cerebellar sign).

## VASCULAR MALFORMATIONS

- **Cerebral aneurysms** represent abnormal focal dilatations of an artery that may be associated with numerous clinical syndromes and conditions. The most common type of intracranial aneurysm is the saccular or "berry" aneurysm, which reflects an outpouching from a parent vessel, usually at a vessel branch point (Fig. 3.29). They can occur because of damage to the endothelium, thinning of tunica media, and fragmentation of the internal elastica secondary to shear forces on the vessel wall, magnified at vessel branch points.

**TEACHING POINTS**

Disorders Associated With Intracranial Aneurysms

Alkaptonuria
Anderson-Fabry disease
Autosomal dominant polycystic kidney disease
Behçet disease
Coarctation of the aorta
Collagen vascular disease
Ehlers-Danlos syndrome type IV
Familial idiopathic nonarteriosclerotic cerebral
    calcification syndrome
Fibromuscular dysplasia
Hereditary hemorrhagic telangiectasia
Homocystinuria
Marfan syndrome
Moyamoya disease
Neurofibromatosis type I

Noonan syndrome
Pseudoxanthoma elasticum
Sickle cell disease
Systemic lupus erythematosus
Takayasu disease
Tuberous sclerosis
Wermer syndrome
α-Glucosidase deficiency
α1-Antitrypsin deficiency
3 M syndrome

- Given the proposed etiology of shear forces on the vessel wall contributing to weakness points, it is not surprising that we do not see saccular aneurysms arise in children or young adults unless there is a predisposing factor. Such predisposing factors include fibromuscular dysplasia, polycystic kidney disease, or collagen disorders, such as Marfan syndrome or Loeys-Dietz syndrome.
- A fusiform aneurysm is a diffuse long-segment enlargement of a vessel. These are most often the result of severe atherosclerosis but may also be seen in traumatic and spontaneous arterial dissection or in association with vasculopathies and congenital conditions, including collagen disorders, HIV infections, or neurofibromatosis type I.
- Septic emboli lead to the development of mycotic aneurysms, which involve distal vessels, most commonly in the MCA distribution and M2 and M3 segments. These tend to bleed into the parenchyma with or without subarachnoid space blood.
- On noncontrast CT imaging, SAH is the typical finding associated with a ruptured aneurysm, with patients presenting with the "worst headache of their life." The pattern of SAH will typically be a good indicator for the site of potential aneurysm. For

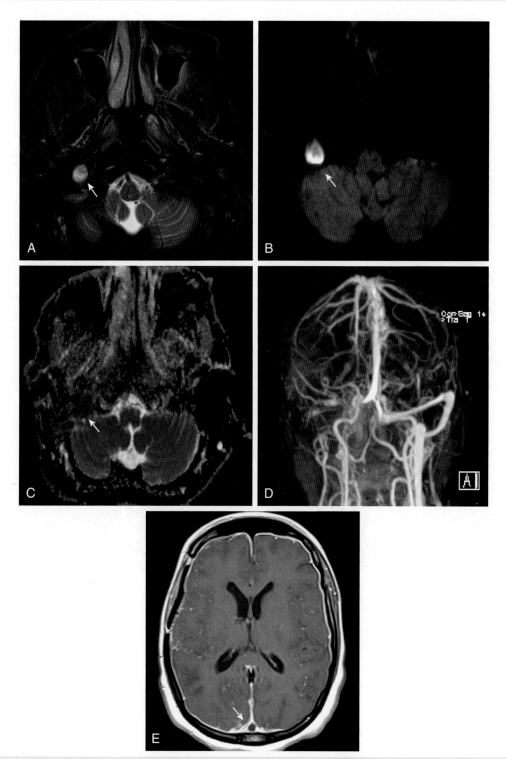

**Fig. 3.26 Venous sinus thrombosis on magnetic resonance imaging (MRI).** (A) Axial T2-weighted image (T2WI) shows abnormally hyperintense T2 signal in the right jugular vein *(arrow)*. (B) Diffusion-weighted imaging and (C) apparent diffusion coefficient (ADC) maps show diffusion restriction in this same location *(arrows)*. (D) Contrast-enhanced magnetic resonance venogram shows absence of opacification within the right transverse and sigmoid sinuses, as well as the right jugular vein, indicating occlusive venous sinus thrombosis. (E) Contrast-enhanced T1-weighted image (T1WI) in a different patient shows the MRI correlate of the "empty delta sign" indicating thrombosis *(arrow)*.

instance, a ruptured anterior communicating artery (ACoA) aneurysm will produce SAH centered in the suprasellar cistern, anterior interhemispheric fissure, and cistern of the lamina terminalis (Fig. 3.30). Posterior communicating artery (PCoA)/anterior choroidal and carotid terminus aneurysms will produce hemorrhage centered in the suprasellar cistern,

ipsilateral sylvian fissure, and anterior perimesencephalic cistern. MCA aneurysms (most common at the M2 bifurcation) produce hemorrhage more localized at the ipsilateral sylvian fissure. Basilar tip aneurysms produce hemorrhage in the interpeduncular and surrounding perimesencephalic and suprasellar cisterns. Presence of isolated intraventricular

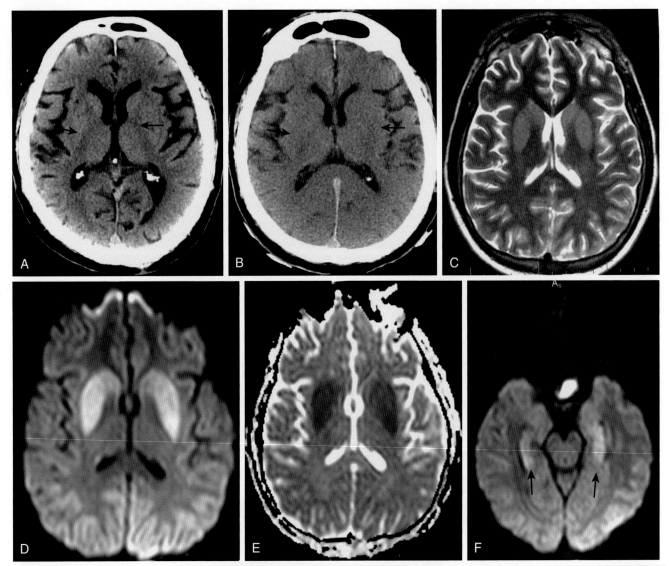

**Fig. 3.27  Anoxic injury.** (A) Computed tomography (CT) scan obtained 8 hours after cardiac arrest reveals normal density of basal ganglia, thalamus, and cortex with good visualization of the normal hypodense internal capsules *(arrows)*. (B) Repeat examination at 36 hours reveals hypodensity in the basal ganglia and thalami (note inability to identify the internal capsule, *arrows*). Diffuse brain edema is present with early loss of gray matter density and some sulcal effacement. (C–F) Magnetic resonance (MR) scan at 6 hours in a different patient. CT scan 1 hour before MR was normal. Mild T2 hyperintensity (C) is present in the basal ganglia bilaterally. Diffusion-weighted image (DWI) hyperintensity (D) and restriction on ADC (E) is present. Hippocampal DWI hyperintensity is also present *(arrows)* (F).

hemorrhage within the fourth ventricle should raise suspicion for a posterior inferior cerebellar artery (PICA) aneurysm.

- CTA imaging should follow and allows for angiographic delineation of the aneurysm, as well as mapping of the neck and intracranial vasculature for intervention. Treatment options include minimally invasive endovascular therapies of embolization and/or stenting versus surgical craniotomy and vascular clipping. Clinical factors may influence surgical candidacy, and aneurysm features such as size and location may also dictate the feasibility of treatment options. Large size, complex morphology (wide neck, multilobed, irregular), peripheral, and MCA aneurysms are often treated surgically so these aneurysm characteristics should be included in the imaging report.

**TEACHING POINTS**

Descriptive Aneurysm Features

- Size including maximum diameter and width
- Aneurysm neck morphology—narrow or broad-based
- Shape and contour—multilobed or irregular
- Associated thrombus or calcification
- Wall thickness
- Relationship to adjacent vessels
- Anatomic variations
- Additional aneurysms

- Vasospasm of the adjacent vessels can also be seen as a complication of SAH occurring within a few days after the bleed and may require medical intervention to maintain blood pressures. In the case of vasospasm contributing to neurologic deficit or stroke, endovascular interventions with intra-arterial calcium channel blockers, angioplasty, or possibly stenting may be needed. CTA can be performed in conjunction with CT perfusion to assess for vasospasm and perfusions deficits, to guide treatment (Fig. 3.31).

▪ It is important to assess treated aneurysms for regrowth. Artifact from the aneurysm clips or coils can limit assessment for residual aneurysm filling on CTA or MRA. Catheter angiography is performed when aneurysm regrowth is suspected. Small (<3 mm) unruptured aneurysms, particularly those that are extradural, can be expectantly managed with serial angiographic imaging.

▪ SAH without detectable aneurysm on initial angiographic imaging (approximately 10% of cases) commonly requires a short interval repeat angiographic study (typically cerebral angiogram) at 1 week and often subsequently again at 1 month to evaluate the possibility of an occult vascular lesion.

   ▪ An exception to this is benign perimesencephalic nonaneurysmal subarachnoid (Fig. 3.32). In the presence of a negative CTA, the following imaging criteria for nonaneurysmal perimesencephalic SAH can negate the need for DSA: (1) SAH located in the perimesencephalic cisterns anterior to midbrain; (2) SAH extension into the medial sylvian fissure and proximal anterior interhemispheric fissures but not lateral sylvian or distal interhemispheric fissures; (3) layering intraventricular extension without direct dissection of hemorrhage through brain tissue into the ventricles; and, (4) no intraparenchymal hemorrhage.

   ▪ Imaging of the spine can also be performed if a spinal vascular anomaly (AVM or AVF) is a suspected source of the SAH.

▪ Some vessels, in particular the posterior communicating arteries, may have a somewhat dilated origin mimicking an aneurysm, but, in fact, represent an infundibulum, or focal prominence at the vessel origin. These are typically less than 2 mm in size, conical in shape, and have the branch vessel exiting from its apex (Fig. 3.33).

▪ A **dissection** is a tear and weakening in the wall of the blood vessel that allows for blood to enter into and separate the inner (tunica intima), medial (tunica media), or outer (adventitia) walls of the blood vessel. Dissections can be seen in the setting of trauma or in patients with underlying vascular predispositions.

   ▪ Angiographic imaging shows abrupt tapered narrowing of the vessel that may be distally occluded (see Fig. 3.1A). This is a prothrombotic situation so it is important to look beyond the affected segment for distal thrombi. A tear in the vessel wall that leads to an outpouching with collection of blood between the intima and media reflects a dissecting aneurysm.

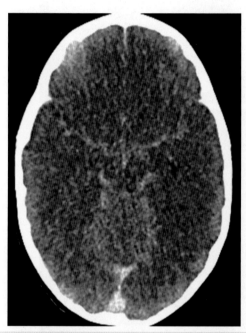

**Fig. 3.28 Pseudosubarachnoid hemorrhage.** Diffuse cerebral edema and global parenchymal hypoattenuation along with cisternal effacement results in increased conspicuity of the vessels in the subarachnoid space, mimicking the appearance of subarachnoid hemorrhage.

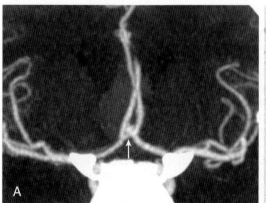
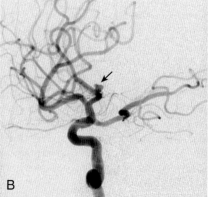
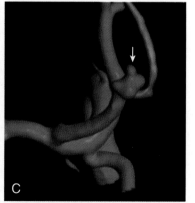

**Fig. 3.29 Aneurysm work-up.** (A) Coronal maximum intensity projection from computed tomography angiography examination in this patient presenting with diffuse subarachnoid hemorrhage shows a lobulated aneurysm arising from the anterior communicating artery complex *(arrow)*. (B) Conventional catheter angiogram redemonstrates the aneurysm to better advantage *(arrow)*, with (C) rotational three-dimensional reconstructed images better depicting the lobulated morphology of the aneurysm *(arrow)*.

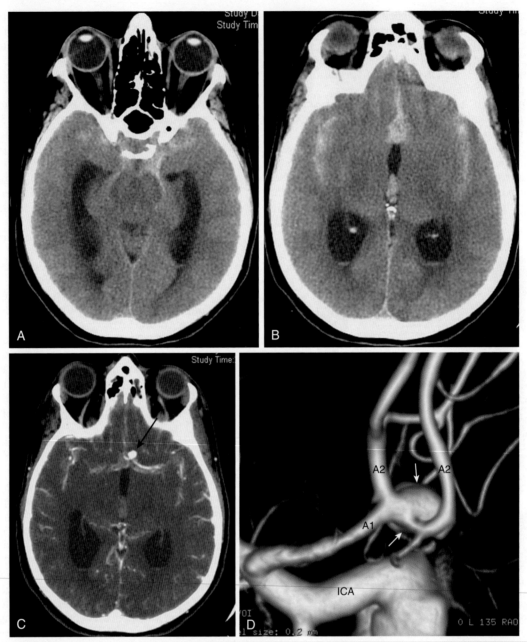

**Fig. 3.30 Aneurysmal subarachnoid hemorrhage.** (A–B) Computed tomography (CT) scans at the level of the suprasellar cistern and inferior third ventricle reveal diffuse hyperdensity in the suprasellar cistern, sylvian fissures, and anterior interhemispheric fissure. Intraventricular hemorrhage and hydrocephalus are present. (C) CT angiography source image reveals left-sided anterior communicating aneurysm *(arrow)*. (D) Three-dimensional reconstruction from catheter angiogram reveals relationship between aneurysm neck *(arrows)* and adjacent *A1* and *A2* segments of the anterior cerebral artery and anterior communicating artery. *ICA*, Internal carotid artery.

When the tear goes through the inner two layers and the outpouching of blood is only contained by the adventitia and surrounding soft tissues, this reflects a dissecting pseudoaneurysm or false aneurysm. Discerning between these two types of aneurysms can be difficult on conventional noninvasive angiographic imaging.

■ These injuries may require antiplatelet agents, anticoagulation, or stenting/embolization, depending on the location of the insult and risk of vessel rupture. Once treated, it is reasonable to expect follow-up imaging; some of these injuries have happy endings with improved vessel patency, but other times the injury can progress to frank vessel occlusion.

■ **Capillary telangiectasias** are slow-flow capillary malformations found most commonly as a solitary lesion within the pons, although they can be seen in other regions of the brain or as multiple lesions when associated with congenital disorders such as hereditary hemorrhagic telangiectasia (HHT) or ataxia telangiectasia or when radiation is induced. They can vary in size but average about 3 mm in diameter.

■ These lesions are typically occult on noncontrast CT and conventional angiography. On MRI, capillary telangiectasias are appreciated as lesions with faint

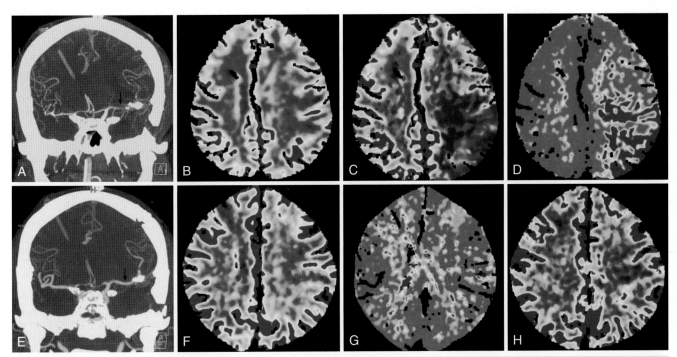

**Fig. 3.31 Postsubarachnoid hemorrhage vasospasm.** (A) Coronal maximum intensity projection (MIP) reconstruction from computed tomography angiography (CTA) performed on patient with treated left middle cerebral artery (MCA) aneurysm shows severe narrowing with beaded appearance of the left M1 segment *(arrow)*, indicating vasospasm. (B) Symmetric appearance of cerebral blood volume (CBV) map from computed tomography perfusion study suggests that there is no infarcted tissue. However, cerebral blood flow (CBF) map and mean transit time (MTT) maps (C, D, respectively) show at-risk brain tissue in the left MCA distribution. (E) After medical therapy, coronal MIP reconstruction from repeat CTA shows improved patency of the left M1 segment *(arrow)*. Not surprisingly, the CBV, MTT, and CBF maps (F, G, H, respectively) show no asymmetries, indicating restored perfusion to this region.

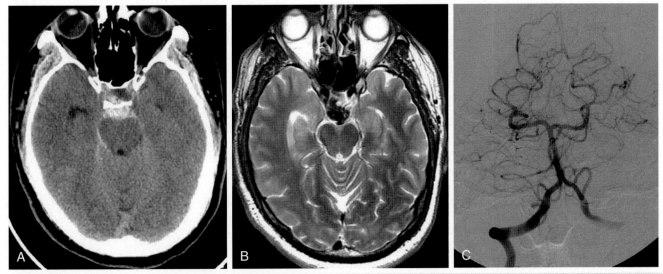

**Fig. 3.32 Perimesencephalic subarachnoid hemorrhage.** (A) Computed tomography scan reveals focal subarachnoid clot posterior to the clivus anterior to the brain stem. (B) T2-weighted image reveals acute hypointense clot in the interpeduncular cistern. (C) Right vertebral artery anterior posterior view from catheter angiogram is normal. There is no evidence of posterior circulation aneurysm.

stippled enhancement, associated decreased signal on SWI or GRE imaging (because of vessel stasis with deoxyhemoglobin and not hemorrhage), and with normal to increased T2/FLAIR signal. They are clinically asymptomatic and often an incidental, serially stable MRI finding.

■ **Cerebral cavernous malformations** are grouped under the International Society for the Study of Vascular Anomalies system into slow-flow venous malformations. It has been argued to eliminate the use of cavernous hemangioma or cavernoma to describe these lesions because they are not neoplastic. They are composed of dilated thin-walled capillaries with surrounding hemosiderin and no intervening normal brain tissue.

■ There are varying degrees of thrombosis and calcification within the lesion, which can be identified on CT imaging as hyperdensity or frank calcification. In

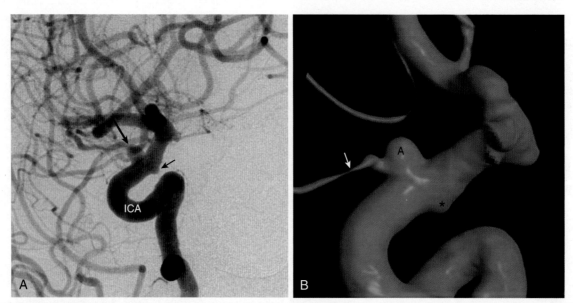

**Fig. 3.33 Conventional angiogram in the work-up of aneurysm.** (A) After suspicion for aneurysm on time-of-flight magnetic resonance angiography head (not shown), selective internal carotid artery (ICA) injection in the lateral projection shows the ICA, a small outpouching along the posterior aspect of the ICA reflecting infundibular origin of the posterior communicating artery *(small arrow)*, and an aneurysm arising from the paraophthalmic segment of the ICA *(large arrow)*. (B) Three-dimensional reconstruction from rotational angiogram beautifully depicts the aneurysm (A), with the ophthalmic artery *(arrow)* arising from the base of the aneurysm, which will add complexity to the patient's treatment options. Infundibular origin of the posterior communicating artery is indicated by an *asterisk*.

the absence of edema and mass effect on CT, recent hemorrhage is less likely.

- On MRI, areas of internal thrombosis of the lesion leads to the characteristic "popcorn" appearance with mixed hyper-/hypointensity on T2WI and intrinsic T1 shortening, and with surrounding rim of peripheral hemosiderin staining (Fig. 3.34). Absence of enhancement is common, although mild enhancement of the lesion is possible. The presence of new deoxyhemoglobin and/or surrounding edema are suggestive of recent hemorrhage. Similar to capillary telangiectasias, these lesions are also angiographically occult.
- Developmental venous anomalies are often not too far in location from a cavernous malformation and can provide a good diagnostic clue to look for these lesions.
- Multiple cavernous malformations can be seen in the setting of familial multiple cavernous malformation syndrome or in the years following brain radiation.
- **Developmental venous anomaly** (DVA, venous angioma) is a slow-flow venous malformation that consists of a network of dilated medullary veins converging in a radial fashion to a larger vein that drains into either deep or superficial veins. This radial converging pattern gives rise to the "caput medusa" appearance (see Fig. 3.34D) on postcontrast CT or MRI. In the absence of postcontrast imaging, these lesions can also be identified as linear-branched signal abnormalities on SWI or GRE MRI.
  - These lesions are now recognized to be the most common cerebral vascular malformations, accounting for 55% of these lesions. DVAs are most commonly incidental findings and asymptomatic clinically. Rarely, hemorrhage occurs in conjunction with a cavernous malformation.
  - These lesions drain normal brain parenchyma, and thus surgical resection or rarely idiopathic thrombosis can lead to venous hypertension and possibly infarct

and hemorrhage in the parenchyma drained by the DVA. They are the classic "leave me alone lesion." The absence of an accompanying vascular nidus and arterial component distinguishes them from draining veins of a true AVM.

- **AVMs** are characterized by an abnormal growth of vessels (i.e., a nidus) that allows for abnormal arterial to venous connections and shunting of blood. These are one of the causes of spontaneous parenchymal hemorrhage in adults (20–50 years of age). There is a 2% to 3% annual risk of hemorrhage of an untreated AVM because of rupture of a feeding vessel, intranidal aneurysm, or (rarely) venous thrombosis.
  - Risk of surgical resectability can be graded by the Spetzler-Martin criteria, which focuses on lesion size,

**TEACHING POINTS**

Spetzler-Martin Arteriovenous Malformation Classification

| Feature | Score |
| --- | --- |
| **Size** | |
| <3 cm | 1 |
| 3–6 cm | 2 |
| >6 cm | 3 |
| **Eloquent brain involvement** | |
| No | 0 |
| Yes | 1 |
| **Venous drainage** | |
| Superficial only | 0 |
| Any deep | 1 |

(From Spetzler RF, Martin NA. A proposed grading system for arteriovenous malformations. *J Neurosurg.* 1986;65:476–483.)

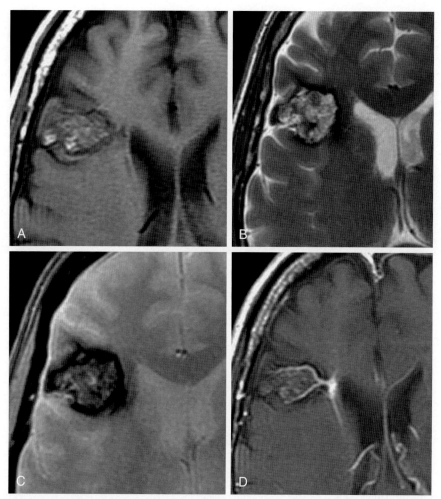

**Fig. 3.34 Cavernous malformation and developmental venous anomaly (DVA).** (A) T1-weighted image (T1WI) reveals a mixed-intensity lesion with small foci of hyperintensity and mild peripheral hypointensity. (B) T2-weighted image (T2WI) reveals a peripheral hypointense margin with central foci of both hypointensity and hyperintensity. (C) Gradient-echo scan reveals marked peripheral hypointensity that extends into and "stains" the adjacent parenchyma. (D) Enhanced T1WI reveals linear enhancing DVA that surrounds the cavernous malformation and drains into the subependymal venous system.

location, and drainage pattern to prognosticate surgical outcome.

- On CT, dilated vessels (mostly draining veins) associated with the lesions are mildly hyperdense, have a serpentine configuration, and may demonstrate scattered calcifications. Surrounding hypodensity and mass effect may indicate edema in the setting of acute hemorrhage. Surrounding hypodensity and volume loss more likely indicates encephalomalacia because of vascular shunting (i.e., parenchymal steal phenomenon) or the residua from a prior bleed.
- Conventional MRI tends to show a low T2 signal abnormal cluster of vessels, reflecting prominent "flow voids." This tangle of vessels will have correlating susceptibility on SWI/GRE imaging and enhancement on postcontrast imaging.
- Dedicated cerebral angiographic imaging or multiphase dynamic imaging with CTA and/or MRA is essential to document the arterial contributions to the nidus and the venous drainage (Fig. 3.35). Care should be made to identify and describe any intranidal

aneurysms, which are typically venous in nature, because of arterialized pressure within draining veins.

- **Dural AVFs (dAVFs)** are usually acquired lesions that are the consequence of dural sinus thrombosis with subsequent recanalization of the sinus resulting in direct communication between the small dilated arteries in the sinus wall and the sinus lumen. The direct communication results in high pressure within the sinus and can result in venous hypertension with impaired venous outflow of the brain parenchyma drained by the sinus. These are commonly idiopathic, but other causes include trauma or previous surgery. Inherited prothrombotic conditions (i.e., protein C and S, and antithrombin deficiencies) have also been associated with the development of dAVFs. Symptoms depend on the location, size of the malformation, and venous drainage pattern.
- Resultant complications include parenchymal hemorrhage, SAH, and venous infarct. Increased risk of neurologic deficit is associated with dural fistulas that (1) drain the deep venous system, (2) have associated retrograde venous flow, (3) have venous aneurysms,

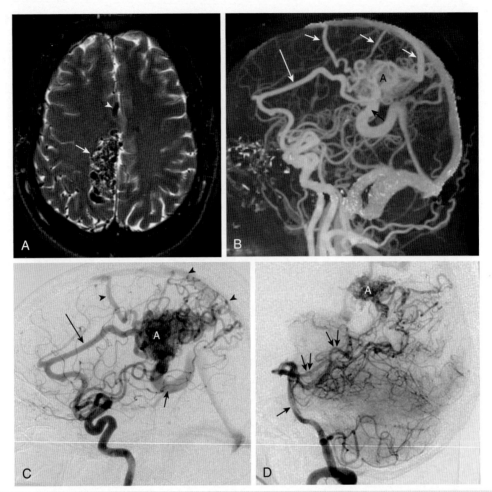

**Fig. 3.35 Arteriovenous malformation (AVM).** (A) Axial T2-weighted image shows large tangle of vessels *(arrow)* representing the nidus of an arteriovenous malformation in the right parietal lobe. Large caliber vessels are seen around the AVM *(arrowhead)*, which may reflect arterial supply or venous drainage for this lesion. (B) Three-dimensional maximum intensity projection reconstruction from subsequently performed computed tomography angiography (CTA) head shows the nidus (A). The major arterial supply from an enlarged pericallosal artery *(white arrow)* and both superficial *(small white arrows)* and deep *(black arrow)* venous drainage are depicted. (C) Selective internal carotid artery injection from conventional catheter angiogram in the lateral projection again shows arterial supply from an enlarged pericallosal artery *(large arrow)* to the AVM nidus (A), with both early superficial *(arrowheads)* and deep *(small arrow)* venous drainage. (D) The superiority of conventional angiography over techniques in diagnosing AVMs is shown with this selective vertebral artery injection in the lateral projection. The posterior aspect of the AVM nidus (A) is also supplied by bilateral posterior cerebral arteries *(double arrows)*, which was not appreciated on magnetic resonance or CTA. Basilar artery is indicated by *single arrow*.

(4) have stenotic channels through which they must drain, and (5) are complex.

■ Catheter angiography is the key for diagnosis. The initial internal carotid or vertebral artery injections may be unrevealing; however, selective injection of the external carotid arteries (ECAs) can demonstrate the dilated meningeal arteries, the site of the fistulae, and delayed filling of cortical veins. Dural malformations can be treated by embolization (arterial and/or venous) or stenting procedures to restore flow in previously thrombosed sinuses.

■ One special type of fistula to consider is the cavernous-carotid fistula (CCF), which can present acutely (in the trauma setting) with chemosis, and pulsatile exophthalmos or subacutely with progressive visual loss, subconjunctival hemorrhage, as a result of pathologic communication between the cavernous ICA and the adjacent cavernous sinus. There

are several proposed classification systems, but the bottom line is that there will be either direct connection between the cavernous ICA and sinus, or indirect connection between cavernous ICA and/or ECA branches with the sinus. Angiographic imaging of carotid-cavernous fistulas reveals enlargement of the cavernous sinus and superior (and inferior) ophthalmic vein (Fig. 3.36), with attenuation similar to the arterial vascular structures. Conventional CT or MRI may also show associated stranding of the intraorbital fat, enlargement of the extraocular muscles, and proptosis.

■ Fistulae arising from the sigmoid sinus can present with tinnitus and bruit over the temporal bone. Transverse sinus and superior sagittal sinus fistulae may present with parenchymal hemorrhage and increased intracranial pressure associated with sinus stenosis—this can be seen with pseudotumor cerebri

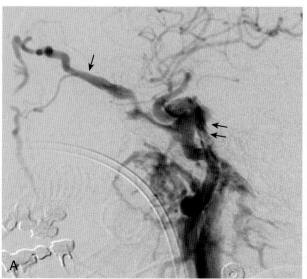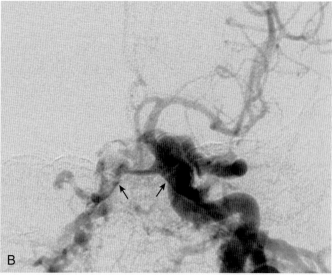

**Fig. 3.36 Cavernous carotid fistula.** (A) Lateral projection from conventional catheter angiogram with left internal carotid artery (ICA) injection shows abnormal opacification and enlargement of the superior ophthalmic vein *(single arrow)* and abnormal enhancement of the cavernous sinus *(double arrows)*, petrosal sinuses, and jugular vein in the arterial phase because of the presence of a cavernous-carotid fistula. (B) Frontal projection from left ICA injection shows similar early enhancement of major inferior venous sinuses, including bilateral cavernous sinuses *(arrows)*, which communicate at the midline. This fistulous connection was subsequently coiled.

(i.e., idiopathic intracranial hypertension). These fistulae may be difficult to diagnosis, but conventional and angiographic imaging may reveal prominent, dilated vessels in the region of the malformation and adjacent sinus stenosis or occlusion.

■ "Vein of Galen" aneurysmal malformations (VGAMs), more appropriately termed *median prosencephalic arteriovenous fistulas*, have a higher prevalence in the pediatric population, accounting for approximately 30% of vascular malformations in this age group. At 6 to 11 weeks of gestation, the median prosencephalic vein (MPV), a precursor to the Vein of Galen, forms a fistula and fails to regress. The MPV becomes aneurysmal and drains into the straight sinus or a persistent falcine sinus, and subsequently into the transverse/sigmoid sinuses. A true VGAM has no nidus, and the Vein of Galen does not form. Affected neonates most commonly present with high output cardiac failure. Rapid shunting across the lesion can limit CT delineation of the malformation with contrast. MRA represents an alternative cross-sectional method of delineation. The dilated feeding and draining vessels also appear as prominent flow voids on conventional T2 MRI sequences. Venous and arterial embolization is the mainstay of therapy.

## OTHER VASCULOPATHIES

■ *Vasculopathy* is an umbrella term that encompasses any pathology that affects the blood vessel.
■ *Vasculitis* is a more specific term used when the vessel wall disease has an inflammatory component. Causes of vascular injury may be intrinsic to the vessel wall on an immunologic basis, such as in the setting of endothelial

damage and thrombosis produced by circulating antigen-antibody complexes and inflammatory cells. In other cases, the insult may be extravascular (e.g., brain parenchyma or leptomeninges resulting in compression of the vessel leading to spasm and mural inflammation). Many of the vasculopathies are part of a systemic process, and therefore laboratory, clinical, and imaging evidence of other organ involvement provide clues as to the correct diagnosis.

■ CTA and MRA are noninvasive angiographic techniques that have evolved, with comparable sensitivity and specificity to catheter angiography in detecting vessel wall abnormalities. The integration of specialized black-blood and postcontrast MRI/MRA has further enhanced the sensitivity of detection of thickening and enhancement of vessels in the setting of vasculitis or at-risk plaque.

■ Evaluation of the secondary and tertiary intracranial branches may be limited, however, with these modalities, and catheter angiography remains the imaging "gold standard" for detection and characterization of vasculopathy.

■ In cases where the angiographic studies are normal or nonspecific and the clinical and laboratory findings do not yield a definitive diagnosis, brain/meningeal biopsy may be the final diagnostic option.

■ Broadly, the vasculopathies can be said to affect: (1) extracranial arteries, (2) arteries at the skull base at or near the circle of Willis, (3) secondary and tertiary branches of the carotid and/or basilar arteries (e.g., sylvian and convexity branches of the middle cerebral artery), and (4) small perforating arteries (e.g. lenticulostriate arteries). The following section is a summary of this topic.

## TEACHING POINTS

Vasculopathy: Clinical and Imaging Features

| Disease | Age (years) | Sex | Etiology | Special Features |
|---|---|---|---|---|
| **Extracranial** | | | | |
| Fibromuscular dysplasia | >50 | F > M | Unknown | Extracranial internal carotid artery (C2) and vertebral arteries; multiple vessels |
| Giant cell arteritis | 70 | F > M | Associated with polymyalgia rheumatica | Extracranial vessels in particular superficial temporal artery |
| **Skull Base—Circle of Willis** | | | | |
| Moyamoya disease | 10–30 | M = F | q25.3, on chromosome 17 | Childhood and adult variants |
| Sickle cell disease | 10–20 | M = F | Sickle cell | More common in children; transfusions reduce risk; may mimic moyamoya disease |
| Basal meningitis | 5–15 | M = F | Tuberculosis and fungal disease, among other infectious agents | Also affects basilar artery; deep collaterals less common |
| Cocaine abuse | 20–40 | M = F | Chronic vasospasm leads to fibrosis | Rare |
| **Secondary and Tertiary Vessels** | | | | |
| *Inflammatory Granulomatous* | | | | |
| (1) Primary angiitis of the central nervous system (PACNS) | 50 | F = M | Autoimmune | Brain involvement can coexist |
| (2) Polyarteritis nodosum | 30–50 | M > F | Autoimmune | |
| (3) Granulomatosis with polyangiitis | 20–60 | M > F | Unknown | |
| (4) Sarcoidosis | 20–40 | F > M | Unknown | |
| (5) Behçet disease | 20–30 | M > F | Autoimmune—HLA-B51? | |
| *Infectious* | | | | |
| (1) Herpes zoster | >50 | F = M | Spread along fifth nerve from facial zoster infection | Often immune compromised (e.g., HIV) |
| (2) Tuberculosis and fungal | 20–40 | M = F | Often in association with basal meningeal disease | |
| (3) Neurosyphilis | >50 | M > F | Late tertiary phase of disease | |
| *Noninflammatory* | | | | |
| (1) Drug-related | 20–50 | M > F | Vasospasm and mural edema; inflammation late, vaso-spasm edema, eclampsia | Acute hypertension may produce PRES |
| (2) Pregnancy, puerperium, birth control pills | 20–40 | F (duh) | | Cocaine, amphetamines, sympathomimetic amines (e.g., Ephedrine) |
| Lymphomatoid Granulomatosis | >50 | M > F | Epstein Barr–induced lymphoma | |
| **Small Vessel** | | | | |
| *Collagen Vascular Diseases* | | | | |
| (1) Systemic lupus erythematosus (SLE) | 20–50 | F > M | Autoimmune | Relative sparing of periventricular white matter |
| (2) Anticardiolipin and antiphospho-lipid antibody syndrome | 20–50 | F > M | With or without SLE | Cortical infarcts because of emboli (Libman-Sacks endocarditis) |
| (3) Sjögren syndrome | 40–60 | F > M | Autoimmune | |
| (4) Radiation change | Any | M = F | Fibrinoid necrosis | Confluent white matter disease; months to years after treatment; focal mass like lesions less common |
| (5) Migraine headache | 20–50 | F > M | Vasospasm | Few lesions, subcortical frontal lobes |
| (6) HIV encephalitis | <15 | M = F | Inflammatory vasculitis | Deep gray; basal ganglia calcification in children |
| (7) Susac syndrome | 20–40 | F > M | Idiopathic | Corpus callosum involvement frequent; lesions smaller than in MS; microinfarcts in cortex |
| Cerebral Autosomal Dominant Arteriopathy with Subcortical Infarcts and Leukoencephalopathy (CADASIL) | 30–50 | M = F | NOTCH 3 gene on chromosome 19 | Predilection for the anterior frontal and temporal lobes |

*HIV,* Human immunodeficiency virus; *MS,* multiple sclerosis; *PRES,* posterior reversible encephalopathy syndrome.

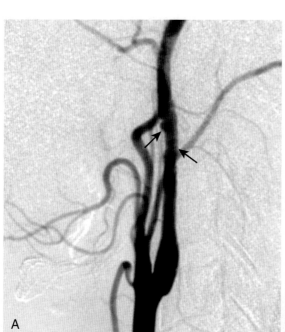 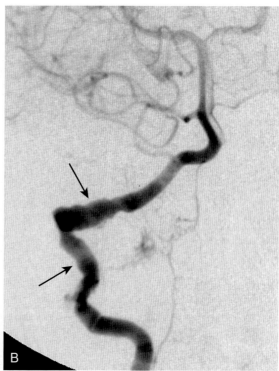

**Fig. 3.37 Fibromuscular disease.** "String of beads" appearance of both the internal carotid (A) and vertebral (B) arteries on conventional catheter angiogram. Abnormal segments are indicated with *arrows*. (Courtesy Philippe Gailloud, MD.)

## EXTRACRANIAL AND EXTRADURAL ARTERIES

■ **Fibromuscular dysplasia (FMD)** is a nonatheromatous fibrous and muscular thickening alternating with dilatation of the arterial wall of unknown etiology. FMD most commonly affects the renal arteries at a prevalence of 4% to 6%, and next most commonly the cervicoencephalic arteries at a prevalence of 0.3% to 3%. The condition has a marked female predominance (4:1) with a mean age of 50 years. Symptoms and findings such as headache, TIAs, stroke, vascular dissection, or subarachnoid hemorrhage have been reported. There may also be systemic vessel involvement, most commonly of the renal arteries.

   ▪ The classic angiographic appearance is characterized as a "string of beads" in type 1 FMD (Fig. 3.37). Less common appearances include unifocal or multifocal tubular stenosis (type 2) or lesions confined to only a portion of the arterial wall (type 3). Although all layers of the artery may be involved, the media is most commonly affected, with hyperplasia producing segmental arterial narrowing and thinning associated with disruption of the internal elastic lamina producing saccular dilatations.

   ▪ The ICA, approximately 2 cm from the bifurcation (around C2), is most commonly affected (90% of cases). The vertebral artery is involved in approximately 12% of cases, usually at the C2 level. Bilateral carotid involvement occurs in 60% of cases. Intracranial involvement of FMD is rare.

   ▪ Carotid webs are considered to be a variant form of fibromuscular dysplasia and are thrombogenic due to associated stasis, turbulence and ultimately platelet activation. These appear as shelf-like projections into the carotid lumen (see Fig. 3.1D). Thrombus formed at the level of the web can embolize distally, and can be a cause of stroke and/or TIA, particularly in younger patients. For treatment and prevention of future events, patients may require antiplatelet medication, carotid stenting, or endarterectomy.

■ **Giant cell arteritis** is a chronic granulomatous arteritis generally affecting older populations (>50 years old) and with a propensity for involvement of the extracranial carotid branches, particularly the superficial temporal artery. Clinical presentation are myriad, including headache, jaw pain, and visual changes. High spatial resolution contrast-enhanced MRI techniques such as black-blood MRI can elucidate the segmental vessel involvement with wall thickening and mural enhancement in affected segments. Such imaging can be useful for targeted biopsy, which remains the gold standard for diagnosis. However, most often imaging is performed to exclude other etiologies for the patient's presenting symptoms.

## CIRCLE OF WILLIS

■ **Moyamoya syndrome** encompasses the numerous vasculopathies that lead to proximal artery stenoses, including neurofibromatosis, radiation vasculopathy, severe atherosclerosis, and sickle cell disease. The idiopathic form of the condition is designated as Moyamoya *disease*. This type of vasculopathy is characterized by progressive stenosis and occlusion of the distal ICAs and their proximal first segment branches (A1 and M1 branches

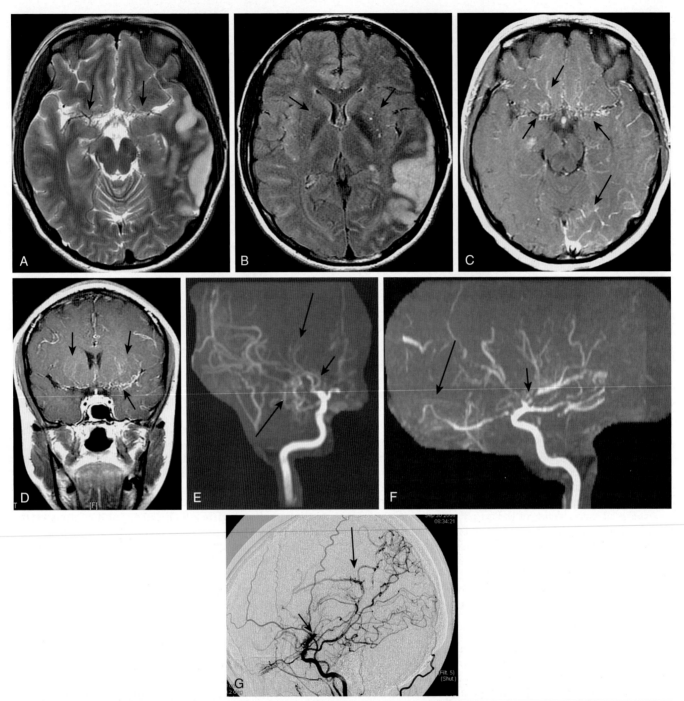

**Fig. 3.38 Moyamoya.** (A) Axial T2-weighted image (T2WI) at the level of the suprasellar cistern reveals absence of normal flow voids of the distal internal carotid arteries. Small arterial branches along the sylvian fissures are present instead of the expected dominant M1 segment flow voids *(arrows)*. (B) Axial fluid-attenuated inversion recovery image at the level of the basal ganglia demonstrates multiple T2 hyperintense foci within the basal ganglia, representing slow flow within dilated lenticulostriate arteries *(arrows)*. Axial (C) and coronal (D) contrast-enhanced T1-weighted imagery (T1WI) demonstrate multiple small vascular structures along the expected course of the bilateral proximal middle cerebral arteries (MCAs). Small serpentine enhancing vessels along the gyrus rectus and dilated lenticular arteries are present *(small arrows* in C and *arrows* in D). Leptomeningeal enhancement is present in the occipital lobes *(long arrow* in C). Frontal (E) and lateral (F) magnetic resonance angiography images of the right carotid artery demonstrate occlusion of the distal internal carotid artery *(short arrows)* with numerous small collateral branches in the region of the M1 segment of the MCA *(long arrows* in E). Note enlarged ophthalmic artery *(long arrow* in F) and poor filling of distal MCA branches. (G) Catheter angiogram confirms occlusion of the distal internal carotid artery *(short arrow)* with filling of the right posterior cerebral artery and retrograde filling of the pericallosal artery via leptomeningeal collaterals *(long arrow)*. Note acute left MCA infarct in A and B.

of the circle of Willis) (Fig. 3.38). Clinically, moyamoya has a progressive course, with patients presenting with symptoms of stroke and TIA. Over time, dementia develops because of progressive compromise of the vascular system and chronic hypoxia.

- Extensive collaterals often develop in the progression of disease to supply the brain distal to the circle of Willis. These collaterals include dural vessels (e.g., ECA and orbital branches of the internal maxillary artery to transethmoid collaterals to the inferior frontal ACA branches), leptomeningeal collaterals from the posterior cerebral artery (splenial branch to pericallosal artery to distal ACA and MCA territory), and deep perforating lenticulostriate arteries. The collateral lenticulostriate vessels produce a classic hazy appearance on angiography termed *moyamoya*, which from Japanese translates to "puff of smoke."
- Revascularization procedures are the basis of therapy. Most commonly, the ECA branches within the temporalis muscles are used as a source for peripheral leptomeningeal collateralization of the MCA distribution (pial synangiosis).
- Perfusion imaging can be used to evaluate the extent of vascular compromise (by assessing brain tissue at risk; i.e., penumbra) and, in the posttherapy stage, to evaluate the effects of vascular reperfusion.

- **Reversible cerebral vasoconstriction syndrome** (RCVS) describes a migratory phenomenon of vasospasm in cerebral arterial vessels presenting most commonly among young adult and middle-aged females presenting with recurrent "thunderclap" headaches. There are a number of predisposing conditions including pregnancy, eclampsia, drug use, or recent head trauma/

neurointervention, although most cases are idiopathic. About 20% of affected patients have SAH on CSF analysis. Angiography during symptomatic periods can show beaded narrowing of the vessels of the circle of Willis (Fig. 3.39). These areas of narrowing can spontaneously resolve on the order of weeks to months; resolution of findings helps to confirm the "reversible" diagnosis.

- The brain parenchyma findings may resemble posterior reversible encephalopathy syndrome (PRES) with confluent white matter lesions predominantly affecting the posterior brain parenchyma (that can resolve in a matter of weeks with antihypertensive medications) and peripheral cortical or sulcal-based hemorrhages.

- **Lymphomatoid granulomatosis** (neoplastic angioendotheliosis) is a very rare malignant lymphoma that is restricted to the intracranial vessels. It presents with recurrent strokes or stroke-like symptoms, encephalopathy, and seizures. There are multiple high-signal intensity lesions on T2WI and FLAIR imaging in the cerebral white matter often extending along the perivascular spaces, with associated enhancement. Angiography shows evidence of medium-sized vessel occlusions. Brain biopsy is needed to establish the diagnosis.

- **Infectious vasculitis** can occur in the setting of meningitis or skull base infection (e.g., osteomyelitis, invasive fungal sinusitis). Patients with severe basal cisternal meningeal inflammation (e.g., tuberculosis) may develop proximal stenosis and occlusion because of arterial constriction and spasm, which may lead to massive catastrophic infarction. In chronic granulomatous meningitis (e.g., tuberculosis), stenosis and occlusion may develop slowly and persist for long periods. In these diseases, involvement of the basilar artery and its branches is common, and therefore posterior circulation changes occur. Skull base meningitis may also affect the small perforating arteries that arise within the leptomeninges, leading to deep gray matter (basal ganglia and thalamus) infarcts. The combination of communicating hydrocephalus (because of inflammatory meningeal obstruction of CSF flow) and deep infarctions is suggestive of a skull base meningitis.

## SECONDARY AND TERTIARY BRANCH VESSELS

- A large number of disease processes can produce the class findings of "cerebral vasculitis." Patients may present with nonfocal symptoms, such as headache and/or seizure, but focal deficits may also occur when there is a secondary infarction or hemorrhage (parenchymal or subarachnoid) and are location dependent.
- There is typically circumferential tapered stenosis in arteries alternating with regions of normal vessel caliber. Multiple short segments of narrowing may produce a "string of beads" appearance. Typically, vessels in multiple vascular territories are involved often within the distal portions of a vascular territory. Focal occlusion may lead to leptomeningeal collateral filling of portions of a vascular territory distal to the occlusion.
- CTA and MRA can reveal vascular involvement or can be normal. Catheter angiography remains the gold standard for detecting and characterizing the extent of vasculitis.
- **Primary angiitis of the central nervous system** (PACNS) is a rare form of vasculitis with unknown cause

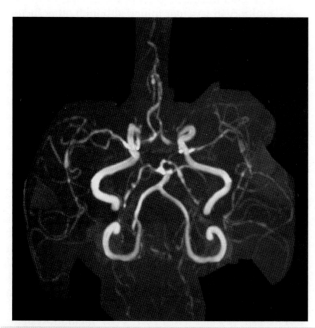

**Fig. 3.39 Reversible cerebral vasoconstrictive syndrome.** Three-dimensional time-of-flight magnetic resonance angiography (MRA) of the circle of Willis shows beaded appearance of the proximal and distal anterior cerebral arteries, middle cerebral arteries, and posterior cerebral arteries and distal branches bilaterally. MRA returned to normal several months later, confirming the diagnosis.

that affects parenchymal and leptomeningeal arteries with a predilection for small arteries and arterioles. This can be a rapidly progressive, frequently fatal disease. Median age of onset is 50 years and males are twice as often affected as females.

- Imaging findings are variable and nonspecific. Multiple infarcts in different vascular territories of varying ages and stages of healing are most common. T2 FLAIR hypertense lesions throughout the cerebral white matter are also common, however nonspecific.
- Leptomeningeal enhancement and subarachnoid and parenchymal hemorrhages can occur.
- PACNS may also present as a solitary mass-like lesion in 5% of cases.
- Vessel wall imaging may be useful in detailing arterial wall enhancement that distinguishes vasculitis from other vasculopathies in the differential, such as reversible cerebrovascular constriction syndrome (RCVS).
- Evaluation for malignancy, system vasculitis, and connective tissue disorders, as well as immunologic (antineutrophil cytoplasmic antibody [ANCA] and antinuclear antibody [ANA]) and infectious (varicella zoster virus [VZV], human immunodeficiency virus [HIV], hepatitis B virus [HBV], hepatitis C virus [HCV], and tuberculosis) testing are part of the workup to exclude secondary causes. Symptoms or serologic markers related to system inflammation are uncommon. For example, the sedimentation rate is elevated in less than 25% of patients. CSF does, however, demonstrate elevated protein and pleocytosis in more than 80% of cases.
- A diagnosis can also be established by brain biopsy.
- Treatment is immunosuppressive, with high-dose steroids and cytotoxic agents.
- **Granulomatosis with polyangiitis** (formerly Wegener's granulomatosis) is a necrotizing systemic vasculitis that affects the kidneys and upper and lower respiratory tracts. It can affect the brain producing stroke, visual loss, and other cranial nerve problems. The peak incidence is in the fourth to fifth decade with a slight male predominance. History plus positive c-antineutrophil cytoplasmic antibody (c-ANCA) tests help make the diagnosis.
- **Polyarteritis nodosa** is a multisystem disease characterized by necrotizing inflammation of the small and medium size arteries with CNS involvement occurring late in the disease in more than 45% of cases. It is an immune-mediated disease with about 40% of patients having hepatitis B surface antigen. Polyarteritis is closely related to allergic angiitis and granulomatosis (Churg-Strauss). Aneurysms, which more commonly involve the renal and splanchnic vessels in this disease, are unusual in the CNS.
- **Neurosarcoidosis** can produce a CNS vasculitis characterized by frank granulomatous invasion of the walls of the arteries with or without ischemic changes in the supplied brain parenchyma. These patients usually have a history of systemic sarcoid, although sarcoid can rarely affect only the CNS. Sarcoidosis may also cause inflammation of the small vessels and lead to microinfarcts from the venous side.
  - On MRI, enhancing parenchymal lesions or smooth or nodular leptomeningeal enhancement, particularly along the basal aspects of the brain and circle of Willis, can be seen. Enhancement can extend superiorly into the brain to involve the perivascular spaces, mimicking parenchymal lesions. Pituitary, hypothalamic, and cranial nerve involvement (facial and optic nerve most common) can be seen. Intracranial microhemorrhages may also be noted along the perivascular spaces.

- **Infectious vasculitis**, such as in the setting of tuberculosis and *Haemophilus influenzae* infections, may on occasion affect secondary and tertiary arteries.
  - Neurosyphilis can cause an acute syphilitic meningitis and a meningovascular syphilis that affects both arteries and veins, particularly in the middle cerebral distribution, and can lead to stroke and parenchymal neurosyphilis. There are two types of arteritis associated with syphilis. The endarteritis obliterans type affects the medium and large arteries (i.e., Heubner arteritis), and Nissl-Alzheimer arteritis type affects small arterial vessels.
  - More recently reported are the neurologic manifestations of coronavirus disease 2019 (COVID-19) caused by severe acute respiratory syndrome coronavirus 2 (SARS-CoV-2) infection. Encephalopathy, stroke from large vessel occlusion, and supra- and infratentorial patchy enhancing ischemic lesions in the subcortical, periventricular, and deep white matter; basal ganglia; cerebellar peduncles and hemispheres; and corpus callosum in a pattern mimicking small vessel vasculitis have all been described.
    - SARS-CoV-2 infects a host through its CoV spike glycoprotein that binds to angiotensin converting enzyme 2 (ACE 2) receptors expressed on the most targeted organs of this disease—lungs, heart and kidneys—and also on endothelial cells. The resultant endotheliitis is a proposed mechanism of the multiorgan vascular injury, although other factors, such as hypercoagulable/prothrombotic state or cytokine storm, implicated in COVID-19 infection may also be at play.
  - Herpes zoster infections may spread to the cavernous sinus from the face along the trigeminal nerve branches and then produce an extensive vasculitis with multiple areas of infarction, mimicking PACNS.
  - Fungal sinusitis from aggressive mucor or aspergillosis may also affect the cavernous sinuses, causing ICA stenosis or occlusion and cavernous sinus thrombosis.
- **Small vessel diseases** include several disease processes, with involvement of small perforating arteries and arterioles. Because of the small caliber of the vessels involved, angiographic studies are virtually always normal. Imaging features consist of deep gray matter, white matter, and subcortical infarcts. Lesions tend to be irregular and parallel the periventricular white matter, differentiating these chronic ischemic lesions from multiple sclerosis lesions, which tend to be flame-shaped and perpendicular to the periventricular white matter.
  - *Collagen vascular diseases* (CVDs) include systemic lupus erythematosus and anticardiolipin and antiphospholipid antibody syndromes. Cerebral vasculitis is rarely associated with CVD. More commonly, the causes of stroke in patients with CVD include cardiac valvular disease (Libman-Sacks aortic and mitral

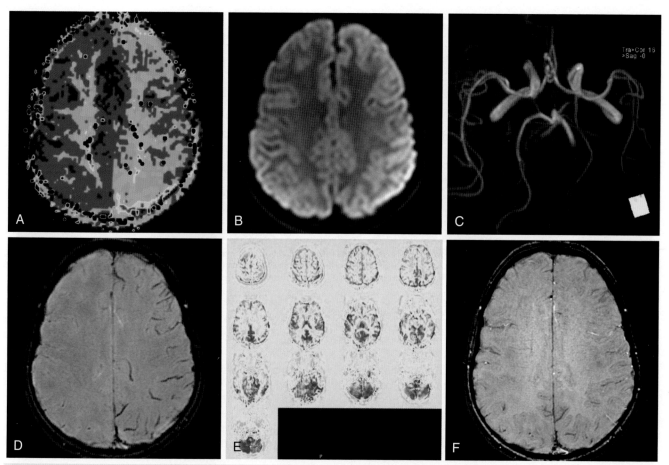

**Fig. 3.40 Migraine-related vasospasm.** (A) Marked asymmetry with prolonged relative mean transit time (rMTT) is seen in the left cerebral hemisphere on this contrast-enhanced magnetic resonance perfusion study in a young patient presenting with acute right-sided weakness in conjunction with her usual migraine headache. Although no diffusion abnormality is seen (B) and three-dimensional time-of-flight magnetic resonance angiography appears normal (C), the susceptibility-weighted imaging (SWI) scan shows increased prominence of cortical vessels over the left cerebral hemisphere, suggesting venous engorgement (D). Her symptoms improved over the next several hours and (E) arterial spin labeling perfusion imaging performed the following day shows resolution of the perfusion deficit involving the left cerebral hemisphere. (F) SWI scan shows symmetric appearance of distal vessels on the follow-up exam as well.

valve vegetations in lupus), an increased tendency toward thrombosis (or reduced thrombolysis) related to antiphospholipid antibodies such as lupus anticoagulant and/or anticardiolipin antibodies, and atherosclerosis accelerated by hypertension or long-term steroid use. Venous thrombosis is also a risk. Atrophy, related to either encephalopathy or chronic steroid use, may also be found in these patients.

- *Sjogren syndrome* is characterized by focal or confluent lymphocytic infiltrates in the exocrine glands producing clinical features of dry eyes and dry mouth. However, 25% of these patients have CNS complications including infarction. The etiology of the stroke may be a small vessel vasculitis; however, these patients also have antiphospholipid antibodies (another risk factor).

- White matter T2 hyperintensities can be seen in 10% to 25% of patients with *migraine* headaches. Lesions are typically few in number and have a predilection for the subcortical white matter of the frontal lobes. These are felt to be the result of spasm in small arteries associated with migraine attaches. Rarely, patients with migraines

will present with clinical findings of stroke syndrome (hemiplegic migraine), usually in the distribution of the anterior or middle cerebral arteries. There can be correlating territorial abnormalities seen on susceptibility weighting imaging (vessel engorgement) and perfusion imaging (arterial territory blood flow deficits) during acute hemiplegic migraines (Fig. 3.40). Females with migraine auras are at highest risk for subsequent development of migraine-associated strokes.

- *Cerebral autosomal dominant arteriopathy with subcortical infarcts and leukoencephalopathy* (CADASIL) is a rare disease with a genetic causation: a mutation on chromosome 19p12.12 involving the NOTCH3 gene. It results in small vessel and arteriole stenosis secondary to fibrotic thickening of the basement membrane of the vessels. On imaging, the disease manifests as multiple subcortical white matter and lacunar infarcts within the basal ganglia, thalami, and pons, with a predilection of confluent white matter hyperintensity on FLAIR to involve the anterior temporal lobes and external capsules (Fig. 3.41). This extent of involvement in a typically young patient

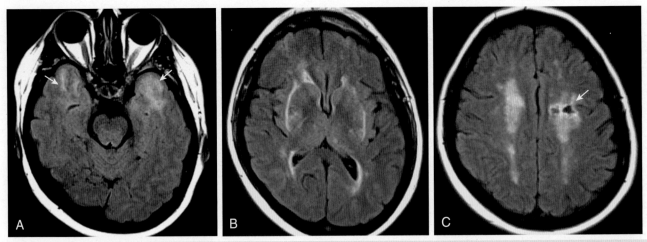

**Fig. 3.41 Cerebral autosomal dominant arteriopathy with subcortical infarcts and leukoencephalopathy (CADASIL).** (A–C) Axial fluid-attenuated inversion recovery images show characteristic features of CADASIL, including subcortical infarct in the left superior frontal lobe (*arrow* in C) as well as confluent T2 hyperintensity in the superior frontal lobes, external capsule, and anterior temporal lobes (*arrows* in A).

(between 30–50 years old) is a clue for diagnosis. Microhemorrhages are also present in the majority of cases seen on GRE or SWI MRI sequences. As the disease progresses, involvement becomes more widespread and confluent.

- *Cerebral amyloid angiopathy* (CAA) represents its own subset of vascular pathology, more commonly in patients over 50 years of age. Sporadic and familial forms exist, and there is a strong association with Alzheimer disease with more than 80% of Alzheimer patients demonstrating CAA changes on autopsy. It results from deposition of amyloid (an eosinophilic, insoluble, extracellular protein), in the media and adventitia of small- and medium-sized vessels of the superficial layers of the cerebral cortex and leptomeninges, resulting in vascular fragility.
  - The resulting hemorrhages are usually peripheral and lobar, typically involving the frontal and parietal lobes, including the subjacent white matter, and may be multiple. There is a propensity for recurrent hemorrhage in the same location and/or multiple simultaneous hemorrhages. GRE or SWI imaging typically highlights susceptibility from hemosiderosis related to cortical and subarachnoid-based hemorrhages of the superficial vessels involved in CAA (Fig. 3.42).
  - In many cases, CAA is accompanied by white matter changes which tend be periventricular, extending to the subcortical white matter, unifocal or multifocal, and with posterior predominance.
- In 2022, Boston 2.0 criteria were proposed to distinguish definite and probable CAA with supporting pathology (both requiring presence of CAA in pathologic specimen) from probable (multiple intracranial

hemorrhagic foci and/or white matter changes) and possible CAA (single intracranial hemorrhagic focus or white matter change).

- In more rare instances, there can be an active inflammatory component (i.e., CAA-related inflammation), on the basis of perivascular (cerebral amyloid angiopathy-related inflammation) and/or intramural inflammatory destruction (Aβ-Related Angiitis or ABRA). Clinical presentation may be acute or subacute with declining cognition, seizures, headache, and stroke-like symptoms. In such cases, there are large regions of vasogenic edema in a background of CAA related microhemorrhages (Fig 3.42E-F). Leptomeningeal enhancement can coexist and multifocal vessel narrowing, wall thickening and perivascular enhancement may be seen on MR vessel wall imaging. Patients respond to treatment with corticosteroids and immunosuppressants.
- Separate but related, Amyloid-Related Imaging Abnormalities (ARIA) consisting of parenchymal edema and sulcal FLAIR non-suppression (ARIA-E) and/or parenchymal/leptomeningeal hemorrhage (ARIA-H), can be seen (often incidentally) among Alzheimers patients treated with anti-amyloid immunotherapy agents. The imaging findings are very similar to inflammatory CAA; awareness of the medication history can help narrow the differential diagnosis.

Take it all in, and enjoy the moment of having made it through the chapter! Lots more interesting things to come, but a break to refresh the blood flow to the brain may be in order.

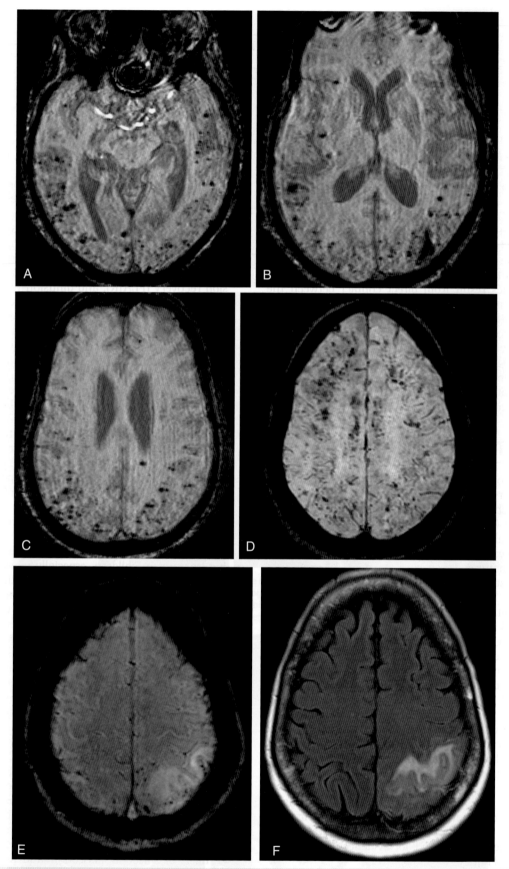

**Fig. 3.42 Cerebral amyloid angiopathy.** (A–C) Susceptibility-weighted imaging (SWI) scans in an 89-year-old woman show innumerable foci of signal loss predominantly in cortical/subcortical parenchyma indicating microhemorrhages. Note absence of such signal changes in basal ganglia and brain stem, as might be seen in the setting of chronic hypertension. This distribution of microhemorrhage in a patient of this age is most compatible with cerebral amyloid angiopathy. (D) Be aware there is a differential for such microhemorrhages based on clinical context and patient demographics. In this young adult patient with sickle cell disease, the innumerable microhemorrhages on SWI ("*starfield*" *pattern*) are a consequence of chronic fat embolic infarcts occurring secondary to avascular necrosis of long bones. (E) Axial SWI and (F) FLAIR images in a different patient with cerebral amyloid angiopathy-related inflammation shows numerous peripheral microhemorrhages in the parietal regions, with large area of cerebral edema on the left.

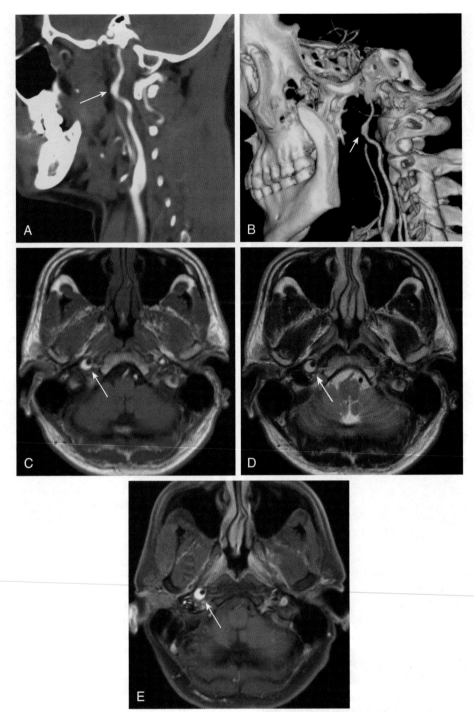

**Fig. 4.20 Dissection on computed tomography angiography (CTA) and magnetic resonance imaging (MRI).** (A) Sagittal maximum intensity projection and (B) surface-rendered reconstructions of the left cervical carotid artery system from CTA performed in setting of trauma shows abrupt focal enlargement of the caliber of the internal carotid artery (ICA) below the skull base *(arrows)*, indicating dissection with associated pseudoaneurysm. The dissection is not flow limiting because contrast opacifies the vessel beyond the level of caliber change. On MRI, in a different patient, axial T1-weighted image (T1WI) (C) and axial T2WI (D) show crescentic mural hematoma within the wall of the right ICA at the skull base *(arrows)*. Fat-suppressed postcontrast T1WI (E) confirms presence of T1 hyperintense intramural hematoma *(arrow)*. Note preservation of the flow void within the residual ICA lumen on these MRI images (target sign).

- MRA is an excellent tool for identifying dissection, although intraluminal intensity changes secondary to turbulent and in plane-flow artifacts may be difficult to differentiate from flaps and false lumens. On MRI, the mural hematoma is commonly T1 hyperintense and T2 hypointense to hyperintense (see Fig. 4.20C–E). Within the expanded T1 hyperintense artery wall the small hypointense residual lumen is often present (target sign).

Fat-suppressed T1WI sequences may be useful to distinguish periarterial fat from intramural hematoma, particularly in the neck. Because the mural hematoma is typically hyperintense, care must be taken in evaluating MRA sequences to make sure that hyperintense mural clot is not mistaken for hyperintense normal flow. The mural clot is typically less hyperintense than the lumen and has an amorphous appearance.

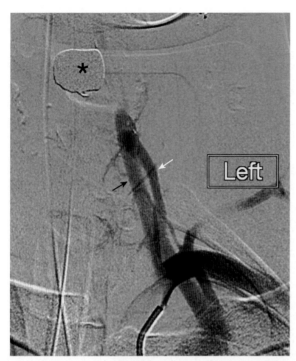

**Fig. 4.21 Post traumatic arteriovenous (AV) fistula.** Conventional catheter angiogram in a patient status post gunshot wound to left neck shows opacification of the proximal left vertebral artery *(white arrow)*. This vessel occludes abruptly, and there is direct communication with draining vein *(black arrow)* which opacifies in the arterial phase, indicating AV fistula. *Asterisk* indicates bullet fragment in the neck.

- Mural clot is less often visualized in vertebral artery dissections. Black-blood MRA is more sensitive for detection of intramural hematoma. MR is also useful for following the dissection to visualize when the hemorrhage is reabsorbed, when the normal lumen dimensions are reestablished, and if there is progression to pseudoaneurysm or occlusion.
- The principal complications of extracranial vascular dissection, infarcts, and transient ischemic attacks result from luminal compromise and, more commonly, embolic phenomena. Ischemic infarction is usually the result of distal embolization from the cervical dissection. Embolic infarction typically occurs several hours to days after the onset of the dissection but may be delayed for several weeks. Treatment (anticoagulation) is directed toward preventing recurrent emboli. Most dissections of the neck heal spontaneously.
- Other terrifying sequelae of traumatic vascular injury include laceration, extravasation, occlusion, pseudoaneurysm, and arteriovenous fistula (Fig. 4.21).
- Trauma to the cavernous carotid artery can produce direct communication between the carotid artery and cavernous sinus, resulting in the dreaded cavernous-carotid fistula (see Fig. 3.36) discussed in Chapter 3.

## DIFFUSE AXONAL INJURY

- DAI is the injury responsible for coma and poor outcome in most patients with significant closed head injury resulting from automobile accidents (although it can result from other kinds of trauma as well). At the time of injury, the stress induced by rotational acceleration/deceleration movement of the head causes some regions of the brain to accelerate or decelerate faster than other regions, resulting in axonal shearing injury. Axons may be completely disrupted together with adjacent capillaries, or some axons may be incompletely disrupted, the so-called injury-in-continuity. Patients with severe DAI are unconscious from the moment of injury and may remain in a persistent vegetative state or be severely impaired.
- DAI characteristically involves the corpus callosum, brain stem, internal capsule, and gray-white interface. Rotationally induced shear-strain may also produce cortical contusion and lesions in the deep gray matter. The unbending falx, which is broader posteriorly, prevents the cerebral hemispheres from moving across the midline, whereas anteriorly the falx is shorter so that the brain can transiently move across the midline. The fibers of the splenium and posterior corpus callosum are thus under greater risk of shearing than the anterior fibers.
- Lesions may be ovoid or elliptic, with the long axis parallel to fiber bundle directions. CT is not as sensitive as MR in detecting DAI in the brain (Fig. 4.22). On CT, one may visualize focal punctate regions of high density that may be surrounded by a collar of low density edema. These are hemorrhagic shearing injuries most likely associated with complete axonal disruption. On CT, it may be difficult to detect nonhemorrhagic shearing injury early and initial CT may appear normal. When DAI is clinically suspected and CT is unrevealing, MRI should be performed because it has a much higher sensitivity for detecting shear injuries. MRI reveals high intensity on T2WI/FLAIR at injured sites, which, through the magic of SWI sequences, are shown to frequently be associated with hemorrhage. DWI may be positive, reflecting the hemorrhagic lesions or nonhemorrhagic shearing injuries. Splenial lesions in particular seem to restrict diffusion.

## TRAUMATIC BRAIN INJURY IN THE LONG TERM

- Cognitive deficits include decreased speed in information processing, poor attention, concentration, and memory, and impaired logical reasoning skill, as well as more focal deficits, including impairment of language or constructional abilities.
- TBI is now considered a risk factor in the development of Alzheimer disease.
- Long-term sequela of TBI include:
  - Loss of brain parenchymal volume, particularly involving the caudate nucleus, corpus callosum, hippocampus, fornix, and thalamus
  - Enlargement of the ventricles
  - Post traumatic thalamic atrophy in the presence of cortical and subcortical (but nonthalamic) lesions
  - Hypertrophic olivary degeneration (see Chapter 7) may result from traumatic injuries affecting the red nucleus, dentate nucleus, central tegmental tract, or cerebellar peduncles
  - Wallerian degeneration of the corticospinal tract will often be seen after contusions/shears of the motor

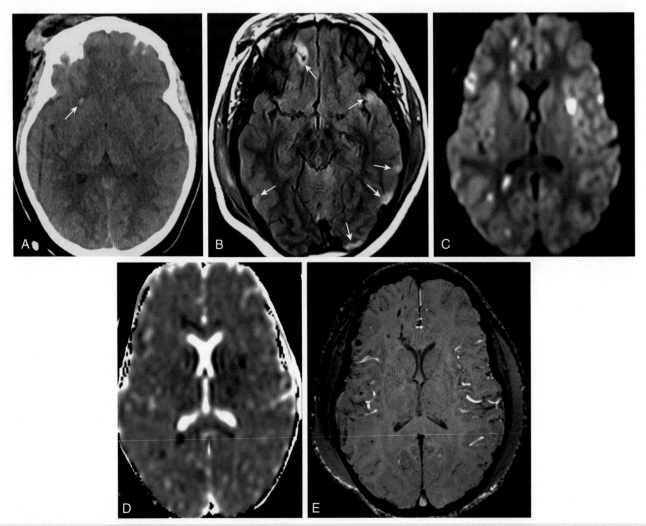

**Fig. 4.22 Diffuse axonal injury (DAI).** (A) Axial noncontrast computed tomography (CT) image shows small focus of hemorrhage with surrounding edema in the right external capsule *(arrow)*. (B) Axial fluid-attenuated inversion recovery (FLAIR) image performed on subsequent magnetic resonance imaging shows numerous additional lesions that are not appreciable by CT, which lie at the gray-white interface *(arrows)*. (C) Diffusion-weighted imaging and (D) apparent diffusion coefficient map show numerous additional lesions also at gray-white interface and at/near the splenium of the corpus callosum. (E) Axial susceptibility-weighted imaging is the most sensitive in picking up tiny hemorrhages and confirming the diagnosis of DAI. Every dark spot on this image indicates a focus of shear injury.

area of the frontal cortex or white matter tracts, respectively
- Increased prevalence of cavum septum pellucidum
- Hydrocephalus

## HERNIATION SYNDROMES

- The brain lives in a rigid container (the skull) and is compartmentalized by inelastic dural reflections (tentorium, falx cerebri, falx cerebelli). Herniations of brain from one region to another can produce both brain and vascular damage. Five basic patterns can be encountered (Fig. 4.23): inferior tonsillar and cerebellar herniation, superior vermian herniation (e.g., upward, ascending transtentorial or supratentorial herniation), temporal lobe/uncal herniation, descending transtentorial herniation, and subfalcine herniation. It is important to alert the clinical teams caring for the patient with incipient herniation because these are potentially life-threatening situations. In the setting of herniation syndromes, death

is a very likely outcome unless urgent surgical decompression is performed. The neurosurgeon's decision to decompress is based on both clinical and imaging parameters (Table 4.5).
- **Tonsillar herniation** occurs in the setting of space-occupying lesions in the posterior fossa. The fourth ventricle is compressed, producing obstructive supratentorial hydrocephalus (dilated temporal horns are particularly sensitive indicators of such hydrocephalus). The cerebellar tonsils and cerebellum are usually pushed inferiorly through the foramen magnum. Absence of the normal CSF around the foramen magnum and the presence of tonsillar and cerebellar tissue in that site should raise suspicion for tonsillar herniation (Fig. 4.24).
- **Upward/ascending transtentorial herniation** occurs when superior cerebellar mass effect produces upward herniation of the vermis (Fig. 4.25). Cerebellar tissue obliterates the superior vermian, ambient, and quadrigeminal cisterns. Compression of the aqueduct by such mass effect can lead to obstructive hydrocephalus.

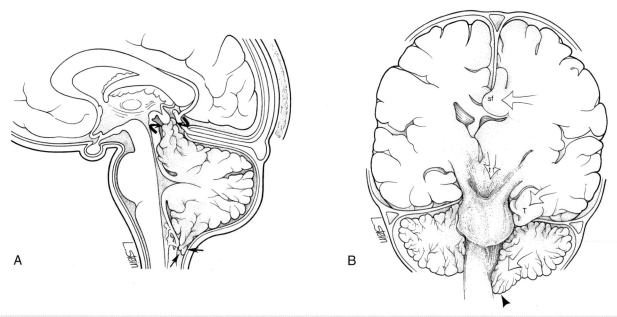

**Fig. 4.23 Herniations of the brain.** (A) Sagittal diagram of cerebellar herniation, with *curved arrows* demonstrating upward herniation of the superior cerebellum and superior vermis and *straight arrows* demonstrating tonsillar and inferior vermian herniation. (B) Coronal diagram with temporal lobe herniation *(T)*, central transtentorial herniation *(tt)*, tonsillar herniation *(arrowhead)*, and subfalcine herniation *(sf)*. Lines of force are demonstrated by *large open arrows*. Note the pressure on the brain stem from these herniation patterns.

**Table 4.5** Clinical and Imaging Indications for Surgical Intervention Versus Observation in Patients with Intracranial Hemorrhage

| Lesion | Indications for Surgery—Clinical | Indications for Surgery—Imaging | Nonsurgical Management (close clinical monitoring, serial imaging) |
|---|---|---|---|
| Parenchymal hemorrhage | Progressive neurologic deterioration<br>Refractory intracranial hypertension<br>GCS 6–8 | Signs of mass effect<br>Midline shift >5 mm<br>Cisternal effacement<br>Hematoma volume > 50 mL (temporal contusion >20 mL) | No neurologic compromise<br>Controlled ICP<br>No mass effect on imaging |
| Acute EDH | Focal deficit<br>GCS <8 | Volume >30 mL<br>Volume <30 mL *and* >15 mm thickness<br>*or* >5 mm midline shift *and* clinical indications for surgery | Volume <30 mL *and* <15 mm thickness *and* <5 mm midline shift *and* GCS >8 without focal deficit |
| Acute SDH | GCS <9<br>Decrease in GCS by 2 points<br>Asymmetric, fixed, dilated pupils<br>ICP >20 mm Hg | Thickness >10 mm *or* >5 mm midline shift<br>Thickness <10 mm and <5 mm shift *and* GCS <9 *and* clinical indications for surgery | No neurologic compromise |
| Posterior fossa lesions | Neurologic deterioration | Signs of mass effect (displacement/effacement of fourth ventricle, effaced basal cisterns, obstructive hydrocephalus) | No mass effect on CT<br>No neurologic compromise |
| Depressed open (compound) skull fracture | Clinical evidence of dural penetration | Depression > thickness of skull | No clinical/imaging evidence of dural penetration<br>No significant intracranial hemorrhage<br><1 cm depression<br>No frontal sinus involvement<br>No significant cosmetic deformity<br>No wound infection<br>No pneumocephalus |

CT, Computed tomography; *EDH*, epidural hematoma; *GCS*, Glasgow Coma Scale; *ICP*, intracranial pressure; *SDH*, subdural hematoma.
(Modified from Winn HR. *Youmans Neurological Surgery*. Elsevier; 2011.)

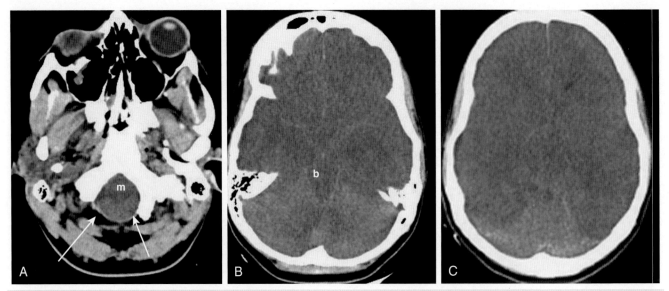

**Fig. 4.24 Cerebral edema.** (A) The cerebellar tonsils *(arrows)* have herniated through the foramen magnum in this patient with global anoxic injury. No surrounding cerebrospinal fluid (CSF) is seen and the medulla *(m)* is displaced anteriorly. (B) Note the elongated squeezed midbrain (b) and the absence of gray-white differentiation and CSF in the basal cisterns. Often the relatively denser vessels will simulate subarachnoid hemorrhage. (C) Further superiorly, things are equally tight with compressed lateral ventricles. Note the relatively preserved density of the cerebellum compared to the cerebral hemispheres (white cerebellum sign.)

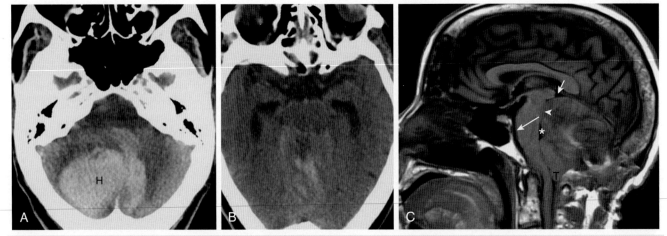

**Fig. 4.25 Ascending transtentorial herniation.** (A) Axial computed tomographic image through the posterior fossa shows a large hematoma *(H)* in the right cerebellar hemisphere resulting in leftward shift of posterior fossa structures and complete effacement of sulci. (B) More superiorly, there is effacement of the quadrigeminal plate cistern from superior migration of the vermis because of mass effect in the posterior fossa. Note enlarged temporal horns of the lateral ventricles, indicating early hydrocephalus. (C) Despite urgent suboccipital craniectomy for decompression, the fourth ventricle *(asterisk)* remains nearly completely effaced, the quadrigeminal plate cistern *(arrowhead)* is effaced, and the superior vermian cistern *(small arrow)* is partially effaced. The pons is flattened against the clivus *(large arrow)* and there is crowding of structures at the craniocervical junction because of downward descent of the cerebellar tonsils *(T)*.

- **Uncal and descending transtentorial herniation** are seen with mass lesions whose vector force is directed inferiorly and medially, best detected on coronal images. In uncal herniation, the temporal lobe uncus shifts over the tentorium, compressing the oculomotor nerve and its parasympathetic fibers (with ipsilateral pupillary dilatation). Compression of the posterior cerebral and anterior choroidal arteries against tentorium or petroclinoid ligament may result in ischemia/infarction (Fig. 4.26).
    - Transtentorial herniation is more severe with compression of the contralateral cerebral peduncle against the edge of the tentorium producing ipsilateral motor weakness (Kernohan-Woltman notch phenomenon or false localizing sign). It is associated with high intensity on T2WI in the midbrain from compression and occlusion of perforating arteries at the tentorial notch.
- Small hemorrhages in the tegmentum of the pons and the midbrain caused by transtentorial herniation have been termed Duret hemorrhages.
- Transtentorial herniation results in ipsilateral ambient cistern widening and contralateral cisternal obliteration, contralateral temporal horn dilatation, rotation, and/or contralateral sliding of the brain stem.

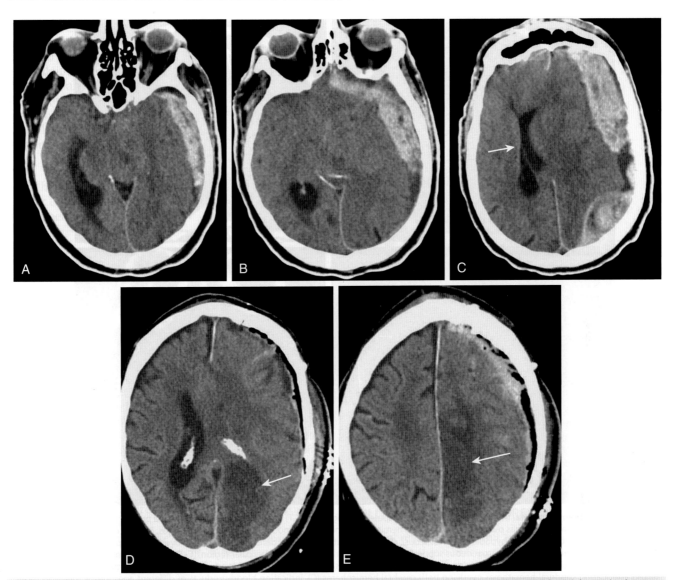

**Fig. 4.26 Herniation complications.** (A) This patient had a large subdural hematoma. Note the compression of the uncus from *left* to *right*, the contralateral temporal horn dilation of the right lateral ventricle, and rotation of the midbrain indicative of transtentorial herniation. (B) Basal cisterns are effaced and the brain stem is distorted. (C) More superiorly, the lateral ventricles *(arrow)* are displaced across the midline with subfalcine herniation. (D) Two days later, after evacuation of the hematoma, one can see a left occipital lobe infarct *(arrow)* from the compression of the left posterior cerebral artery associated with the downward transtentorial herniation. (E) A left anterior cerebral artery infarction *(arrow)* is also present, likely from the stretching by the subfalcine herniation.

- Supratentorial mass effect can be directed medially, causing the cingulate gyrus to shift beneath the falx cerebri, resulting in **subfalcine herniation**. In this situation, compression of the anterior cerebral artery (see Fig. 4.26) or internal cerebral veins can result in ischemia. The frontal horns are shifted and rotated to one side, and the septum pellucidum deviates over at the level of the foramen of Monro.

## HYDROCEPHALUS

- Hydrocephalus, as a secondary complication of TBI, may occur from numerous causes.
- Noncommunicating hydrocephalus (NCH) can occur as a result of herniations (obstruction at the foramen of Monro because of subfalcian herniation; obstruction of the third ventricle because of upward herniation of the cerebellar vermis; or parenchymal hemorrhages in basal ganglia, thalamus, or dentate nucleus obstructing the lateral, third, and fourth ventricles, respectively).
- NCH because of clots lodging in the aqueduct or fourth ventricle occurs more commonly than in the lateral ventricles and third ventricle.
- Communicating hydrocephalus results from obstruction of the arachnoid villi from subarachnoid hemorrhage, inhibiting resorption of CSF.

## BRAIN DEATH

- Brain death is defined as the irreversible cessation of all cerebral and brain stem functions. The absence of cerebral blood flow (from increased ICP) is generally accepted as a definite sign of brain death. In the clinical setting of

- Skull base injuries, including fractures of the carotid canal, jugular foramen, cavernous sinus walls, and skull fractures adjacent to major venous sinuses, should prompt angiographic evaluation to assess integrity of housed arterial or venous vascular structures. Clival and central skull base fractures can be associated with extra-axial hematomas along the craniocervical junction, so when such fractures are seen, a careful review of soft tissues to exclude associated hemorrhage should ensue. Identification of temporal bone fractures should prompt a review of middle and inner ear structures addressing integrity of ossicles and otic capsule structures (see Chapter 11).

- In children, most linear skull fractures heal in time, whereas in adults evidence of these fractures is present for years after injury, although the margins are less distinct. When the dura is torn with the skull fracture, the arachnoid can insinuate itself into the cleft of the fracture. Rarely, the pulsations of the CSF enlarge the cleft between the fracture fragments, producing either linear widening of the fracture margins or multiloculated cysts with smooth, scalloped margins. This appearance has been termed a *growing fracture* or "leptomeningeal cyst" and is seen more commonly in children.

## FACIAL AND ORBITAL TRAUMA

- CT is the most efficient imaging modality for visualizing facial fractures. Axial MDCT thin (less than or equal to 1 mm) sections with coronal and sagittal reconstructions are essential for detecting the full extent of the injury. Certain classic fracture eponyms have attained historical notoriety and at times are useful in describing what tends to be a complex of fractures. What is more important is that these mechanistic descriptions allow you to raise your suspicion for associated fractures elsewhere. "Simple" fractures are those without displaced fragments, whereas "complex" ones are associated with displaced and rotated fracture fragments that may produce secondary airway compromise, trismus, or vascular injury. Open fractures breach the skin surface. Depressed fractures are inwardly displaced.

- Signs of facial and orbital trauma include soft-tissue swelling about the face or orbit, and fluid and blood in the maxillary or paranasal sinuses. In orbital fractures, note the location of the fracture, its extent, whether muscle or fat is entrapped in the fracture site, and whether associated orbital hemorrhage, including subperiosteal hematomas, is present (see Fig. 4.1). It is important to keep in mind that nasal, zygomatic, and mandibular bone fractures are commonly seen facial injuries in elder abuse;, an unfortunate problem that is becoming increasingly prelancent worldwide. Orbital fractures inconsistent with reported mechanism can raise suspicion for elder abuse.

- The **orbital blow-out fracture** is the most common fracture caused by a direct (blunt) injury resulting in fracture of the orbital wall and entrapment of the orbital contents.
  - This injury can involve the orbital floor, with the fracture usually through the orbital plate of the maxilla medial to or involving the infraorbital canal (Fig. 4.29). The fracture is commonly hinged on the medial side, appearing on coronal CT as a "trapdoor." Rectus muscles and orbital fat may be displaced through the fracture site. This can result in clinically apparent entrapment syndromes with limitation of movement of the globe.
  - The injury may be associated with enophthalmos, diplopia (on upgaze), and ocular injuries and may or may not involve the orbital rim. Superior orbital rim fracture is a more severe injury, and may be associated with intracranial injury. The weakest portion of the roof is near the superior orbital fissure and optic canal, and fracture of the orbital roof can predispose to pseudomeningocele (Fig. 4.30).

- **Medial orbital blow-out fractures** involve the lamina papyracea of the ethmoid bone. Medial rectus muscle (and/or fat) herniation and entrapment can lead to diplopia. Orbital emphysema or air-fluid level in sinuses may indicate associated subtle sinus fracture.

- Rarely, **upward blow-out** can occur into the frontal sinus.

- A direct blow to the maxillary sinus can cause an **orbital "blow-in" fracture**, with elevation of the orbital floor into the orbit. These fractures cause proptosis and restrict ocular motility. Blow-in fractures with superior orbital rim fractures are associated with frontal lobe contusion and EDH.

- Ocular trauma can result in perforation of the globe and ocular hypotony (flat tire sign). Orbital hemorrhage can occur in the intraconal space, within the nerve sheath (subdural), or in the extraconal space, subperiosteal space, and sub-Tenon space (between the sclera and Tenon capsule, which is a fibrous membrane adjacent to the orbital fat). Hemorrhage within the globe can be seen in the anterior segment (anterior chamber hyphema) and posterior segment (where vitreous fluid resides). Posterior segment hemorrhages can be centered in the vitreous or can be seen with retinal or choroidal detachments. Lens dislocations or acute traumatic cataracts (low in density) can be seen in the setting of ocular trauma. Corneal lacerations are seen as defects in the dense border of the anterior segment margin.

- Foreign bodies may be seen within the orbit and within the globe. Presence of air and/or foreign body material within the globe in the trauma setting implies globe rupture, even if globe morphology appears preserved (Fig. 4.31). Certainly, a collapsed, misshapen globe in the setting implies globe rupture. These findings are critical to report to the clinical service because such findings may be difficult to appreciate on physical exam when the eye is swollen shut. Open globes are often treated surgically and accompanied by aggressive antibiotics.

- MR can have a special role in detecting optic nerve sheath hematomas. These tend to be more obvious on MR than on CT. Diagnosis is important because vision can be rapidly lost and operative nerve sheath decompression can be restorative. On MR, hemorrhage can be observed along the nerve sheath, which may be swollen and irregular. On CT, the nerve sheath complex may be enlarged.

- **Zygomaticomaxillary (ZMC) complex** (tetrapod) fracture includes:
  - Fracture of the lateral wall of the orbit, usually as diastasis of the zygomaticofrontal suture

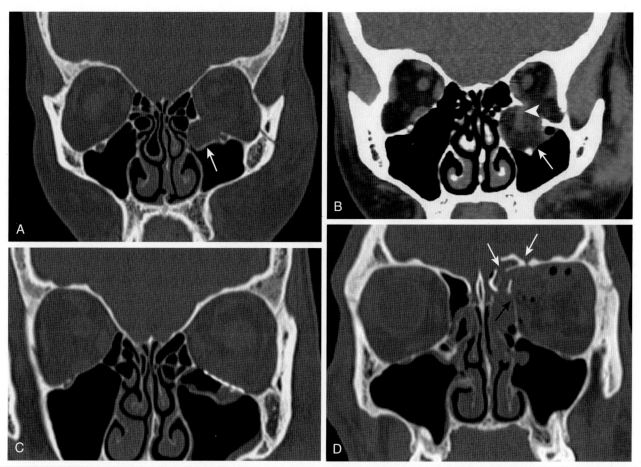

**Fig. 4.29  Orbit fractures.** (A) Coronal computed tomographic image in bone window shows orbital floor fracture fragment *(arrow)* projecting inferiorly (trap door appearance), also taking out the inferomedial orbital wall. (B) The fat *(arrow)* and muscular *(arrowhead)* herniation through the fracture gap led to restriction of motion. (C) Subsequent repair with plate and screws of the orbital floor led to anatomic alignment. (D) This patient was stabbed in the eye and incurred a combination of orbital roof *(white arrows)* and medial orbital wall *(black arrow)* fractures. Note the air and hematoma and traumatized muscles in the superomedial orbit.

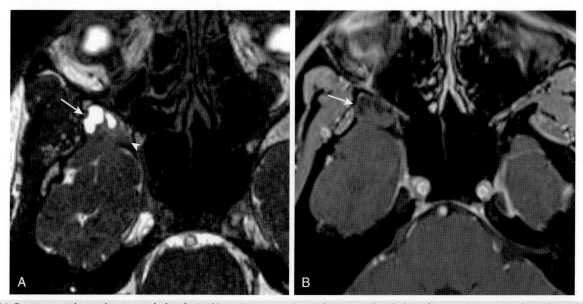

**Fig. 4.30  Post traumatic meningoencephalocele.** In this patient presenting with recurrent headaches after a recent motorcycle crash, axial T2 constructive interference in steady state (CISS) (A) image shows a meningoencephalocele *(arrow)* extending through a defect in the sphenoid wing. Note fluid and brain *(arrowhead)* contents within the herniation. (B) As expected, the meningoencephalocele does not enhance on postcontrast T1-weighted image *(arrow)*.

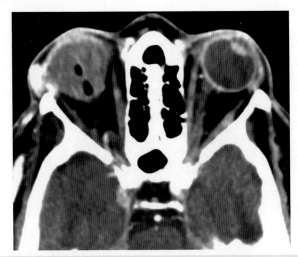

**Fig. 4.31 Ocular injury.** Axial-unenhanced computed tomographic image through the orbits shows heterogenous attenuation of fluid in the posterior segment of the globe indicating vitreous hemorrhage. Presence of air within the globe and loss of normal globe morphology indicates globe rupture.

- Fracture of the inferior orbital rim and floor, at times injuring the infraorbital nerve
- Fracture of the zygomatic arch
- Fracture of the zygomaticomaxillary strut (see Fig. 4.33).
- The zygoma can be displaced posteriorly and medially, causing difficulty with the normal motion of the jaw. When this occurs, the lateral wall (at times the anterior and posterior walls as well) of the maxillary sinus is involved in addition to the floor of the orbit.
- The **naso-orbital-ethmoid complex (NOE) fracture** typically involve the nasal bones, medial maxillary buttresses, nasal septum, ethmoid sinuses, and medial orbital walls because of direct trauma to the midface and nasal bones. Clinical consequences include telecanthus (widening of the interorbital distance caused by rupture of the medial canthal ligament), transection of the nasolacrimal system associated with epiphora or lacrimal mucocele, and CSF rhinorrhea.
- LeFort has classified maxillary fractures into three basic forms of **LeFort injuries** based on laboratory experiments on skulls (Fig. 4.32). Although these individual injuries may exist in isolation, more commonly, combinations of the ZMC and LeFort I, II, or III fractures occur (Fig. 4.33).
  - **LeFort I** (transmaxillary fracture) extends across maxillary antra, through the nasal septum and the pterygoid plates. The maxilla is free from the rest of the facial bones (floating palate) and is usually displaced posteriorly. LeFort fractures more commonly occur bilaterally. This fracture spares the orbit.
  - **LeFort II** (pyramidal fracture) starts at the bridge of the nose and extends obliquely lateral to the nasal cavity, traversing the medial wall of the orbit, the floor of the orbit, the inferior orbital rims, the maxillary antra, and the pterygoid plates. It results in disarticulation (usually posteriorly) of the nose and maxilla from the remainder of the face. This fracture is characterized by involvement of the floor and medial wall of the orbit.
  - **LeFort III** (cranial-facial separation) fracture lines run from the nasofrontal area across the medial, posterior, and lateral orbital walls, the zygomatic arch, and through the pterygoid plates. The nose, zygoma, and maxilla are disarticulated from the skull. This fracture is distinguished by the lateral orbital wall involvement.
- In the trauma setting, **mandible injuries** can be single or multiple, unilateral or bilateral with presence of fractures and/or dislocations. Fractures can range from nondisplaced to severely displaced and comminuted. If the mandibular (inferior alveolar) canal, which conveys the inferior alveolar nerve, is involved by fracture, this should be reported. Additionally, injury to adjacent teeth, including loosening and/or fracture, should be commented on, because in the obtunded patient, these can be aspirated and result in future complications. The temporomandibular joint should be assessed for displacement, keeping in mind physiologic anterior subluxation of the condylar head relative to the glenoid fossa in the open mouth position. A 3D surface-rendered reformation can be very useful to the clinician when surgical reconstruction is being planned (see Fig. 4.33).

## TRAUMATIC CRANIAL NERVE INJURY

- Cranial nerve injury occur after head trauma, and knowledge of the anatomy is useful in the search for the lesion. This may present on imaging as focal absence of or edema within the affected nerve or may be implied with edema within adjacent soft tissues.
- The olfactory bulb and tract can be injured in frontal brain trauma or from surgery. This can result in anosmia. Associated gyrus rectus injury from gliding trauma along the anterior cranial fossa floor can be seen.
- Fractures of the optic canal/orbital apex or direct injuries to the optic nerve result in visual loss (injury to the optic nerve). Chiasmal injury has been reported secondary to mechanical, contusive, compressive, or ischemic mechanisms. Fractures of the sella, clinoid processes, sphenoid sinus walls, or facial bones should initiate a careful evaluation of the optic nerve and chiasm. Also, be mindful of associated pituitary stalk or hypothalamic injuries.
- Third nerve injury can occur in the absence of skull fracture from rootlet avulsion and distal fascicular damage secondary to a shearing type mechanism. It is also stretched during downward transtentorial herniation (DTTH). Hemorrhage at the exit site of the nerve and high intensity in the midbrain can be identified by MR. Horner syndrome from traumatic carotid dissection should also be considered with third nerve symptoms. Duret hemorrhages in the brain stem may injure the third nerve nucleus.
- Isolated fourth nerve palsy is common after TBI. The trochlear nerve may be compressed with DTTH as it runs through the perimesencephalic cistern.
- The trigeminal nerve can be injured in orbital floor, roof, or apex fractures as well as central skull base injuries.

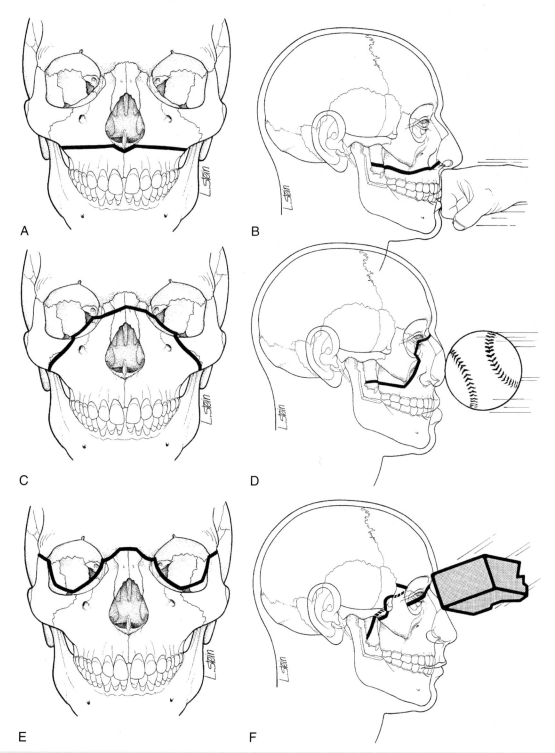

**Fig. 4.32 LeFort fractures.** (A) Frontal view of LeFort I fracture. (B) Lateral view of LeFort I fracture. (C) Frontal view of LeFort II fracture. (D) Lateral view of LeFort II fracture. (E) Frontal view of LeFort III fracture. (F) Lateral view of LeFort III fracture.

The pterygopalatine fossa, with its branches of the maxillary nerve (V-2), may be injured with the pterygoid plate fractures seen in the LeFort classification.

■ The sixth cranial nerve can be affected from basilar skull fractures (Dorello canal), and injuries to the cavernous sinus/orbital apex or secondary to increased intracranial pressure/hydrocephalus. It has been acknowledged to be particularly sensitive to injury because of its long intracranial course.

■ The seventh nerve can also be injured from otic capsule violating fractures through the petrous bone involving the facial canal (see Chapter 11). Associated injuries will

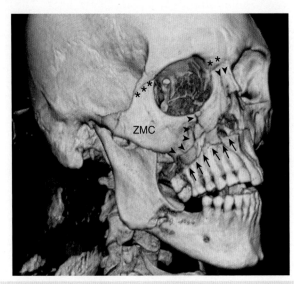

**Fig. 4.33 Facial smash.** Three-dimensional surface-rendered reconstruction of the face says it all and shows coexistence of multiple facial injuries simultaneously. LeFort I injury is indicated by *black arrows*, LeFort II injury is indicated by *black arrowheads*, and LeFort III injury is indicated by *black asterisks*. Zygomaticomaxillary complex (ZMC) fracture is present, with the separated fragment indicated by ZMC. There is a comminuted displaced fracture of the mandible as well.

include disruption of the ossicular chain, hematotympanum, otorrhea, and injury to the temporomandibular joint. Mechanisms of posttraumatic peripheral facial nerve palsy include transection, extrinsic compression by bony fragment or hematoma, or intrinsic compression within the facial canal secondary to intraneural hematoma/edema.

■ Cochlear nerve avulsion after head trauma is extremely rare but has been reported in the literature.

■ Fractures of the jugular foramen and hypoglossal canal, although uncommon, are frequently associated with IX to XI and XII injuries, respectively. Carotid dissection may lead to sheath hematomas that may also injure these nerves. PICA injury during downward cerebellar herniation can lead to lateral medullary infarcts, which may affect the lower cranial nerve nuclei.

# 5 Infectious and Noninfectious Inflammatory Disease of the Brain

KAREN BUCH

## Relevant Anatomy

- Infectious and inflammatory diseases of the brain often involve the meninges that overly the brain. There are three membrane layers covering the brain (from outer to inner layer): dura mater, arachnoid mater, and pia mater (Fig. 5.1).
- Dura mater is also referred to as the pachymeninges.
  - There are two layers of tough connective tissue: the outer layer adheres to the skull (periosteum); the inner layer reflects to give rise to the tentorium cerebelli, falx cerebri, diaphragma sellae, and falx cerebelli, which contain the venous sinuses.
- The space between the inner table of the skull and the dura mater is epidural space.
- The subdural space sits between the dural covering and arachnoid and contains bridging veins.
- Beneath the subdural space are two layers called arachnoid mater and pia mater, which make up the leptomeninges.
  - Arachnoid is a delicate outer layer and parallels the dura.
  - Subarachnoid space separates arachnoid mater from pia mater, with cerebrospinal fluid (CSF) in-between.
  - Pia adheres to the brain and spinal cord and carries a vast network of blood vessels.

## Imaging Techniques/Protocols

### MAGNETIC RESONANCE IMAGING

- Magnetic resonance imaging (MRI) is the preferred imaging modality if central nervous system (CNS) infection is suspected because of its far greater sensitivity for detecting meningeal disease. If MRI is not an option, computed tomography (CT) with and/or without contrast could be a reasonable alternative.
- Contrast enhancement is very useful in detecting the extent of infection and inflammation at the meninges or parenchyma on T1-weighted images (T1WI) or postcontrast fluid-attenuated inversion recovery (FLAIR) sequences.
- Diffusion restriction within brain lesions and extra-axial spaces can be a very useful finding in determining whether a fluid collection is purulent or not. Some forms of encephalitis lead to cytotoxic edema, which also restricts diffusion.
- FLAIR images can also be very useful in detecting parenchymal signal changes of infection/inflammation. High signal in the CSF on FLAIR may be because of blood products or infection.

## Pathology

### EPIDURAL ABSCESS

- Epidural abscesses arise from infection from operative beds or from inflammation arising from the mastoid bones, paranasal sinuses, infected skull, or by direct open wound inoculation. Infections can extend into the overlying scalp, and complications can include cerebral venous sinus thrombosis and adjacent encephalitis.
- Imaging findings include an extra-axial collection, lentiform in shape and confined by sutures (Fig. 5.2). The collection may have a mass effect on the subjacent brain parenchyma.
- On CT, you can appreciate a focal epidural mass of low to intermediate density, which can show rim enhancement if contrast is administered.
- On MRI, the collection will show low intensity or isointensity on T1WI, iso-high intensity on T2/FLAIR, diffusion restriction, and peripheral enhancement on postcontrast T1WI.

### SUBDURAL EMPYEMA

- This consists of a purulent infection in the potential subdural space with numerous potential causes (Box 5.1).
- Proposed mechanisms for formation include a rupture of infectious material from the arachnoid villus into the subdural space, extension from phlebitic bridging veins (in the setting of meningitis), hematogenous dissemination and seeding, direct extension from the subarachnoid space or extracranial infections, or by iatrogenic means (e.g., surgeries, ventriculostomy catheters, pressure bolts, subdural grids).
- Clinical signs and symptoms include fever, vomiting, meningismus, seizures, and signs of increased intracranial pressure. Mortality is high, reported between 12% and 40%.
- As with epidural hematoma, there are dangerous complications, including venous thrombosis or brain abscess (develops in about 10% of patients), and outcome depends on prompt treatment with antibiotics and drainage.
- Imaging features include an extra-axial collection overlying cerebral convexities, with associated mass effect on subjacent brain parenchyma if large enough.
- On CT, you can see a low to isodense extra-axial fluid collection conforming to the shape of the adjacent brain parenchyma, which can show rim enhancement if contrast is administered (Fig. 5.3).

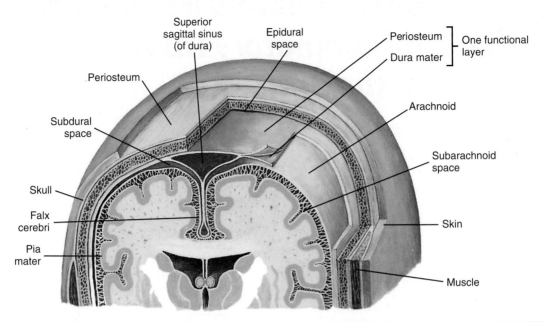

**Fig. 5.1 Meninges.** Schematic demonstrates major meningeal layers, including dura, arachnoid, and pia mater, and their anatomic relationships with each other. (From Thibodeau GA, Patton KT. *Anatomy and Physiology.* 5th ed. St. Louis: Mosby; 2003:376, 379.)

- On MRI, the collection will show low intensity or isointensity on T1WI, iso-high intensity on T2/FLAIR, diffusion restriction, and peripheral enhancement on postcontrast T1WI.

## LEPTOMENINGITIS

- This is an infection of pia and arachnoid mater, developing from hematogenous seeding from distant infectious focus or from direct extension from sinusitis, orbital cellulitis, or mastoiditis.
- Clinical signs and symptoms relate to patient age.
- Infants/neonates can show fussiness or poor feeding, and it may occur because of delivery, chorioamnionitis, immaturity, or iatrogenic infections (e.g., catheters, inhalation therapy equipment), with causative organisms including gram-negative bacilli, group B *Streptococcus*, and *Listeria monocytogenes*.
- Young children and adults present with fever, headache, photophobia, neck pain, and cranial neuropathies, with *Streptococcus pneumoniae* and *Neisseria meningitidis* as the most common organisms.
- Elderly patients may present with confusion, depressed levels of consciousness, and stupor.
- Imaging may be normal on CT and MRI in the early stages or with early treatment.
- On MRI, sometimes congestion and hyperemia of pia and arachnoid mater can be seen. Sterile subdural effusions may develop (more often in very young children), which will not show diffusion restriction or prominent rim enhancement.
- Diffusion-restricting material within the sulci and incomplete fluid suppression in the subarachnoid spaces on FLAIR can reflect purulent material, and leptomeningeal enhancement can be seen on postcontrast T1WI or FLAIR (Fig. 5.4). Leptomeningeal enhancement should not be confused with pachymeningeal enhancement; the latter refers to enhancement along the dural reflections overlying the cerebral and cerebellar convexities and the tentorial leaflets

(Fig. 5.5). There are several clinical considerations for the two patterns of enhancement.

---

**TEACHING POINTS**

Conditions That Produce Pachymeningeal and Leptomeningeal Enhancement

**Pachymeningeal**

Cerebrospinal fluid leak
Idiopathic hypertrophic pachymeningitis
Sarcoidosis
Metastases, including those involving the skull
Shunting
Postsurgical reactive change
Spontaneous intracranial hypotension

**Leptomeningeal**

Acute stroke
Leptomeningeal infection
Metastases
Sarcoidosis
Subarachnoid hemorrhage

---

- Complications (Box 5.2) include cerebritis (infection of subjacent brain parenchyma with or without abscess), cerebral edema resulting in herniation syndromes, vasculitis with or without infarctions, venous sinus thrombosis, infected pseudoaneurysm, communicating hydrocephalus from impaired CSF drainage, and hearing loss related to labyrinthitis ossificans from the spread of infection to involve endolymph.

## PYOGENIC BRAIN ABSCESS

- Most commonly, brain abscesses arise from hematogenous dissemination from a primary infectious site, such as in the setting of intravenous (IV) drug abuse,

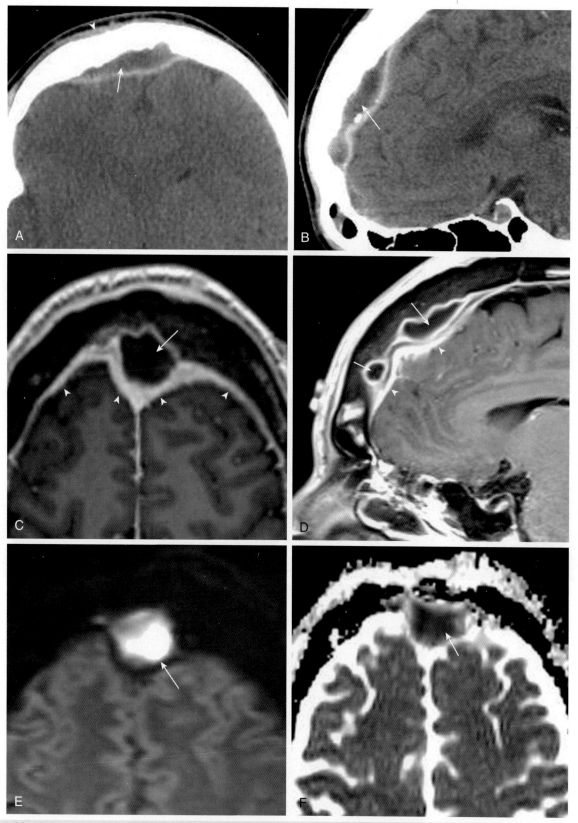

**Fig. 5.2 Epidural abscess resulting from frontal skull osteomyelitis.** On (A) axial and (B) sagittal contrast-enhanced computed tomography, a rim-enhancing fluid collection *(arrow)* that crosses the midline is noted, indicating organized abscess in the epidural compartment. There is overlying scalp swelling *(arrowhead)*. (C) On axial and sagittal (D) postcontrast T1, the abscess *(arrows)* is again demonstrated. The location above the dura is confirmed *(arrowheads)*. (E) Diffusion restriction reflecting purulent material within the collection is shown on diffusion-weighted imaging (DWI) and (F) apparent diffusion coefficient (ADC) map *(arrows)*.

## Box 5.1    Causes of Subdural Empyema

Hematogenous dissemination
Osteomyelitis of calvarium
Otomastoiditis
Paranasal sinusitis
Postcraniotomy infection/calvarial osteomyelitis
Posttraumatic
Purulent bacterial meningitis
Thrombophlebitis

endocarditis, and sepsis, but can also occur from direct adjacent spread of infection from otologic and paranasal sinus infections (Box 5.3). That said, in up to 25% of cases, no predisposing factors are identified.

- Infection progresses in stages: (1) early cerebritis (1–3 days), (2) late cerebritis (4–9 days), (3) early capsule formation (10–13 days), (4) late capsule formation (14+ days).
- Complications include dissemination of abscess throughout the brain parenchyma, development of meningoencephalitis and/or ventriculitis, herniation from mass effect from abscess and surrounding edema, and obstructive hydrocephalus.

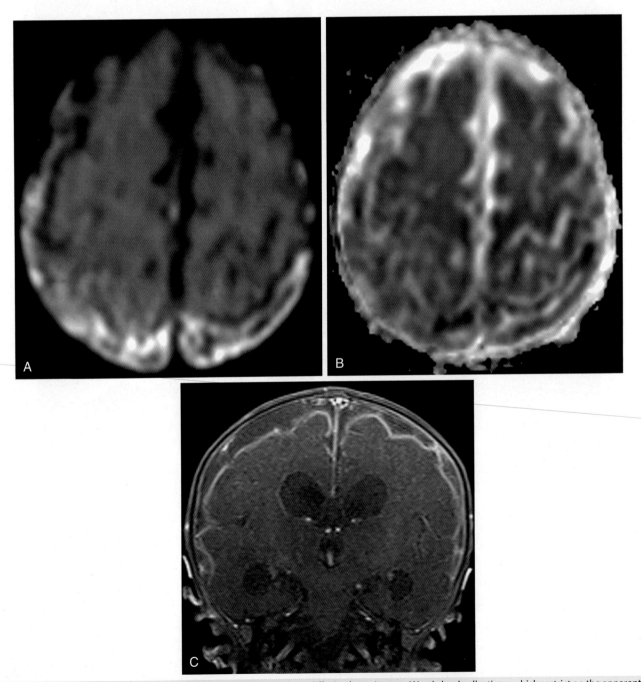

**Fig. 5.3  Subdural empyema.** In this newborn with meningitis, there are diffusion hyperintense (A) subdural collections, which restrict on the apparent diffusion coefficient (*ADC*) map indicating purulent material (B). On coronal T1 postcontrast image (C), the subdural collections show rim enhancement, confirming bilateral subdural empyemas. Note leptomeningeal enhancement, indicating concomitant leptomeningitis.

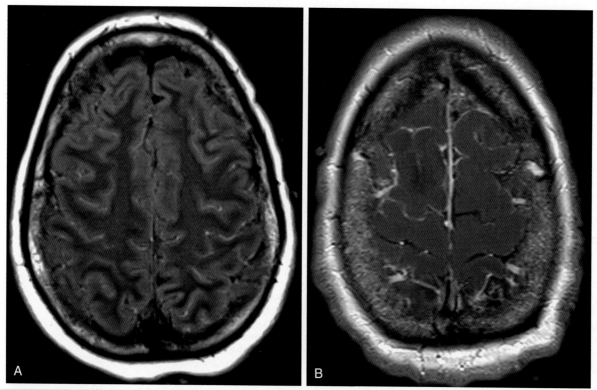

**Fig. 5.4 Leptomeningitis.** (A) Fluid-attenuated inversion recovery (FLAIR) scan shows incomplete suppression of cerebrospinal fluid (CSF) signal within frontoparietal sulci which can be seen when blood, purulent material, or tumor reside within the leptomeninges. (B) Postcontrast T1 image shows enhancement in these sulci. In the context of headache, fever, and elevated white blood cell count, these findings are consistent with meningitis.

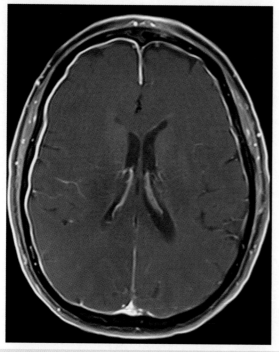

**Fig. 5.5 Pachymeningitis.** Note the smooth thick enhancement of the dura mater over both cerebral convexities, right more so than left, distinct from the leptomeningeal pattern shown in Fig. 5.4. This was biopsy proven IgG4-related pachymeningitis.

## Box 5.2    Complications of Leptomeningeal Infection

Arterial infarction
Atrophy (late)
Basilar adhesions
Encephalitis
Epidural empyema
Focal abscess formation
Hydrocephalus
  Communicating
  Obstructive
Subdural empyema
Subdural hygroma
Vasculitis
Venous thrombosis/venous infarction
Ventriculitis

surrounding edema and peripheral enhancement on postcontrast imaging.

- On MRI, early cerebritis can manifest as high T2 signal within the involved parenchyma, usually with patchy diffusion restriction. As the abscess organizes, the lesion will show low T1 signal intensity and high T2/FLAIR signal intensity centrally while the developing abscess capsule shows hypointensity (Fig. 5.6) with adjacent high signal from surrounding edema. The organized abscess shows diffusion restriction and peripheral enhancement. Keep in mind there is a broad differential for rim-enhancing lesions (Box 5.4).

- Head CT can appear normal in early cerebritis, but later, low density with irregular rim enhancement can develop. With time, the collection organizes and can appear as a low density, rounded intra-axial lesion, with

- The double rim sign described on susceptibility-weighted imaging (SWI) and T2WI can indicate an abscess. It consists of two concentric rims surrounding the abscess cavity, with the outer one being hypointense and the inner one hyperintense. This feature may help distinguish abscesses from necrotic glioblastomas.

## VENTRICULITIS/EPENDYMITIS

- This is an infection of the ependymal lining from meningitis, occurring as a postoperative complication, direct inoculation from trauma/penetrating injury, or an extension of a leptomeningeal infection.
- On CT, ventricular enlargement including either the entire ventricular system or parts of it can be seen. If acutely obstructed, transependymal CSF flow can be seen in the periventricular white matter as low density along the margins of the entrapped ventricle.

---

### Box 5.3    Causes of Cerebral Abscess

**Direct Extension**
Meningitis
Otomastoiditis
Paranasal sinusitis
Via dermal sinus tracts

**Hematogenous Dissemination**
Arteriovenous shunts (Osler Weber Rendu)
Cardiac (endocarditis, infected thrombi)
Drug abuse
Pulmonary infection
Sepsis

**Trauma**
Penetrating injury
Postsurgical
Immunosuppression

---

### Box 5.4    Differential Diagnosis of Ring Enhancement

Metastasis
High-grade astrocytoma
Demyelinating plaque
Abscess
Radiation necrosis
Tuberculoma
Infarction
Lymphoma
Subacute parenchymal hematoma
Thrombosed aneurysm

---

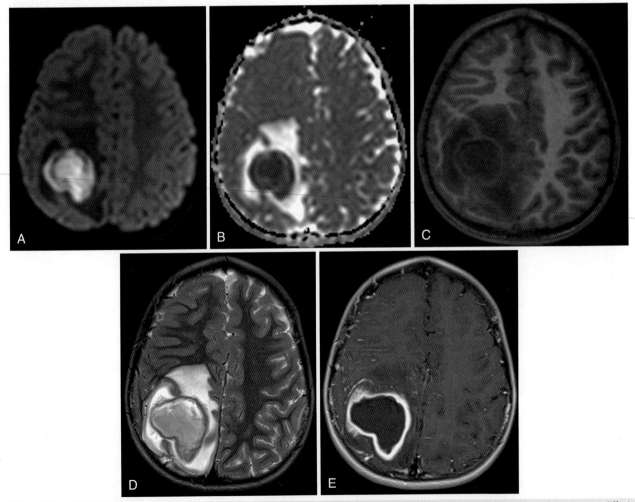

**Fig. 5.6  Mature abscess.** There is a large diffusion hyperintense (A) mass in the right parietal lobe showing restriction (B) on the apparent diffusion coefficient (ADC) map. High precontrast T1 (C) and dark T2 signal (D) are noted along the rim of the mass, and on the (E) postcontrast T1-weighted image (T1WI), there is thick rim enhancement, characteristic features of an organized abscess.

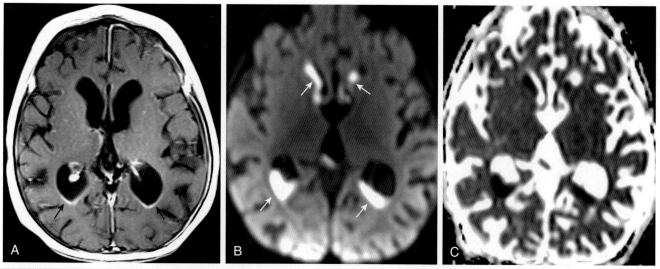

**Fig. 5.7 Ependymitis.** (A) Enhancement of the ependyma *(arrows)* on postcontrast T1-weighted imaging (T1WI) is accompanied by (B) the diffusion-weighted image and (C) apparent diffusion coefficient (ADC) map showing proteinaceous material layering in the ventricles *(arrows)*.

**Table 5.1** Location and Favored Pathogen

| Location | Favored Pathogen | Useful Hint |
|---|---|---|
| Cerebellum/brain stem | *Listeria* | Hard to culture |
| Perivascular spaces | *Cryptococcus* | AIDS host |
| Deep gray matter | Tick/mosquito borne | Very sick |
| Basal meninges | TB | Endemic locale |
| Periventricular | TORCH | Neonate, calcifications |
| Cavernous sinus | Fungi | Spread from sinusitis |
| Subdural space | *H. flu* | Effusions with meningitis |

*AIDS,* Acquired immunodeficiency syndrome; *H. flu, Haemophilus influenzae; TB,* tuberculosis; *TORCH,* toxoplasmosis, other infections, rubella, cytomegalovirus, herpes simplex.

- On MRI, generalized or partial ventriculomegaly can also be seen. Periventricular high signal on T2 images indicate transependymal flow of CSF. On diffusion-weighed imaging (DWI), restricted-diffusion layering in the ventricles reflects purulent material. On postcontrast T1WI, curvilinear enhancement along the ependymal surface of the ventricles with or without choroid plexus enhancement can be seen (Fig. 5.7). On SWI in neonates, you may see periventricular calcifications after ventriculitis.

## Specific Types/Patterns of Intracranial Infections

There are innumerable pathogens that affect the CNS, and it is often not possible to identify the infectious pathogen by imaging. We will discuss the most commonly seen infections and those with recognizable imaging patterns to help narrow your differential diagnosis when intracranial infection is suspected (Tables 5.1 and 5.2).

**Table 5.2** Characteristic Targets of Viral Encephalitides

| Location | Favored Virus | Useful Hint |
|---|---|---|
| Medial temporal lobe, insula, cingulum | HSV I | May bleed, bilateral |
| Holohemispheric, cortical | HSV 2 | Neonatal, cystic encephalomalacic |
| MCA infarcts | VZV | Vasculitis |
| Brain stem and cerebellum | EBV | Mono symptoms, nodes, nasopharyngeal cancer |
| Brain stem, deep gray matter | EEE | Whinny |
| Deep gray matter, brain stem | Japanese | Giant panda sign |
| White matter, atrophy | HIV | Opportunistic infections |
| Periventricular, ependymitis | CMV | Congenital migrational anomalies |
| Subcortical white matter | JC virus | Immune compromised |
| Small vessel infarcts in white matter | Nipah | Bat-borne |
| Myelitis, central brain and deep gray matter | West Nile virus | |
| Substantia nigra | St Louis encephalitis | |
| Basal ganglia, brain stem | Rabies | Tick bite |
| Cortical edema, basal ganglia disease | Measles | Rash |

*CMV,* Cytomegalovirus; *EBV,* Epstein-Barr virus; *EEE,* eastern equine encephalitis; *HIV,* human immunodeficiency virus; *HSV,* herpes simplex virus; *MCA,* middle cerebral artery; *VZV,* varicella zoster virus.

### SEPTIC EMBOLI

- Showering emboli produce infarcts from infected material usually from infective endocarditis (usually *S. aureus*), IV drug use, thrombophlebitis with right to left cardiac shunts, or infected catheters. Although the imaging

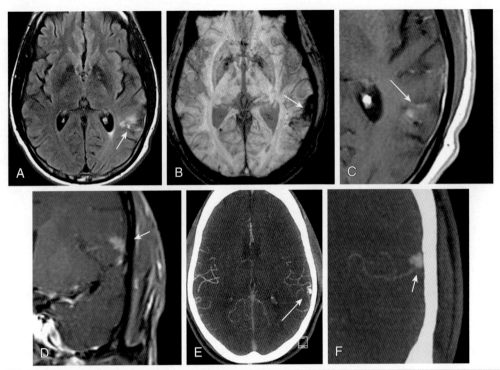

**Fig. 5.8** *Streptococcus viridans* **bacterial endocarditis with septic aneurysm.** (A) Fluid-attenuated inversion recovery (FLAIR) shows a wedge-shaped abnormality in the temporal lobe *(arrow)*. (B) Hemorrhagic component is confirmed on susceptibility-weighted imaging *(arrow)*. (C) Postgadolinium, there also is meningeal enhancement *(arrow)*, (D, *arrows*) which is confirmed on the coronal T1-weighted imaging (T1WI). (E) Axial and (F) magnified axial computed tomography (CT) angiography images show middle cerebral artery distal mycotic aneurysm *(arrows)*.

features of the infarcts are similar to infarcts of other causes on CT and MRI, the distribution involving multiple vascular territories, infarcts of different ages, with or without enhancement should raise concern for an embolic source. Sometimes rim enhancement is superimposed.

- Disease can progress with developed cerebral abscess, mycotic aneurysms (distal vessels; Fig. 5.8), and obliterative vasculitis.

## HERPES SIMPLEX ENCEPHALITIS

- As opposed to cerebritis (a precursor to abscess formation) encephalitis refers to inflammation of the brain due to viral, autoimmune, or paraneoplastic causes. Herpes simplex viral encephalitis is the most common cause of fatal endemic encephalitis in the United States, with high mortality of 70% if untreated. Symptoms include acute confusion, coma, seizures, fevers, viral prodrome, and focal neurologic deficits (<30% cases).
- Infections occur from both the oral strain (herpes simplex virus 1 [HSV1]) and genital strain (herpes simplex virus 2 [HSV2]).
- HSV1 presents as fulminant necrotizing encephalitis in children and adults with a predilection for temporal lobes, insula, the orbitofrontal region, and the cingulate gyrus. Although hypoattenuation in these regions might be appreciable by CT, parenchymal changes are best seen on MRI as T2 FLAIR hyperintensity and swelling, with or without contrast enhancement (Fig. 5.9). These regions develop encephalomalacia in the chronic phase.
- HSV2, on the other hand, affects neonates, on the basis of transplacental infection or infection from the birth canal. Microcephaly, microphthalmia, and retinal

dysplasia can be seen (Box 5.5) with long-term sequela of seizures and motor and cognitive deficits. There may be gross destruction of the brain in a variety of diffuse patterns.

- CSF sampling with viral polymerase chain reaction (PCR) assays is an important component of diagnosis.
- On CT, you can see geographic hypodensity early and parenchymal calcifications late. There may be hyperdense components from intracranial hemorrhage.
- On MRI, you can see high T2 signal in affected parenchyma with swelling and associated geographic-restricted diffusion, which may be confounded by superimposed ictal-related changes. Enhancement, either meningeal and parenchymal, can be seen. On SWI, areas of intracranial hemorrhage can be visualized.
- On CT/MRI, late stages of disease show marked volume loss and/or multicystic encephalomalacia.

## EASTERN EQUINE ENCEPHALITIS

- This is a mosquito-borne arboviral infection. Patients present with a short typical viral prodrome followed by altered mental status and seizures.
- On MRI, high-intensity T2WI lesions in the basal ganglia, thalamus, and brain stem have been observed early in the course of the disease (Fig. 5.10). Usually the disease is bilateral, but it may be asymmetric. Other less common areas of involvement are the periventricular and cortical regions. Meningeal enhancement can be seen.
- Imaging findings are not specific for eastern equine encephalitis and have been described in Japanese encephalitis, measles, mumps, echovirus 25 encephalitis, and even Creutzfeldt-Jakob disease.

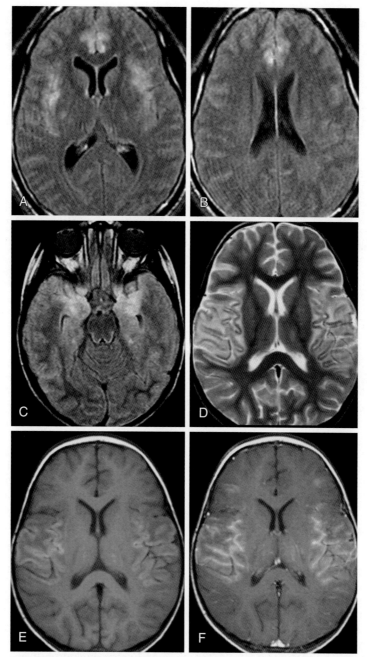

**Fig. 5.9 Herpes simplex I gallery.** Case 1 (A and B): There is high signal in both temporal lobes, in bilateral insula and cingulum, on fluid-attenuated inversion recovery (FLAIR). (C) More inferiorly, we can see the amygdala involved on FLAIR as well. Case 2: (D) Later on in the disease process in a different patient, on T2-weighted imaging (T2WI), in both temporal lobes, high signal is present. The brightness pregadolinium suggests laminar necrosis (E), and there is leptomeningeal enhancement on postgadolinium T1-weighted imaging (T1WI).

## Box 5.5  Features of Neonatal Herpes Simplex Infection

Atrophy
Encephalomalacia with cysts (late)
Hydrocephalus
Increased density in cortical gray matter
Intracranial calcification from punctate to gyriform
Microcephaly
Microphthalmia
Multiple cysts

## JAPANESE ENCEPHALITIS

■ This disease occurs throughout Asia, usually in the summer and early fall, with viral vector transmitted by mosquito. Patients present with fevers and headache with rapid progression to encephalitis and coma.

■ On MRI, classic T2WI/FLAIR high-intensity, bilateral lesions in the thalami and putamina are typically reported, as well as tegmental disease, which spares the red nuclei and corticospinal tract, resulting in a "giant panda sign" in the brain stem (Fig. 5.11). Signal

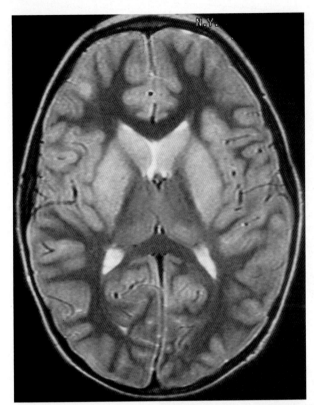

**Fig. 5.10 Eastern equine encephalitis.** The T2-weighted image (T2WI) demonstrates increased intensity in the deep gray structures. (Courtesy R. Zimmerman, MD.)

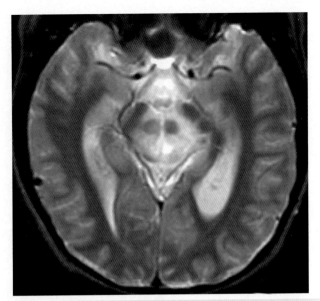

**Fig. 5.11 Giant panda sign in Japanese encephalitis.** Abnormal signal in the brain stem is seen on the fluid-attenuated inversion recovery (FLAIR). Can you make out the giant panda bear? (Courtesy Mai-Lan Ho, UCSF.)

change may also involve the brain stem, hippocampus, thalamus, basal ganglia, and white matter. Usually no enhancement is observed.

## AIDS/HUMAN IMMUNODEFICIENCY VIRUS

- Human immunodeficiency virus (HIV) infects and disrupts function of the immune system, and HIV disease progresses to acquired immunodeficiency syndrome (AIDS) in later stages. Approximately 40% of patients with AIDS have neurologic symptoms during life. CNS complications of HIV/AIDS include infections, neoplasms, neurodegenerative disease, vascular disease, and inflammatory and treatment-related changes.

### Neurodegenerative: AIDS Dementia Complex/HIV Encephalopathy

- Clinically manifested by a subcortical dementia with cognitive, motor, and behavioral deficits, resulting from HIV infection itself or HIV-induced vasculopathy, HIV encephalopathy is seen in patients during the end stage of their disease.
- On MRI, periventricular high signal abnormalities on T2WI/FLAIR in periventricular white matter and deep gray matter and global atrophy are the typical imaging findings (Fig. 5.12). The periventricular predilection is in contradistinction to the subcortical white matter involvement favored by progressive multifocal leukoencephalopathy (PML; see later). No mass effect or enhancement is seen in the involved regions.

- There is no significant correlation between the imaging findings and the state of immunosuppression, the severity of histopathologic white matter changes, atrophy, and the severity of AIDS dementia.
- Protease inhibitor therapy as part of a combination highly active antiretroviral (HAART) drug therapy can result in regression or stabilization of periventricular and subcortical white matter signal intensity abnormalities seen in HIV encephalopathy (see Figs. 5.12D–E).
- HIV encephalopathy can coexist with infectious, inflammatory, and neoplastic manifestations of HIV/AIDS.

### Infectious: Opportunistic Pathogens

- Opportunistic pathogens take advantage of the host's compromised immune response and, in the early days of the HIV pandemic, were commonly the cause of patient demise. In the more recent past, at least in developed countries, opportunistic infections in the CNS are becoming less common, thanks to HAART. Opportunistic pathogens include but are not limited to toxoplasmosis (most commonly), cryptococcosis, tuberculosis, and cytomegalovirus (CMV). These are discussed individually later in this chapter.

### Inflammatory: Progressive Multifocal Leukoencephalopathy

- This is a demyelinating process in which the reactivated JC virus infects myelin sheaths of oligodendrocytes. The key finding in PML is non–masslike, typically nonenhancing high signal intensity on T2WI/FLAIR in the peripheral white matter (although PML can involve the cortex). Occasionally, lesions are noted to cross the corpus callosum. Diffusion restriction may be seen at sites of active demyelination.
- PML characteristically involves the subcortical U-fiber as opposed to HIV or CMV, which tend to involve the white matter more centrally.

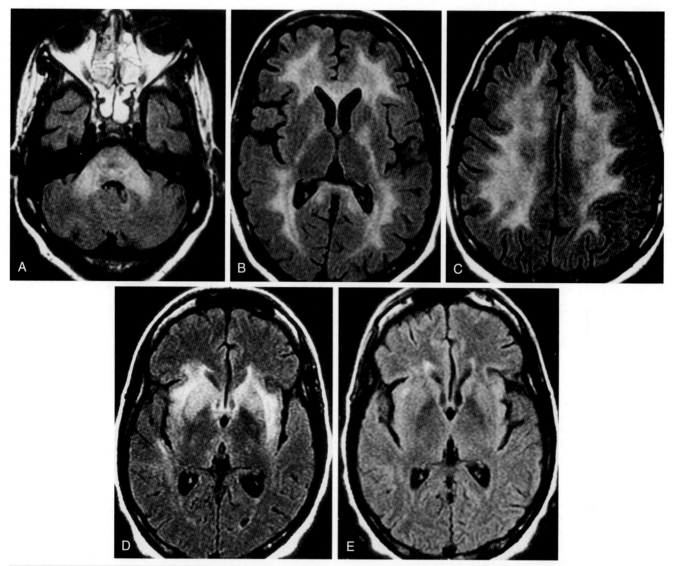

**Fig. 5.12 Pastiche of acquired immunodeficiency syndrome (AIDS).** Case 1: (A) Brain stem abnormal signal intensity is well seen on the fluid-attenuated inversion recovery. (B) Diffuse bilateral symmetric white matter involvement is present in both cerebral hemispheres. (C) Centrum semiovale disease generally spares subcortical U-fiber white matter. Case 2: (D) Basal ganglia involvement was present in this woman with dementia from AIDS. (E) After highly active antiretroviral therapy (HAART), note that the gray matter disease has improved dramatically.

## Inflammatory: Immune Reconstitution Inflammatory Syndrome (IRIS)

- Immune reconstitution inflammatory syndrome (IRIS) can occur among HIV/AIDS patients within 2 months of initiating HAART treatment and appears as a fulminant inflammatory immune reconstitution response or may occur secondary to subclinical opportunistic infection. Symptoms progress despite improvement in immune function. On MRI, enhancing lesions with mass effect are seen or imaging stigmata of underlying opportunistic infection may be evident. This is most commonly seen in the scenario of a PML-like picture which, complicated by IRIS, develops masslike enhancing disease that is more aggressive. Upon cessation of HAART, the imaging picture stabilizes (Fig. 5.13). Interestingly, IRIS is now increasingly seen in other clinical scenarios such as multiple sclerosis patients treated with immunomodulators like natalizumab.

## Vascular: Cerebral Infarction

- Frequency of clinical cerebral infarction in AIDS is between 0.5% to 8%, whereas the autopsy frequency is between 19% and 34%.
- The causes for infarction in HIV/AIDS are numerous and include altered vasoreactivity from HIV in combination with drug use (particularly cocaine), HIV vasculitis, infection (varicella-zoster, CMV, tuberculosis, cryptococcosis, syphilis, and toxoplasmosis), marantic endocarditis, disseminated intravascular coagulopathy, or hypoxia.

## Neoplasm: Lymphoma

- Primary CNS lymphoma of the brain has an incidence in AIDS patients of about 6%, although the condition is also seen in other types of immunosuppressed patients, particularly allograft recipients (heart, kidney).
- On CT, lymphoma may be isodense, hyperdense, or hypodense (in AIDS) on unenhanced CT. It is unusual

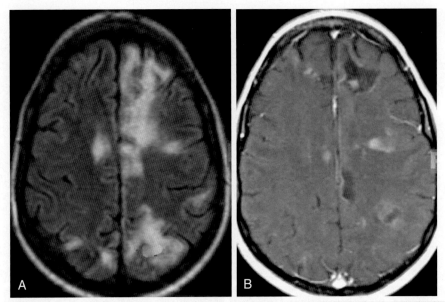

**Fig. 5.13  Immune reconstitution inflammatory syndrome.** (A) This patient with progressive multifocal leukoencephalopathy was undergoing treatment with HAART (highly active antiretroviral therapy), and the axial fluid-attenuated inversion recovery (FLAIR) image shows multiple foci of increased signal. On postcontrast T1-weighted imaging (T1WI) (B), there is associated enhancement.

for this lesion to demonstrate central necrosis except in AIDS. Most lesions enhance in a solid or ring fashion, although nonenhancing lymphoma has been reported. Lesions often show restricted diffusion.

- Imaging features can overlap with toxoplasmosis. Both processes may present with multiple lesions of various sizes (although toxoplasmosis abscesses tend to be more numerous and smaller than lymphoma), and either ring enhance or display solid enhancement.
- Distinguishing between lymphoma and toxoplasmosis is important because of the differences in treatment strategies. Lymphoma patients benefit from radiation therapy with more than a fourfold increase in survival rates over the untreated and delaying radiation to embark on a trial of antitoxoplasmosis therapy diminishes the benefit of radiation therapy. Of course, both conditions can coexist, making the diagnosis that much more complicated.
- High-density masses on noncontrast CT (not as frequent in AIDS lymphoma) and periventricular lesions with subependymal disease burden are findings suggestive of lymphoma. On MRI, lymphoma has a tendency to be isointense to hypointense relative to white matter on T2WI/FLAIR, whereas toxoplasmosis is more likely to be hyperintense on T2WI/FLAIR.
- Toxoplasmosis can have a low-intensity ring surrounded by high-intensity on T2WI/FLAIR with ring enhancement (Fig. 5.14). Toxoplasmosis has a propensity for the basal ganglia and a predilection for hemorrhage, particularly in the healing phase, which is not the case with CNS lymphoma (except after steroids or radiation therapy).
- Magnetic resonance perfusion measurement is another technique that has been suggested to differentiate lymphoma (increased perfusion) from toxoplasmosis (decreased perfusion). Thallium-201 single-photon emission CT (SPECT) has been reported to show abnormal uptake in lymphoma but not in toxoplasmosis. Similarly, CNS fluorodeoxyglucose (FDG) positron

emission tomography (PET) has shown uptake ratios that are significantly lower in infections, including toxoplasmosis, compared with lymphoma.

## PEDIATRIC AIDS

- Although only 1% to 2% of AIDS occurs in the pediatric population, 80% of these cases have CNS involvement, including acquired microcephaly, diffuse cerebral atrophy, calcifications, and HIV encephalitis. This is usually because of in utero or peripartum infections.
- On CT, calcifications are uncommon before the age of 1 among the general population but are a prominent feature of HIV infection in children (but not in adults). The calcifications are located in the basal ganglia, periventricular, frontal white matter, and cerebellum (Fig. 5.15).
- On MRI, vascular disease on the basis of hypoperfusion, thromboembolic disease, and infectious vasculitis can be seen. On magnetic resonance angiography (MRA), vascular ectasia, stenoses, and aneurysmal dilatation of the circle of Willis occurs with neonatal AIDS.
- Infections and lymphoma are uncommon in pediatric patients, whereas cerebral atrophy, basal ganglia calcification, white matter high-intensity on T2WI/FLAIR, and hemorrhage are the predominant findings in this population.
- Sinusitis and mastoiditis are common coexisting infections in HIV-positive children. Adenopathy and adenoidal hypertrophy, as one would expect, are seen on the scans too.

## CYTOMEGALOVIRUS

- Of the so-called perinatal TORCH infections (toxoplasmosis, other [syphilis, varicella zoster, parvovirus B19], rubella, CMV, and herpes), CMV is the most frequent

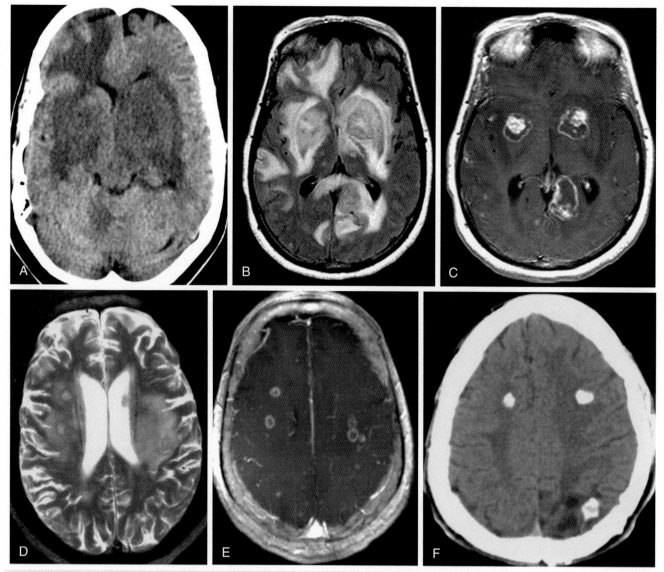

**Fig. 5.14** (A) Acute toxoplasmosis on computed tomography (CT) with basal ganglia low density seen on fluid-attenuated inversion recovery (B) as hyperintensity. Lesions show central nodular and rim enhancement on postgadolinium T1-weighted imaging (T1WI) (C). (D) In a different patient, lots of edema, seen associated with these lesions on T2, show postgadolinium ring enhancement (E). (F) Burnt-out, healed toxoplasmosis appear as numerous parenchymal calcifications on CT.

cause of fetal and neonatal viral infection. Transplacental CMV transmission occurs as a result of either recurrent or primary maternal infection. The mechanism of injury is ischemia because of insufficient fetal circulation, probably secondary to placentitis and secondary chronic perfusion insufficiency.

- CNS abnormalities associated with CMV include microcephaly, ocular defects, and deafness. Injury before 18 weeks results in agyria, and injury between 18 and 24 weeks results in polymicrogyria.
- Other findings in infants with CMV include atrophy, cerebellar hypoplasia, focal white matter lesions, hippocampal abnormalities, ventriculomegaly, hydranencephaly, porencephaly, paraventricular cysts, and gyral anomalies, including complete lissencephaly, pachygyria, microgyria, and localized cortical dysplasia (Fig. 5.16).

- CMV calcifications are usually limited to the subependymal region, whereas neonatal toxoplasmosis has calcifications not only in the periventricular region but also throughout the brain, especially the basal ganglia.
- Periventricular low density on CT or high-intensity on T2WI/FLAIR, although nonspecific, has also been reported in CMV.

## ZIKA VIRUS

- Zika is a flavivirus (transmitted to humans by mosquito bite) that has gained recent worldwide attention and may end up joining the ranks of the TORCH club.
- There is increasing evidence that pregnant women, when infected by Zika virus, can transmit it transplacentally to the fetus; a dramatic rising incidence of infants born with microcephaly in Brazil in 2015 was linked to the Zika virus infection in utero.

■ Although nonspecific to Zika, imaging findings can include parenchymal calcifications, ventriculomegaly, white matter hypoattenuation, disruption in cortical gyral development, and cerebellar hypoplasia.

## MYCOBACTERIAL/TUBERCULOSIS

■ Tuberculosis (TB) is caused by *Mycobacterium tuberculosis*, which typically infects the lungs but can spread systemically as well. Incidence has increased in recent years, in conjunction with AIDS and the emergence of drug-resistant strains of the bacillus. Approximately 5% to 10% of cases of tuberculosis have CNS involvement because of hematogenous dissemination of seeds in the leptomeninges and brain parenchyma, resulting in tuberculous meningitis and parenchymal tuberculomas (Fig. 5.17).

■ With tuberculous meningitis, the basal cisterns are most affected by exudative meningitis demonstrated by thick nodular enhancement on postcontrast T1WI. The enhancement can extend into the hemispheric fissures and over the cortical surfaces. In severe cases, this is evident even on CT. There is associated incomplete suppression of CSF signal on FLAIR and diffusion restriction, reflecting purulent material. Obstruction to normal CSF flow results in hydrocephalus, and leptomeningeal inflammation may also produce cranial nerve palsies, arteritis, and brain infarctions.

■ Tuberculomas are, in fact, the most common brain stem lesion in underdeveloped countries, although tuberculomas can present anywhere within the brain parenchyma. Tuberculomas may rupture into the subarachnoid space, resulting in tuberculous meningitis and meningoencephalitis.

■ The typical tuberculoma appears as a nodule with a small central area of high signal on T2WI/FLAIR or low density on CT. These nodules may be solitary but are commonly multiple and are associated with mass effect and edema. Small nodules (1–3 mm in diameter) can coalesce to form a large lesion.

■ On MRI, high-intensity may be observed in the wall of tuberculomas on T1WI and low intensity on T2WI/FLAIR (see Fig. 5.17F). Surrounding the nodule is high-intensity on T2WI/FLAIR or low density on CT. Ringlike enhancement (with irregular walls with variable thickness, leading

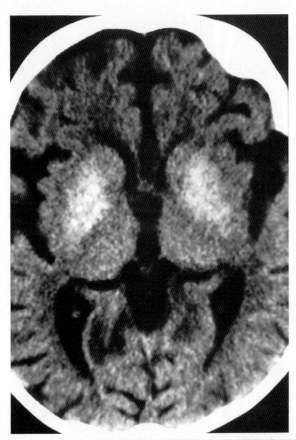

**Fig. 5.15 Pediatric acquired immunodeficiency syndrome (AIDS).** Calcification in the basal ganglia and atrophy on computed tomography, in a child with AIDS contracted neonatally.

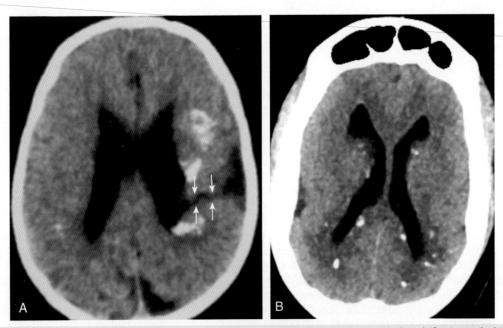

**Fig. 5.16 Congenital cytomegalovirus (CMV) infection.** (A) Computed tomography (CT) shows periventricular calcification and schizencephalic cleft *(arrows)*. (B) In a different patient, CMV calcifications, pachygyria, and hydrocephalus are present.

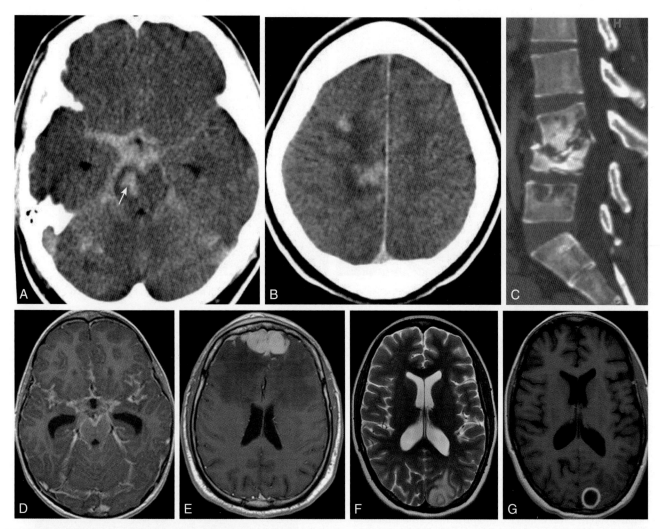

**Fig. 5.17 The many faces of tuberculosis (TB).** Case 1: (A) Note the coating of enhancement of the cisterns and midbrain on the postcontrast computed tomography (CT) image. A focus in right brain stem also enhances *(arrow)*. (B) Above this level are additional foci of parenchymal and leptomeningeal enhancement. Although the findings are nonspecific, when taken with the findings in the spine (C), with discitis-osteomyelitis and vertebral body collapse at L3-5 (Pott disease), TB in the brain is the most likely diagnosis. Case 2: (D) Different patient with leptomeningeal enhancement on magnetic resonance imaging (MRI), on this postcontrast T1-weighted image (T1WI). Note abnormal dilatation of the temporal horns, indicating hydrocephalus. Case 3: (E) Another patient with human immunodeficiency virus (HIV) and TB. In this case, there is masslike meningeal disease with significant edema in the adjacent brain. Case 4: Axial T2 (F) shows dark wall and postcontrast T1WI (G), showing ringlike enhancement in this patient with parenchymal tuberculoma.

to a "crenated" look) or nodular enhancement (which may have punctate nonenhancing centers) can be seen. As it enlarges, the tuberculoma may adhere to dura, causing hyperostosis and thus masquerading as a meningioma.

■ Follow-up imaging after appropriate antibiotic therapy shows that the tuberculous nodules decrease in size with residual small areas of punctate calcification on CT at the tuberculoma site.

## LISTERIA MONOCYTOGENES

■ This infection is a food-borne illness from uncooked meats and vegetables, unpasteurized milk and cheese, and smoked seafood.

■ CNS involvement occurs in the form of meningitis, meningoencephalitis, and, rarely, brain abscess. There is a particular predilection for involvement of the posterior fossa with abscess formation or rhombencephalitis (inflammation of the brain stem and cerebellum).

**TEACHING POINTS**

Differential Diagnosis of Rhombencephalitis

Acute disseminated encephalomyelitis
Brain stem tumor
Coccidioidomycosis
Legionnaire disease
*Listeria monocytogenes*
Lyme disease
Mycoplasma infection
Rickettsia
Tuberculosis
Viral diseases
    Adenovirus
    Arbovirus
    Influenza A

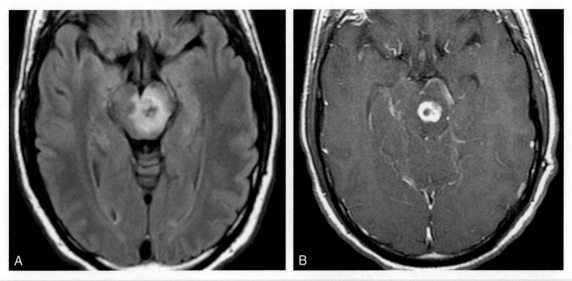

**Fig. 5.18** (A) *Listeria monocytogenes* rhombencephalitis. Fluid-attenuated inversion recovery (FLAIR) with high-intensity in brain stem is present in this patient. (B) A thick rim-enhancing abscess is present in the midbrain on postcontrast T1WI.

- Diagnosis of *Listeria* infection should be considered in patients with impaired cellular immunity (including chemotherapy and other related predisposing conditions, such as diabetes, alcoholism, renal transplantation, and AIDS) with meningitis or abscess (Fig. 5.18). Prompt initiation of antimicrobial therapy is critical because of high morbidity and mortality.

## LYME DISEASE

- This is an inflammatory disease that can involve multiple organ systems and is caused by spirochete (*Borrelia burgdorferi*) and transmitted most commonly by the deer tick (*Ixodes dammini*).
- There are three clinical stages: (1) constitutional symptoms and an expanding skin lesion (erythema chronicum migrans) (2) cardiac and neurologic problems (meningitis, radiculoneuropathy) occurring weeks to months after the initial infection, and (3) arthritis and chronic neurologic problems that are noted from months to years after infection. The stages may overlap or occur alone.
- Approximately 10% to 15% of patients with Lyme disease have CNS involvement, most commonly presenting with facial nerve palsy. In endemic areas (northeastern United States), it may account for two-thirds of childhood facial nerve palsy. Lyme disease may be associated with optic neuritis. Lyme encephalopathy has been characterized as a cognitive disturbance of mild to moderate memory and learning problems, sometimes accompanied by somnolence months to years after the onset of infection.
- Diagnosis is based on clinical findings and serology, although the yield of culture is very low.
- On MRI, the most common findings include: (1) normal scan, (2) high signal abnormalities in the white matter on T2WI/FLAIR, which can vary in size from punctate to large mass lesions, and (3) a contrast-enhancing lesion within the parenchyma, meninges, labyrinth, and cranial nerves (Fig. 5.19). Of the

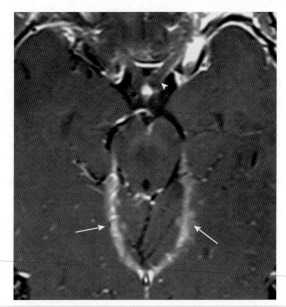

**Fig. 5.19 Lyme disease.** Enhancement of the optic nerve sheath *(arrowhead)*, pituitary stalk *(black arrow)*, and meninges *(white arrows)* should suggest the possibility of infection by *Borrelia burgdorferi*.

cranial nerves, those in the internal auditory canal are affected most, with clinical manifestations of facial palsies and/or labyrinthitis/hearing loss. Look for VII or VIII enhancement or inner ear cochleovestibular enhancement. Other abnormalities reported include hydrocephalus and high-intensity in the pons, the thalamus, and basal ganglia. There may be a predilection for subcortical high-intensity abnormalities on MRI in the frontal and parietal lobes.

## CRYPTOCOCCOSIS

- This is a yeast with a polysaccharide capsule that ranks third behind HIV and Toxoplasmosis in causes of CNS

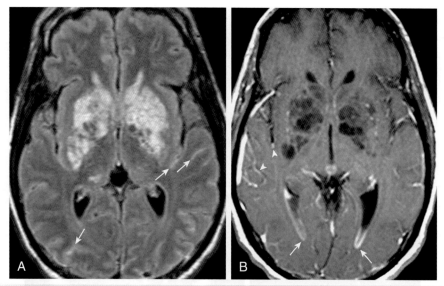

**Fig. 5.20** (A) Cryptococcal meningitis. The axial fluid-attenuated inversion recovery (FLAIR) image demonstrates enormous hyperintense Virchow-Robin spaces. (B) Axial contrast-enhanced T1 scan shows few foci of associated enhancement within the enlarged spaces. If enlarged and masslike, think gelatinous pseudotumors of cryptococcal infection. Bonus findings: *Arrows* in (A) indicate nonsuppression of cerebrospinal fluid signal, implying meningeal disease in the sulci. Abnormal enhancement along sulci and ventricular margins (*arrowheads* and *arrows* in B, respectively) indicate meningitis and, you guessed it, ventriculitis!

infection among AIDS patients (up to 11%), manifesting in the CNS as meningitis or granuloma formation, usually from hematogenous dissemination from an occult pulmonary focus.

- MRI may be normal but can also have a spectrum of abnormalities, including dilated Virchow-Robin spaces (Fig. 5.20) filled with gelatinous cysts ("pseudotumor"), in and adjacent to the basal ganglia and the corticomedullary junction, which may or may not enhance. There may be numerous bilateral small foci of high signal intensity on T2WI/FLAIR along the perivascular spaces. Gumming up of arachnoid villi by cryptococcal infection leads to hydrocephalus. Diffuse confluent basal cisternal-leptomeningeal enhancement is not usually present in cryptococcal meningitis (unlike tuberculosis or bacterial meningitis). Rarely, involvement of the spinal cord and spinal nerve roots can be seen.

## COCCIDIOIDOMYCOSIS

- This is an endemic fungus infection in the southwestern United States and northern Mexico. After spore inhalation and the development of a primary pulmonary focus, hematogenous dissemination to CNS can occur within a few weeks, months, or even years.
- Intracranial infection may be manifested pathologically by a thick basilar meningitis with meningeal and parenchymal granulomas. Intra-axial granulomas have a propensity for cerebellum. Vasculitis producing occlusion has also been noted.
- On MRI, dilated Virchow-Robin spaces similar to cryptococcus (see previous discussion) can be identified. On PDWI/FLAIR, there is increased signal in the cisterns. Enhancement is noted in the basal meninges, cisterns, and sulci. When ependymitis is present,

enhancement is noted along the ventricular margin. Focal areas of infarction secondary to vasculitis and enhancing parenchymal nodules can occasionally be observed.

- On CT or MRI with contrast, basal arachnoiditis with obliteration and distortion of the cisterns can be seen. Meningeal disease may show increased density on CT even before contrast. Associated with this active arachnoiditis is communicating hydrocephalus.

## MUCORMYCOSIS

- This fungus is usually inhaled and rapidly destroys nasal mucosa, forming black crusts (classic eschar). It can then spread into the paranasal sinuses (with or without bone destruction), orbit, and the base of the skull or may extend through the cribriform plate, resulting in involvement of the anterior cranial fossa.
- Prognosis is directly related to early recognition of the disease. The infection more commonly affects patients with altered cellular immunity (e.g., diabetic patients with ketoacidosis or debilitated patients with burns, uremia, or malnutrition). It is also seen in immunocompromised patients, such as those with HIV or cancer patients undergoing bone marrow transplant.
- Presenting symptoms include facial pain, bloody nasal discharge, dark swollen turbinates, chemosis, exophthalmos, and cranial nerve palsy, progressing rapidly to stroke, encephalitis, and death.
- On CT, sinus or nasal cavity opacification, air-fluid levels, increased density or calcification, and obliteration of the nasopharyngeal tissue planes can be seen. The infection has a propensity to creep out of the sinonasal cavity into the premaxillary soft tissue, infratemporal fossa, pterygopalatine fossa, orbits, or skull base, with bone dehiscence or destruction in its wake (Fig. 5.21).

formation are seen. Presence of true ring enhancement argues against the most aggressive meningoencephalitic variety of aspergillosis.

## CANDIDIASIS

- This fungus is the most common cause of autopsy-proved non-AIDS cerebral mycosis. There is a propensity for neutropenic patients who are receiving steroids, in whom it reaches the CNS by hematogenous dissemination through respiratory or gastrointestinal tracts.
- Intracranial manifestations include hydrocephalus (leptomeningeal disease), enhancing nodules with edema (granuloma), calcified granuloma, infarction, and (micro)abscess formation.

## *TOXOPLASMOSIS GONDII*

- This ubiquitous protozoan parasite (20%–70% of the American population is seropositive) infects the CNS in approximately 10% of patients with AIDS and in those with compromised cellular immunity. Acute toxoplasmosis in immunocompromised patients often occurs from reactivation of remotely acquired latent infection.
- Lesions have a propensity for the basal ganglia, corticomedullary junction, white matter, and periventricular regions. As opposed to congenital toxoplasmosis, calcification is not common, although it has been reported after therapy. Occasionally, these lesions may be hemorrhagic.
- On MRI, multiple lesions of high-intensity on T2WI/FLAIR, associated with vasogenic edema and ring or nodular enhancement, are seen on T1WI (see Fig. 5.14). Prompt response to appropriate antibiotic therapy can distinguish toxoplasmosis from lymphoma.
- Congenital toxoplasmosis occurs during maternal infection. Its manifestations include bilateral chorioretinitis associated with hydrocephalus (secondary to ependymitis producing aqueductal stenosis) and intracranial calcifications, particularly in the basal ganglia and cortex.

## CYSTICERCOSIS

- This parasite is endemic in parts of Mexico, Central and South America, Asia, Africa, and Eastern Europe. Humans are the only known definitive hosts (in whom the parasite undergoes sexual reproduction) for the adult tapeworm (*Taenia solium*) and the only known intermediate hosts (in whom the larval or asexual stage is present) for the larval form (*Cysticercus cellulosae*), which prospers in the CNS even years after initial infection.
- Infected patients present most commonly with seizures and headaches. It is not until the larvae die that an acute inflammatory reaction is incited and patients become symptomatic.
- The parasite is acquired by ingestion of insufficiently cooked pork containing the encysted larvae or by fecal-oral transmission. Larvae develop into adult tapeworms in the human intestinal tract to ultimately reach the bloodstream, which carries them to the CNS and to other regions, where they form cysticerci.
- The cysticerci vary in size from a pinpoint to 6 cm in diameter and are located in the brain parenchyma,

subarachnoid space, ventricles, or, rarely, intraspinal locations. Parenchymal cysts have a propensity for cortical and deep gray matter, whereas the subarachnoid cysts can produce basal meningitis and hydrocephalus. Cerebral arteritis (in over 50% of cases with subarachnoid lesions) with subsequent infarction may follow, usually in the middle cerebral or posterior cerebral distribution. Intraventricular cysts (most commonly seen in the fourth ventricle) may be free or attached to the wall and become symptomatic when ventricular drainage is obstructed.

- A spectrum of MRI and CT findings is associated with active cysticercosis (Fig. 5.24), which parallel the four stages of cyst formation. The time it takes for the parasite to evolve through all of the different stages is from 2 to 10 years, with an average of approximately 5 years. The dead cyst often elicits a lot of edema despite its small size.
  - In the vesicular stage, the larvae are alive and the cyst contains clear fluid. Edema is minimal, and the cyst is surrounded by a thin capsule. On MRI, the fluid appears isointense to CSF on all pulse sequences, and the eccentric scolex (which appears as a mural nodule) can be identified. CT in this stage shows a circumscribed cyst with a density similar to CSF and a denser scolex.
  - In the colloidal vesicular stage, the fluid in the cysts becomes turbid and the larvae die, with associated thickening of the capsule. In some cases, there is a strong inflammatory reaction and encephalitis can occur as the cysts move into the colloidal vesicular stage.
  - In the granular nodular stage, the cyst shrinks in size and begins to calcify. In patients without significant reaction to the parasite, no enhancement may occur and edema can be minimal.
  - The cyst in the colloidal and granular stages can be isointense to hyperintense on T1WI. On T2WI/FLAIR, the fluid is isointense to high-intensity and the cyst wall is difficult to identify or may be hypointense. The lesions uniformly enhance as dense nodules or small ring areas. Enhancement is thought to be the result of larval death, reaction to antigen, and release of metabolic products, with associated blood-brain barrier abnormality.
  - In the nodular calcified stage, focal calcifications are seen on CT. On MRI, the lesion is seen as a hypointense nodule with susceptibility artifact on T2WI and SWI.

## ECHINOCOCCOSIS (HYDATID DISEASE)

- Echinococcosis is another parasitic disease brought to you by the dog tapeworm. It is endemic in the Middle East, South America, Eurasia, and Australia and is caused by ingestion of dog feces that include ova of the dog tapeworm (*Echinococcus granulosus*). The ova hatch in the gastrointestinal tract, and embryos are spread throughout the body. The embryo matures into a cystic larva (hydatid cyst), which is commonly large and unilocular, although other cystic configurations may be seen.
- Cerebral involvement is seen in 2% to 5% of cases. Clinical signs and symptoms include seizures, raised intracranial pressure, and focal neurologic deficits.

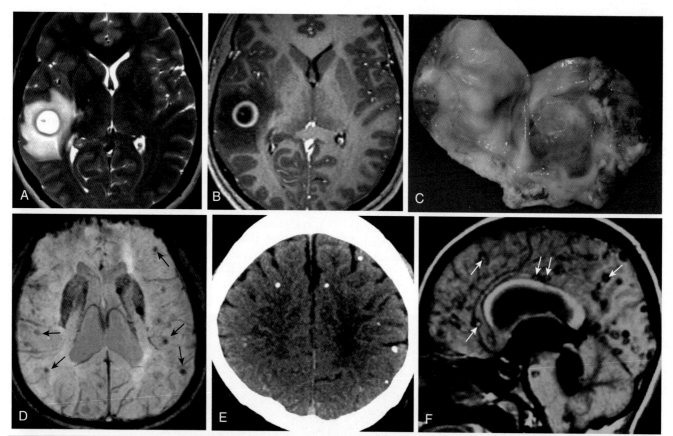

**Fig. 5.24 Cysticercosis.** Case 1: (A) Live cyst with scolex on T2-weighted imaging (T2WI) scan. (B) Postgadolinium ring and scolex enhancement is noted on postcontrast T1-weighted imaging (T1WI). (C) Check out cysticercus in the pathology pan. Case 2: (D) Multifocal parenchymal signal loss *(arrows)* on susceptibility-weighted imaging (SWI) compatible with calcified lesions. (E) Multiple calcifications seen on computed tomography (CT). (F) Innumerable lesions *(arrows)*, including one in the fourth, suggests cysticercosis.

- On MRI, the cystic component has an intensity similar to CSF. Severe inflammatory reaction in the brain occurs if the cyst ruptures (surgeons need to be careful here).

## PRION DISEASE

- This term encompasses a number of disease processes thought to be caused by prions, which are abnormally folded proteins that accumulate in the CSF, resulting in rapid neurologic decline and, ultimately, death. Although confirmatory diagnosis requires biopsy (which is technically difficult because of issues related to equipment sterilization), suffice it to say that Creutzfeldt-Jacob disease and Bovine spongiform encephalopathy, the most common of these disorders, are being diagnosed serologically or through CSF markers more readily these days.

- Not much is seen on CT, but the imaging features on MRI of bilateral deep gray matter and superficial cortical gray matter areas of restricted diffusion with or without FLAIR signal intensity abnormalities are becoming sufficiently well-described that we neuroradiologists may be the ones suggesting investigation for these CSF and serologic markers (see Fig. 7.15).

## COVID-19

- At the time of this writing, the COVID-19 pandemic has become front and center in the lives of everyone on this planet, and its impact on humanity continues to be devastating and merciless. Although the infection primarily affects the ventilatory system, a systemic inflammatory syndrome can also occur with this infection. The syndrome facilitates thrombus formation, and, as a result, thromboembolic infarct (arterial or venous) is the most common manifestation of this infection in the CNS. Outside of stroke, the infection can cause a hemorrhagic necrotizing encephalitis or a leukoencephalopathy, sometimes in a posterior reversible leukoencephalopathy pattern, but not always.

- Although imaging findings are by themselves nonspecific, some more commonly reported patterns on MRI include diffuse white matter signal changes and extensive white matter microhemorrhages. Leptomeningeal contrast enhancement and cortical signal changes have also been reported. To date, it remains unclear if these signal changes are a direct result of COVID infection or a secondary effect of a COVID-related phenomena, such as hypercoagulability.

- Curiously, clinical presentation can often include abrupt onset of anosmia; however, elevated signal without caliber change of the olfactory bulb on postcontrast FLAIR images is variably present in patients both with and without anosmia.

- Although the long-term sequelae of CNS involvement remains to be seen, our current understanding is that the presence of microhemorrhages portends a poorer prognosis.

# NONINFECTIOUS INFLAMMATORY DISEASES

There are numerous noninfectious inflammatory disease processes that affect the brain and meninges, some of which are extremely rare. Here we will focus on the relatively more common conditions you might encounter in daily practice.

## Sarcoidosis

- This is a systemic granulomatous disease of unknown etiology, which primarily occurs in the third and fourth decades of life, affecting the nervous system clinically in approximately 5% of cases of systemic sarcoid and up to 16% in autopsy series. A very small percentage of patients have only the CNS disease without systemic manifestations. Intracranial sarcoid disease has several imaging appearances.

- The more common presentation is a chronic basilar leptomeningitis with involvement of the hypothalamus, pituitary stalk, optic nerve, and chiasm. The convexities may also be involved. Patients may have unilateral or bilateral cranial nerve (particularly nerve VII) palsy or endocrine or electrolyte disturbances. In these patients, hydrocephalus develops and signs of meningeal irritation may be present. The granulomatous process frequently spreads from the leptomeninges to the Virchow-Robin spaces (Fig. 5.25), invading and thrombosing affected blood vessels (arteries and/or veins) and producing a granulomatous angiitis similar to primary angiitis of the CNS. Nonenhancing parenchymal edema adjacent to fulminant leptomeningeal sarcoidosis is a common manifestation of sarcoidosis.

- Another pattern is parenchymal based, with granulomatous nodules or masses throughout the brain parenchyma, with a marked predilection for the skull

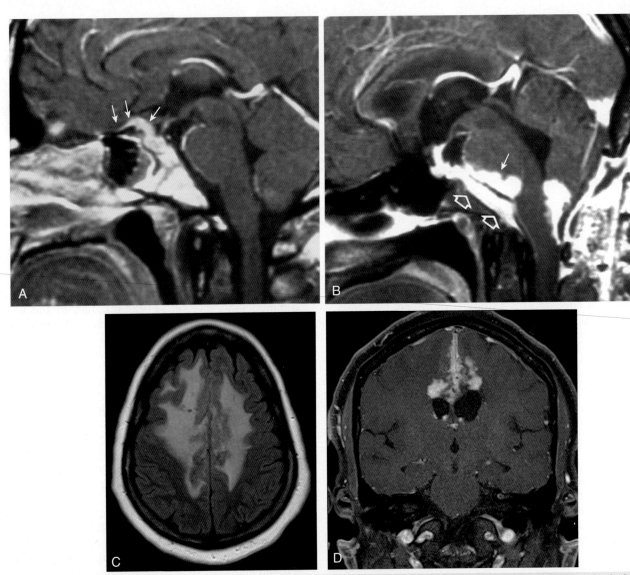

**Fig. 5.25  A mélange of sarcoidosis.** Case 1 (A): Sagittal-enhanced T1-weighted imaging (T1WI) scan of the sella region shows a mass that looks like a meningioma lesion *(arrows)*. However, leptomeningeal enhancement along the ventral pons should give us pause to consider alternate diagnoses. Case 2 (B): With leptomeningeal *(arrow)*, dural *(open arrows)*, and nodular enhancement at the fourth ventricular outlet, this case begs the diagnosis of sarcoidosis. Case 3 (C): Abnormal intensity to the bifrontal white matter along with avid bulky nodular enhancement (D) of the adjacent leptomeninges, again urges us to consider sarcoid.

base regions, pituitary, pons, hypothalamus, and periventricular region, usually associated with extensive arachnoiditis. These masses may be calcified and nonenhancing. High-intensity white matter on T2 and FLAIR can be observed in sarcoid, and this can be indistinguishable from multiple sclerosis.

- Dural-based sarcoid is a mimic of the more common meningioma, with a dural-based mass, occasional hyperostosis, and meningeal enhancement.
- Up to 25% of patients can have ophthalmic manifestations, including anterior uveitis (most common manifestation), posterior uveitis, lacrimal gland infiltration, optic nerve/sheath involvement, retrobulbar masses, exophthalmos, and extraocular muscle thickening. Infiltration of the orbit can also occur by direct extension from the cavernous sinus along the superior orbital fissure, from the suprasellar cistern to the optic canal, or at the inferior orbital fissure from the pterygopalatine fossa.
- Sarcoid may affect the spinal cord with leptomeningeal coating of the cord or appear as an intramedullary mass. Sarcoid can inflame the cauda equina, causing a polyradiculopathy and demonstrating nodularity and thickening of the nerve roots . There is a differential diagnosis for this finding of course (Box 5.6)!

## Granulomatosis With Polyangiitis

- The term *granulomatosis with polyangiitis* (GPA), also called *antineutrophil cytoplasmic antibody* (ANCA)–associated granulomatous vasculitis, has supplanted the term *Wegener granulomatosis*. In this condition, necrotizing granulomas affect multiple organs of the body (upper and lower respiratory tracts, kidneys, orbits, heart, skin, and joints) and can produce a vasculitis that results in peripheral neuropathy and myopathy. In 2% to 8% of cases, the meninges and brain can be affected.
- Imaging findings in the CNS are varied and may be focal or diffuse. On MRI, you can see meningeal thickening and enhancement. In the brain and spinal cord, infarction, nonspecific white matter abnormalities on T2WI/FLAIR, parenchymal granulomas, and atrophy can be seen. You may also see parenchymal and subarachnoid hemorrhage, as well as arterial and venous thrombosis. GPA can involve the pituitary gland and stalk, either from direct extension of extracranial disease or as an isolated focus of disease. Mucosal ulceration and bone destruction may be evident on CT of the paranasal sinuses.

## Autoimmune Encephalitis

- Autoimmune encephalitis is becoming an increasingly recognized diagnostic consideration in the workup of otherwise unexplained altered mental status, psychosis and seizures and requires serum antibody testing for definitive diagnosis. Although the list of causative antibodies is broad and ever growing, generally speaking it is the antibody-mediated inflammation of the brain that is the underlying basis of this condition.
- Antibody-mediated encephalitis can be characterized as paraneoplastic (in the setting of known malignancy) or non-paraneoplastic. There are also two subtypes of

**Box 5.6   Differential Diagnosis of Nerve Root Enhancement**

Arachnoiditis
Charcot-Marie-Tooth
CSF metastases
Dejerine Sottas
Disc herniation with root inflammation
Guillain-Barré
Infection
  CMV
  Herpes zoster
  Lyme
  TB
Neurofibroma
Sarcoid and other granulomatous diseases
Schwannoma

*CMV*, Cytomegalovirus; *CSF*, cerebrospinal fluid; *TB*, tuberculosis.

antibodies: group 1 antibodies target intracellular antigens and group 2 target cell surface antigens. The distinction is important with respect to treatment response and prognosis; Group 1 antibodies are more often associated with malignancy and poorer prognosis compared to group 2.

- Among group 1, Anti-Hu antibody is the most commonly implicated in paraneoplastic autoimmune encephalitis, most often seen in the setting of small cell lung cancer and has the poorest prognosis. Anti-Ma1 and Ma2 autoimmune encephalitis is seen in setting of testicular tumors and Anti-CV2 encephalitis can be seen in the setting of small cell carcinoma and malignant thymoma. Glutamic acid decarboxylase (GAD) encephalitis is not associated with malignancy but rather is seen in non-neoplastic conditions such as type 1 diabetes. Other less common group 1 antibodies include anti-amphiphysin and anti-Ri (lung and breast cancer), as well as anti-Yo (ovarian and breast cancer).
- Among group 2, anti-N-methyl D-aspartate receptor (NMDAr) antibodies are associated with the best understood of the autoimmune encephalidities. Patients with NMDAr encephalitis are typically young women and children who present with psychiatric symptoms. Uniquely, brain MRI in patients with NMDAr encephalitis is typically normal or with minimal signal abnormalities in affected areas. Voltage-gated potassium channel (VGKC) encephalitis is also common, typically presenting with intractable seizures and limbic encephalitis (based on high concentration of potassium channels in the limbic system). Less common group 2 encephalidities include voltage gated calcium channel (VCGG) encephalitis seen in women and young children with migratory extralimbic involvement, γ-aminobutyric acid (GABAr) encephalitis more often seen in setting of malignancy, alpha-amino-3-hydroxy-5-methyl-4-isoxazolepropionic acid receptor (AMPAr) encephalitis with predominant hippocampal involvement, and glutamate receptor 3 (GluR3) encephalitis implicated in Rasmussen encephalitis.

**TEACHING POINTS**

Rasmussen Encephalitis

- This condition is seen more commonly among pediatric population (mean age 6-8 years), with patients presenting initially with focal motor seizures and subsequently with loss of ipsilateral motor function and cognitive decline.
- The etiology remains unknown, but presence of anti-GluR3 receptor antibodies suggests the condition reflects an antigenic driven inflammatory response. Viral etiology has been postulated as well, and there may also be a genetic component at play resulting in abnormal inflammatory response to otherwise minor antigen.
- Early in the process, imaging can be normal or unilateral cerebral swelling may be seen. Subsequently, T2 hyperintense lesions can be seen in the basal ganglia on the affected side with or without diffusion restriction. Enhancement is typically not seen. In later stages, unilateral cortical atrophy predominates (although bilateral involvement has been reported), with ex vacuo dilatation of the ventricular system (Fig 5.26).
- Symptoms are typically resistant to anti-seizure medication but high dose steroid and IV immunoglobulin treatment can help with seizure control. Functional hemispherectomy provides the most definitive means of seizure control.

- Finally, systemic autoimmune disease processes can also manifest with encephalopathy, with antiphospholipid antibodies and anti-glutamate receptor antibodies demonstrated in patients with systemic lupus erythematosus. Patients can present with stroke symptoms with multifocal hemorrhages throughout the brain on hemosiderin sensitive MRI sequences. Patient with autoimmune thyroid dysfunction (for example in the setting of Graves or Hashimoto's disease) can present with autoimmune encephalitis with multifocal regions of increased FLAIR signal within the white matter.
- Clinical and imaging features can vary depending on the particular antibody in question and the region(s) of the brain involved. Signal changes in the limbic system are most commonly observed on MRI, but basal ganglia,

cortex, brainstem, cerebellum, cord and peripheral nerves can also be affected. Findings are not readily apparent by CT unless significant brain edema is present. On MRI, the affected regions will show elevated T2 and FLAIR signal (Fig 5.27). Microhemorrhage, diffusion restriction, and contrast enhancement are less commonly seen. PET-CT may show increased FDG uptake in the affected regions. Findings may be reversible depending on the culprit antibody and timing of therapy initiation.

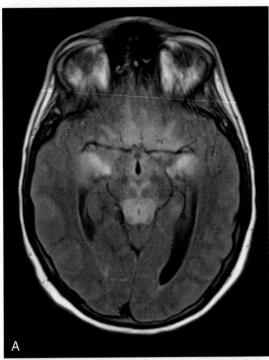

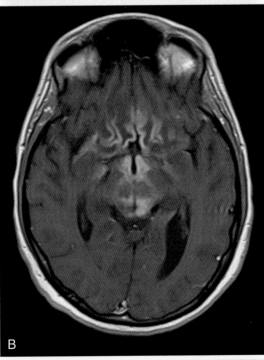

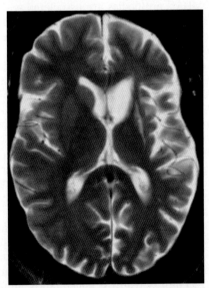

**Fig. 5.26 Rasmussen encephalitis.** Axial T2WI shows atrophy of the left cerebral hemisphere, including caudate and lentiform nucleus with ex vacuo dilatation of the left frontal horn.

**Fig. 5.27 Anti-Ma2 paraneoplastic encephalitis.** A. Axial FLAIR and (B) post contrast axial T1 weighted images show abnormal signal and patchy enhancement in the mesial temporal lobes, cingulate gyri, hypothalamus and midbrain in this patient presenting with altered mental status and lethargy in setting of seminoma.

# 6 | *White Matter Disease*

DORIS D.M. LIN

White matter diseases represent a heterogeneous group of conditions affecting myelin, axons, glial cells, and vascular structures that may result from a myriad of acquired and inherited pathologies. These include (immune-mediated) inflammatory and demyelination, infectious (most often viral), vascular, metabolic, toxic, and traumatic etiologies (Box 6.1). In this chapter, emphasis will be placed on inflammatory demyelinating conditions occurring in both adults and children, and rarer "dysmyelinating" diseases or leukodystrophies, which most frequently manifest in childhood.

## Relevant Anatomy

- White matter refers to the areas of the central nervous system (CNS) predominantly composed of myelinated axonal fiber tracts, which are responsible for connecting neurons by rapid and efficient conduction of electrochemical neural impulses.
- In the CNS, oligodendrocytes form myelin sheaths, which envelop the axons while leaving unmyelinated gaps (nodes of Ranvier) that allow saltatory (from one node of Ranvier to the next node down the full length of an axon in a rapid fashion) propagation of action potentials.
- White matter is so named because lipid-rich myelin produces a paler color compared with that of gray matter, which consists predominantly of neuronal cell bodies.
- In the brain, white matter is situated deep to the cortical gray matter, whereas in the spinal cord, white matter is present in the periphery surrounding the butterfly-shaped central gray matter. White matter fibers also connect the deep gray matter structures (i.e., basal ganglia) of the brain.
- Depending on the groups of neurons being connected, the white matter tracts can serve as association, commissural, or projection fibers. These are described in detail in Chapter 1. However, additional players present in the white matter include vascular structures and other glial cells, such as astrocytes and astrocytic processes, microglia, and oligodendrocytes.

## Imaging Techniques/Protocols

### COMPUTED TOMOGRAPHY

- Computed tomography (CT) of the brain can be useful in depicting white matter lesions associated with calcification or hemorrhage. Otherwise, it does not play a major role in the diagnosis or characterization of white matter diseases.

### MAGNETIC RESONANCE IMAGING

- Magnetic resonance imaging (MRI) is the primary modality to evaluate white matter diseases affecting the brain, optic pathways, and spinal cord. Gadolinium contrast is typically included during the initial diagnostic evaluation, acute phase assessment, and at the time of symptom flares.

### Conventional Imaging Techniques

- Among conventional anatomic images, fluid-attenuated inversion recovery (FLAIR) is most sensitive in depicting white matter disease because pathologic lesions show increased signal intensity. In the posterior fossa and brainstem, standard T2-weighted scans highlight white matter lesions best.
- Particularly useful for multiple sclerosis (MS) is sagittal three-dimensional (3D) FLAIR for the evaluation of characteristic lesions in the calloso-septal junction; 3D FLAIR also provides a global view of the posterior fossa structures and upper cervical cord that may be involved.
- T1-weighted images are important for depicting hypointense demyelinating lesions called "black holes," which represent severely damaged tissues and strongly correlate with clinical disability.
- In children under 2 years of age, dual echo sequences (proton density [PD] and T2-weighted) are preferred because of incomplete or immature formation of myelin. PD is also useful for the evaluation of the posterior fossa in adult MS.
- Double inversion recovery (DIR) sequence can be used to increase lesion conspicuity.
- Typical "MS protocol" is shown in Table 6.1.

### Optional and Advanced Imaging Techniques

- *Susceptibility-weighted images (SWIs)* can be included to delineate the perivenular location of demyelinating plaques and depict accumulation of iron in recruited macrophages at sites of demyelination. Hemorrhagic white matter lesions are characteristic of diffuse axonal injury.
- *Magnetic resonance spectroscopy* or proton magnetic resonance spectroscopy ($^1$H-MRS) is a noninvasive method of interrogating brain biochemistry in vivo.
  - N-acetyl aspartate (NAA), an important metabolite found in neuronal cells and processes, has a peak at 2.0 ppm. NAA is decreased in MS and several dysmyelinating processes, suggesting neuroaxonal loss or dysfunction.
  - Creatine (Cr) and phosphocreatine are energy metabolites found at 3.0 ppm. They may also be decreased in white matter diseases and profoundly low or even absent in patients with creatine deficiency, an inborn error of metabolism.

## Box 6.1   White Matter Diseases Categorized by Presumed Etiology

### Autoimmune (Idiopathic)
- Multiple sclerosis (MS)
- Monophasic demyelination (clinically isolated syndrome [CIS])
- Acute disseminated encephalomyelitis (ADEM)
- Acute hemorrhagic leukoencephalitis
- Neuromyelitis optica spectrum disorder (NMOSD)
- Myelin oligodendrocyte glycoprotein antibody-associated disease (MOGAD)
- Optic neuritis (may also be a manifestation of MS)
- Acute transverse myelitis (may also be a manifestation of MS)

### Viral
- Progressive multifocal leukoencephalopathy (PML)
- Subacute sclerosing panencephalitis
- Human immunodeficiency virus (HIV)–associated encephalitis

### Vascular
- Migraines
- Cerebral autosomal dominant arteriopathy with subcortical infarcts and leukoencephalopathy (CADASIL)
- Cerebral microangiopathy
- Inflammatory cerebral amyloid angiopathy (see Chapter 3)
- Postanoxic encephalopathy
- Posterior reversible leukoencephalopathy (PRES)
- Subcortical vascular dementia (aka subcortical arterio-sclerotic encephalopathy/Binswanger disease/subcortical leukoencephalopathy)

### Metabolic/Nutritional
- Osmotic demyelination
- Marchiafava-Bignami disease
- Combined system disease ($B_{12}$ deficiency)

### Toxic
- Radiation
- Chemotherapy
- Toxins
- Drugs
- Disseminated necrotizing leukoencephalopathy

### Trauma
- Diffuse axonal injury

---

- Elevated choline (Cho), normally found at 3.2 ppm, is associated with membrane (myelin) breakdown, inflammation, and/or remyelination.
- Lactate represents a terminal metabolite in anaerobic glycolysis, has a characteristic doublet peak at 1.33 ppm, and can be present in some lesions, particularly the inherited white matter abnormalities attributable to mitochondrial disorders.
- MRS adds value in the evaluation of leukodystrophies by characterizing the nature of white matter lesions, whether there is hypomyelination, demyelination, or rarefaction.
- MRS diagnostic findings for other neurometabolic disorders are outlined.
- *Magnetization transfer* (MT) results from the transfer of magnetization from protons attached to rigid macromolecules (such as myelin) to free water protons. The effect is observed by noting a decrease in intensity performed with an off-resonance pulse.
  - Injury resulting in demyelination causes a decrease in MT.
  - Usually, MT effects are noted as 1 minus the ratio of the image intensity with a saturation pulse on ($MT_S$) divided by the intensity with the saturation pulse off ($MT_0$), specifically $1 - MT_S/MT_0$, which is termed the magnetization transfer ratio [MTR]).
  - Low MTR equates with myelin loss. There is decreased MT in MS in both plaques and normal-appearing white matter (NAWM), and the decrease is correlated with clinical disability.
- *Diffusion-weighted and diffusion tensor imaging* (DWI/DTI) is an advanced MRI technique interrogating the random Brownian motion of water molecules within the image voxel.
  - In the characterization of white matter diseases, DWI provides a distinction between vasogenic and cytotoxic edema, the latter of which may be seen in acute demyelination.
  - DTI further allows delineation of white matter tracts and provides quantitative assessment of microstructural integrity by measuring fractional anisotropy and mean diffusivity in a selected region of interest. It is useful in quantifying axon loss and demyelination in diseases including MS and posttraumatic injuries.

# Pathology

## IMMUNE-MEDIATED INFLAMMATORY DEMYELINATION

### Multiple Sclerosis

- MS is an autoimmune disease resulting in progressive inflammatory demyelination and neurodegenerative change. Epidemiologically, it has a high prevalence of about 33 out of 100,000 persons, affecting more in Europe and North America (temperate zones). Mean age of onset is 20 to 40 years, but the disease may also begin in childhood and, more often, during the teenage years.
- MS is marked by perivascular infiltrate of mononuclear inflammatory cells, demyelination with remyelination or axonal loss, and gliosis in the chronic stage. The process can affect the supratentorial brain, optic nerves, brainstem, and cerebellum, resulting in related symptoms. Although there is a distinct predilection for periventricular white matter presenting as "Dawson's finger" lesions, MS has also been well demonstrated to affect the cortical and subcortical gray matter.
- Diagnosis is established by a combination of clinical and paraclinical tests with demonstration of dissemination in space (DIS) and time (DIT). The full slate of possibilities for diagnosing MS is described in Table 6.2 according to the revised 2017 McDonald criteria. Before the new version, there were consensus recommendations to upgrade the imaging criteria for MS, known as MAGNIMS criteria (Box 6.2), published in 2016 by a European collaborative research network called the MRI in Multiple Sclerosis (MAGNIMS). MRI is important in supporting the clinical diagnosis, excluding

**Table 6.1**  Typical Brain MRI Protocol for Follow-Up Examination of Multiple Sclerosis

| Recommended | Optional |
| --- | --- |
| 2D or 3D FLAIR | 3D T1-weighted MPRAGE isotropic |
| Axial dual echo (PD + T2-weighted) | 2D or 3D DIR |
| Axial DWI | |
| 2D or 3D T1-weighted + Gd | |

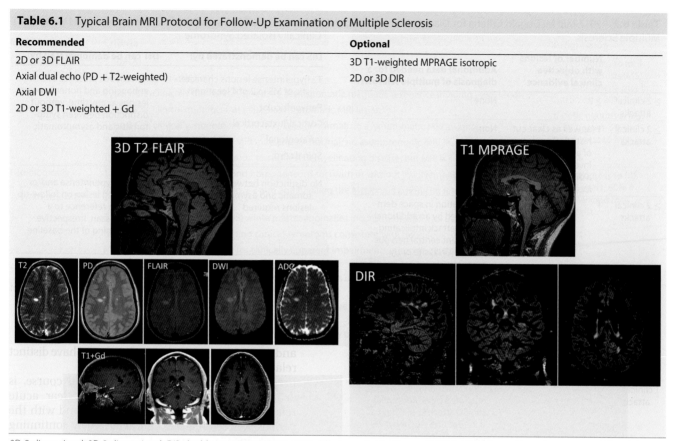

*2D,* 2-dimensional; *3D,* 3-dimensional; *DIR,* double inversion recovery; *DWI,* diffusion-weighted image; *FLAIR,* fluid-attenuated inversion recovery; *Gd,* gadolinium; *MPRAGE,* magnetization-prepared rapid acquisition gradient echo; *PD,* proton density.

other mimicking processes, and, in some cases, replacing other paraclinical findings for establishing the diagnosis. If two or more of four possible locations of plaques are identified (periventricular region, juxtacortical region, infratentorial region, and spinal cord), the magnetic resonance (MR) scan meets the criteria of DIS (2017 McDonald criteria). If nonenhancing plaques and enhancing plaques coexist on the same scan or a second scan shows new enhancing or nonenhancing plaques, DIT criteria have been satisfied.

- Clinically isolated syndrome (CIS) clinically isolated syndrome denotes a single (or inaugural) episode that may be unifocal clinically. The updated 2017 McDonald criteria for the diagnosis of CIS is shown (Table 6.3).
  - Eighty percent of patients with CIS at 15 years will meet diagnostic criteria for MS if they have positive MR findings, but only 20% at 15 years get diagnosed with MS if they have a normal MR when staged as CIS.
  - Seventy-seven percent of patients presenting with isolated brainstem syndrome have been reported to have asymptomatic supratentorial white matter abnormalities. Progression to MS occurs in about 57% of patients with isolated brainstem syndrome and 42% of patients with spinal cord syndrome.
- In radiologically isolated syndrome (RIS), patients clinically have not experienced an MS episode but imaging features fulfilling McDonald criteria are incidentally

discovered on brain and spinal cord imaging performed for other reasons. In this situation, one-third progress to a diagnosis of MS in 3 years, and the rate increases significantly if there are enhancing plaques. Table 6.4 summaries the diagnostic criteria for CIS versus RIS and differences in rates of disease progression.

- Laboratory tests for MS, including visual, auditory, and somatosensory evoked responses, can also contribute to confirm the presence of lesions, but they are nonspecific and provide no clue to the cause of abnormal findings. Approximately 70% of patients with MS have elevated cerebrospinal fluid (CSF) levels of immunoglobulin G (IgG), and approximately 90% have elevated oligoclonal bands.
- MS is a disease characterized by a variety of clinical courses.
  - Relapsing remitting (RR) MS is the most common form, initially occurring in up to 85% of cases. In the beginning, exacerbations are followed by remissions. However, over years, additional exacerbations result in incomplete recovery.
  - Within 10 years, 50% (and within 25 years, 90%) of these cases enter a progressive phase, termed secondary progressive (also termed relapsing progressive) MS. During this phase, deficits are progressive without much remission in the disease.
  - Less commonly, the disease is progressive from the start, termed "primary progressive MS." These

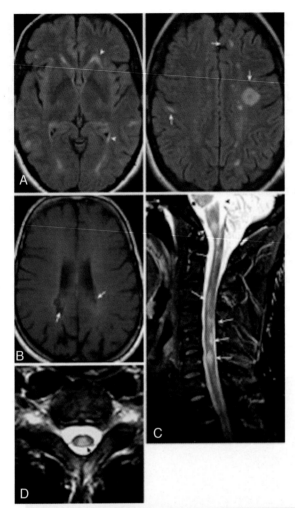

**Fig. 6.2 Magnetic resonance imaging (MRI) manifestations of multiple sclerosis.** (A) Axial fluid-attenuated inversion recovery (FLAIR) scan shows multiple hyperintense periventricular (*arrowheads*) and subcortical white matter lesions (*arrows*). (B) The T1-weighted image shows low-intensity lesions in periventricular sites (*arrows*) indicative of the so-called "black holes" that correlate well with disability scores. The rim of high signal, thought to be because of paramagnetic deposition, is also sometimes seen in MS. (C) Infratentorial brainstem (*arrowheads*) and cord demyelinating plaques (*arrows*) are evident. (D) Lesions favor the posterior cord (*arrows*).

This includes the cortex (6%), where white matter fibers track up to the superficial cortical cells, and in the deep gray matter (5%), best seen on FLAIR.

- On T1WI, plaques are isointense or hypointense regions, whereas on T2WI, the lesions are hyperintense. Uncommon hypointense lesions on T1WI that approximate CSF intensity have been termed "black holes" (see Fig. 6.2B) and are reported to be associated with areas of greatest myelin loss. The volume of black holes correlates most closely with disability as determined by the EDSS.
- FLAIR imaging does not detect lesions in the posterior fossa, brainstem, and spinal cord as well as T2WI scans. Also, very hypointense lesions on T1WI (black holes) may look similar to CSF on FLAIR and thereby be overlooked.
- Studies suggest high-intensity lesions at the callosal-septal interface visualized with proton density (PD) or

FLAIR sagittal MR have 93% sensitivity and 98% specificity in differentiating MS lesions from vascular disease (see Fig. 6.1). The shape of plaques in this location may be variable; however, ovoid lesions are believed to be more specific for MS. Their morphology has been attributed to inflammatory changes around the long axis of a medullary vein (so-called Dawson fingers; Fig. 6.3); the detection of the "central vein sign" on SWI, best shown on high magnetic field strength such as 7 Tesla, has been found to offer increased diagnostic accuracy of differentiating MS from small vessel disease.

- Postcontrast MR images in patients with plaques may show no enhancement, or a wide variety of patterns of enhancement indicative of active demyelination, including solid nodular, solid linear, complete ring, open ring/arcs, and punctate enhancement. These patterns may also coexist (Fig. 6.4). Meningeal irritation near far peripheral areas of demyelination can cause meningeal enhancement as well. Superficial enhancement along cranial nerves (excluding the optic nerve) and brain stem can also occur in MS (Fig. 6.5). The normal window of enhancement is from 2 to 8 weeks (about 2 months); however, plaques can enhance for 6 months or more.
- MS lesions may be large (2 cm or greater) with contrast enhancement and display mass effect, hence mimicking a neoplasm ("tumefactive MS"; Fig. 6.6). (Of note, a "tumefactive demyelinating lesion" may be used to describe any CNS demyelinating lesion that is tumor-like, resulting from inflammatory disorders including but not limited to MS.) There are several clues that aid in suggesting this diagnosis, including patient history, which is usually acute or subacute onset of neurologic deficit(s) in a young adult, and other white matter abnormalities unassociated with the mass lesion but characteristic of MS, such as in the periventricular zone, spinal cord, or callosal-septal interface. Tumefactive MS lesions often have a leading edge of enhancement and an incomplete "horseshoe-shaped" open ring toward the ventricular margin or outward along the subcortical region. Perfusion helps to differentiate between tumor and MS lesions; perfusion usually increases in tumors but not in MS. Additionally, veins are displaced by neoplasms but course through MS lesions.
- Another possible radiologic finding in MS is atrophy of the brain and spinal cord. The greater the loss of myelin and axons, the increased likelihood of atrophy and that the lesion becomes hypointense on T1WI. High intensity on unenhanced T1WI can be observed infrequently, most often in the periphery of the plaque (see Fig. 6.2B). The cause of this phenomenon is unknown, but hypotheses include paramagnetic accumulation from hemorrhage, myelin catabolites including fat, free radical production from the inflammatory response, or focally increased regions of protein.
- With MS, disease also exists within NAWM, which is beyond the resolution of standard imaging and contrast techniques. New MR methods (such as DTI, MT, and MRS, as discussed previously) clearly demonstrate that the NAWM in MS is not normal; that is, there are lesions not depicted by conventional MR. This is important because the extent of disease in MS patients is greater than the visible T2 lesion load.

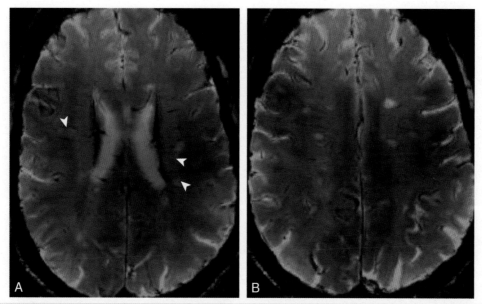

**Fig. 6.3  Perivenular location of multiple sclerosis (MS) plaques depicted on 7 Tesla gradient echo magnetic resonance images.** (A) Note both the ovoid appearance of the MS lesions and the veins (*white arrowheads*) course through the middle of the ovoid lesion. (B) At the ventricular junction, these perpendicular lesions are referred to as Dawson fingers. (Courtesy Robert I. Grossman.)

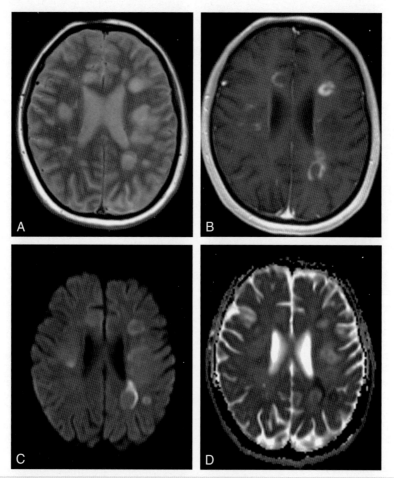

**Fig. 6.4  Imaging patterns in multiple sclerosis (MS).** (A) Axial proton density (PD) image shows numerous rounded or ovoid subcortical and periventricular white matter lesions. (B) Active MS plaques on postcontrast axial T1WI in the same patient show different enhancing patterns including open ring, complete ring, linear, and nodular. (C) Diffusion-weighted imaging (DWI) and (D) the apparent diffusion coefficient (ADC) map show that some of the enhancing lesions also demonstrate restricted diffusion reflecting cytotoxic edema. Note that not all T2 hyperintense lesions show contrast enhancement; hence on this single exam, there is evidence of dissemination in time (DIT).

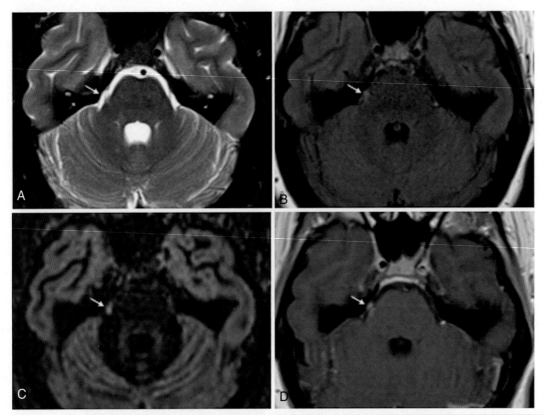

**Fig. 6.5** Active demyelinating lesion involving right trigeminal nerve in a patient presenting with tingling on the right side of the face for 4 days. Note the small T2 hyperintensity along the right pontine surface and the root entry zone of the trigeminal nerve on (A), T2 better seen on (*arrow*) (B), fluid-attenuated inversion recovery (FLAIR) and even better depicted on (arrow) (C), double inversion recovery (DIR), corresponding to contrast enhancement on (*arrow*) (D), postcontrast T1-weighted imaging (T1WI) (*arrow*).

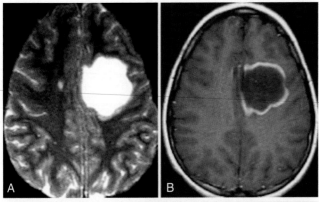

**Fig. 6.6 Tumefactive demyelinating lesion.** (A) Axial T2-weighted imaging (T2WI) with large mass compressing the left medial frontal gray matter presumed to be a glioma. (B) T1WI shows open ring of enhancement medially, classic for tumefactive multiple sclerosis and unusual for glioblastoma, lymphoma, or metastasis. Note also that given its large size, there is very little vasogenic edema and associated mass effect is modest.

## Spinal Cord Disease

- MS can affect the spinal cord alone (5%–24%) or, more commonly, both the brain and the spinal cord. Approximately 60% of spinal cord lesions occur in the cervical region (see Fig. 6.2D). Lesions can be single or multiple. Spinal cord MS tends to affect the cord periphery and often posterolaterally, typically does not involve the entire cord cross-section, and, in 90% of cases, extends less than two vertebral body segments in length.

### Box 6.3    Differential Diagnosis of Spinal Cord Lesions

- Idiopathic acquired transverse myelitis
- Autoimmune demyelination
- ADEM
- MS
- NMOSD
- MOGAD
- Spinal cord tumor (primary or metastatic)
- Syringohydromyelia
- Acute infarction
- Vascular lesions including dural arteriovenous malformation, infarction
- Infectious processes (toxoplasmosis, vacuolar myelopathy in AIDS, herpes zoster)
- SLE
- Trauma (hematomyelia)
- Diffuse leptomeningeal coating of the spinal cord from sarcoid, lymphoma, or other tumors
- Compressive myelopathy (e.g, degenerative spine disease, extramedullary tumors)

*ADEM*, Acute disseminated encephalomyelitis; *MOGAD*, myelin oligodendrocyte glycoprotein antibody-associated disease; *MS*, multiple sclerosis; *NMOSD*, neuromyelitis optica spectrum disorder; *SLE*, systemic lupus erythematosus.
Reprinted with permission from Elsevier. Prof Massimo Filippi MD a, Maria A Rocca MD a, Prof Olga Ciccarelli PhD b c, et al. MRI criteria for the diagnosis of multiple sclerosis: MAGNIMS consensus guidelines. *Lancet Neurol* 2016;15(3):292–303.

- Spinal cord swelling is associated with lesions in 6% to 14% of cases, whereas atrophy ranges from 2% to 40%. Most lesions in the spinal cord do not demonstrate enhancement. Usually, no correlation is found between spinal cord lesion load and EDSS, but clinical disability has been correlated with spinal cord atrophy. Box 6.3 lists the differential diagnosis of an enlarged T2 hyperintense spinal cord lesion.

## Multiple Sclerosis Syndromes

- Balo disease (concentric sclerosis) represents a histologic MS lesion with alternating concentric regions of demyelination and normal brain that may be observed on T2WI scans (Fig. 6.7).
- Diffuse sclerosis (Schilder disease) is an acute, rapidly progressive form of MS with bilateral relatively symmetric demyelination in childhood and rarely after the age of 40 years, characterized by large areas of demyelination that are well-circumscribed, often involving the centrum semiovale and occipital lobes.
- The Marburg variant of MS is defined as repeated relapses with rapidly accumulating disability producing immobility, lack of protective pharyngeal reflexes, and bladder involvement.

## Optic Neuritis

- Optic neuritis may be secondary to infectious (viral usually), inflammatory (e.g., sarcoidosis), or demyelinating disorders (Box 6.4). In the chronic stage, optic neuritis may lead to optic neuropathy. However, the most frequent cause (usually seen in older adults) is acute ischemic optic neuropathy, which occurs in patients with atherosclerotic risk factors, particularly diabetes.
- A person with optic neuritis at first presentation has a 50% chance of carrying the diagnosis of MS in 5 years; this rate increases if there are MS-like plaques on their brain MRI scan but is less if the brain MRI scan is negative. All told, 80% of MS patients have an episode of optic neuritis at some point in their lives. Thus, the entity is considered separate from MS but may overlap MS at the same time (50/50). This may be one manifestation of clinically isolated syndrome.
- For best visualization of optic neuritis, fat-suppressed scans making signal changes in the nerve more conspicuous through the orbit using FLAIR or T2 weighting is best (Fig. 6.8) because these null the orbital fat around the nerve

making signal changes in the nerve more conspicuous. Additional suppression of CSF within the optic nerve sheath can make signal changes in the optic nerve more conspicuous but comes at a cost of decreased signal to noise. That said, there have been studies suggesting that optic nerve

---

**BOX 6.4    Causes of Optic Neuritis**

**Infectious**

- Viral: HSV, CMV, HIV, varicella
- Bacterial: Lyme, syphilis, TB, spread from sinusitis
- Protozoan: toxoplasmosis

**Inflammatory**

- Sarcoidosis
- SLE
- Polyangiitis with granulomatosis
- Idiopathic orbital inflammation ("pseudotumor")

**Demyelination**

- Idiopathic isolated optic neuritis
- Clinically isolated syndrome
- MS
- ADEM
- NMOSD
- MOGAD

---

*ADEM,* Acute disseminated encephalomyelitis; *CMV,* cytomegalovirus; *HIV,* human immunodeficiency virus; *HSV,* herpes simplex virus; *MOGAD,* myelin oligodendrocyte glycoprotein antibody-associated disease; *MS,* multiple sclerosis; *NMOSD,* neuromyelitis optica spectrum disorder; *SLE,* systemic lupus erythematosus; *TB,* tuberculosis.

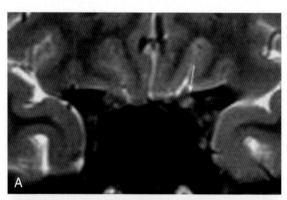
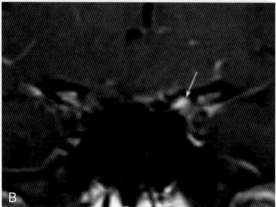

**Fig. 6.8 Optic neuritis.** (A) Coronal T2-weighted imaging (T2WI) shows hyperintensity in the left optic nerve corresponding to contrast enhancement on (B) T1WI (*arrow*).

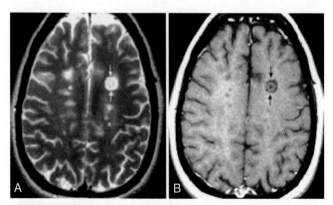

**Fig. 6.7 Balo's concentric sclerosis.** (A) Axial T2-weighted imaging (T2WI) shows alternating rings of different intensities (*arrows*) and (B) postgadolinium T1-weighted imaging (T1WI).

enhancement may precede signal intensity abnormalities on T2WI scans in some cases of optic neuritis.

### Neuromyelitis Optic Spectrum Disorder

- Neuromyelitis optica spectrum disorder (NMOSD), as the name implies, is an immune-mediated inflammatory disease that affects the spinal cord and optic nerves. It was also known as Devic's disease and for a long time was considered a subtype of MS. Since the 2004 discovery of antiaquaporin 4 (AQP4) immunoglobulin G (IgG) as the mediator of NMOSD and further characterization by its clinical course and imaging findings, NMOSD is now recognized as a distinct entity. Neuromyelitis optica spectrum disorder (NMOSD) is a broad term that includes patients seropositive for AQP4 but with only limited manifestations of the disease, as well as those who are seronegative but have characteristic symptoms. Of note, several rheumatological diseases such as systemic lupus erythematosus (SLE) and Sjögren's can have characteristic longitudinally extensive transverse myelitis and clinical findings of NMOSD.

- Compared with MS, NMOSD is more humoral mediated and presents as severe inflammatory episodes of optic neuritis (often long segment and bilateral) and a spinal cord lesion that extends over three or more vertebrae—so-called longitudinally extensive transverse myelitis (LETM; Fig. 6.9). The importance of making this diagnosis is that NMOSD treatment uses monoclonal antibody agents (i.e., rituximab) rather than the typical MS cocktail of steroids and/or interferons (the latter of which may exacerbate NMOSD); in other words, there is a difference in first-line therapy: immunosuppressives in NMOSD versus immunomodulators in MS.

- NMOSD-IgG/AQP4 antibodies are the culprits that attack the astrocytic water channels in the periependymal regions of the brain, contributing to the pathophysiology of the disease.

- The international consensus diagnostic criteria for NMOSD, devised in 2015 by the International Panel for NMOSD Diagnosis, indicated that among individuals with positive AQP4-IgG, diagnosis can be fulfilled by at least one of the core symptoms while excluding alternative diagnoses (Table 6.5). NMOSD diagnosis can also be made in individuals without antibodies or with unknown status by fulfilling a combination of core clinical characteristics and imaging patterns, and exclusion of alternative diagnoses (Table 6.6).

- The clinical and imaging findings supportive of NMOSD in contrast to MS are summarized in Table 6.7. Note that brain findings are often normal or nonspecific in NMOSD, and rare occurrences of brain demyelinating lesions do have a central predilection along the ependymal lining such as around the third and fourth ventricles along the diencephalon and brainstem (particularly pons and medulla), following the anatomic distribution of aquaporin water channels (Fig. 6.10). Of note, the area postrema at the dorsal medulla is particularly rich in AQP4 and hence frequently involved in NMOSD, resulting in the characteristic "area postrema syndrome" presentation of unrelenting hiccups, nausea, and/or vomiting ("area postrema syndrome"). Less

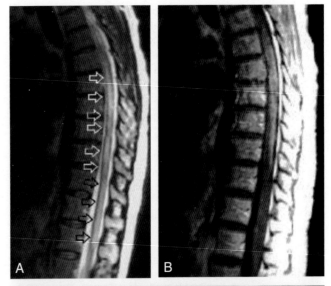

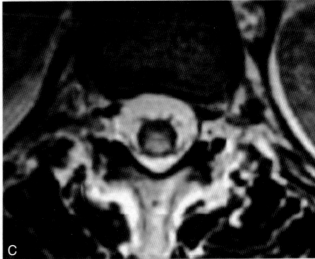

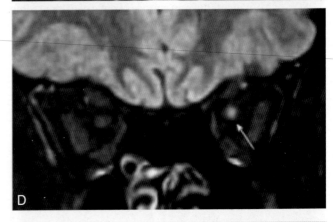

**Fig. 6.9 Neuromyelitis optica (NMO), characterized by longitudinally extensive transverse myelitis and optic neuritis.** (A) Sagittal T2-weighted imaging (T2WI) shows high intensity of the spinal cord involving more than seven vertebral body segments (*open arrows*). (B) Sagittal T1-weighted imaging (T1WI) shows contrast enhancement throughout the upper area of signal abnormality. (C) Axial T2WI shows hyperintensity involving more than two-thirds of cross-section of the spinal cord and predominantly centrally. (D) Fat-suppressed coronal fluid-attenuated inversion recovery (FLAIR) shows bright left optic nerve (*arrow*) representing the optic neuritis element of NMO.

**Table 6.5**  Diagnostic Criteria for Neuromyelitis Optica Spectrum Disorder (NMOSD) With AQP4-IgG

| At least 1 core clinical characteristic: | Positive test for AQP4-IgG using best available detection method (cell-based assay strongly recommended) | Exclusion of alternative diagnoses |
|---|---|---|
| Optic neuritis | | |
| Acute myelitis | | |
| Area postrema syndrome: unexplained hiccups or nausea and vomiting | | |
| Acute brainstem syndrome | | |
| Symptomatic narcolepsy or acute diencephalic syndrome with NMOSD (with typical diencephalic lesions on magnetic resonance imaging [MRI]) | | |
| Symptomatic cerebral syndrome with NMOSD (with typical brain lesions) | | |

From Wingerchuk DM, Banwell B, Bennett JL, et al. International consensus diagnostic criteria for neuromyelitis optica spectrum disorders. *Neurology.* 2015;85(2):177–189.

**Table 6.6**  Diagnostic Criteria for Neuromyelitis Optica Spectrum Disorder (NMOSD) Without or Unknown AQP4-IgG Status

| At least two core clinical characteristics occurring as a result of one or more clinical attacks and meeting all of the following requirements: | (a) At least one core clinical characteristic must be optic neuritis, acute myelitis with longitudinally extensive transverse myelitis (LETM), or area postrema syndrome<br>(b) Dissemination in space (two or more different core clinical characteristics)<br>(c) Fulfillment of additional magnetic resonance imaging (MRI) requirements, as applicable (see below) |
|---|---|
| Negative tests for AQP4-IgG | Using best available detection method or testing unavailable |
| Exclusion of alternative diagnoses | |
| Additional MRI requirements | 1. Acute optic neuritis: requires brain MRI showing<br>(a) Normal findings or only nonspecific white matter lesions<br>(b) Optic nerve MRI with T2-weighted hyperintense lesion or T1-weighted gadolinium-enhancing lesion extending over half the optic nerve length or involving optic chiasm<br>2. Acute myelitis: requires associated intramedullary MRI lesion extending over 3 contiguous segments (LETM) or 3 contiguous segments of focal spinal cord atrophy in patients with history compatible with acute myelitis<br>3. Area postrema syndrome: requires associated dorsal medulla/area postrema lesions<br>4. Acute brainstem syndrome: requires associated periependymal brainstem lesions |

(From Wingerchuk DM, Banwell B, Bennett JL, et al. International consensus diagnostic criteria for neuromyelitis optica spectrum disorders. Neurology. 2015;85(2):177–189.)

**Table 6.7**  Clinical and Imaging Findings of Neuromyelitis Optica Spectrum Disorder (NMOSD) Versus Multiple Sclerosis (MS)

| | NMOSD | MS |
|---|---|---|
| Age | 30–40 | 20–40 |
| Sex | 80%–90% female | 60%–70% female |
| Symptomatic brain involvement | Uncommon | Common |
| Severity of attack | Usually severe | Usually mild |
| Brain magnetic resonance imaging (MRI) | Variable sized lesions; along the ependymal lining, diencephalon and brainstem around fourth ventricle and dorsal brainstem (area postrema); deep white matter, medullary lesions, nodular periventricular; no cortical gray or juxtacortical white matter lesions | Usually ovoid, small lesions, along the calloseptal margin, ovoid in the perivenular distribution; uncommon to involve diencephalon; brainstem often dorsal but also along pial surface; leukocortical lesions common |
| Optic nerve | Often bilateral, longitudinally extensive | Unilateral, short segment |
| Spinal cord | > 3 segments, often one large lesion, centrally located involving gray matter, holo-cord, T1 hypointensity (syrinx-like), variable enhancement (patchy/ring-like)<br><br>"bright spotty lesions"--marked T2 hyperintense (higher than CSF) and T1 hypointense foci in the central grey matter | < 1–2 segments, multifocal, marginal (posterolateral), less than half of spinal cord diameter, isointense on T1, nodular or homogenous enhancement |

frequently involved regions include basal ganglia, corpus callosum, cerebellum, and the periventricular area. When the periventricular zone is involved, the lesion is more typically linear along the ependymal margin or focal nodular. Associated contrast enhancement may occur in about 25% of cases.

## Acute Disseminated Encephalomyelitis

- Acute disseminated encephalomyelitis (ADEM) was originally described as a monophasic immune-mediated demyelinating disease with a self-limited course, more commonly affecting children (median age 5–8 years) than adults.
- The usual history is of a child with recent viral infection, vaccination, respiratory infection, or exanthematous disease. A latency period of 7 to 14 days or even longer has been described. ADEM has in the past been identified most frequently with antecedent measles, varicella, mumps, or rubella infection; nowadays Epstein-Barr virus, cytomegalovirus, or mycoplasma pneumonia respiratory infections are the most common precipitants. Other associated infections include myxoviruses, herpes group, and human immunodeficiency virus (HIV). Most recently with novel coronavirus, severe acute respiratory

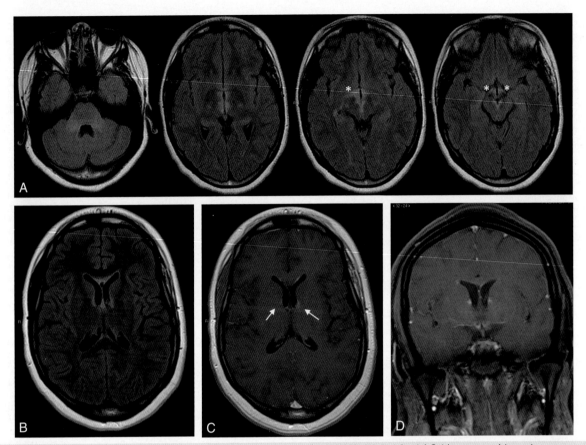

**Fig. 6.10 Brain magnetic resonance imaging (MRI) in neuromyelitis optica (NMO).** (A) Serial axial fluid-attenuated inversion recovery (FLAIR) images show hyperintensity along the surface of the ventral midbrain, periaqueductal gray, and medial thalami outlining the interpeduncular cistern and third ventricle, in addition to the bilateral middle cerebellar peduncles. Note also signal abnormality along the optic tracts bilaterally (*). (B) At another time point in the same patient, increased FLAIR hyperintense signal abnormality in the white matter adjacent to the frontal horns and anterior third ventricle and within callosal genu, accompanied by small nodular enhancement (*arrows*) on (C), axial and (D) coronal T1-weighted imaging (T1WI) reflecting acute inflammatory changes.

syndrome coronavirus 2 (SARS-CoV-2) or COVID-19, ADEM is also found at a high prevalence, particularly hemorrhagic presentation, among a myriad of neurologic manifestations.

- ADEM may also be idiopathic.
- Although rare, at the fulminant end of the spectrum of ADEM is acute hemorrhagic leukoencephalitis (Hurst disease) associated with diffuse multifocal perivascular demyelination and hemorrhage confined to the cerebral white matter with strict sparing of the subcortical U-fibers.
- The suspected etiology is based on immune mediated cross-reaction with a viral protein. Clinical syndromes of acute transverse myelitis, cranial nerve palsy, acute cerebellar ataxia (acute cerebellitis), or optic neuritis are well described, and recent diagnostic criteria also include the acute presentation of encephalopathy.
- The diagnosis is usually made by history and CSF, which may demonstrate an increase in white cells with a lymphocytic predominance and increased myelin basic protein. ADEM may have a mortality rate of up to 30%, and steroid therapy is commonly rendered to manage the disease.
- On T2WI imaging, ADEM lesions, which may be multiple and large, are high intensity and may enhance in a nodular or ring pattern (Fig. 6.11). No new lesions should appear on MR after approximately 6 months from

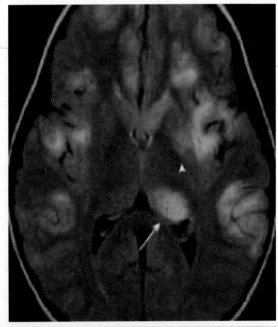

**Fig. 6.11 Acute disseminated encephalomyelitis (ADEM).** Fluid-attenuated inversion recovery (FLAIR) image shows high signal in the thalamus (*arrow*), putamen (*arrowhead*), and multifocal bilateral juxtacortical white matter.

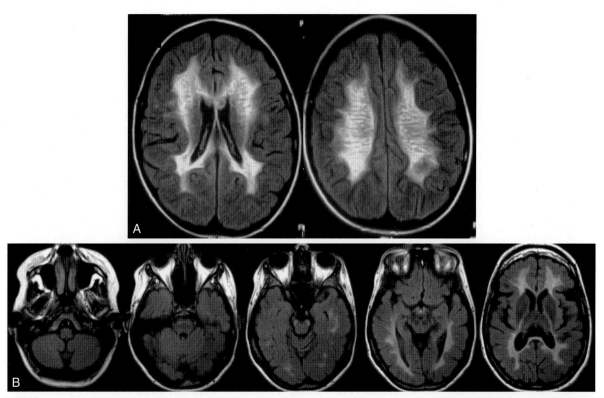

**Fig. 6.19 Metachromatic leukodystrophy (MLD).** (A) Axial fluid-attenuated inversion recovery (FLAIR) images show widespread symmetric high intensity throughout the white matter centrally with sparing of the U-fibers. Note the tiny, black dots and stripes perforating the high signal white matter, termed the "tigroid stripes" of MLD. (B) Serial axial FLAIR images in a different patient show hyperintensity involving the internal capsules and corticospinal tracts in addition to periventricular white matter.

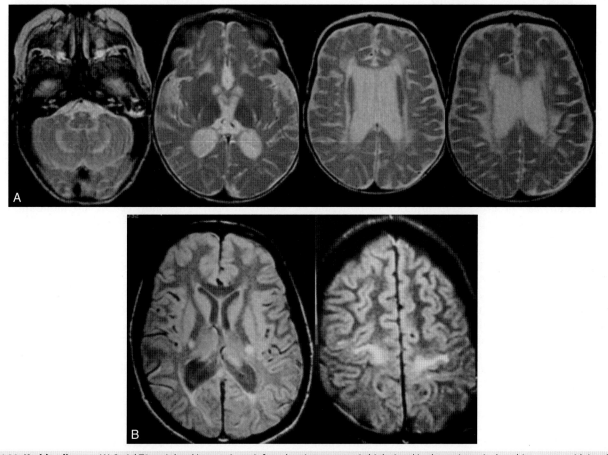

**Fig. 6.20 Krabbe disease.** (A) Serial T2-weighted images in an infant showing symmetric high signal in the periventricular white matter with involvement of the cerebellum and pyramidal tracts. (B) Axial fluid-attenuated inversion recovery (FLAIR) images in a different patient show bilateral hyperintense signal abnormalities involving the corticospinal tracts at the level of the precentral gyri and posterior limbs of the internal capsules.

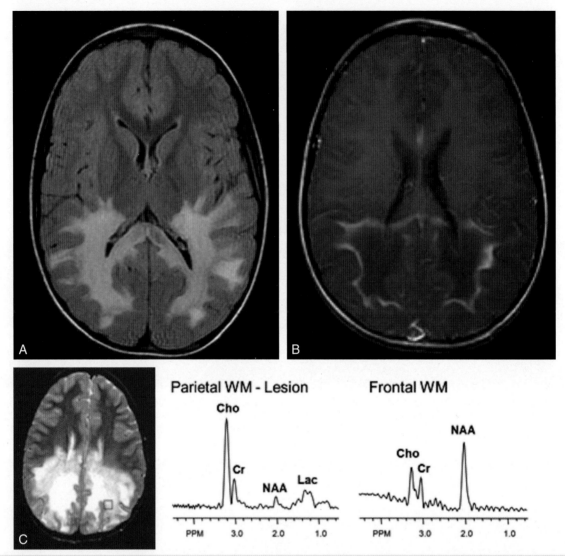

**Fig. 6.21 Adrenoleukodystrophy (ALD) in a 6-year-old boy.** (A) Axial fluid-attenuated inversion recovery (FLAIR) image shows bilateral symmetric hyperintense signal abnormality involving the parieto-occipital white matter and the splenium of the corpus callosum. (B) Postcontrast axial T1-weighted imaging (T1WI) shows enhancement in the margin of white matter signal abnormality, so-called "advancing front," representing areas of active demyelination. (C) ¹H magnetic resonance spectroscopy (¹H-MRS) shows elevated Cho and decreased N-acetylaspartate (NAA) with a Lac doublet peak in the left parietal white matter lesion, consistent with active inflammatory demyelination. Note the normal spectral pattern from the voxel in the normal-appearing left frontal white matter.

disease can also progress from anterior to posterior. The advancing edge of the lesion represents the region of active demyelination and shows contrast enhancement, whereas the nonenhanced regions are gliotic (Fig. 6.21). This active inflammatory demyelination is readily depicted using ¹H-MRS (see Fig. 6.21C), showing a signature elevation of choline (Cho) because of membrane breakdown, and the presence of lactate (Lac).

■ Patients have been described with enhancement of major white matter tracts, including the corticospinal, spinothalamic, visual (including the lateral geniculate body), auditory, and dentatorubral pathways. Other findings include calcifications in the trigone or around frontal horns, mass effect in the advancing region of demyelination, and isolated frontal lobe involvement. On MR, there may be relative sparing of the subcortical U-fibers.

■ Spinal cord disease can be seen with degeneration of the entire length of the corticospinal tracts and cord atrophy. This may be the predominant finding in the adult-onset form of the disease, also known as adrenomyeloneuropathy.

## Sudanophilic Leukodystrophy/Pelizaeus-Merzbacher Disease

■ Sudanophilic leukodystrophy is a degenerative myelin disorder distinguished by the accumulation of sudanophilic material in the brain. It may appear as failure of myelin maturation. This may be related to deficiency of proteolipid apoprotein and reduced production of other myelin proteins necessary for oligodendrocyte survival and differentiation.

■ Sudanophilic leukodystrophy has a variable age at onset, usually within the first months of life (but can emerge from neonatal to late infancy), with slow progression. The disease is divided into three subgroups, which differ in onset and clinical severity: classic (slowly progressive with death in young adulthood), connatal (more severe, with death in the first decade of life), and transitional (less severe than connatal, with average age at death of 8 years).

■ Pelizaeus-Merzbacher disease (PMD) may present as an x-linked form of sudanophilic leukodystrophy arising because of a mutation of the proteolipid protein (PLP) gene. Clinical findings of this type of sudanophilic leukodystrophy include bizarre eye movements and rotatory nystagmus, head shaking, psychomotor retardation, hypotonia, and cerebellar ataxia.

■ On CT, atrophy, low density in the white matter, and pinpoint periventricular calcifications have been reported. MR may be normal early on, but later they reveal cerebral, cerebellar, brainstem, and upper cervical cord atrophy. Further, there is diffuse symmetric abnormal signal in the white matter, which extends to the U-fibers because of the complete lack of myelination or hypomyelination (Fig. 6.22). In addition, there is low intensity on T2WI in the lentiform nucleus, substantia nigra, dentate nuclei, and thalamus, probably related to increased iron deposition. A "tigroid" pattern has been noted within the diffusely abnormal white matter, which corresponds to histopathologic findings of scattered, small regions of normal neurons and myelin sheaths. The corpus callosum is atrophic and undulating. Because of the lack of inflammatory or demyelinating components, PMD shows normal metabolites on [1]H-MRS (see Fig. 6.22D).

## Alexander Disease

■ Alexander disease can be classified as an astrocytopathy and is caused by a genetic mutation affecting glial fibrillary acidic protein. It is a progressive leukodystrophy characterized by fibrinoid degeneration of astrocytes

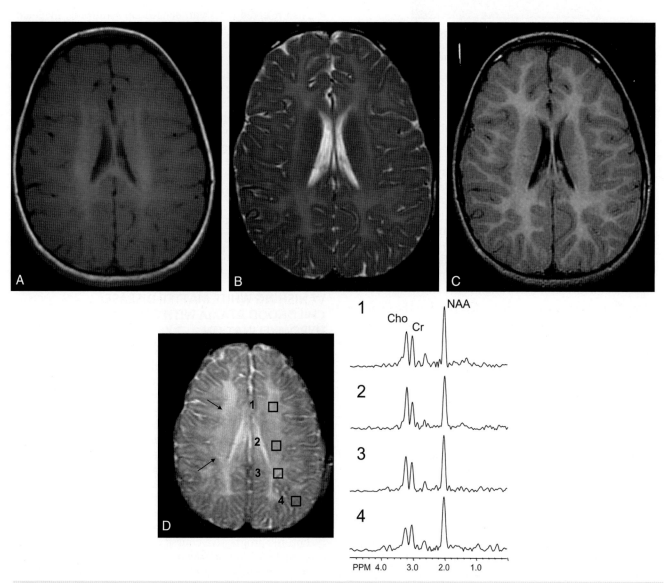

**Fig. 6.22 Pelizaeus-Merzbacher disease.** Magnetic resonance imaging (MRI) of a 6-year-old boy showing absence of normal myelination on (A) T1-weighted imaging (T1WI) and (B) T2-weighted imaging (T2WI). Normal white matter would be more hyperintense compared with the cortical gray matter on T1WI and darker on T2WI. (C) Axial fluid-attenuated inversion recovery (FLAIR) has signal intensity and contrast similar to a T1-weighted scan, which is abnormal for a 6-year-old. (D) Tigroid pattern because of patchy dysmyelination showing pinpoint dots of low intensity (*arrows*) in the white matter on T2WI. [1]H-MRS of 4 voxels in the white matter (*#1–3*) and gray matter (*#4*) shows normal spectral patterns.

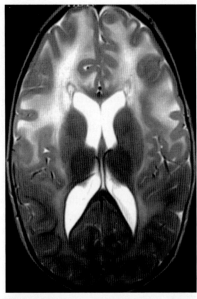

**Fig. 6.23 Alexander disease in a child with macrocephaly.** Axial T2-weighted image (T2WI) show confluent hyperintense signal abnormality preferentially involving the anterior cerebral white matter extending to the capsular regions.

and diffuse Rosenthal fibers in the subependymal, subpial, and perivascular regions.

- The disease has been divided into three clinical subgroups. The infantile type is characterized by symptoms such as seizures, spasticity, psychomotor retardation, and early-onset macrocephaly which are associated with extensive demyelination. The juvenile group (7–14 years old) demonstrates progressive bulbar symptoms with spasticity, and the adult group (second to seventh decades) has normal head size with predominant caudal brainstem and cervical cord atrophy. The latter two groups have preservation of neurons and less myelin loss.

- On CT, hyperdensity has been described in the caudate nucleus and diffuse hypodensity in the white matter and the internal and external capsules. Enhancement may be observed early in the disease course near the tips of the frontal horns. Changes in T2WI signal intensity have frontal predominance (Fig. 6.23) with early, extensive involvement of the subcortical white matter progressing to the capsular regions and edematous deep gray nuclei. In late-stage disease, atrophy ensues and there is cystic formation. Brainstem atrophy and decreased intensity in the basal ganglia have also been reported.

## CANAVAN DISEASE

- Canavan disease (spongiform degeneration) is an autosomal recessive leukodystrophy that results from deficiency in the enzyme N-acetylaspartoacylase from the *ASPA* gene on chromosome 17. The disease causes abnormal accumulation of N-acetylaspartate (NAA) in the urine, brain, and plasma.

- The age at disease onset is during early infancy from 2 to 4 months. Hallmarks include macrocephaly, hypotonia, and failure to thrive, followed by seizures, optic atrophy, and spasticity. Death usually occurs by the age 5.

- On routine MRI, the subcortical U-fiber white matter is most often involved with vacuolization progressing to deep white matter. Symmetric involvement of white matter (high signal on T2WI) and ventriculomegaly have been described (Fig. 6.24). Proton MR spectroscopy (1H-MRS) shows a signature of elevated NAA (see Fig. 6.24B). NAA is synthesized in the mitochondria and may function as a carrier for acetyl groups across the mitochondrial membrane. N-acetylaspartoacylase cleaves NAA into acetate and aspartate in the cytosol, and deficiencies in this enzyme can interfere with the supply of acetate for fatty acid synthesis and myelination.

## MEGALENCEPHALIC LEUKOENCEPHALOPATHY WITH SUBCORTICAL CYSTS

- Also referred to as van der Knaap syndrome, megalencephalic leukoencephalopathy with subcortical cysts (MLC) occurs because of the *MLC* gene isolated to chromosome 22. It is classified as an astrocytopathy, with intramyelin vacuolar changes and disruption of ion-water exchange homeostasis.

- Clinical manifestations are seizures, ataxia, macrocephaly, spasticity, and mental retardation presenting in the first year of life. There are two phenotypes: the classic progressive phenotype related to autosomal recessive mutation of the *MLC1* or *MLC2A* gene is the most common; the other phenotype, related to *MLC2B*, has the typical early clinical features but improvement of symptoms over time.

- MRI shows cysts at the temporal tips, which may become extreme in size, and frontoparietal regions with white matter disease (Fig. 6.25). Rarely, there is absence of macrocephaly.

## VANISHING WHITE MATTER DISEASE/ CHILDHOOD ATAXIA WITH CENTRAL HYPOMYELINATION

- Vanishing white matter (VWM) disease, also known as childhood ataxia with central hypomyelination (CACH), was initially believed to only occur in children and teenagers but has more recently been recognized in individuals of any age, ranging from prenatal to senescence, although most commonly 2 to 6 years, with variable clinical severity. It is a disorder related to autosomal recessive mutation in 1 of 5 genes encoding the subunits of eukaryotic translation initiation factor 2B.

- Clinical findings consist of prominent ataxia, spasticity, optic atrophy, and relatively preserved mental capabilities in young patients and presenile dementia, psychiatric symptoms, and migraine in adults. The disease follows a chronic progressive course with decline associated with episodes of minor infections and head trauma. The cortex is relatively normal. However, beneath the cortex, the white matter is largely destroyed, with the exception of some sparing of the U-fibers. There is progressive rarefaction of white matter to cystic degeneration from the frontal to occipital regions with the temporal lobe least

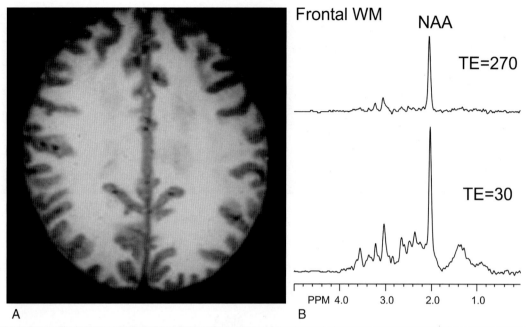

**Fig. 6.24 Canavan disease.** (A) T2-weighted image (T2WI) shows markedly hyperintense signal throughout the entire white matter reflecting myelin vacuolization. (B) ¹H-magnetic resonance spectroscopy (¹H-MRS) shows elevated N-acetylaspartate (NAA) peak at both high and low TE values. Note that choline and creatine (peaks at 3.2 and 3.0 ppm, respectively) are markedly low in comparison. *ppm*, Parts per million.

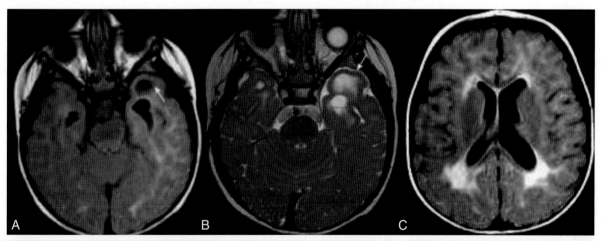

**Fig. 6.25 Megalencephalic leukoencephalopathy with subcortical cysts.** As the name implies, this child with this vacuolating leukodystrophy is characterized by subcortical cysts in the bilateral temporal lobes (*arrows*) on (A), axial fluid-attenuated inversion recovery (FLAIR), and (B) axial T2-weighted imaging (T2WI). (C) Axial FLAIR scan also shows bilateral white matter hyperintense signal abnormality.

involved. In noncystic regions of the brain, there is diffuse and severe myelin loss.

■ MR demonstrates regions of white matter that have a signal intensity similar to CSF on all pulse sequences, and the brain has a swollen appearance with cystic degeneration around the periventricular region (Fig. 6.26). Radial stripes in the white matter reflect spared tissue. There is no contrast enhancement. Cerebellar atrophy is present and may be severe, particularly in the vermis. Symmetric high intensity in the pontine tegmentum, cerebellar white matter, and central tegmental tract on T2WI has also been observed. ¹H-MRS findings included decreased metabolites, and the presence of lactate (see Fig. 6.26B).

## AICARDI-GOUTIERES SYNDROME

■ Aicardi-Goutières syndrome is a rare disorder related to autosomal recessive mutation of the *TREX1* gene located on chromosome 3p21.

■ Consistent with chronic lymphocytosis, the immune system and skin are also affected in addition to the brain. Clinically there is early encephalopathy followed by stabilization of neurologic symptoms.

■ Imaging findings show microcephaly and marked cerebral atrophy with dystrophic calcification (Fig. 6.27), mimicking congenital infections even though no infection is involved.

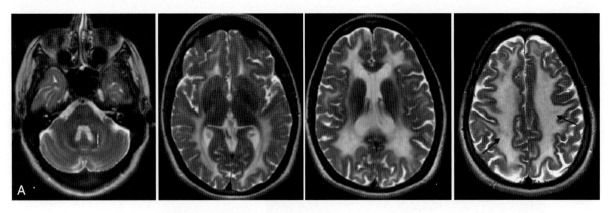

White Matter

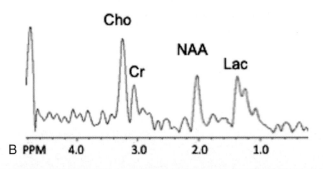

**Fig. 6.26  Vanishing white matter (VWM)/childhood ataxia with central nervous system hypomyelination (CACH) in a 36-year-old.** (A) Serial axial T2-weighted images show extensive white matter signal abnormality reflecting rarefaction, which leads to cystic degeneration. Note the radial stripes (*arrows*) within the T2 hyperintense white matter representing spared tissue. Cerebellar white matter also shows T2 hyperintense signal abnormality without cystic degeneration. (B) ¹H-magnetic resonance spectroscopy (¹H-MRS) shows decreased level of N-acetylaspartate (NAA) and creatinine (Cr), and an abnormally elevated Lac doublet at 1.33 ppm.

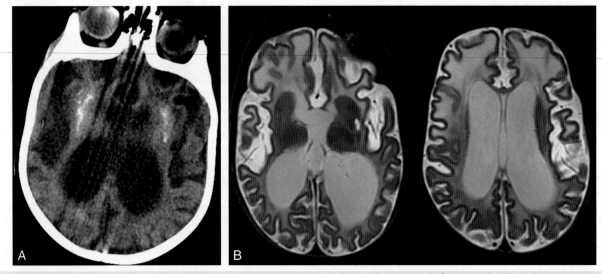

**Fig. 6.27  Aicardi-Goutières syndrome.** (A) Head computed tomography (CT) best depicts dystrophic calcification in the bilateral putamina, which are small. (B) Axial T2-weighted images show large ventricles and sulci indicative of volume loss, and extensive hypomyelination with T2 hyperintensity in the white matter, particularly confluent in the frontal and temporal regions.

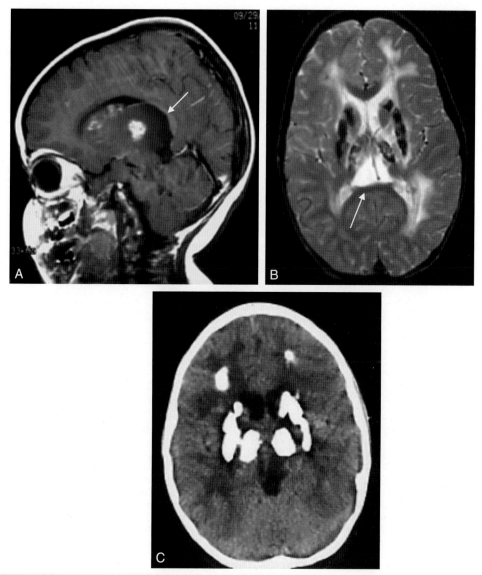

**Fig. 6.28  Labrune syndrome, or leukoencephalopathy with calcifications and cysts (LCC).** (A) Sagittal T1-weighted imaging (T1WI) shows globular T1 hyperintensity in the thalamus and basal ganglia, along with cavum vellum interpositum cyst (*arrow*). (B) T2-weighted imaging (T2WI) depicts T2 dark signal reflecting coarse calcifications in the deep gray nuclei bilaterally. A cystic lesion is present posteriorly in the region of cavum vellum interpositum (*arrow*). Note also periventricular T2 hyperintense signal abnormality. (C) Axial head CT best demonstrates multifocal coarse calcifications.

## LEUKOENCEPHALOPATHY WITH CALCIFICATIONS AND CYSTS/LABRUNE SYNDROME

- As the name implies, leukoencephalopathy with calcifications and cysts (LCC) presents with white matter disease, progressive cerebral calcifications, and parenchymal cysts (Fig. 6.28). Like Aicardi-Goutières syndrome, LCC presentation may mimic infection. The condition was first described in three unrelated children in 1996 by P. Labrune et al. Hence it is also known as "Labrune syndrome."

- Affected individuals present with cognitive decline, seizures, and movement disorder with pyramidal, extrapyramidal, and cerebellar signs. Brain biopsy reported by Labrune from one patient revealed microangiomatous change, including vessel wall thickening and calcification. Subsequently, genetic mutation was localized to *SNORD118* on chromosome 17, with autosomal recessive inheritance pattern.

- A very similar phenotype in the brain can be seen in Coats plus syndrome (Fig. 6.29), which is an inherited disorder characterized by retinal telangiectasia (i.e., Coats disease) plus abnormalities of the brain indistinguishable from LCC, as well as other systemic manifestations including osteopenia, gastrointestinal bleeding, anemia, thrombocytopenia, and hair and skin changes. Coats plus syndrome is, however, caused by distinctly different gene mutations (*CTC1*, *STN1*, or *POT1* genes). Before the localization of genetic mutations, Coats plus and LCC were referred to collectively as cerebroretinal microangiopathy with calcifications and cysts (CRMCC).

## CEREBRAL AUTOSOMAL DOMINANT ARTERIOPATHY WITH SUBCORTICAL INFARCTS AND LEUKOENCEPHALOPATHY

- Cerebral autosomal dominant arteriopathy with subcortical infarcts and leukoencephalopathy (CADASIL) is

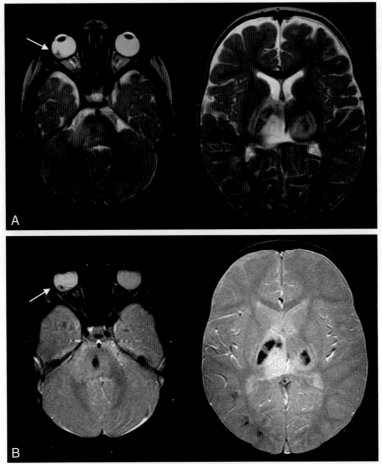

Fig. 6.29 **Coats plus syndrome has parenchymal cysts and calcifications indistinguishable from Labrune syndrome (see Fig. 6.28) but is caused by different genetic mutations, has other systemic manifestations, and is characterized by retinal telangiectasia (Coats disease) that is depicted in this patient's right eye** (*arrows*). **(A) Axial T2 images show high intensity in the pons, right middle cerebellar peduncle, and bilateral thalamocapsular regions. A parenchymal cyst can be seen in the right thalamic region. (B) Axial susceptibility-weighted images (SWI) show multifocal dark foci in the pons, bilateral thalami, and right parieto-occipital subcortical white matter, representing dystrophic calcifications.**

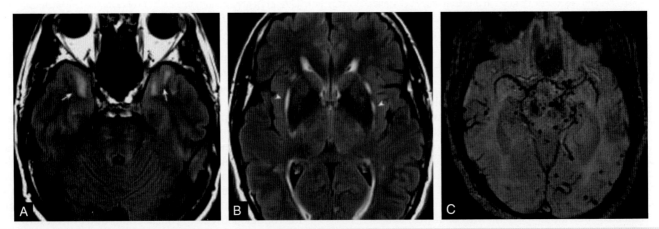

Fig. 6.30 **Cerebral autosomal dominant arteriopathy with subcortical infarcts and leukoencephalopathy (CADASIL).** (A) Axial fluid-attenuated inversion recovery (FLAIR) shows diffuse high intensity in the white matter of the anterior temporal lobes (*arrows*). (B) Higher image section in the same patient showing involvement of the external capsules (*arrowheads*). (C) Axial susceptibility-weighted imaging (SWI) in an older (62-year-old) individual with CADASIL shows innumerable microhemorrhages scattered throughout the deep structures and cortical and subcortical regions.

an inherited arterial disease caused by mutations of the *Notch 3* gene on chromosome 19.

- Distinctly different from most other leukodystrophies described in this section, its onset is predominantly in adulthood in the fourth decade of life; however, presentation in childhood as young as 3 years of age has been reported. As the most common form of an inherited stroke disorder, the disease is characterized by migraines, recurrent transient ischemic attacks, strokes, dementia, depression, pseudobulbar palsy, and hemiplegia or quadriplegia.
- MRI typically shows extensive, confluent white matter T2/FLAIR hyperintense signal abnormality, particularly in the periventricular and deep white matter, basal ganglia, and brainstem with subcortical lacunar infarcts. Most characteristically, CADASIL involves the anterior inferior temporal lobes and external capsules (Fig. 6.30). Diffusion tensor measurements have revealed increased diffusivity and concomitant loss of fractional anisotropy in CADASIL patients that can be correlated with clinical impairment, hypothesized to be the result of neuronal loss and demyelination. Microhemorrhages are reported in 25% to 69% of individuals with CADASIL depending on series, with increased frequency associated with age but not vascular risk factors. The common sites include the basal ganglia, deep structures, and cortical and subcortical regions.

In summary, inherited leukodystrophies are rare disorders that are ever expanding and challenging to diagnose, often requiring a combination of clinical, biochemical, pathologic, genetic, and neuroimaging approaches. Nevertheless, several imaging patterns can help narrow down the differential diagnosis in the currently well-defined leukodystrophies, which are listed in Box 6.8.

---

## Box 6.8    Imaging Patterns of Leukodystrophies

**Frontal Predominance**

- Alexander disease
- Frontal variant of X-ALD (17% of X-ALD)

**Parieto-occipital Predominance**

- Classic form of X-ALD

**Periventricular Predominance**

- Metachromatic leukodystrophy (MLD)
- Krabbe disease
- Leukoencephalopathy with brainstem and spinal cord involvement and lactate elevation (LBSL)

**Subcortical White Matter Involvement**

- Kearns-Sayre syndrome
- Canavan disease
- Alexander disease
- Vanishing white matter (VWM)/childhood ataxia with central nervous system hypomyelination (CASH)
- Pelizaeus-Merzbacher disease (PMD)

**Diffuse White Matter Involvement**

- Megalencephalic leukoencephalopathy with subcortical cysts (MLC)
- VWM/CACH

**Corticospinal Tract Involvement**

- MLD
- Krabbe
- ALD
- PMD

**Large Head**

- Alexander disease
- Canavan
- MLC
- VWM/CACH

**Small Head**

- Aicardi-Goutières

**Parenchymal Calcification**

- Aicardi-Goutières
- Leukoencephalopathy with calcifications and cysts (LCC)
- Krabbe disease

**Parenchymal Cysts**

- MLC
- LCC

# Neurodegenerative Diseases and Hydrocephalus

MEMI WATANABE

## Anatomic Considerations: Hydrocephalus versus Atrophy

- Atrophy and hydrocephalus often share the finding of dilatation of the ventricular system; however, the implications as far as prognosis and treatment are vastly different between the two. Whereas generally there is no treatment for atrophy, hydrocephalus can often be treated with well-placed ventricular or subarachnoid space shunts and/or removal of the obstructing or overproducing lesion. Therefore accurate distinction between atrophy and hydrocephalus is essential.
- Hydrocephalus reflects expansion of the ventricular system from increased intraventricular pressure, which is, in most cases, caused by abnormal cerebrospinal fluid (CSF) hydrostatic mechanics. Hydrocephalus may be because of three presumed causes:
  - overproduction of CSF
  - obstruction at the ventricular outlet level (noncommunicating hydrocephalus)
  - obstruction at the arachnoid villi level, leading to poor resorption of CSF back into the intravascular space (communicating hydrocephalus)
- Computed tomography (CT) or magnetic resonance imaging (MRI) findings that suggest hydrocephalus over atrophy are summarized in Table 7.1. Periventricular smooth high signal (best seen on fluid-attenuated inversion recovery [FLAIR]) (Fig. 7.1) is because of transependymal CSF migration into the adjacent white matter, leading to interstitial edema (dark on diffusion-weighted imaging [DWI]). This is most commonly seen at the angles of the lateral ventricles and, because of its smooth and diffuse nature, can usually be distinguished from the focal periventricular white matter abnormalities associated with atherosclerotic small vessel ischemic disease. Be aware that there may normally be mild high intensity at the angles of the ventricle (ependymitis granulosa) in middle-aged patients. Evan's index (ratio of width of frontal horns and maximal inner table of skull on same image) can be used as an approximate marker for ventricular enlargement, with ratio >3 indicating ventriculomegaly. Variabilities in measurement however make it less reliable indicator than other imaging features.

## Imaging Techniques and Protocols

- In addition to routine brain imaging, isovolumetric T1- and T2-weighted images (T1WI and T2WI, respectively) can provide higher resolution images that can be reconstructed in any plane:
  - T1 spoiled gradient echo sequences can provide greater anatomic detail, especially when evaluating change in size of anatomic structures, which is an important feature in workup of neurodegenerative processes.
  - Steady-state free precession three dimensional (3D) sequences (constructive interference in steady state) are part of a fluid-sensitive technique that provides high contrast resolution between fluid and adjacent soft tissues, enabling diagnosis of aqueductal stenosis or other causes of hydrocephalus.
- There are several phase contrast CSF flow study techniques, with the most common being the time-resolved two-dimensional (2D) phase contrast with velocity

**Table 7.1** Differentiation of Hydrocephalus and Atrophy

| Characteristic | Hydrocephalus | Atrophy |
|---|---|---|
| Temporal horns | Enlarged | Normal except in Alzheimer disease |
| Third ventricle | Convex | Concave |
| | Distended anterior recesses | Normal anterior recesses |
| Fourth ventricle | Normal or enlarged | Normal except with cerebellar atrophy |
| Callosal angle (measured coronally perpendicular to the anterior commissure-posterior commissure plane) | More acute | More obtuse |
| Mamillo-pontine distance | <1 cm | >1 cm |
| Corpus callosum | Thin, distended, rounded elevation | Normal or atrophied |
| | Increased distance between corpus callosum and fornix | Normal fornix-corpus callosum distance |
| Transependymal migration of cerebrospinal fluid | Present acutely | Absent |
| Sulci | Flattened | Enlarged out of proportion to age |
| Aqueductal flow void | Accentuated in normal-pressure hydrocephalus | Normal |
| Choroidal-hippocampal fissures | Normal to mildly enlarged | Markedly enlarged in Alzheimer disease |
| Sella | Remodeling of floor and ballooning of sella | Normal |

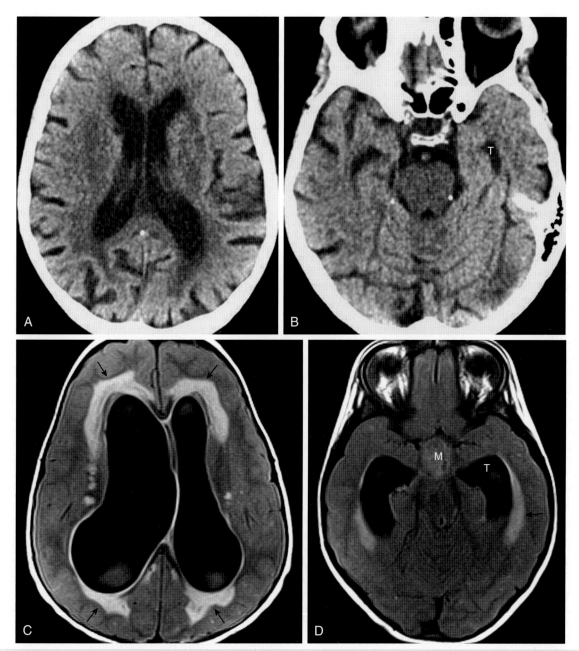

**Fig. 7.1 Atrophy versus hydrocephalus?** (A) Axial computed tomography (CT) image from an 85-year-old patient shows moderate enlargement of the lateral ventricles, with commensurate moderate dilatation of the cerebral sulci, indicating atrophy. Central white matter ischemic injury and right caudate lacune coexist. (B) In this same patient, the temporal horns (T) are relatively nondilated compared with the remainder of the lateral ventricles. (C) Axial fluid-attenuated inversion recovery (FLAIR) image in a different patient shows marked enlargement of the lateral ventricles but with effacement of the cerebral sulci, indicating hydrocephalus. Note the rounded margins of the frontal horns. There is increased signal *(arrows)* around the margins of the lateral ventricles, indicating transependymal flow of cerebrospinal fluid (CSF). (D) Axial FLAIR image in same patient shows marked enlargement of the temporal horns (T) further supporting diagnosis of hydrocephalus. Transependymal flow of CSF is again demonstrated. The cause of the hydrocephalus is a large mass (M) within the third ventricle with suprasellar extension.

encoding. In this technique, signal from moving protons is limited to the flow rate of CSF only (excluding vascular flow), which can be evaluated qualitatively and quantitatively. This is particularly useful at the level of the cerebral aqueduct and foramen magnum where CSF flow obstruction might be suspected. It may also be employed to assess the patency of third ventriculostomies.

■ Quantitative volumetric techniques from various vendors can also provide precise volumetric data, which can aid in diagnosis of neurodegenerative processes.

## Pathology

### OVERPRODUCTION OF CEREBROSPINAL FLUID

■ It has been theorized that patients with choroid plexus papillomas and choroid plexus carcinomas have hydrocephalus based on the overproduction of CSF. Increasingly, this hypothesis has come into question because it is believed that some cases of hydrocephalus may, in fact, be because of obstruction of the arachnoid villi or other CSF channels secondary to adhesions from tumoral hemorrhage, high-protein levels, or intraventricular debris. This is particularly true with fourth ventricular choroid plexus papillomas, which generally tend to obstruct the sites of egress of the CSF in the foramina of Luschka and Magendie. In the cases of lateral ventricle choroid plexus papillomas (particularly in the pediatric population), the overproduction of CSF may be the cause of hydrocephalus.

## NONCOMMUNICATING (OBSTRUCTIVE) HYDROCEPHALUS

- Noncommunicating forms are because of abnormalities at the ventricular outflow levels, which includes aqueductal stenosis, masses/tumors, clots, synechiae, or ventricular compression by parenchymal lesions, like tumors, hematomas, and infarcts. It is useful to identify the cause of the hydrocephalus because noncommunicating types often need brain surgery to remove offending agents; communicating types respond best to shunts.

### Colloid Cyst

- The classic cause of obstruction at the foramina of Monro is the colloid cyst (Fig. 7.2). This is typically located in the anterior region of the third ventricle. On unenhanced CT, the lesion is high in density. Magnetic resonance (MR) often shows a lesion that is high intensity on T1WI and T2WI. However, the signal of colloid cysts is variable, depending on the protein concentration, presence of hemorrhage, and other paramagnetic ion effects.

### Aqueductal Stenosis

- Aqueductal stenosis is a common cause of the congenital obstructive hydrocephalus, showing dilatation of the lateral and third ventricles, but with a normal-appearing fourth ventricle. The etiology is multifactorial, including both genetic/congenital and acquired causes. Of the genetic causes, this is most commonly an X-linked recessive disorder seen in early childhood, although it can present at any age. As intrinsic causes, aqueductal webs, septa, or diaphragms may obstruct the exit of CSF from the third ventricle (Fig. 7.3). Clots and synechiae from intraventricular hemorrhage (IVH) or infection are acquired intrinsic sources. Brainstem, tectal, extraaxial, and pineal lesions can also result in aqueductal stenosis caused by extrinsic mass effect on the aqueduct (Fig. 7.4).
- Sagittal MR is very helpful for distinguishing extrinsic mass compression from an intrinsic aqueductal abnormality. Aqueductal stenosis may also be diagnosed on CSF flow (phase contrast) MRI. Phase contrast MR with a velocity encoding set to 10 to 15 cm/sec may be the best way to assess aqueductal patency. The technique is also useful to establish CSF flow at third ventriculostomy sites as an alternative CSF outflow pathway (Fig. 7.5).

### Trapped Ventricles

- The so-called "trapped ventricle" may occur when the egress of CSF is obstructed, either from intrinsic or extrinsic masses. For example, in the trauma setting, a large subdural hematoma (SDH) can compress the ipsilateral lateral ventricle, but because of midline shift and outflow obstruction at the foramen of Monro, the contralateral lateral ventricle can abnormally dilate. Not uncommonly, transependymal edema around the margins of the trapped ventricle can be seen.
- Trapping of the third ventricle is uncommon. Selective enlargement of the third ventricle must be distinguished from the presence of an intraventricular ependymal/arachnoid cyst and third ventricle squamopapillary craniopharyngiomas.
- Isolation of the fourth ventricle may occur when the aqueduct of Sylvius, and foramen of Magendie and Luschka are occluded. The fourth ventricle becomes "trapped" and will expand as CSF production by the choroid plexus continues unabated (Fig. 7.6). This expansion may compress the cerebellum and brain stem and lead to posterior fossa symptoms. Many of these cases are because of fibrous adhesions with or without earlier hemorrhage.

## COMMUNICATING HYDROCEPHALUS

Communicating hydrocephalus is because of abnormalities at the level of the arachnoid villi, blockage at the incisura of the foramen magnum, or shunt failure, while CSF can still flow between the ventricles.

### Obstruction at the Arachnoid Villi Level

- The arachnoid villi are sensitive, delicate structures that may get gummed up by insults of several causes, resulting in communicating hydrocephalus. The most common causes of obstruction include infectious meningitis, ventriculitis, ependymitis, subarachnoid hemorrhage, and carcinomatous meningitis. As the CSF becomes more viscous with a higher protein concentration, the arachnoid villi lose their ability to reabsorb the fluid.
- It is not uncommon to see dilated lateral and third ventricles but a normal-sized fourth ventricle in communicating hydrocephalus. The fourth ventricle is the last ventricle to dilate, possibly because of its relatively confined location in the posterior fossa, surrounded as it is by the thick calvarium and sturdy petrous bones. The hunt for a source of the ventricular dilatation should not stop at the aqueductal level with this pattern.

### Normal-Pressure Hydrocephalus

- Normal-pressure hydrocephalus (NPH) or adult hydrocephalus has a classic triad of clinical findings: gait apraxia, dementia, and urinary incontinence. Half of patients have no known prior insult (idiopathic NPH), whereas the other half carry a remote history of prior infection or hemorrhage (nonidiopathic NPH).
- Hydrocephalus may respond to shunting or endoscopic third ventriculostomy procedures with amelioration of clinical symptoms, making this a treatable cause of dementia (although the gait disturbance is more readily responsive to treatment and occurs earlier in the course). Because there is a chance at the possibility of return of function with a shunt, it is important to at least consider the diagnosis of NPH when ventricles appear larger than expected. The most accurate predictors of a positive response to shunting is clinical improvement following large volume lumbar tap. From an imaging standpoint, some positive predictors of response to shunting include

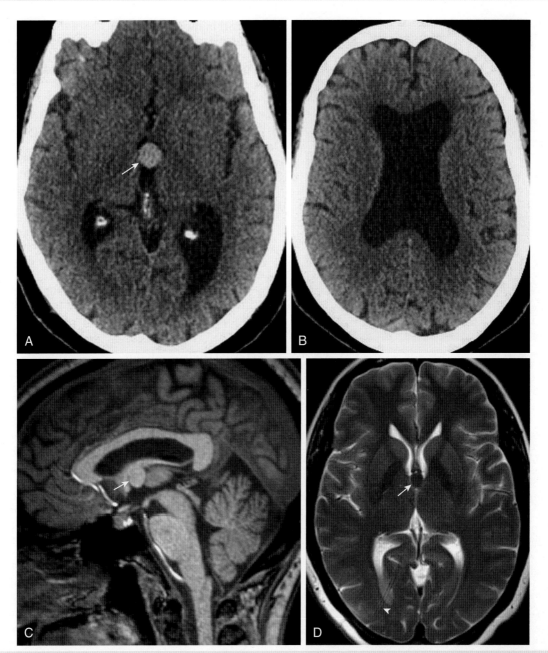

**Fig. 7.2  Colloid cyst.** (A) Axial computed tomography image shows classic appearance of a colloid cyst as a rounded hyperattenuating lesion within the anterior aspect of the third ventricle *(arrow)*. (B) More superiorly, there is enlargement of the lateral ventricles because of obstructive hydrocephalus by the colloid cyst. (C) Sagittal T1-weighted image (T1WI) in a different patient shows a hyperintense rounded mass in the anterior aspect of the third ventricle *(arrow)*. (D) The same lesion is hypointense on T2WI *(arrow)*. Note that the patient has been shunted *(arrowhead)* to decompress the lateral ventricles, which now appear normal in size.

(1) absence of central atrophy or ischemia, (2) upward bowing of the corpus callosum with flattened gyri and ballooned third ventricular recesses, (3) prominent intraventricular CSF pulsations.

■ Imaging features on CT and MRI may also include enlarged ventricles with particular enlargement of the temporal horns, upward bowing of the corpus callosum, disproportionate prominence of the sylvian fissures (disproportionally enlarged subarachnoid space hydrocephalus [DESS or DESH]) and smaller sulci at the vertex, acute callosal angle (<90 degrees), Evans' index greater than 0.3 (maximum width of the frontal horns of the lateral ventricles divided by the maximal internal diameter of the skull at the same level), enlarged convex appearance of the infundibular and chiasmatic recesses of the third ventricle, and transependymal CSF leakage (Fig. 7.7). Stroke volume, the mean CSF volume through the aqueduct during systole and diastole of the cardiac cycle over several minutes, can be assessed quantitatively using phase contrast technique. Volumes greater than 42 microliters have been described in patients with NPH.

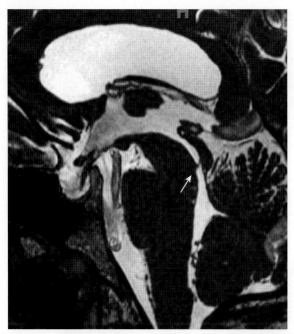

**Fig. 7.3 Aqueductal web.** This high-resolution sagittal constructive interference steady-state T2-weighted image shows a fine web *(arrow)* crossing the inferior aqueduct. The ventricles are not tremendously enlarged, because of the lateral ventriculostomy catheter (not shown).

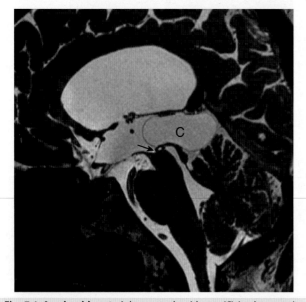

**Fig. 7.4 Arachnoid cyst.** A large arachnoid cyst (C) in the superior vermian cistern focally occludes the superior aspect of the cerebral aqueduct *(arrow)* and causes hydrocephalus of the lateral and third ventricles, seen as upward bowing of the corpus callosum and dilatation of the third ventricle's anterior recesses.

---

**TEACHING POINTS**

Normal-Pressure Hydrocephalus (NPH)

- The term "disproportionately enlarged subarachnoid space hydrocephalus" (DESH) can be used when imaging shows enlarged ventricles, widening of the sylvian fissures, and crowded sulci at the vertex. These findings might support good response to shunt treatment.

- DESH in the setting of absence of the clinical features of NPH can be called "asymptomatic ventriculomegaly with features of idiopathic NPH on MRI" (AVIM) and is felt by some to represent a preclinical form of NPH.

---

- Although infrequently performed, there is abnormal indium 111-DTPA (diethylenetriaminepentaacetic acid) distribution (Fig. 7.8). Normally, the tracer, which is instilled in the CSF through a lumbar puncture, is resorbed over the convexities without ventricular reflux within 2 to 24 hours. In cases of communicating hydrocephalus and NPH, reflux of the tracer into the ventricles is seen with lack of tracer accumulation over the convexities 24 to 48 hours after instillation. Patients who demonstrate this scintigraphic appearance allegedly have a better response to shunting than patients with normal or equivocal indium findings.
- A diagnostic large volume (40–60 cc) CSF withdrawal via lumbar puncture or lumbar drain showing improvement in gait is the best study that predicts improvement with shunting in NPH.

## External Hydrocephalus

- Another benign cause of hydrocephalus from arachnoid villi malfunction is "external hydrocephalus," also referred to as "benign enlargement of the subarachnoid spaces in infants" (BESS). This may be because of immaturity of the arachnoid villi with a decreased capacity to absorb CSF. BESS is typically seen in children younger than 2-years-old who have a rapidly enlarging head circumference. Transient developmental delay may be present at the time of presentation; however, the clinical and imaging findings usually resolve by the time the child is 3 to 4 years old, and the head circumference returns to normal. Prematurity, a history of IVH, and some genetic syndromes predispose to this condition.
- CT and MR show dilatation of the subarachnoid spaces over the cerebral convexities and normal or slightly enlarged ventricular system (Fig. 7.9). Sulcal dilatation and vessels coursing through the subarachnoid spaces indicate enlarged subarachnoid spaces, whereas displacement of vessels toward the surface of the brain implies the more concerning finding of subdural collection. Atrophy is not usually associated with an enlarging head circumference.
- Patients with BESS have an increased rate of SDHs, presumably because the enlarged subarachnoid space causes stretching of the bridging veins in the subdural space. If nonaccidental trauma (NAT) is suspected in these patients, SDHs of different ages would suggest NAT—along with additional findings of retinal hemorrhages and fractures (see Chapter 4).
- It has been suggested that patients with NPH as adults may suffer the same issue (decreased resorption of CSF) as children with BESS, and the two may be related.

## IDIOPATHIC INTRACRANIAL HYPERTENSION

- Idiopathic intracranial hypertension (aka pseudotumor cerebri), is a disorder related to elevated intracranial pressure (ICP). Patients with this disorder are typically

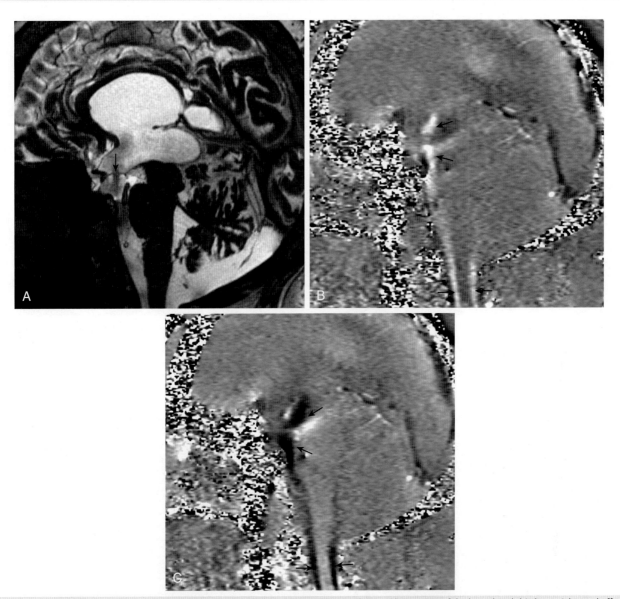

**Fig. 7.5  Biphasic flow of cerebrospinal fluid (CSF).** (A) Sagittal T2-weighted image shows enlargement of the lateral and third ventricles and efface-ment of the cerebral aqueduct in this patient with aqueductal stenosis. The patient underwent a third ventriculostomy procedure, whereby a defect is intentionally created at the floor of the third ventricle to allow for CSF flow between the third ventricle and suprasellar cistern (*arrow*). Note CSF pulsa-tion artifact through the defect, indicating patency and absence of flow related signal at the cerebral aqueduct. Phase contrast magnetic resonance imaging CSF flow study shows bright (B) and dark (C) signal indicating robust biphasic CSF flow at the level of the ventriculostomy defect and ventrally and dorsally at the foramen magnum (*arrows*).

obese, female and young (presenting from late childhood to first few decades of life). They have frequent head-aches, cranial nerve VI palsies, papilledema, or visual field deficits on examination. The disease may occur in association with pregnancy, endocrine abnormalities, medications, or intracranial venoocclusive disease.

- Diagnosis is confirmed when lumbar puncture dem-onstrates extreme elevations of CSF pressure, and treatment consists of repetitive lumbar punctures to drain fluid, but often the disease remits spontaneously. Ventriculoperitoneal shunting can be useful in keeping symptoms at bay.
- The role of imaging is to exclude secondary causes of elevated ICP, such as a brain tumor, hydrocephalus, a dural venous malformation, venous stenosis, or venous thrombosis (Fig. 7.10).

- CT and MRI findings that support this disorder include:
  - Flattened transverse sinuses
  - Papilledema
  - Normal or slightly small ventricles
  - Larger cerebral subarachnoid space volume
  - Expanded, empty sella
  - Other areas of spontaneous CSF-filled outpouchings of the dura (meningoceles), both frequently around the Meckel cave and the petrous apex
  - An enlarged and more tortuous optic nerve sheath complex
- Most MR studies in patients with pseudotumor cerebri show normal brain parenchyma.
- The venous sinuses and veins may be small and may enlarge after spinal fluid drainage. In some cases, venous sinus stenosis or thrombosis demonstrated on MR

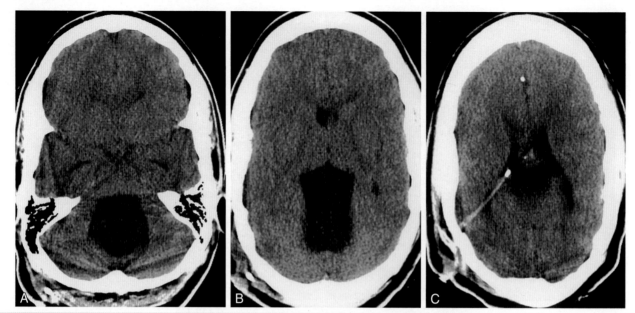

**Fig. 7.6 Trapped fourth ventricle.** (A) The fourth ventricle is markedly enlarged with effacement of cerebellar sulci. Note, however, how small the temporal horns and frontal horns are. (B) A more superior cut shows the ballooning upward of the fourth. Did you catch the edge of the skull film finding? (C) Yes, there was a shunt present that decompressed the ventricles above, but the aqueductal obstruction coupled with Magendie and Luschka outflow occlusion trapped the fourth ventricle.

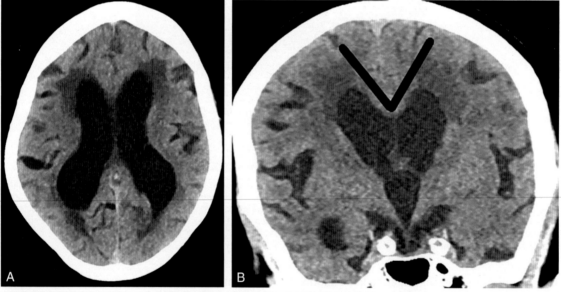

**Fig. 7.7 Normal-pressure hydrocephalus (NPH).** (A) Axial computed tomography (CT) image shows ventricular enlargement out of proportion to sulcal dilatation without an obstructing lesion, the sine qua non of NPH. B, Coronal reconstruction from this same patient shows an acute callosal angle (*dark black lines*). Note the narrowed sulci at the vertex compared with sulci elsewhere, also consistent with NPH.

venography (MRV) or CT venography (CTV) may yield the underlying cause of the condition. Some researchers wonder whether the increased ICP is the primary issue, and the venous sinus stenosis is because of collapse from the high pressure. In any case, stenting of the "stenosed" sinuses that show pressure gradients across the stenosis, can be curative.

- Spontaneous intracranial hypotension, on the other hand, is a condition characterized by low intracranial pressures, due to dural tears and CSF leakage. Patients present with postural headaches, relieved when lying down. On imaging, subdural collections, brainstem sagging with tonsillar descent, venous sinus distention and pachymeningeal enhancement (see Chapter 4).

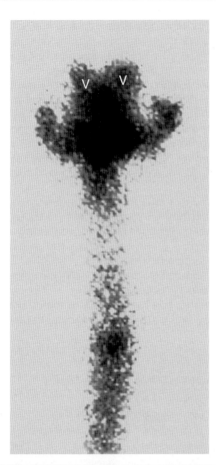

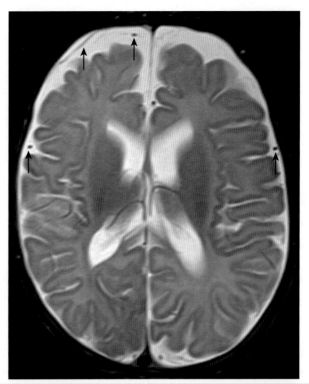

**Fig. 7.9 Benign enlargement of the subarachnoid spaces (BESS).** Note the prominence of the extraaxial spaces overlying the frontal lobes in this infant with external hydrocephalus. The sulci are not effaced, as would be seen in the setting of bilateral subdural collections. Cortical vessels *(arrows)* cross the extraaxial spaces, not displaced toward the surface of the brain (as would be seen with subdural fluid collections). The ventricular system is also prominent, not uncommonly seen in this condition.

**Fig. 7.8 Indium-DTPA (diethylenetriaminepentaacetic acid) study in a patient with normal-pressure hydrocephalus.** Coronal indium-labeled study shows lack of ascension of the radiotracer over the convexities with reflux of the tracer into the lateral ventricles (V). This study was taken 48 hours after intrathecal tracer insertion.

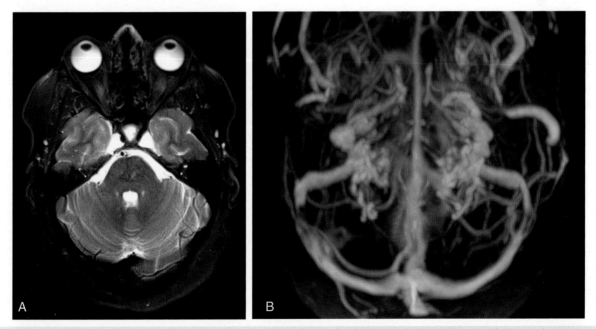

**Fig. 7.10 Idiopathic intracranial hypertension.** (A) Axial T2W image in a patient with headaches and elevated intracranial pressure shows empty sella and large Meckel cave meningoceles bilaterally. Bulging of optic nerve heads bilaterally, which correlated with papilledema on fundoscopy was also noted (not shown) as shown in Figure 9-18. (B) Contrast enhanced MR venogram in a different patient shows marked focal narrowing of the transverse sinuses bilaterally.

# Atrophy

- Atrophy reflects the loss of brain tissue, be it cortical, sub-cortical, or deep. With the loss of cell bodies in the cortex (gray matter), axonal Wallerian degeneration occurs with white matter atrophy or demyelination. Selective atrophy of the white matter may also occur with perivascular small-vessel insults. Remember that certain drugs (steroids) or metabolic states (dehydration, alcoholism) may cause an appearance of increased CSF spaces (suggesting atrophy) but are potentially reversible.

## NEURODEGENERATIVE DISORDERS

See Table 7.2.

## Alzheimer Disease

- The term *dementia* is less frequently used nowadays after the *Diagnostic and Statistical Manual of Mental Disorder*, Fifth Edition (DSM-5) revised the terminology. *Neurocognitive disorder (NCD)* is the new DSM-5 terminology replacing dementia and suggesting abnormalities in one or more of six cognitive domains: complex attention, executive function, learning and memory, language, perceptual motor, or social cognition. Major NCD implies interference with independence in daily activities (dementia), whereas mild NCD does not and was formerly likened to "mild cognitive impairment (MCI)."

- Alzheimer disease (AD) is one of the most common neurodegenerative disorders, accounting for 60% to 90% of the dementing disorders with progressive memory loss, often with personality changes, impaired cognition, and depression.

- AD affects 2 to 4 million Americans and 8% of the population older than 65 years and 30% of those older than over 85 years. Females are more commonly affected by a 2:1 margin. Late in the course, the patient becomes severely impaired, myoclonic, vegetative, and weak. Current treatments are limited in effectiveness and focus on slowing progression of disease.

- Senile plaques, seen as amorphous material in the cerebral cortex, and neurofibrillary tangles in the nerve cells

**Table 7.2** Neurodegenerative Causes of Atrophy

| Entity | Distinguishing Anatomic Imaging Findings | Distinguishing Clinical Findings |
|---|---|---|
| Alzheimer disease | Temporal lobe predominance | Severe memory loss |
| | Increased hippocampal-choroidal fissure size | Speech and olfaction affected early |
| | Hippocampal and amygdala atrophy, global atrophy | No early myoclonus or gait disturbance |
| | | Course in years |
| Frontotemporal dementias | Behavioral variant: anterior temporal and frontal atrophy, hemispheric asymmetry | Behavioral variant: prominent changes in personality and interpersonal relationships |
| | Primary progressive aphasia variant: perisylvian and insular atrophy, especially of superior temporal gyrus | Primary progressive aphasia variant: word-finding difficulties, difficulties with writing and comprehension |
| Creutzfeldt-Jakob disease | Abnormal intensity in basal ganglia and thalami | Transmission of prion |
| | | Rigidity |
| | | Myoclonus |
| | | Course in months |
| Parkinson disease | Substantia nigra decreased in size | Rigidity, bradykinesia, tremor |
| Lewy body dementia | Brain stem, substantia nigra, cortical atrophy | Cognitive difficulties, hallucinations |
| Multisystem atrophy | Variants include olivopontocerebellar degeneration with olive, pons, cerebellar; and putaminal atrophy, striatonigral degeneration with smaller midbrain | Parkinsonism, autonomic dysfunction, cerebellar gait disorders |
| Progressive supranuclear palsy | Midbrain, collicular atrophy, increased putaminal iron | Ophthalmoplegia, pseudobulbar palsy, rigidity |
| Corticobasal degeneration | Atrophy of the paracentral structures, superior parietal lobule knife blade atrophy, dilated central sulcus asymmetry characteristic | Rigidity of limbs |
| | | Alien limb phenomenon |
| | | Personality disorders |
| | | Myoclonus |
| AIDS | Atrophy | Young age |
| | High intensity in basal ganglia | Risk factors |
| | Superimposed infection | Positive HIV |
| | PML and lymphoma | |
| Multi-infarct dementia | White matter and deep gray lacunae | Stuttering course with discrete events |
| | Strokes of different ages | Stroke risk factors |
| | Central pontine infarcts | Early gait disturbance |
| Amyotrophic lateral sclerosis | Hypointensity in motor cortex (T2WI) | Weakness |
| | Hyperintensity in corticospinal tract (T2WI) | Atrophy |
| | Anterior horn cell atrophy | Spasticity |
| | | Preserved cognition |

*AIDS*, Acquired immunodeficiency syndrome; *PML*, progressive multifocal leukoencephalopathy; *T2WI*, T2-weighted image.

in the form of tangled loops of cytoplasmic fibers, are the diagnostic histopathologic features of AD. Disease progression from the entorhinal cortex to the hippocampus to the neo-cortex is the rule. Other pathophysiological processes, such as vascular disease, may contribute to the AD pathogenesis

■ Studies suggest that the amyloid deposition, which is imaged with amyloid biomarkers (amyloid positron emission tomographic [PET] findings and CSF amyloid-$\beta_{42}$ [A$\beta_{42}$]), comes decades before the first clinical symptoms appear. Elevated CSF tau and fluorodeoxyglucose [FDG]

PET findings can be seen early in the disease process. The typical atrophy on structural MRI becomes apparent during the clinically symptomatic phase of the disease. For both MCI and AD criteria, clinical diagnosis is of most importance and biomarkers are complementary. The roles of neuroimaging include (1) detection of early AD, (2) prediction of conversion from MCI to AD, (3) differential diagnosis between AD and other dementias, and (4) understanding of underlying pathophysiology.

■ The main imaging findings of AD include diffuse cortical atrophy, often more prominent in the mesial temporal lobes (Fig. 7.11). The subiculum and entorhinal cortex of the parahippocampal region appears to be most severely affected in AD. On longitudinal studies, the rate of atrophic change in patients with AD is much faster than in normal persons. There may be, in fact, a continuum of progressive hippocampal atrophy between normal elderly people, those with MCI, and those with AD.

■ The Medial Temporal Lobe Atrophy Score may be appropriately reported in patients suspected of neurodegenerative disorders, with score (0-4) based on age and qualitative assessment of choroid fissure width, temporal horn width, and hippocampal height on coronal images (CT or MRI). An abnormal score is 2 or higher in

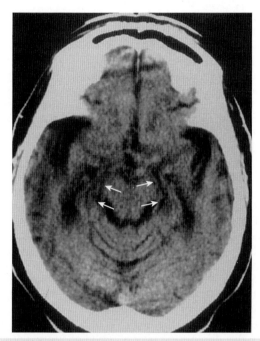

**Fig. 7.11 Alzheimer Disease.** Axial unenhanced computed tomography (CT) scan shows dilation of the choroidal-hippocampal fissure complex *(arrows)* with dilation of the adjacent temporal horns caused by temporal lobe atrophy.

**TEACHING POINTS**

Mesial Temporal Lobe Atrophy Score

| Score | Observations |
|-------|--------------|
| 0 | Normal appearance of choroid fissure |
| 1 | Slightly widened choroid fissure |
| 2 | Moderately widened choroid fissure, mild prominence of temporal horns, mild hippocampal atrophy |
| 3 | Severely widened choroid fissure, moderate prominence of temporal horns, moderate hippocampal atrophy |
| 4 | Severely widened choroid fissure, severe prominence of temporal horn, severe hippocampal atrophy |

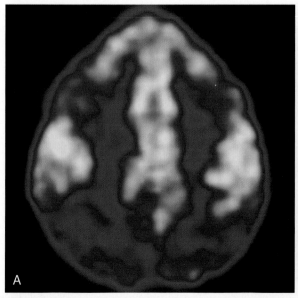
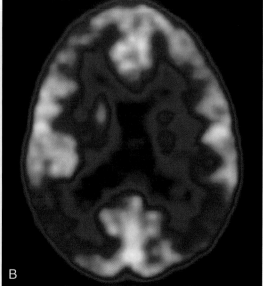

**Fig. 7.12 Alzheimer Disease.** Images from fluorodeoxyglucose–positron emission tomography (FDG-PET) show decreased activity in the parietal (A) and temporal (B) regions.

a patient younger than 75-years-old, and 3 or more in a patient 75 years or older.

- There is a stepwise increase in the number of microhemorrhages seen on susceptibility-weighted imaging (SWI) scans between normal, MCI, and AD subjects. People have suggested that the amyloid deposition, the same amyloid in amyloid angiopathy, may be the source of these dark SWI foci.

- FDG PET scanning has demonstrated decreased oxygen utilization and decreased regional cerebral blood flow in the posterior cingulate gyrus, and the posterior temporoparietal lobes in patients with AD (Fig. 7.12). On single-photon emission computed tomography (SPECT) brain studies, patients with AD have reduced cerebral blood flow as measured by parietal-to-cerebellar and parietal-to-mean cortical activity. The severity of symptoms may correspond to the reduction in uptake of technetium hexamethylpropyleneamine oxime (HMPAO).

- Amyloid PET imaging is a molecular imaging technique of specific Aβ ligands, such as $^{11}$C labeled Pittsburgh Compound B ($^{11}$C PiB), and several fluorine$^{18}$ compounds, florbetapir, flutemetamol, and florbetaben. Positive amyloid PET scan strongly suggests the diagnosis of AD. However, abnormal amyloid PET scan can be seen in around 30% of cognitively normal elderly subjects, which matches the proportion of cognitively normal elderly subjects with an autopsy diagnosis of AD. The degree of PiB uptake does not distinguish the cognitively normal elderly from patients with amnesic MCI or AD.

## Frontotemporal Dementia

- Frontotemporal dementia (FTD) is used to classify patients with focal cortical atrophy affecting the frontal and/or temporal lobes. Clinically, patients with FTD have peculiar behaviors (hyperorality, hypersexuality, lack of personal awareness, apathy, and perseverations) with personality shifts, inappropriate social conduct, and psychiatric overtones. FTD occurs in younger age groups compared with AD, usually presenting in the age range of 40 to 75 years and affecting males and females equally.

- CT and MR show symmetric or asymmetric atrophy of the frontal and anterior temporal lobes. In early-onset dementia, radiologic differentiation of FTD and early AD may be challenging because both entities are characterized with medial temporal lobe atrophy. In established FTD cases, affected regions include the frontal lobes, specifically the ventromedial, orbitofrontal, anterior cingulate, anterior insula, and amygdala.

- Anterior hypoperfusion/hypometabolism on SPECT/ FDG PET and frontal lobe hypoperfusion in arterial spin labeling (ASL) MRI may also be seen.

- Further, FTD is subdivided into a number of clinical distinct entities:

  - Behavioral variant FTD (bvFTD) is characterized by changes in personality, behaviors and cognition, such as apathy, abulia, disinhibition, and compulsive behaviors. Patients with bvFTD can develop speech dysfunction as disease progresses. Atrophy is seen in in the prefrontal cortex and anterior temporal lobes. Heterogeneity in patterns of neurodegeneration is also observed.
    - There is more often frontal lobe than anterior temporal lobe predominance to the atrophy (Fig. 7.13).

  - Primary progressive aphasia (PPA) FTD is a rare dementing disorder with language impairment as the dominant deficit (Fig. 7.14). There are three subtypes that have been described based on specific speech and language features. These are: progressive nonfluent aphasia (PNFA) or nonfluent/agrammatic variant PPA (nfvPPA), semantic variant (svPPA), and logopenic PPA.
    - In nfvPPA, the main clinical feature is cognitive diminution over a period of years, with word finding difficulties leading over time to mutism. Behavioral changes are less prominent. Atrophy is seen in dorsolateral frontal lobe and peri-insular regions (often affecting Broca's area) rather than

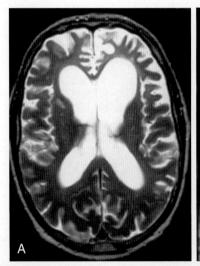
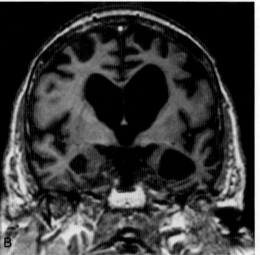

**Fig. 7.13 Frontotemporal dementia (FTD), frontal variant.** (A) Axial T2-weighted image (T2WI) is remarkable for the dilated subarachnoid space over the frontal lobes and compensatory enlargement of the frontal horns, signifying striking frontal predominant atrophy. (B) The coronal T1WI again shows the striking frontal and anterior temporal atrophy. The patient was in his late 50s.

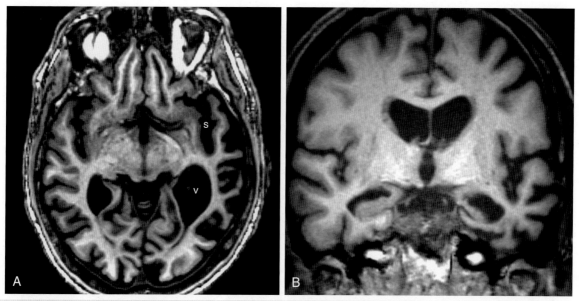

**Fig. 7.14 Primary progressive aphasia (PPA).** (A) Axial T1-weighted image (T1WI) shows generalized volume loss with superimposed marked atrophy of the left temporal lobe in this patient with PPA. Note the expanded sylvian fissure (s) and ex vacuo enlargement of the atrium of the left lateral ventricle (v). (B) Coronal T1W1 in this same patient again demonstrates the striking asymmetry of left-sided temporal volume loss.

the hippocampal region. "Knife blade shaped gyri" (knife blade atrophy) are described in the anterior aspect of the superior temporal gyrus with a widened sylvian fissure and insular atrophy.

- Patients with svPPA have difficulties with naming, word comprehension, object recognition, semantic relatedness of objects, and interrelations between words and meanings. Short-term memory is usually intact, but long-term memory is affected. Anterior, left more than right, temporal lobe atrophy is more dramatic with semantic FTD. The temporal pole and inferolateral gyri (including the parahippocampal gyri) are more affected than the hippocampi, marking a distinction from AD. The technetium SPECT scans show hypoperfusion of one or both temporal lobes, and the PET scan shows reduced uptake of FDG in the left anterior temporal lobe.

- In the logopenic variant of PPA, the major features are word retrieval and sentence repetition deficits, and slow speech with frequent pauses. On imaging, volume loss in the left temporoparietal junction, including posterior temporal, supramarginal, and angular gyri, is seen.

- More recently, motor disorders associated with FTD have been described. These include corticobasal syndrome, progressive supranuclear palsy (PSP), FTD with parkinsonism, and FTD with amyotrophic lateral sclerosis (ALS). Each of these variants of FTD will be characterized by their primary features later in this chapter.

## Creutzfeldt-Jakob Disease

- Creutzfeldt-Jakob disease (CJD) is a rare but fatal degenerative prion disease characterized by rapidly progressive dementia with myoclonus, a characteristically abnormal electroencephalogram (EEG), and 14-3-3 protein, neuron-specific enolase (NSE), and total tau protein (T-tau) in the CSF. CJD progresses rapidly, and

most patients die within 1 year. Definite diagnosis of CJD is based on histopathological findings, although biopsy is rarely performed. CJD often affects a younger population than AD.

---

**TEACHING POINTS**

Four Forms of Creutzfeldt-Jakob Disease (CJD)

- Sporadic: Typically occurs at the ages of 50 to 70 years by unknown causes
- Familial: Mutations of the prion protein gene
- Iatrogenic: Exposure to contaminated medical instruments or transplant of infected tissues
- Variant: Linked to bovine spongiform encephalopathy (BSE), it has different clinical features, such as a tendency to affect a younger age group and lack of periodic electroencephalogram (EEG) changes. Because CJD also involves the lymph nodes, spleen, tonsil, and appendix, a tonsil biopsy may be needed to cinch the diagnosis

---

- DWI and FLAIR hyperintensity confined to the cerebral cortex and/or basal ganglia (usually caudate) is the most specific feature in the early stages (Fig. 7.15). The DWI changes are more sensitive than the FLAIR findings, and cortical involvement is more common than deep gray involvement. With time, cerebral atrophy and symmetric high signal intensity foci in all the basal ganglia, thalami, occipital cortex (the Heidenhain variant), and white matter may develop.

- The Pulvinar sign is highly suggestive of variant CJD. The MR abnormalities are usually limited to bilateral thalamic pulvinar hyperintensity on DWI and FLAIR (hockey stick sign). Additional involvement of the putamen and caudate may be seen as well, and cortical involvement may coexist.

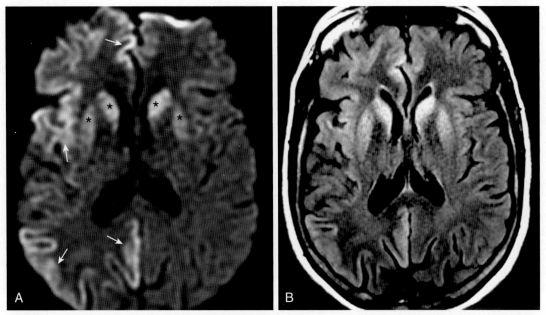

**Fig. 7.15 Creutzfeldt-Jakob disease (CJD).** (A) Diffusion-weighted and (B) fluid-attenuated inversion recovery (FLAIR) magnetic resonance (MR) study reveals peripheral cortical high intensity *(arrows)* reflecting the most common manifestation of CJD on MR. The location may be variable, but all lobes may be involved. In this case the caudate heads and putamina are also involved bilaterally as might be seen in variant CJD *(asterisks)*.

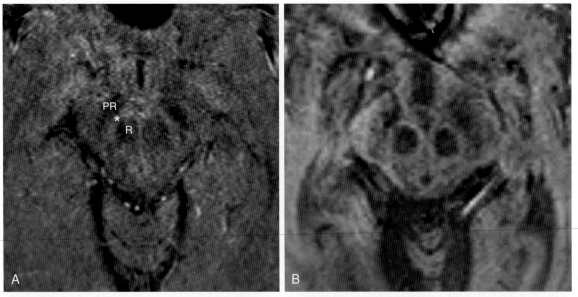

**Fig. 7.16 Parkinson disease.** (A) Normal appearance of the midbrain on susceptibility-weighted imaging shows hypointense signal within pars reticulata (PR) of the substantia nigra and the red nucleus (R). The pars compacta is normal in width *(asterisk)*. (B) In this patient with Parkinson disease, note that the width of the pars compacta is decreased compared with normal, and this appears more pronounced on the right compared with the left (yes, it is subtle).

## Parkinson Disease

- Parkinson disease (PD) is a neurodegenerative disorder that is defined clinically by the presence of bradykinesia and at least one additional motor symptom, such as resting tremor or rigidity. Dementia can be a late phenomenon. If dementia occurs within the first year of onset of the movement disorder, a diagnosis of dementia with Lewy bodies (DLB) is favored. The lesion in PD has been localized to the dopaminergic cells of the pars compacta of the substantia nigra. Treatment consists of dopamine stimulation therapy (levodopa), dopamine receptor agonists (bromocriptine), anticholinergics (benztropine,

trihexyphenidyl), and/or tricyclic antidepressants. Deep brain stimulation may be offered to patients with advanced PD who have unstable medication responses.

- Although no structural abnormalities are appreciable on traditional anatomic imaging in early PD, MRI and CT are performed to exclude underlying cerebrovascular disease or other causes of secondary parkinsonism, such as NPH, frontal neoplasm, or multiple sclerosis. In more advanced stages, a decreased width of the pars compacta has been described (Fig. 7.16).

- Recent studies with susceptibility-weighted and neuromelanin-sensitive sequences have shown increased iron and reduced neuromelanin in the substantia nigra of PD patients. The normal substantia nigra appears as a "V" shape on its side on SWI with apex medially directed; the V itself is dark and space between the V is bright, likened to a "swallow-tail". Loss of normal hyperintensity within the substantia nigra, the so-called "absent swallow tail sign", has been described on SWI as a finding of PD. However, this is often difficult to make out on 1.5T and 3T scanners but can be seen more reliably at 7T if you are lucky enough to have one on hand.

- Reduced uptake in the striatum on dopamine transporter (DAT) SPECT/fluorodopa F[18] (FDOPA) PET. Quantitative assessment in DAT SPECT is an accurate and reproducible tool to identify the presence of presynaptic dopaminergic denervation and can differentiate the presynaptic parkinsonian syndromes (PD, DLB, PSP, and multiple system atrophy [MSA]) from essential tremor or secondary parkinsonism (vascular, drug-induced, and psychogenic parkinsonism).
- Treatment-related findings include:
  - Hemorrhage and edema along the tract of stereotactic pallidotomy, which may extend into the optic tract or internal capsule
  - Stimulator implantation in the globus pallidus internus (GPi) or subthalamic nucleus
  - Abnormal signal in the target, GPi, or ventralis intermedius thalamic nucleus after gamma knife radiosurgery.

## Atypical Parkinson Disease/"Parkinson Plus Syndromes"

Atypical PD includes the entities of DLB, MSA, PSP, and corticobasal degeneration (CBD). In each of these entities, there is a movement disorder.

## Dementia with Lewy Bodies

- DLB is an entity probably related to PD in which Lewy bodies are found not only in deep gray matter structures but also diffusely in the brain, including on the cortex. DLB presents in older subjects than PD and accounts for 25% of dementing disorders. Although dementia may be primarily associated with PD, clinicians distinguish these entities based on the fact that PD dementia shows parkinsonism preceding the dementia by 1 year or more. Dementia preceding or accompanying parkinsonism is DLB.
- PD dementia is termed "subcortical" (psychomotor slowing, difficulty concentrating, impaired retrieval), but DLB is a cortical dementia (aphasia, anomia, apraxia, visuospatial problems, memory deficits). Clinically, patients with DLB show fluctuating cognitive impairment, visual hallucinations, and parkinsonism. Cognitive deficits are usually in memory, attention, executive function, and visuospatial and visuoconstructional abilities.
- Unfortunately, there are no specific anatomic imaging features of DLB, although atrophy of the cortex, substantia innominata, and brainstem can be seen with relative preservation of the mesial temporal structures.
- On metabolic imaging, reduced uptake in the striatum on DAT SPECT/FDOPA PET and generalized decreased uptake on SPECT/FDG PET with low occipital activity can be seen with DLB. Reduced cardiac uptake in the cardiac sympathetic imaging by meta-[123]I-iodobenzylguanidine

(MIBG) myocardial scintigraphy has been reported as an early finding in PD and DLB, before the involvement of the central nervous system (CNS).

## Multiple System Atrophy

- MSA is a rapidly progressive neurodegenerative disease associated with autonomic system dysfunction that presents in middle age and simulates PD (tremors, cogwheel rigidity, bradykinesia, and ataxia) in some respects. MSA-striatonigral type (MSA-P) displays more parkinsonian features (rigidity, bradykinesia, postural instability) and autonomic dysfunction (impotence, incontinence, orthostatic hypotension), whereas MSA-olivopontocerebellar atrophy type (MSA-C) is characterized by dominance of cerebellar dysfunction. Patients may have autonomic abnormalities of temperature regulation, sweat gland function, and maintenance of the blood pressure (orthostatic hypotension). Dementia is usually not a prominent component of MSA.
- On CT and MRI, atrophy of the putamen, pons, middle cerebellar peduncle, or cerebellum may be seen. Profound putaminal atrophy and T2 hypointensity, equal to or greater than pallidal hypointensity, is visible, correlating with severity of rigidity, and more common in MSA than PD. This finding may be combined with a slit-like hyperintense band lateral to the putamen, which is specific for MSA-P. As the disease progresses, pontocerebellar atrophy is seen with central cruciform T2 hyperintensities as the characteristic "hot cross bun" sign in the pons (Fig. 7.17).
- Hypometabolism on FDG PET in the putamen, brainstem, or cerebellum can be seen in patients with MSA, as well as presynaptic nigrostriatal dopaminergic denervation on SPECT or PET (MSA-C).

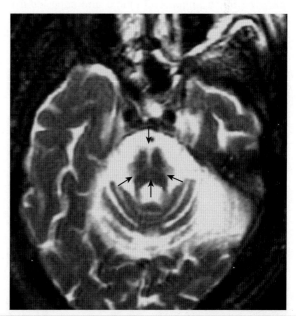

**Fig. 7.17  Hot cross buns sign.** On this axial T2-weighted image, note the four quadrants of dark signal *(between arrows)* that make up the hot cross buns sign in the pontine region in this patient with multisystem atrophy. Note the marked atrophy of the pons and included cerebellum.

## Progressive Supranuclear Palsy

- PSP resembles PD in its manifestations (rigidity, brady-kinesia) but also expresses a severe supranuclear ophthalmoplegia (impaired downward gaze), gait disorder, dysarthria, postural instability, and pseudobulbar palsy a few years after the onset of parkinsonian symptoms. Patients present with hyperextension of the neck and contracted facial muscles, giving a "surprised look" to the face. PSP is another dementing disorder associated with personality changes of uncontrolled emotions, social withdrawal, and depression.
- On CT and MRI, dilatation of the third ventricle, atrophy of the midbrain, and enlargement of the interpeduncular cistern is seen. Volume loss in the midbrain contributes to the "hummingbird sign" or "penguin sign" on sagittal imaging of the brainstem (Fig. 7.18). MR may show decreased width of the pars compacta of the substantia nigra, reduced anteroposterior (AP) diameter of the midbrain, and atrophy of the superior colliculi. Putaminal T2 hypointensity may be seen because of increased iron, more hypointense than the globus pallidus on T2WI (the opposite of normal patients). Atrophy of the superior cerebellar peduncle is a sensitive parameter for PSP—the width is reduced to 2 mm in greater than 80% of patients with the disease.
- Presynaptic nigrostriatal dopaminergic denervation can be seen on SPECT or PET.

## Corticobasal Degeneration

- CBD is a rare degenerative disorder characterized by parkinsonism, dystonia, and dementia. This disease demonstrates neuronal loss in the substantia nigra, frontoparietal cortex, and striatum.
- MR shows symmetric or asymmetric thinning of precentral and postcentral gyri with central sulcus dilatation. The superior parietal lobule and superior frontal gyrus seem to be at particular risk for volume loss as well, whereas the temporal and occipital lobes are less

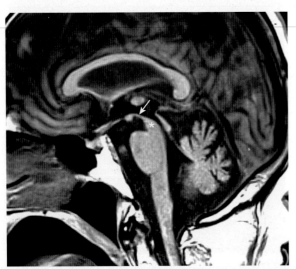

**Fig. 7.18 Progressive supranuclear palsy.** Sagittal T1-weighted image shows atrophic midbrain, with characteristic configuration of a hummingbird head in profile. The *arrow* indicates the beak, and the *asterisk* indicates the head of the hummingbird.

involved. Atrophy of the basal ganglia and midbrain may be subtle.
- Subcortical gliosis seen as high intensity on T2WI may be a clue to this diagnosis.
- High signal on T1WI of the subthalamic nuclei may also suggest CBD.
- Asymmetric hypometabolism/hypoperfusion in the superior parietal and superior frontal cortex and ipsilateral basal ganglia on FDG PET and SPECT can support the diagnosis.

## Acquired Immunodeficiency Syndrome Dementia Complex

- The acquired immunodeficiency syndrome (AIDS) dementia complex (ADC) has remained a concern for human immunodeficiency virus (HIV) patients. The term "HAD" is sometimes employed for HIV-associated dementia and "HAND" for HIV-associated neurocognitive disorder.
- Young patients with cerebral atrophy and mild to marked white matter T2 hyperintensity without mass effect may well have AIDS dementia complex (Fig. 7.19).
- A diffuse decrease in N-acetyl aspartate (NAA) and elevated choline on MR spectroscopy (MRS) may precede mental status deterioration and are present in children and adults with AIDS.
- Treatment-related findings: Protease inhibitors may cause reversal in the cognitive decline associated with HIV encephalopathy and may also result in the regression of periventricular white matter and basal ganglia signal intensity abnormalities. However, the MR imaging response to the highly active antiretroviral therapy (HAART) is often delayed compared with the clinical response. In fact, the MR findings may progress for the first 6 months before regressing or stabilizing with time. Basal ganglia and brainstem manifestations seem to respond to the greatest degree.

## Vascular Dementias

- Multiinfarct dementia (MID) is characterized clinically by a progressive, episodic, stepwise downward course. There may be intervals of clinical stabilization or even limited recovery. Some neurologists distinguish the stepwise decline and combined gray and white matter disease (MID) from Binswanger (subcortical leukoencephalopathy and subcortical arteriosclerotic encephalopathy; Fig. 7.20), which they claim is slowly progressive and exclusively involves white matter. Even if there really is a clinical difference between Binswanger disease and MID, pathophysiologically, the mechanism is the same: arteriolosclerosis. Lacunar infarcts and central pontine ischemic foci may coexist. MID is characterized on imaging studies by multiple areas of white matter infarction accompanied by severe deep gray matter lacunar disease caused by atherosclerosis of deep penetrating arteries.
- Cerebral autosomal dominant arteriopathy with subcortical infarcts and leukoencephalopathy (CADASIL) is a hereditary arteriopathy leading to recurrent cerebral infarcts and dementia. This disorder, linked to the *notch* gene on chromosome 19, presents with severe lacunar

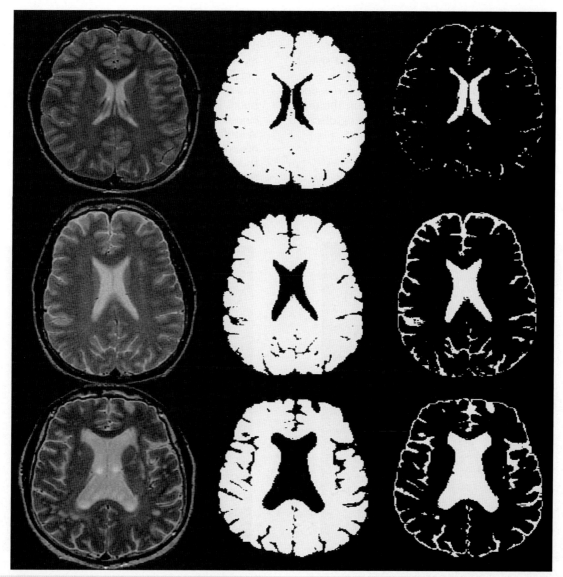

**Fig. 7.19** Spectrum of human immunodeficiency virus (HIV) brain, *Top* row (from *left* to *right*) T2-weighted image, brain parenchymal segmentation, and cerebrospinal fluid (CSF) segmentation. The *top* row is from a normal patient. *Middle* row is in an asymptomatic HIV patient, and *lower* row is in acquired immunodeficiency syndrome (AIDS) dementia complex. Observe how the CSF spaces increase and the parenchyma volume decreases.

disease and subcortical white matter ischemic changes in the frontal and anterior temporal lobes and reduced perfusion to affected areas. Clinically, the patients present with presenile dementia and migraine headaches in the third to fourth decade of life. CADASIL shows a striking pattern of subcortical lacunar infarcts and confluent high signal on FLAIR in the frontal and anterior temporal lobes; the involvement of the subcortical and deep white matter of the temporal lobes just behind the greater wings of the sphenoid bone bilaterally and symmetrically is rarely seen in any other entities and suggests this unusual diagnosis (see Fig. 3.41). Chronic microhemorrhages on SWI can be seen in about half of patients with CADASIL, although in no particular distribution.

### Amyotrophic Lateral Sclerosis

- ALS is a degenerative disease of upper motor neurons, generally manifested in the spinal cord, but also affecting the full extent of the corticospinal tract. The disease causes relentless loss of motor strength in facial, limb, and diaphragmatic musculature with atrophy and hyperreflexia. Death usually occurs from pulmonary infections as airway competency and respiratory muscle integrity are lost. This disease spares the patient from dementia, which may be more tragic because the patient is cognizant of the deadly downward course, which occurs over years. There are sporadic (95%) and familial forms (5%).
- The most common finding is T2 hyperintensities in the corticospinal tract at the level of the internal capsules. Occasionally, one sees extension of the atrophy or Wallerian degeneration along the full length of the corticospinal or bulbospinal tract into the brainstem, cerebral peduncles, internal capsule, corona radiata, and Betz cells of the cortex (Fig. 7.21).
- Sometimes (around 40%–60% of cases) the signal intensity of the precentral gyrus is decreased on SWI, thought

to be because of iron deposition, but don't hang your hat on this finding because it can be seen in normal patients too (Fig. 7.22).

■ Atrophy of the anterior horn cell region of the spinal cord may be evident.

■ On MRS, reductions in NAA and glutamate levels and increases in choline and myoinositol levels in the precentral gyrus region correlate with increasing disease severity.

## DEEP GRAY NUCLEI DISORDERS

The diseases that affect the deep gray matter nuclei are summarized in Table 7.3.

## Huntington Disease

■ Huntington disease is a progressive neurodegenerative disorder characterized by involuntary choreoathetoid movements, alterations in mood, and severe memory impairment. The disorder has an autosomal dominant inheritance pattern and is expressed in young adulthood. The Huntington gene, which includes CAG (cytosine-adenine-guanine) trinucleotide repeat, has been identified, and there are genetic tests available for this disorder. Histologically, early damage is most evident in the striatum, and analysis may show increased deposition of iron in the caudate and putamen.

■ On imaging, the frontal horns of the lateral ventricles are dilated and rounded because of caudate

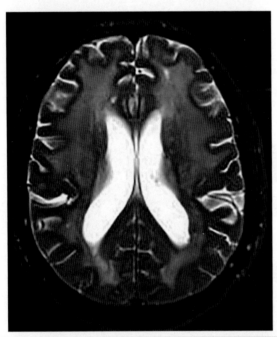

**Fig. 7.20 Subcortical arteriosclerotic encephalopathy.** Confluent hyperintensity in the white matter is shown on this axial T2-weighted image.

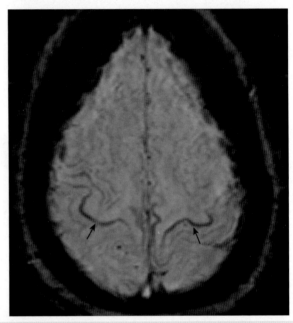

**Fig. 7.22 Amyotrophic lateral sclerosis (ALS).** Axial susceptibility-weighted imaging scan shows signal loss along the cortical margins of the precentral gyrus bilaterally *(arrows)* in this patient with ALS.

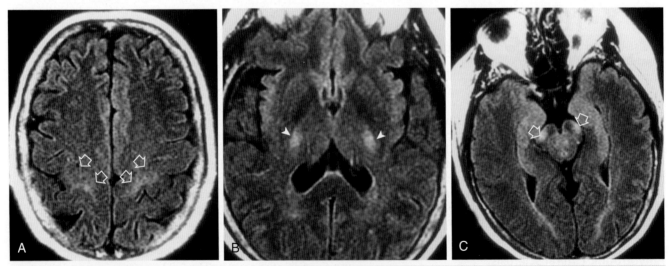

**Fig. 7.21 Amyotrophic lateral sclerosis (ALS).** Follow the high signal on these fluid-attenuated inversion recovery (FLAIR) scans from the white matter of the motor strip anterior to the central sulcus bilaterally *(arrows)* (A), to the posterior limb of the internal capsule *(arrowheads)* (B), to the cerebral peduncles *(arrows)* (C) in this patient with ALS.

**Table 7.3**  Deep Gray Nuclei Disorders

| Disorder | Distinguishing Imaging Features | MRS Features | Distinguishing Clinical Features |
|---|---|---|---|
| Huntington disease | Caudate atrophy | Increased lactate | Familial transmission, autosomal dominant |
|  | Abnormal signal in lentiform nuclei |  | Choreiform movements |
| Wilson disease | Abnormal intensity in basal ganglia | Decreased NAA/Cho | Kayser-Fleischer copper rings in globes |
|  | Cerebellar atrophy | Increased lactate/NAA | Coexistent liver disease |
|  |  |  | Ataxia, dysarthria |
| Pantothenate kinase-associated neurodegeneration | Basal ganglia, red nuclei low-intensity | Increased glutamate-glutamine/Cr | Dementia in young adults |
|  | Globus pallidus atrophy | Decreased PME | Rigidity, bradykinesia, toe-walking, hyperreflexia |
|  |  | Increased PCr/Pi | Familial transmission, autosomal recessive |
| Leigh syndrome | Favors putamen, other basal ganglia structures, brain stem tegmentum | Increased lactate | Childhood onset |
|  |  |  | Failure to thrive |
|  |  |  | Lactic acidosis |
| Fabry | Dense symmetric calcifications and atrophy in basal ganglia, thalami, dentate nuclei, subcortical white matter |  | Autosomal dominant and autosomal recessive inheritance patterns |
|  |  |  | Presents in midlate adulthood |
|  |  |  | Psychosis, dementia, cognitive impairment, gait abnormality, movement disorders |

*Cho*, Choline; *Cr*, creatine; *MRS*, magnetic resonance spectroscopy; *NAA, N*-acetyl aspartate; *PCr*, phosphocreatine; *Pi*, inorganic phosphate; *PME*, phosphomonoester.

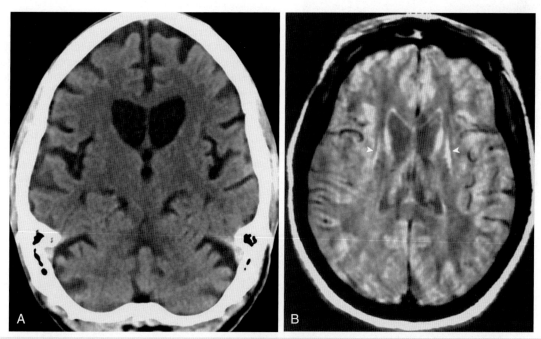

**Fig. 7.23  Huntington disease.** (A) Axial unenhanced computed tomography demonstrates caudate atrophy with ballooning of the frontal horns of the lateral ventricles. (B) Proton density–weighted image in a different patient shows high signal intensity in the caudate nuclei bilaterally and in the putamina *(arrowheads)*. Again seen is frontal horn dilatation caused by the atrophy of the caudate nuclei.

atrophy (Fig. 7.23). On MRI, signal intensity changes (low-to-high T2 signal) in the putamen and globus pallidus are observed, which may reflect complicated pathologic processes (neuronal loss accompanied by loss of myelin, gliosis, and copper and iron accumulation).

■ Hypometabolism in the caudate on PET and hypoperfusion on SPECT can also be seen.

### Neurodegeneration with Brain Iron Accumulation

■ Neurodegeneration with brain iron accumulation (NBIA) is a group of rare genetic disorders, characterized by iron accumulation, especially in the basal ganglia,

which results in abnormal involuntary movements, spasticity, and progressive dementia. The most common gene defect causes the disorder called pantothenate kinase-associated neurodegeneration (PKAN; formerly Hallervorden-Spatz syndrome), a familial autosomal recessive disorder, which presents in children and young adults, whereas another type of NBIA, neuroferritinopathy, may not become apparent until adulthood.

■ Characteristic accumulation of iron-containing compounds in the globus pallidus, red nuclei, and substantia nigra is seen as decreased intensity on T2WI. The presence of dramatic iron deposition within the basal ganglia with a central spot of high signal in the globus pallidus seen on T2WI should suggest the diagnosis of PKAN (Fig. 7.24). This pattern is that of the "eye of the tiger," although this has a limited differential diagnosis.

### TEACHING POINTS

"Eye of the Tiger" Differential Diagnosis

Carbon monoxide poisoning
Leigh disease
Neurofibromatosis
Pantothenate kinase-associated neurodegeneration (PKAN) syndrome
Parkinson disease
Progressive supranuclear palsy
Senescent basal ganglia calcification
Shy-Drager syndrome
Toxins
Wilson disease

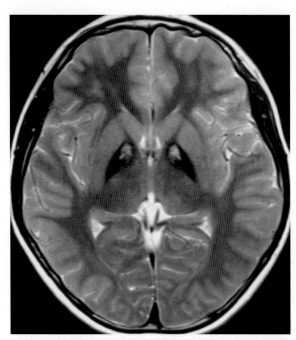

**Fig. 7.24** Pantothenate kinase-associated neurodegeneration (PKAN). Axial T2-weighted image at the basal ganglia level shows excess iron deposition within the globus pallidus bilaterally (dark signal), with central high T2 signal, the "eye of the tiger" sign.

## Wilson Disease

- Wilson disease (hepatolenticular degeneration) is an autosomal recessive disorder caused by abnormal ceruloplasmin metabolism with deposition of copper in the liver and brain. Patients are seen in early adulthood with dysarthria, dystonia, and tremors. Rigidity and ataxia may follow. Copper deposition in the cornea accounts for the classic Kayser-Fleischer rings seen on slit-lamp ophthalmologic examination.
- The most common initial MR findings are increased T1 signal in the globus pallidus, putamen, and midbrain, bilaterally and symmetrically. There may be T2 hypointensity in the lentiform nucleus and thalami possibly caused by a paramagnetic form of copper and/or associated iron deposition.
- In patients with neurologic symptoms, bilateral and symmetric deep gray areas of T2 hyperintensities, in the outer rim of the putamen (Fig. 7.25), ventral nuclear mass of the thalami, the globus pallidus, and the brainstem are seen. The findings may resolve as the symptoms improve.
- Scattered high T2 signal intensity foci in the white matter, pathologically correlating to demyelination, may be seen, particularly in the corticospinal, dentatorubrothalamic, and pontocerebellar tracts.
- In cases of copper toxicosis, one may see bright hypothalami and a bright anterior pituitary gland on T1WI.
- Atrophy is common, especially in the caudate nuclei.

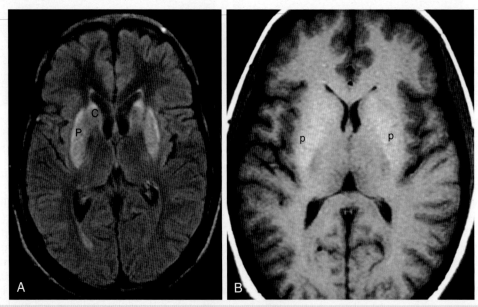

**Fig. 7.25 Wilson disease.** (A) Fluid-attenuated inversion recovery (FLAIR) images are particularly valuable in showing the bright signal in the caudate heads (C) and putamina (P) in this patient with Wilson disease. (B) The T1-weighted (T1WI) scan also shows high signal intensity in the putamen (P). Although the differential diagnosis is quite broad, the presence of Kayser-Fleischer rings in this individual clinched the diagnosis of Wilson disease.

## Fabry Disease

- Fabry disease (familial cerebral ferrocalcinosis) is an inherited disorder with both autosomal dominant and recessive inheritance patterns. The condition is characterized by calcium deposition in arterial, capillary, and venous walls, without abnormality of calcium metabolism. Patients present in mid-to-late adulthood with progressive symptoms, including psychosis, movement disorders, cognitive decline, and dementia (Fig. 7.26). Unfortunately, there is no treatment available.
- On CT, dense symmetric calcification and atrophy in the basal ganglia, thalami, dentate nuclei, and subcortical white matter is seen. These areas can show high T1 and low T2 signal on MRI. Additional areas of T1 and T2 hyperintensity in the white matter of the centrum semiovale separate from calcified regions may also be seen.

### TEACHING POINTS

#### Causes of Basal Ganglia Calcifications

Although most commonly physiologic, these may also be seen in other conditions:

#### Endocrinologic/Metabolic
Hyperparathyroidism
Hypoparathyroidism
Pseudohypoparathyroidism
Hypothyroidism

#### Mitochondrial
Kearns-Sayre Syndrome
Mitochondrial encephalopathy, lactic acidosis and stroke-like episodes (MELAS)
myoclonic epilepsy with ragged red fibers (MERRF)

#### Idiopathic
Fabry disease

#### Congenital
Cockayne syndrome
Down Syndrome

#### Phakomatoses
Neurofibromatosis
Tuberous Sclerosis

#### Infectious (most common but there are others)
Toxoplasmosis, Rubella, Cytomegalovirus, Herpes Simplex [TORCH] infections
Cystercerosis
HIV

#### Traumatic
Ischemic
Anoxia
Carbon monoxide poisoning

#### Iatrogenic

## METABOLIC AND TOXIC DISORDERS

### Hepatic Failure

- High signal intensity in the basal ganglia on T1WI has been described in patients with chronic liver disease, hepatic encephalopathy, portosystemic shunting without hepatic encephalopathy, and disorders of calcium-phosphate regulation, and in patients receiving parenteral nutrition therapy (Figs. 7.27 and 7.28). Increased signal intensity may be also seen in the midbrain and the anterior pituitary gland. Deposition of

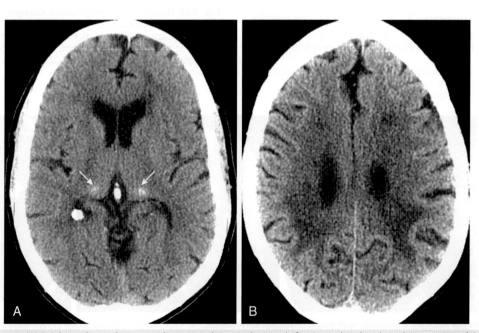

**Fig. 7.26 Fabry disease.** (A) Axial unenhanced computed tomography scan shows calcification isolated to the pulvinar region of the thalami *(arrows)*, which is felt to be a characteristic imaging feature of this condition. (B) More superiorly, chronic ischemic changes are present in the periventricular white matter. (Courtesy K. Chang, MD.)

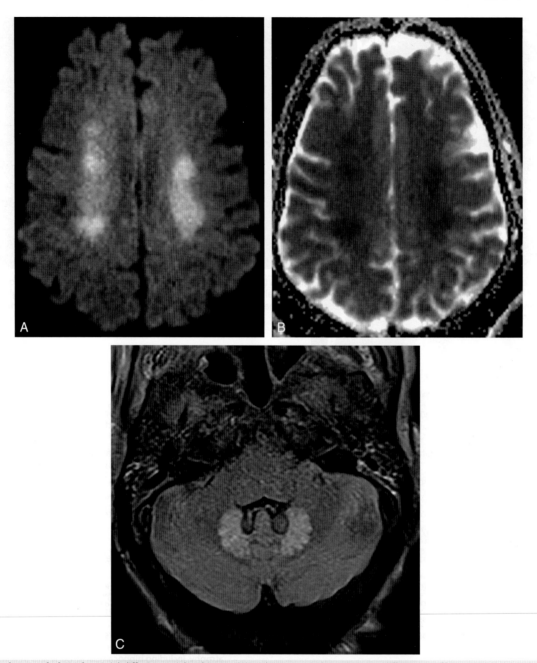

**Fig. 7.30 Toxic encephalopathy.** Axial diffusion weighted image (A) with corresponding apparent diffusion coefficient (ADC) map (B), shows relatively symmetric diffusion restriction in the bilateral centrum semiovale. In this patient who recently received intrathecal methotrexate for leukemia treatment and subsequently developed aphasia, these findings are consistent with methotrexate toxicity. (C) Axial fluid-attenuated inversion recovery (FLAIR) image in a different patient with altered mental status shows symmetric hyperintense signal in the dentate nuclei. The patient had recently been started on metronidazole for infection management, and these findings are consistent with metronidazole toxicity.

even higher rate of drug-induced ischemic strokes, secondary to vasoconstriction, platelet dysmetabolism, and episodic hypertension. Heroin inhalation ("chasing the dragon") can result in toxic spongiform encephalopathy with high T2 signal in the posterior cerebral and cerebellar white matter, cerebellar peduncles, splenium of the corpus callosum, and posterior limbs of the internal capsules.

■ Some patients are susceptible to medication-induced toxic encephalopathies (Fig. 7.30). Intrathecal methotrexate, for example, often used in treatment of CNS involvement by lymphoma, can cause symmetric diffusion restriction and confluent T2/FLAIR hyperintensity in centrum semiovale, which can be reversible. Metronidazole toxicity has a predilection for the dentate nuclei, although signal changes in the corpus callosum and midbrain can occasionally be seen.

## CEREBELLAR ATROPHY

Atrophy of the cerebellum has many causes. We review the most common below.

Causes of Cerebellar Atrophy

**Toxic**
Alcohol abuse
Long-term use of phenytoin (Dilantin), phenobarbital, high-dose cytarabine
Mercury poisoning
Poor nutrition
Steroid use
Thallium poisoning

**Vascular**
Strokes
Vertebrobasilar insufficiency

**Hereditary**
Ataxia-telangiectasia
Dandy-Walker complex
Down syndrome
Friedreich ataxia
Hereditary ataxia
Joubert syndrome
Olivopontocerebellar degeneration
Shy-Drager syndrome
Vermian hypoplasia

**Infectious**
Creutzfeldt-Jakob disease
Cytomegalovirus/rubella

**Treatment Related**
Postoperative
Radiation therapy

## Alcohol Abuse

■ Chronic ingestion of excessive amounts of alcohol is probably the most common cause of cerebellar atrophy. The vermis appears to be more commonly involved than other parts of the brain with alcohol abuse, but the whole cerebellum suffers (Fig. 7.31).

## Thiamine Deficiency

■ When one adds poor nutrition and thiamine deficiency to the alcohol abuse, the midbrain, mammillary bodies, and basal ganglia are damaged. This condition is known as Wernicke encephalopathy. By that point, the patient has tremors, delusions, confabulation, ophthalmoparesis, ataxia, and confusion. When severe amnesia accompanies Wernicke encephalopathy, Korsakoff syndrome is invoked. Although chronic alcoholism is the most common cause of Wernicke encephalopathy, other possible etiologies include bariatric surgery, gastric bypass, hyperemesis gravidarum, prolonged infectious-febrile conditions, carcinoma, anorexia nervosa, and prolonged voluntary starvation.
■ High signal intensity areas in the periaqueductal gray matter of the midbrain (40%), the paraventricular thalamic regions (46%), the mammillary bodies and/or mamillothalamic tract, and in the tissue surrounding the third ventricle on T2WI can be seen (Fig. 7.32).

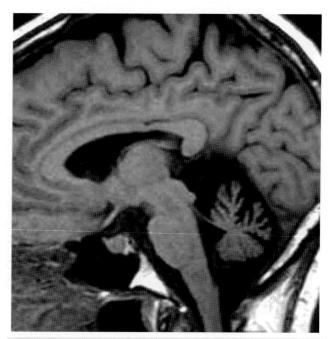

**Fig. 7.31 Cerebellar atrophy.** Sagittal T1-weighted image shows enlargement of the cerebellar sulci and decrease in the size of the cerebellum.

Those areas may have high signal on DWI scans. Reversible thalamic/pulvinar lesions in the dorsal medial nuclei have also been reported. These areas may or may not enhance (in some cases the enhancement may be dramatic, almost sarcoid-like). Mammillary body enhancement and/or abnormal signal on DWI and/or FLAIR may be the sole manifestation of Wernicke encephalopathy.

## Long-Term Drug Use

■ Phenytoin (Dilantin) and phenobarbital are the classic drugs that produce cerebellar atrophy after long-term use. Patients may have reversible nystagmus, ataxia, peripheral neuropathies, and slurred speech. The cerebellar degeneration becomes irreversible after long-term administration. Phenytoin may also cause thickening of the skull when used early in life for a long period.

## Olivopontocerebellar Atrophy

■ Olivopontocerebellar atrophy is a group of progressive neurodegenerative disorders that is associated with cerebellar and brainstem atrophy and characterized by truncal and limb ataxia, dysarthria, tremors, nystagmus, rigidity, brainstem dysfunction. It may be transmitted in an autosomal dominant inheritance and overlap with spinocerebellar ataxia. The sporadic form is considered in the spectrum of multisystem atrophy.
■ On imaging, the pons and inferior olives are strikingly small, as are the cerebellar peduncles (Fig. 7.33). Cerebellar atrophy, particularly of the vermis, is marked.

## Friedreich Ataxia

■ Friedreich ataxia is a progressive neurodegenerative disorder inherited in autosomal recessive pattern. Patients

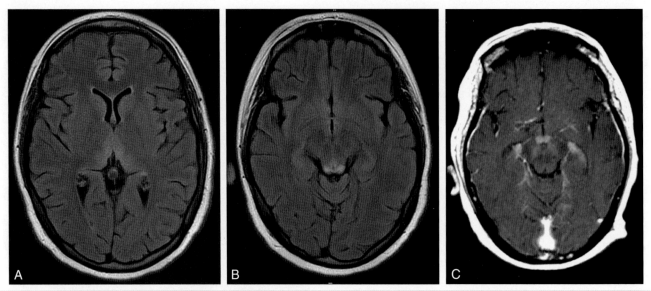

**Fig. 7.32  Wernicke encephalopathy.** Fluid-attenuated inversion recovery (FLAIR) images show high signal in medial thalami (A) and periaqueductal gray matter (B). (C) Postcontrast T1-weighted image (T1WI) in a different patient shows enhancement in the mamillary bodies bilaterally.

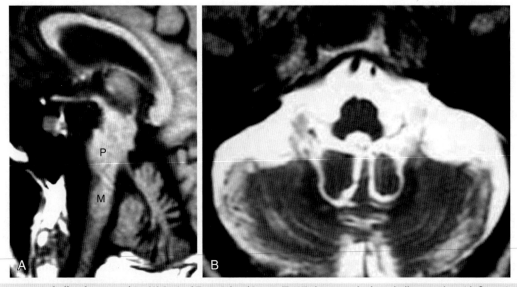

**Fig. 7.33  Olivopontocerebellar degeneration.** (A) Sagittal T1-weighted image (T1WI) shows marked cerebellar atrophy with flattening of the belly of the pons and the enlarged inferior cerebellar cistern. (B) Axial T2-weighted image (T2WI) reveals atrophy of the pons as it swims in the prepontine cistern.

are usually seen in late childhood with lower extremity ataxia, kyphoscoliosis, and tremors of the upper extremity. Areflexia in the lower extremities, scoliosis, deafness, optic atrophy, and dysarthria may occur. Cardiac anomalies may coexist. In addition to cerebellar volume loss, atrophy of the cervicomedullary junction with a decreased anteroposterior diameter of the upper part of the cervical cord has been reported. Signal intensity in the cerebellum and cord is normal.

## Ataxia Telangiectasia

■ Ataxia telangiectasia (Louis-Bar syndrome) is a rare autosomal recessive disorder characterized as one of the phakomatoses. Hallmarks of the disease include

cerebellar vermian and hemispheric atrophy and telangiectatic lesions on the face, mucosa, and conjunctiva. An associated abnormality of the immune system (predominantly affecting immunoglobulin A) causes recurrent sinus and lung infections. Leukemia or non-Hodgkin lymphoma may develop, and the patients usually die of the disease in childhood. If the patients survive to adulthood, they may be besieged by breast, gastric, CNS, skin, and liver malignancies. Increased sensitivity to radiation effects and progeria are manifestations of the disorder as well.

■ The typical imaging findings are vermian/holocerebellar atrophy and increased T2 white matter signal intensity. Rarely, intracranial occult cerebrovascular malformations may be present. These are manifest as dark foci of hemosiderin on T2* scans of the brain and may be because of perivascular hemorrhages.

### Hypertrophic Olivary Degeneration

- Hypertrophic olivary degeneration (HOD) occurs because of ischemic, traumatic, neoplastic, or vascular insult to the components of the "triangle of Guillain and Mollaret," that is, the red nucleus, inferior olivary nucleus, and contralateral dentate nucleus. These structures are connected by the superior cerebellar peduncle (dentate to red nucleus), the central tegmental tract (red nucleus to inferior olivary nucleus), and the inferior cerebellar peduncle (inferior olivary nucleus to dentate nucleus—the olivodentate tract). Lesions in the first two tracts can lead to neuronal degeneration of the inferior olivary nucleus. Patients typically present with palatal myoclonus or tremors, ataxia, and vision blurring.
- Initially this leads to high T2 signal (first 2 months) and then hypertrophy with increased T2 signal (6 months to 3–4 years) of the inferior olivary nucleus of the medulla (Fig. 7.34). In the later stages, olivary hypertrophy resolves and increased T2 signal persists. Contralateral cerebellar atrophy can occur, although this is more commonly seen with involvement of the olivodentate fibers. Look for the cause of the lesion along the triangle, but keep in mind that recent literature reports that the cause of HOD is not always evident on imaging.

### Paraneoplastic Syndromes

- Cerebellar atrophy is one of the manifestations of paraneoplastic syndromes (see Chapter 5). These may be associated with neuroblastoma, Hodgkin disease, and ovarian, gastrointestinal, lung, and breast cancers. An autoimmune mechanism is implicated because antibodies (anti-Yo antibodies) to cerebellar antigens (predominantly directed against Purkinje cells) may be identified. The cerebellar degeneration precedes discovery of the primary tumor in up to 60% of cases.

## Metabolic Disorders

The number of metabolic disorders that affect the brain is probably in the hundreds. We touch on the major metabolic disorders and general imaging manifestations here.

### MUCOPOLYSACCHARIDOSES

- Clinically, the mucopolysaccharidoses (MPS) represents a heterogeneous group of inherited lysosomal storage disorders. The clinical manifestations are diverse, resulting from multisystem involvement including the CNS (Table 7.5). The diagnoses of these disorders are usually based on biochemical and/or chromosomal evaluation.
- MR reveals diffuse cribriform or cystic-appearing areas of abnormal signal intensity in the white matter (low on T1WI, high on T2WI) and hypodensity in the white matter on CT (Fig. 7.35). There often is dilatation of the perivascular spaces that are seen in the striatocapsular regions and occasionally in the corona radiata white matter.
- It is presumed that build-up of glycosaminoglycans in the leptomeninges account for the arachnoid membrane obstruction and ball valve effect that can lead to communicating hydrocephalus and arachnoid cysts, as well as optic nerve sheath dilation.
- At the foramen magnum, thickening of the dura (or mucopolysaccharide deposition) may cause medullary compression in some of the mucopolysaccharidoses.

### LIPIDOSES AND OTHER STORAGE DISEASES

- The gangliosidoses are diseases that manifest white matter abnormalities and cortical atrophy (Table 7.6). Lacunar and white matter small vessel infarctions may occur in Fabry and Gaucher disease. Of the lipidoses, cerebellar ataxia and cerebellar atrophy are more common in Tay-Sachs disease and Niemann-Pick disease. Bilateral thalamic abnormalities with hyperdensity on CT are characteristic of Sandhoff

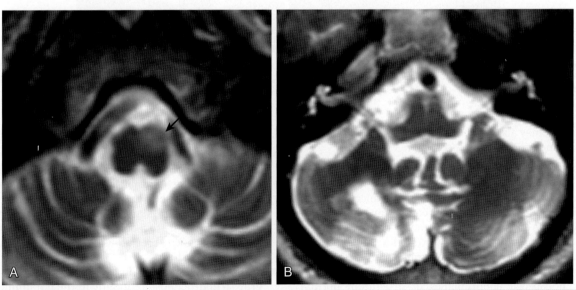

**Fig. 7.34  Hypertrophic olivary degeneration.** (A) On this axial T2-weighted image, there is focal increased signal and slight enlargement within the left ventral medulla *(arrow)* at the level of the inferior olivary nucleus. (B) The hypertrophic olivary degeneration has occurred because of insult in the right dentate nucleus.

**Table 7.5**   Imaging Findings in Mucopolysaccharidoses

| Eponym | Deficient Enzyme | Inheritance | CNS Findings |
|---|---|---|---|
| Hurler (MPS I) | α-l-Iduronidase | AR | Thickened meninges, atrophy, kyphosis, atlantoaxial subluxation, ligamentous thickening causing cord compression, cribriform or cystic areas within white matter or basal ganglia, delayed myelination, hydrocephalus, vertebra plana |
| Scheie (MPS IS)* | α-l-Iduronidase | AR | Pigmentary retinopathy |
| Hunter (MPS II) | Iduronate sulfatase | XR | Macrocrania; enlarged Virchow-Robin spaces; cribriform or cystic areas within white matter, corpus callosum, or basal ganglia; delayed myelination; thickening of dura matter, especially in the spine; communicating hydrocephalus |
| Sanfilippo (MPS III) | Sulfamidase | AR | Atrophy, cribriform or cystic areas within white matter or basal ganglia, delayed myelination, retinal degeneration |
| Morquio (MPS IV) | Galactosamine-6-sulfate sulfatase | AR | Ligamentous thickening leading to cord compression, odontoid hypoplasia, atlantoaxial subluxation, vertebra plana, white matter high intensity |
| Maroteaux-Lamy (MPS VI) | N-Acetyl galactosamine-sulfatase B | AR | Meningeal thickening, hydrocephalus, perivascular gliosis, cord compression from ligamentous thickening, atlantoaxial subluxation |
| Sly (MPS VII) | Glucuronidase | AR | None or hydrocephalus, white matter high intensity |

*AR*, Autosomal recessive; *CNS*, central nervous system; *MPS*, mucopolysaccharidosis; *XR*, X-linked recessive.
*Initially classified as MPS V.

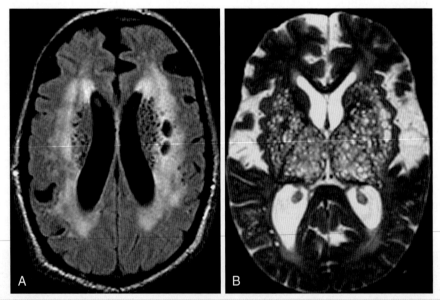

**Fig. 7.35 Hunter mucopolysaccharidosis.** (A) Axial fluid-attenuated inversion recovery (FLAIR) scan shows dilated perivascular spaces (dark) and abnormal corona radiata white matter (bright). (B) On T2-weighted image, the perivascular spaces of the deep gray matter are highlighted in a cribriform pattern.

disease but may also be seen with Tay-Sachs disease, Fabry disease, and toxic exposures (see Fig. 7.35).

## MITOCHONDRIAL DEFECTS

■ Mitochondrial enzymatic disorders are a clinically heterogeneous group of disorders that can be caused by mutation of genes encoded by either nuclear deoxyribonucleic acid (DNA) or mitochondrial DNA. Most patients with mitochondrial disorders demonstrate neurologic symptoms and CNS findings, which include disease-specific features, nonspecific abnormalities, or structurally normal brain (Table 7.7).

## Leigh Disease

■ Leigh disease (subacute necrotizing encephalomyelopathy) is the prototype of the mitochondrial disorders caused by mitochondrial DNA or nuclear DNA mutations, which present with global developmental delay, dystonia, and ophthalmoplegia, typically in infants. The disease may relate to a deficiency in the enzymes associated with pyruvate breakdown; its accumulation leads to lactic acid build-up.

■ MR shows bilateral T2 high signal intensity of the deep gray structure, most frequently in the putamina, globus pallidi, and caudate nuclei, showing necrotic lesions

**Table 7.6** Imaging Findings in Lipidoses, Gangliosidoses, and Other Storage Diseases

| Disorder | Deficiency | Inheritance | CNS Findings |
|---|---|---|---|
| Ceroid lipofuscinosis (Batten disease) | Several proteins and enzymes identified | AR | Cerebellar or less often cortical atrophy, periventricular gliosis, optic atrophy, thickened dura, thick skull |
| Fabry disease | α-Galactosidase A | XR | Multiple infarcts, vascular stenoses, and thromboses; basal ganglia lacunae |
| Farber disease (lipogranulomatosis) | Acid ceramidase | AR | Atrophy, hydrocephalus |
| Fucosidosis | α-l-Fucosidase | AR | Demyelination, gliosis, atrophy, high-intensity TI in basal ganglia, thickened skull, craniostenosis, poorly developed sinus, short odontoid, platyspondyly, anterior beaking, scoliosis, vacuum disk, square vertebrae |
| Gaucher disease | Acid β-glucosidase | AR | Minimal to no atrophy, vertebral body collapse, dementia, infarcts |
| GM₁ gangliosidosis | β-Galactosidase | AR | White matter disease, late atrophy, macroglossia, organomegaly, dementia (1–3 yr), seizures, gibbus deformity, beaked vertebrae, bright putamen caudate atrophy on T2WI |
| Krabbe disease (globoid cell leukodystrophy) | Galactocerebroside β-galactosidase | AR | Increased CT attenuation in cerebellum, thalami, caudate nuclei; decreased signal on T2WI of cerebellum; optic atrophy; small atrophic brain, demyelination, and intracranial optic nerve enlargement |
| Mannosidosis | α-Mannosidase | AR | Low density in parieto-occipital white matter, atrophy, thickened skull, lenticular opacities, brachycephaly, craniostenosis |
| Niemann-Pick disease | Sphingomyelinase | AR | Normal vs areas of demyelination, gliosis, slight atrophy, small corpus callosum |
| Pompe disease | Acid maltase | AR | Gliosis, macroglossia |
| Sandhoff disease | Hexosaminidase A and B (gangliosidase) | AR | Atrophy, thalamic hyperdensity on CT, possibly caused by calcification; diffuse white matter disease |
| Tay-Sachs disease (GM₂ gangliosidosis) | Hexosaminidase A (gangliosidase) | AR | Megalencephaly early; atrophy late, especially of optic nerves and cerebellum; demyelination; high-density thalami, deep gray abnormal signal, large caudate |

*AR*, Autosomal recessive; *CNS*, central nervous system; *CT*, computed tomography; *GM₁*, monosialotetrahexosylganglioside; *T2WI*, T2-weighted imaging; *XR*, X-linked recessive.

**Table 7.7** Imaging Findings in the Mitochondrial Disorders

| Disorder | Inheritance | Deficient Enzyme/Mutated Gene | CNS Findings |
|---|---|---|---|
| MELAS syndrome | Maternal | *A3243G* mutation | Pseudostrokes, demyelination in cord |
| MERRF syndrome | Maternal | *A8344G, T8356C* | White matter demyelination, especially superior cerebellar peduncles, posterior columns, gliosis |
| Kearns-Sayre syndrome | Spontaneous | MtDNA | Diffuse white matter disease, calcified basal ganglia, more cerebellar than cortical atrophy, retinopathy, ophthalmoplegia, microcephaly |
| Alpers disease | AR | Cytochrome c-oxidase | Microcephaly, posterior cortical encephalomalacia, atrophy |
| Leigh disease | AR | Pyruvate dehydrogenase | Periaqueductal gray and putaminal abnormal signal intensity, swollen caudate, low density in putamina on CT, demyelination, lactate peak on MRS |
| Menkes kinky hair disease | XR | Copper metabolism ATPase, *Menkes/OHS* gene | Subdural effusions, irregular vascular atrophy, gliosis, increased wormian bones, infarcts, tortuous dilated vessels |
| Zellweger syndrome (cerebrohepatorenal syndrome) | AR | Peroxisome assembly, *PXR1* gene | Abnormal neuronal migration (polymicrogyria, heterotopias, pachygyria), white matter disease, optic atrophy, decreased *N*-acetyl aspartate level, macrocephaly, open sutures, ventricular dilatation |
| Refsum disease | AR | Phytanic acid-2-hydroxylase | Demyelination of spinal cord tracts, atrophy, abnormal signal intensity, dentate nucleus |

*AR*, Autosomal recessive; *CNS*, central nervous system; *CT*, computed tomography; *MELAS*, mitochondrial encephalomyopathy, lactic acidosis, and stroke-like episodes; *MERRF*, myoclonic epilepsy with ragged red fibers; *MRS*, magnetic resonance spectroscopy; *XR*, X-linked recessive.

associated with demyelination, vascular proliferation, and gliosis (Fig. 7.36). Diffuse supratentorial white matter T2 hyperintensity may accompany. Atrophy can be seen over time.

- Lower brainstem involvement correlates with loss of respiratory control, a potentially fatal complication of the disease.
- The telltale laboratory finding is metabolic acidosis with increased lactate levels; the lactate may be detectable with proton or phosphorous MR spectroscopic examination.

## Mitochondrial Encephalomyopathy, Lactic Acidosis, and Stroke-like Episodes Syndrome

- Mitochondrial encephalomyopathy, lactic acidosis, and stroke-like episodes (MELAS) syndrome presents before the age of 40 with headache, seizures, and stroke-like events. The patients may have cortical blindness.
- Imaging studies demonstrate multiple areas of high T2 signal intensity abnormality affecting predominantly gray matter, which often crosses a traditional cerebral artery distribution (Fig. 7.37). Although the lesions may be bright on DWI scans, they usually do *not* show reduced ADC values and are therefore not acute infarcts. Contrast enhancement may be present.
- The abnormality is associated with serologic and spectroscopic evidence of elevated lactic acid levels.
- Strangely enough, these lesions may disappear with time, leaving only minimal sulcal dilatation in their place. Although resolution of the lesions is the expected course, one may see new lesions appearing as well.

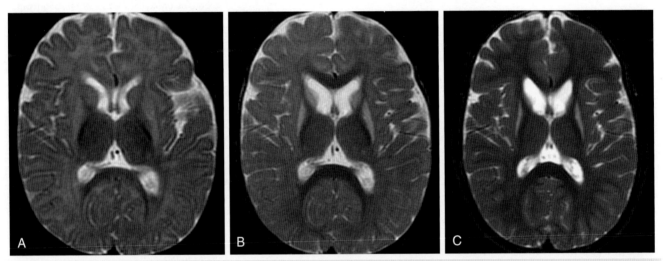

Fig. 7.36  **Leigh disease.** Axial T2-weighted images in the same child at approximately aged 3 months (A), 8 months (B), and 2 years (C) show bilateral symmetric putaminal and caudate high signal intensity, with progressive volume loss of these structures over time.

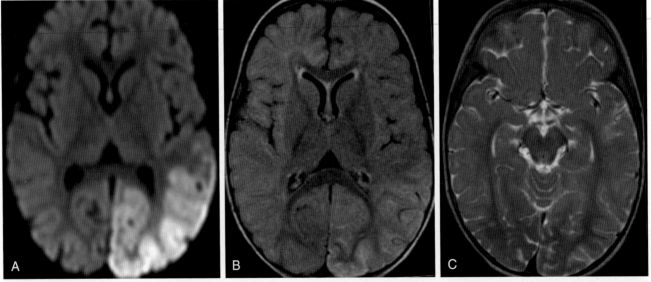

Fig. 7.37  **Mitochondrial encephalomyopathy, lactic acidosis, and stroke-like episodes (MELAS) syndrome.** (A) Axial diffusion-weighted image shows cortically based diffusion hyperintensity in the left occipital and posterior temporal lobe. (B) Axial fluid-attenuated inversion recovery (FLAIR) and (C) axial T2-weighted imaging show high signal intensity in the swollen cortex in the region of diffusion abnormality. Note that the abnormality is not confined to a single vascular territory but rather spans the left middle cerebral artery and posterior cerebral artery distributions without affecting the basal ganglia.

**Table 7.8**   Imaging Findings in Amino Acid Disorders

| Disorder | Inheritance | Deficient Enzyme | Brain Findings |
|---|---|---|---|
| Hyperglycinemia | AR | Glycine metabolism | Microcephaly, atrophy, dysmyelination, corpus callosum anomalies |
| Maple syrup urine disease | AR | Branched-chain amino acid decarboxylase | Abnormal neuronal migration, acute edema after birth followed by atrophy at few months, demyelination of posterior white matter, dorsal midbrain edema, deep gray matter swelling, deep cerebellum edema; MRS shows branched-chain amino acids |
| Methylmalonic academia | AR | CoA carboxylase or mutase | Early swelling then atrophy, decreased density in white matter, basal ganglia (especially globus pallidus) injury, delayed myelination |
| Phenylketonuria | AR | Phenylalanine hydroxylase | White matter demyelination posteriorly (often optic radiations), neuronal migrational abnormalities, atrophy, cerebellar and brainstem high signal foci, basal ganglia calcification, atrophy |
| Propionic acidemia | AR | CoA carboxylase | Atrophy, decreased density in white matter |
| Glutaric acidemia type II | AR | Acyl CoA dehydrogenase | Globus pallidus and white matter hyperintensities on T2WI, macrocephaly, atrophy (frontal/temporal), hydrodense basal ganglia, bat-wing dilatation of sylvian fissures, temporal arachnoid cysts, subdural hematomas |

*AR*, Autosomal recessive; *MRS*, magnetic resonance spectroscopy; *T2WI*, T2-weighted imaging.

## AMINOACIDOPATHIES AND OTHER ENZYME DEFICIENCIES

- As a group, the amino acid metabolic disorders (Table 7.8) are usually seen in children and are manifested neurologically by developmental delay, seizures, and vomiting (when not diagnosed early by screening tests). The normal maturation of the brain is often delayed, and myelination may be affected. Brain atrophy is seen in later stages. Usually, dietary manipulations and/or replacement therapies are effective in gaining some return of function and control of the disease.

## Krabbe Disease

- Also referred to as globoid cell leukodystrophy (GLD), this is an autosomal recessive lysosomal storage disease, characterized by galactocerebroside–beta-galactocerebrosidase deficiency, which disrupts myelin metabolism in both central and peripheral nerve system. When the disease presents before age 2 (the infantile form), the pyramidal tracts, cerebellar white matter, deep gray matter, posterior corpus callosum, and parietooccipital white matter are usually involved (as they are the first areas to myelinate). The U-fibers are generally spared.
- Hyperdensity of the thalami may be seen on CT.
- MRS findings include abnormally elevated choline and myoinositol (thought to be secondary to myelin breakdown products or phospholipid membrane metabolism).There is a marked decrease in relative anisotropy of the affected white matter tracts identified on DWI. Atrophy ultimately develops. In the late-onset group, the same locations may be involved except for the cerebellar white matter and deep gray matter. The corticospinal tract is involved consistently. Splenial disease is also common in this form.

- The upper motor tract, corresponding to the lower extremity region, is affected to a greater extent than the regions that subserve the face and arms. Cerebral atrophy is present in early but not late disease. Involvement of the optic nerve can be seen.

## Glutaric Acidemia

- Among patients with glutaric acidemia, a progressive macrocephaly can often be the only initial presentation. Patients may present with an acute encephalitis-like encephalopathy in infancy or childhood.
- MR findings may help diagnosis, revealing open opercula and abnormally high signal in the basal ganglia, especially the globus pallidus. In the later stage, atrophy and subarachnoid space dilatation may be seen, increasing the propensity for subdural hematomas. Beware: these hematomas may mimic appearance of nonaccidental trauma injury.

## Homocystinuria

- This is an autosomal recessive disorder characterized by cystathionine beta synthase deficiency. The resultant high plasma levels of homocysteine result in multiple thrombotic events, including strokes. Premature atherosclerosis occurs. The thromboses may be either arterial or venous. The presence of lens subluxations might suggest a diagnosis of Marfan syndrome, but those with homocystinuria are "up and in" and those with Marfan disease are "down and out."
  - Other neuroradiologic findings may include optic atrophy, osteoporosis, cataracts, scoliosis, and biconcave vertebral bodies.

# 8 Congenital Anomalies of the Central Nervous System

AYLIN TEKES AND MELIKE GURYILDIRIM

## Relevant Embryology

- Understanding development of the central nervous system (CNS) aids in understanding congenital brain and spine anomalies and the coexistence of multiple anomalies.
- With some overlap, the CNS goes through six major developmental events during which a myriad of malformations can develop:
  - Primary neurulation (3–4 weeks of gestation)
  - Secondary neurulation (5–6 weeks of gestation)
  - Promesencephalic development (2–3 months of gestation)
  - Neuronal proliferation (3–4 months of gestation)
  - Neuronal migration (3–5 months of gestation)
  - Organization (5 months of gestation to postnatal years)
  - Myelination (birth postnatal years)

### PRIMARY NEURULATION

- Neurulation is a series of inductive events that takes place in the dorsal aspect of the embryo and results in the development of the brain and spinal cord.
- Primary neurulation involves events that are related to formation of the brain and spinal cord exclusive of its most caudal region. The first fusion of neural folds occurs in the lower medulla. Closure generally proceeds rostrally and caudally, although it is not a simple zipper-like process.
- Disorders of primary neurulation are cranioschisis, anencephaly, myeloschisis, encephalocele, myelomeningocele, and Chiari II malformations. Various malformations of neural tube closure are accompanied by axial skeleton, meningovascular, and dermal covering abnormalities.

### SECONDARY NEURULATION

- Secondary neurulation occurs later than primary neurulation, with sequential processes of canalization and retrogressive differentiation.
- Disorders of secondary neurulation result in malformations of the lower sacral and coccygeal segments of the neural tube affecting the conus medullaris, filum terminale, and cauda equina. Lipomas of the filum, short-thickened tethered fila and tethered cords, and caudal regression syndrome with sacral agenesis are listed under this category.

### PROMESENCEPHALIC DEVELOPMENT

- The primary inductive relationship is between the notochord-prechordal mesoderm and forebrain and takes place ventrally in the rostral end of the embryo (ventral induction). Formation of the face and forebrain occur during this event, so malformations of the brain are usually accompanied by facial anomalies (such as cyclopia and probosci).
- The spectrum of malformations can range in severity from aprosencephaly to clinically occult callosal malformations.
- Three major sequential events (and related malformations) are promesencephalic development (atelencephaly), premesencephalic cleavage (holoprosencephaly), and midline promesencephalic development (agenesis of corpus callosum, agenesis of septum pellucidum, septo-optic dysplasia, hypothalamic dysplasia).

### NEURONAL PROLIFERATION

- All neurons and glia are derived from the ventricular and subventricular zones of the germinal matrix. Disorders of neuronal proliferation can result in a small or large brain (microcephaly or macrocephaly).
- Neurocutaneous syndromes must be kept in mind when assessing macrocephaly or hemimegalencephaly (see Phakomatoses section in this chapter).

### NEURONAL MIGRATION

- The neurons migrate through the developing cerebral hemispheres from the ventricular and subventricular zones of the subependymal region to the cortex. Initially, neurons migrate by translocation followed by two basic varieties of cell migration: radial and tangential.
- Radial migration leads to projection neurons of the cerebral cortex and deep nuclei in the cerebrum and Purkinje cells in the cerebellum.
- Tangential migration leads to interneurons of the cerebral cortex and internal granule layer of the cerebellar cortex.
- The layering of the neurons is inside out: early arriving neurons are deep, whereas late arriving neurons are in the superficial aspect of the cortex.
- Disorders of neuronal migration include heterotopia, schizencephaly, lissencephaly, pachygyria, polymicrogyria, and focal cortical malformations. Tip: Commissural anomalies (e.g., corpus callosum agenesis partial or complete) and septum pellucidum anomalies can accompany these disorders, so keep a look out!

### NEURONAL ORGANIZATION

- A series of complex processes take place: subplate neuron differentiation; alignment, orientation, and layering of cortical neurons; establishment of synaptic contacts; cell death; and proliferation and differentiation of glia.

- Primary disorders include intellectual disability and syndromes such as Fragile X, Rett, Down, and Angelman. Potential disturbances, such as those seen in premature infants (germinal matrix hemorrhage spectrum, periventricular leukomalacia), can affect neuronal organization.

## MYELINATION

- The structure of myelin is rich in lipid and protein. In the CNS, myelin is primarily found in white matter, although it is also present in gray matter in smaller quantities.
- Myelination of the brain begins during the fifth fetal month, progresses rapidly for the first 2 years of life, and then slows markedly after 2 years.
- Fibers to and from the association areas of the brain continue to myelinate into the third and fourth decades of life. In general, myelination has a predictable maturation, with progression from caudal to cephalad, dorsal to ventral, and central to peripheral.
- Myelination progresses from the brain stem to the cerebellum and basal ganglia and then to the cerebral hemispheres. In any particular location, the dorsal region tends to myelinate before the ventral regions.
- The process of myelination also relates to functional requirements such that the somatosensory system in neonates myelinates earlier than the motor and association pathways.
- A rapid growth of the myelinated white matter volume is observed between birth and 9 months of age.
- Myelination can be assessed using the milestones outlined in Table 8.1.

## CEREBELLAR DEVELOPMENT

- Cerebellar development also occurs at the 5- to 15-week period of fetal development. Cerebellar development is dependent on the germinal matrix about the fourth ventricle.

**Table 8.1**  Timing of Myelination

| Anatomic Structure | T1WI | T2WI |
| --- | --- | --- |
| PLIC (posterior portion) | 36 GW | 40 GW |
| Median longitudinal fasciculus | 25 GW | 29 GW |
| Superior cerebellar peduncles | 28 GW | 27 GW |
| Middle cerebellar peduncles | Birth | Birth–2 mo |
| PLIC (anterior portion) | Birth–1 mo | 4–7 mo |
| Anterior limb internal capsule | 2–3 mo | 5–11 mo |
| Cerebellar white matter | Birth–4 mo | 3–5 mo |
| Splenium of corpus callosum | 3–4 mo | 4–6 mo |
| Genu of corpus callosum | 4–6 mo | 5–8 mo |
| Occipital white matter (central) | 3–5 mo | 9–14 mo |
| Frontal white matter (central) | 3–6 mo | 11–16 mo |
| Occipital white matter (peripheral) | 4–7 mo | 11–15 mo |
| Frontal white matter (peripheral) | 7–11 mo | 14–18 mo |
| Centrum semiovale | 2–4 mo | 7–11 mo |

*GW,* Gestational weeks; *PLIC,* posterior limb of internal capsule; *T1WI,* T1-weighted imaging; *T2WI,* T2-weighted imaging.

- Because hemispheric development occurs before vermian development, and the superior vermis forms before the inferior vermis, it is rare to see hemispheric anomalies without vermian maldevelopment or superior vermian lesions without associated inferior vermian anomalies.
- Those entities associated with vermian maldevelopment include the Dandy-Walker malformation, Joubert syndrome, and rhombencephalosynapsis.
- Inferior vermian hypoplasia can be an isolated finding.
- Disorders of hemispheric development include hemispheric hypoplasia, which can be seen in isolation or associated with vermian hypoplasia, brainstem hypoplasia, or other supratentorial anomalies.

# Imaging Techniques/Protocols

## ULTRASOUND

- Ultrasound is the initial examination of choice in the fetus and neonates, particularly premature infants, because of its portability, lack of radiation, and cost effectiveness.
- Transfontanel ultrasonography with high-frequency transducers is efficient for the detection of intracranial edema, hemorrhage, and hydrocephalus.
- Small fontanel size may limit visualization of the peripheral regions of the brain.
- Ultrasound evaluation of the spine is most ideal in the first 3 months of life. Scanning of the spine should start from the sacrococcygeal region in the sagittal plane, and numbering of the vertebrae should be performed caudocranially.

## MAGNETIC RESONANCE IMAGING

- In terms of assessment of myelination, T1-weighted images (T1WI; inversion recovery, magnetization prepared rapid gradient echo [MP-RAGE]) are most helpful during the first year of life, with myelin hyperintensity related to lipid content in the myelin sheath. T2-weighted images (T2WI) are most useful after the first year of life consequent to reduction in brain water content with developing white matter T2 hypointensity. Conventional spin echo or fast spin echo (FSE) techniques may both be implemented; however, FSE techniques demonstrate myelin maturation at an earlier age. T2-weighted fluid-attenuated inversion recovery (FLAIR) imagery is most helpful after myelin maturation has reached its adult appearance.

---

**TEACHING POINTS**

Myelinate On This!

- Anatomic magnetic resonance imaging (MRI) sequences (T1- and T2-weighted) are very helpful in assessment of myelination.
- There is reduction in T1 and T2 relaxation times with continued white matter maturation that corresponds with reduction in tissue water as well as the interaction of water with myelin lipids.
- On T1-weighted imaging (T1WI), most of the white matter in the newborn brain is hypointense compared with gray matter.

- Some of the exceptions include the dorsal brain stem pathways (medial lemnisci, medial longitudinal fasciculi) and the posterior limb of the internal capsules, which are myelinated at birth and show hyperintensity on T1.
- In general, the white matter myelinates earlier on T1WI than on T2-weighted imaging (T2WI) for reasons having to do with water content versus lipid content.
- Diffusion tensor imaging (DTI) can visualize and quantify neural tracts relating to their myelination: fractional anisotropy (FA) increases with age (myelination), whereas apparent diffusion coefficient (ADC), axial diffusivity (AD), and radial diffusivity (RD) decreases, with a turning point around 6 years of age. Note that developmental stages differ by topography and tract of interest, and changes on T1WI and T2WI differ.

- Diffusion tensor imaging (DTI) can help axonal mapping in the brain and identify absent or abnormally coursing white matter bundles.
- Cerebrospinal fluid (CSF) flow disorders are best evaluated by addition of three-dimensional (3D), high-resolution T2WI and phase-contrast imaging. CSF imaging is especially helpful in aqueductal stenosis and Chiari I deformity.
- Magnetic resonance (MR) evaluation of the spine should include FSE T1WI and T2WI in sagittal planes with a slice thickness of 3 to 4 mm. High-resolution, heavily T2-weighted sequences, such as 3D–constructive interference in steady state (CISS) or 3D-T1 MP-RAGE can allow depiction of tiny structures by multiplanar reconstruction.

## COMPUTED TOMOGRAPHY

- In children, computed tomography (CT) is largely replaced by fast MR sequences, like single-shot FSE or half-Fourier acquisition single-shot turbo spin echo (HASTE), such as in the setting of trauma follow-up or ventricular caliber change among shunted patients. Black bone sequences and susceptibility weighted imaging (SWI) are added to fast trauma MR protocols for the detection of fractures and hemorrhage. However, black bone MR is limited in the detection of linear fractures and fractures through aerated bone compared with CT, especially in young children with thinner skulls.
- CT remains the preferred imaging technique for accurate and complete evaluation of craniosynostosis. Slice thickness should be less than or equal to 1 mm; 3D-volume rendered images are especially helpful.

# Supratentorial Congenital Lesions

- It is useful to separate congenital disorders of the brain into those involving the supratentorial structures and those involving the infratentorial structures from an anatomic perspective. Naturally, some disorders can affect both compartments.

Supratentorial Malformations

### Disorders of the Forebrain Development

Holoprosencephaly
Commissural anomalies
Septo-optic dysplasia
Pituitary anomalies

### Cortical Malformations

Proliferation disorders
    Primary microcephaly with simplified gyral pattern
    Hemimegalencephaly
Migrational disorders
    Lissencephaly
        Pachygyria
        Subcortical band heterotopia
    Nodular heterotopia
    Cobblestone brain
    Focal cortical dysplasia
    Hamartomas
Organizational disorders
    Polymicrogyria
    Schizencephaly

Infratentorial Malformations

### Anomalies Limited to the Cerebellum

Dandy-Walker malformation
Blake pouch cyst
Mega cisterna magna
Rhombencephalosynapsis
Other
    Isolated vermian hypoplasia
    Arachnoid cyst in the posterior fossa

### Anomalies Involving the Cerebellum and Brain Stem

Joubert syndrome
Pontocerebellar hypoplasia
Cerebellar disruptions

### Chiari Malformations I–III

- Clinical information is always useful in distinguishing among various congenital abnormalities because several disorders also have associated cutaneous, ocular, or metabolic abnormalities.

## DISORDERS OF FOREBRAIN DEVELOPMENT

### Holoprosencephaly

- *Holoprosencephaly* refers to a constellation of disorders characterized by failure of cleavage or differentiation of the prosencephalon, resulting in a fused appearance of the prosencephalic structures (Fig. 8.1).
- These abnormalities are associated with rather severe intellectual disability, microcephaly, hypotelorism, and abnormal facies. The finding of a solitary median maxillary central incisor is also indicative of holoprosencephaly.

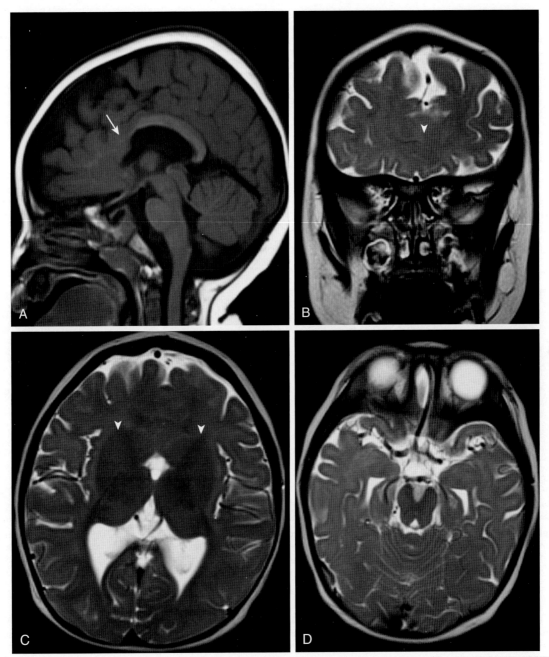

**Fig. 8.1 Lobar holoprosencephaly.** (A) Sagittal T1-weighted imaging (T1WI) shows lack of rostrum and genu of corpus callosum *(arrow)*, whereas the posterior body and splenium are present. (B) Coronal T2-weighted imaging (T2WI) scan shows lack of most anterior portion of the falx cerebri and lack of cleavage in the frontal lobes *(arrowhead)*. (C) Axial T2WI scan shows rudimentary frontal horns *(arrowheads)*. Note normal position of the sylvian fissures. (D) The anterior cerebral artery is azygos as shown in this axial T2WI scan.

The olfactory bulbs and tracts are usually absent, with lack of development of olfactory sulci and flat gyri recti. The range of this disorder is subclassified as alobar, semilobar, lobar holoprosencephaly (with decreasing severity of malformative features; Table 8.2). Syntelencephaly is the middle interhemispheric variant, rarer than the aforementioned.

■ *Lobar holoprosencephaly* presents with near complete cleavage/separation of the frontal lobes (see Fig. 8.1). Formation of the frontal horns of the lateral ventricles can be dysplastic but present. Sylvian fissures are near normal, but formation of an interhemispheric fissure and cerebral falx is incomplete. The deep cerebral nuclei

are fully formed. Tip: A fully formed third ventricle, at least partially present frontal horns, and presence of the posterior body and splenium of corpus callosum classifies the anomaly under lobar holoprosencephaly. Absence of anterior segment of the corpus callosum is associated with lobar holoprosencephaly

■ *Alobar holoprosencephaly* is the most severe and most common form (Fig. 8.2), yet it is rarely encountered in clinical practice because most infants are stillborn. No interhemispheric fissure, falx, or significant separation of the hemispheric structures is identified. A crescentic/horseshoe-shaped monoventricle continuous with a large dorsal cyst usually occupies most of the cranium.

**Table 8.2    Holoprosencephaly Variants**

| Feature | Lobar | Semilobar | Alobar |
|---|---|---|---|
| Facial deformities (cyclopia) | None | None to minimal | Yes |
| Falx cerebri | Anterior tip missing or dysplastic | Partially formed | Absent |
| Thalami | Separated | Partially fused | Fused |
| Interhemispheric fissure | Formed | Present posteriorly | Absent |
| Dorsal cyst | No | Yes, if thalamus is fused | Yes |
| Frontal horns | Yes, but unseparated | No | No |
| Septum pellucidum | Absent | Absent | Absent |
| Vascular | Normal | Normal except rudimentary deep veins | Azygos anterior cerebral artery, absent venous sinuses and deep veins |
| Splenium of corpus callosum | Present | Present without genu or body | Absent |
| Third ventricle | Normal | Small | Absent |
| Occipital horns | Normal | Partially formed | Absent |

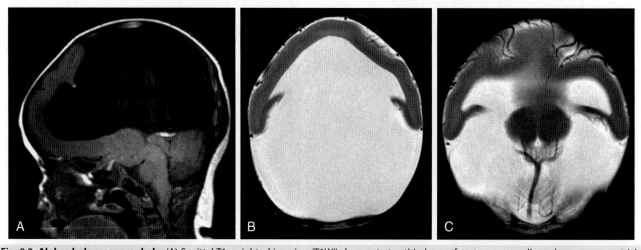

**Fig. 8.2  Alobar holoprosencephaly.** (A) Sagittal T1-weighted imaging (T1WI) demonstrates thin layer of cortex surrounding a large monoventricle which communicates with a large dorsal cyst. (B) Axial T2-weighted imaging (T2WI) scan shows the crescentic shaped monoventricle communicating with the dorsal cyst. Septum pellucidum and falx cerebri are absent. (C) The basal ganglia and thalami are a small mass of fused gray matter that also fuses with the cerebral peduncles.

The basal ganglia and thalami are fused, and the septum pellucidum and corpus callosum are absent. The anterior cerebral arteries in these cases are nearly always azygos (The two A1 segments of the anterior cerebral artery [ACA] join to form a single ACA trunk; i.e., there is no anterior communicating artery.).

- *Semilobar holoprosencephaly* presents with partial development of the falx and the interhemispheric fissure (with partial separation of the lateral ventricles). The basal ganglia and thalami are at least partially fused.
- *Syntelencephaly* ("middle interhemispheric variant") is the least common form. The posterior frontal and parietal lobes are fused, with the interhemispheric fissure being formed anteriorly and posteriorly and absent in between. The sylvian fissures appear as abnormal vertical clefts and meet in the midline. The body of the corpus callosum is absent. Deep gray nuclei are not fused. There is an association with parietal cephaloceles (Fig. 8.3).
- Common differential diagnoses include hydranencephaly and severe congenital hydrocephalus. If no cortical mantle is discernible around the dilated CSF space centrally,

the diagnosis is hydranencephaly, especially if all that can be seen is a nubbin of occipital or posterior temporal cortex remaining with a falx present (Fig. 8.4). If you see a well-formed falx, cortical mantle, and separated ventricles with a septum pellucidum, suggest severe hydrocephalus. If the thalami are fused, septum pellucidum or falx is absent, a cortical mantle is seen, and the ventricles have lost their usual shape, diagnose holoprosencephaly. Holoprosencephalies can be associated with a number of clinical syndromes.

**TEACHING POINTS**

Associations With Holoprosencephaly

Caudal agenesis
DiGeorge syndrome
Fetal alcohol syndrome
Kallmann syndrome
Maternal diabetes
Trisomy 13, 15, 18

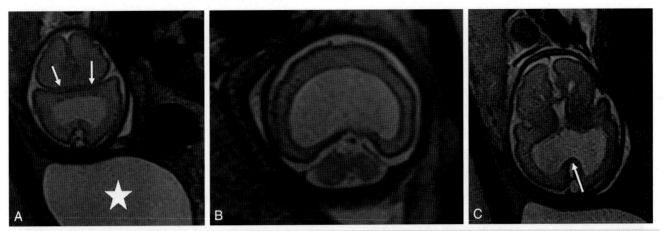

**Fig. 8.3 Syntelencephaly.** (A) Axial T2 half-Fourier-acquisition single-shot turbo spin-echo (HASTE) image from fetal magnetic resonance imaging (MRI) shows lack of cleavage ("fused" appearance) of the bilateral posterior frontal lobes with communication of the abnormal sylvian fissures across the midline at the level of the vertex *(arrows)*. The maternal urinary bladder is partially included in the field of view *(star)*. (B) "Fusion" of the part of the posterior parietal lobes is noted in coronal T2 HASTE image. (C) The corpus callosum is present at the genu and splenium *(arrow)* only. The septum pellucidum is absent. The interhemispheric fissure is formed partially: anteriorly and posteriorly.

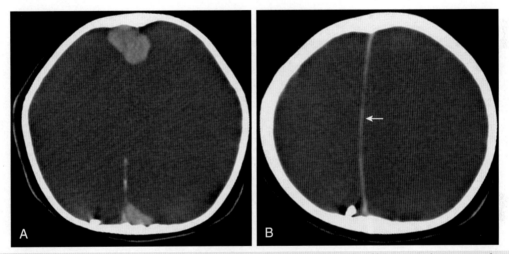

**Fig. 8.4 Hydranencephaly.** (A) Axial computed tomography image shows near complete absence of brain parenchyma except for small portions of anteroinferior frontal lobes and medial occipital lobes. (B) The falx cerebri is present *(arrow)*.

## Commissural Anomalies

- The corpus callosum is the largest of the three midline commissures; the others are the anterior commissure and the hippocampal commissure.
- Agenesis of the corpus callosum is one of the most commonly observed features in malformations of the brain and is a part of many syndromes.
- The classic, more descriptive callosal segments include the lamina rostralis (rostrum), genu, body, isthmus, and splenium. However, from a functional and developmental anatomic point of view, the corpus callosum is divided into two segments by the isthmus: a prominent anterior frontal segment that carries the commissural fibers of the entire anterior frontal lobe, which are called forceps minor, and a smaller posterior splenial segment that carries the commissural fibers of the primary visual and posterior parietal and medial occipitotemporal cortices and white matter, collectively called the *forceps major*. This helps with the understanding of two important concepts: (1) myelination proceeds posterior to anterior, reflecting the fact that myelination of the primary cortical areas connected through the isthmus and splenium precedes myelination of the body, genu, and rostrum, and (2) in holoprosencephalies, the posterior callosum is present because the temporal and occipital lobes are separated in those cases.

- The septum pellucidum forms in close association with the anterior corpus callosum. The cavum is not truly apparent before 20 gestational weeks. This is important to understand partial agenesis of the genu of the corpus callosum in cases with septo-optic dysplasia. The interhemispheric glial bridge provides a support for the first pioneer axons to cross at about gestational weeks 12 to 13. The corpus callosum develops within a very short time during week 13; at week 14, it is virtually complete, although still short. The shape of the corpus callosum is essentially final by week 20; however, its sagittal cross-sectional area is only 5% of what it will be in a mature brain (Fig. 8.5). The corpus callosum enlarges together with the connectivity and the tangential growth of the cortex.

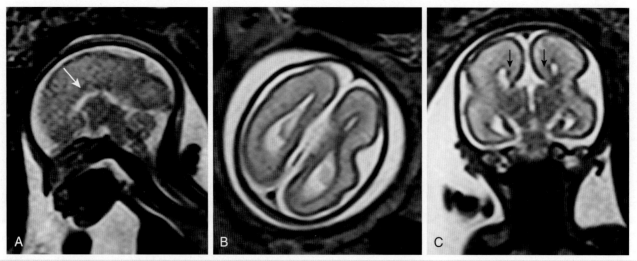

**Fig. 8.5 Agenesis of corpus callosum in an early second trimester fetus.** (A) Sagittal half-Fourier-acquisition single-shot turbo spin-echo (HASTE) demonstrates lack of corpus callosum in the midline *(arrow)*. (B) Axial HASTE shows the pointed frontal horns and dilated occipital horns of the lateral ventricles (colpocephaly). The lateral ventricles are parallel. (C) Crescentic shape of the frontal horns secondary to medially located bundles of Probst *(black arrows)*. The cingulate gyri are everted.

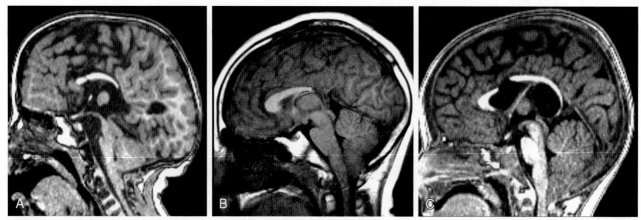

**Fig. 8.6 Examples of partial agenesis/hypogenesis of corpus callosum.** (A) Reduced anteroposterior diameter of the corpus callosum with lack of rostrum, genu, and splenium of corpus callosum. Note the small posterior fossa, effaced fourth ventricle, flattened/elongated brain stem, inferior descent of the tonsils, and tectal beaking in this patient with Chiari II malformation. (B) The splenium of corpus callosum is absent. Note the inferior descent of the cerebellar tonsils below the level of foramen magnum with peg-like configuration in this patient with Chiari I malformation. (C) The anterior and posterior segments of the corpus callosum are disconnected with the lack of isthmus. Note the Chiari II malformation with milder degree of findings described in (A).

- It has long been assumed that the corpus callosum develops from front to back and that partial commissural agenesis, most commonly posterior splenial agenesis, would be lesser forms of agenesis. It is now understood that by determining the missing portions, one cannot reliably predict whether the partial agenesis is a sequela of a destructive event versus a developmental anomaly.
- One needs to evaluate all interhemispheric commissures, the isthmus, the connection of anterior segment to isthmus, and the connection of the posterior segment to isthmus to conclude whether the corpus callosum is developmentally anomalous.
- Sagittal midline T1WI and/or T2WI are ideal in this evaluation. In the most typical partial agenesis, the entire corpus callosum is present, but short in anteroposterior (AP) diameter. Alternatively, along the spectrum of callosal agenesis/hypogenesis, the anterior and posterior segments may be present without the connecting isthmus (no connection of the fornix to the splenium), the splenium may be hypoplastic, or the corpus callosum can be completely absent (Fig. 8.6).
- In classic corpus callosum agenesis, the commissural fibers are not completely genetically absent but rather heterotopic. The noncrossing fibers make an angle and form a parasagittal bundle in the medial aspect of the lateral ventricles, forming the Probst bundles. The lateral ventricles are parallel, frontal horns are pointed and crescentic in shape, and occipital horns are enlarged (colpocephaly), with a high-riding third ventricle (if no corpus callosum, there is nothing to hold the third ventricle in place). The cingulate gyrus is everted, and the cingulate sulcus does not form, resulting in a radiating/disorganized appearance of the sulci in the interhemispheric region (Fig. 8.7).

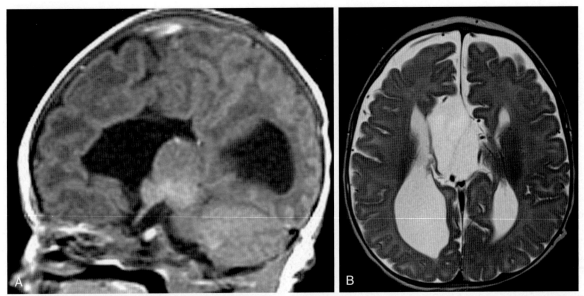

**Fig. 8.7  Agenesis of corpus callosum with interhemispheric cyst.** (A) Sagittal T1-weighted imaging (T1WI) shows agenesis of corpus callosum. Note interhemispheric sulci radiating into the third ventricle with everted cingulate sulcus. (B) Axial T2-weighted imaging (T2WI) scan shows interhemispheric cyst. Lateral ventricles are parallel with asymmetric dilation of the right lateral ventricle.

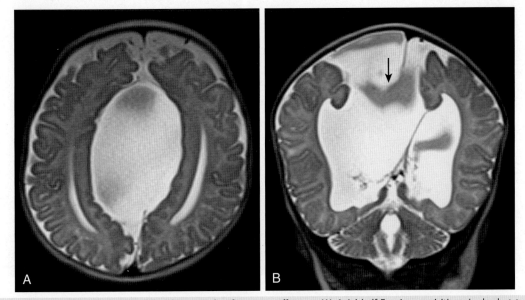

**Fig. 8.8  Large midline interhemispheric cyst with agenesis of corpus callosum.** (A) Axial half-Fourier-acquisition single-shot turbo spin-echo (HASTE) image demonstrates a large midline interhemispheric cyst, which communicates with the right lateral ventricle in the coronal HASTE image. Please note that the right frontal lobe is pushed laterally from the midline by the mass effect of this interhemispheric cyst, which communicates with the right lateral ventricle. This clearly doesn't represent an open lip schizencephaly because there is no cleft with dysplastic gray matter lining. (B) Cerebrospinal fluid flow artifact confirms communication in addition to the displaced septum *(arrow)*.

**TEACHING POINTS**

Findings in Agenesis of Corpus Callosum

Pointed, crescent-shaped frontal horns
Colpocephaly
High-riding enlarged third ventricle
Incomplete development of hippocampal formation
Interhemispheric cyst or lipoma
Medial impingement of Probst bundle on ventricles
No cingulate sulcus
Radially oriented fissures (eversion of cingulate gyrus) into
    the high-riding third ventricle
Septum pellucidum absent or widely separated

- Other midline abnormalities may be associated with agenesis of the corpus callosum, the most common being interhemispheric cysts and less likely being a midline lipoma (both of which are related to meningeal dysplasia).
  - Interhemispheric cysts may be communicating (Fig. 8.8) or noncommunicating with the ventricles; these cysts are important to identify, especially in those cases with ventriculomegaly. Management could differ in noncommunicating cysts and include surgical and endoscopic options, such as placement of shunts or cyst marsupialization versus endoscopic cystoventriculostomy. As expected, the cyst would follow the same

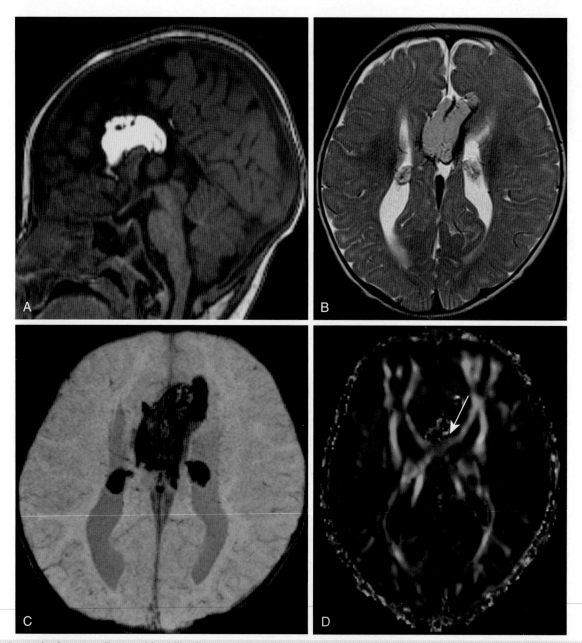

**Fig. 8.9  Agenesis of corpus callosum with midline lipoma.** (A) Sagittal T1-weighted imaging (T1WI) shows T1 bright lobular mass following the same signal as the subcutaneous fat representing a lipoma. (B) Axial T2-weighted imaging (T2WI) scan shows that this lipoma is vascular and extends into the lateral ventricles. (C) Axial minimum intensity projection of susceptibility-weighted imaging shows extensive susceptibility covering the lipomas indicating mineralization/calcification in this lipoma. (D) Fractional anisotropy map demonstrate at least partial presence of genu of the corpus callosum *(arrow).*

density/signal intensity as the CSF, unlike the lipoma, which has fat density/signal intensity (Fig. 8.9).

- Callosal development is closely associated with development of the cortex, so there are associations of complete/partial agenesis with heterotopias, agyria, pachygyria, holoprosencephaly, septo-optic dysplasia, cephaloceles, and Chiari II malformations; Dandy-Walker syndrome is also not uncommon. Trisomy 13, 15, 18; fetal alcohol syndrome; and Meckel syndrome (occipital encephalocele, microcephaly, polycystic kidneys, polydactyly) are also associated with agenesis of the corpus callosum.

- *Aicardi syndrome* is characterized by the triad of agenesis of the corpus callosum, infantile (or even neonatal)

spasms usually without typical hypsarrhythmia (abnormal interictal pattern seen on electroencephalogram [EEG] in patients with infantile spasms), and severe neurologic and mental impairment. The imaging features are partial/total callosal agenesis, an interhemispheric cyst, polymicrogyria, periventricular or subcortical nodular heterotopias, and choroid plexus cysts or papillomas, posterior fossa cyst, choroidal ocular lacunae, and ocular colobomata (Fig. 8.10).

## Septo-optic Dysplasia

- Septo-optic dysplasia (de Morsier syndrome) is a very heterogeneous and usually sporadic condition, defined by any combination of optic nerve hypoplasia, pituitary

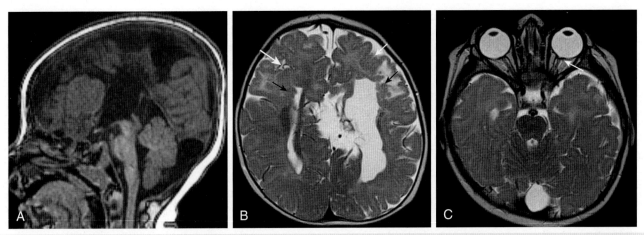

**Fig. 8.10 Aicardi Syndrome.** (A) Agenesis of corpus callosum demonstrated on the sagittal T1-weighted imaging (T1WI) scan. Note the relatively small vermis and small cyst in the posterior fossa confirmed on image (C). (B) Axial T2WI scan shows asymmetric left lateral ventriculomegaly, bifrontal polymicrogyria *(white arrows)*, bilateral subependymal heterotopias *(black arrows)*, and subcortical abnormal myelination. Note the abnormal T2 signal of the subcortical white matter in the region of polymicrogyrias. (C) Note the coloboma *(arrow)* in the left globe on this T2-weighted imaging ( T2WI scan).

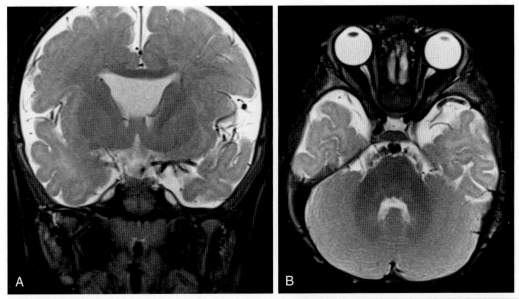

**Fig. 8.11 Septo-optic dysplasia.** (A) Coronal T2-weighted imaging (T2WI) shows absence of septum pellucidum and squared off appearance of the frontal horns. (B) Bilateral hypoplastic optic nerves are demonstrated on this axial T2WI scan.

gland hypoplasia, and midline abnormalities of the ventral and rostral cerebellum.

- Etiology is multifactorial, with the genetic abnormalities identified only in 1% of patients.
- Clinical presentation relies on the extent of the abnormality. Hypothalamic-pituitary dysfunction is seen in two thirds of patients. Effects on the visual pathway may range from blindness to normal vision and from nystagmus to normal eye movements. Seizures may coexist.
- On imaging, congenital absence of the septum pellucidum causes a squared-off appearance to the frontal horns of the lateral ventricles (Fig. 8.11). Low position of fornices on sagittal images is another clue to absence of septum pellucidum.
- MR imaging (MRI) appearances are categorized in two groups, one with a high incidence of malformations of cortical development (especially schizencephaly,

polymicrogyria, and heterotopias) and partial absence of the septum pellucidum with or without incomplete hippocampal rotation; the second with overlapping features of mild lobar holoprosencephaly with complete absence of the septum pellucidum. Hypoplasia of the anterior falx can be seen in the second group.

- When the septum pellucidum is partially absent, usually the anterior portion is present. This is best seen on coronal images.
- Agenesis of the corpus callosum and white matter hypoplasia may be associated with this abnormality.
- In general, patients with septo-optic dysplasia demonstrate small hypoplastic optic nerves and a small optic chiasm resulting from the dysplastic optic pathways. In some cases, dysplasia may be limited to the optic disc, and the nerves/chiasm may not be small.
- Pituitary abnormalities with hormonal changes, such as ectopic posterior pituitary gland, can be seen.

## Isolated Absence of the Septum Pellucidum

- This is a rare structural abnormality that can be asymptomatic or have neurologic manifestations.
- The brain should be carefully evaluated to rule out holoprosencephaly, callosal agenesis, septo-optic dysplasia, schizencephaly, bilateral polymicrogyria, and rhombencephalosynapsis.

## Pituitary Anomalies

- By the third week of gestation, oral ectoderm containing pituitary placode originates from the anterior neural ridge. Between 28 and 32 days of embryonic life, the Rathke pouch or Rathke cleft invaginates from the pituitary placode and comes in contact with the downward extension of the embryonic hypothalamus.
- The Rathke pouch gives rise to the adenohypophysis or anterior lobe of the pituitary, whereas the embryonic hypothalamus forms the neurohypophysis or posterior pituitary lobe. By the sixth gestational week, the Rathke pouch invagination obliterates and disconnects from the oral ectoderm of the buccal cavity. If portions of this connection persist, a persistent craniopharyngeal canal may develop (Fig. 8.12). Absence of the pituitary gland is very rare and fatal at birth. Pituitary hypoplasia is more common, with imaging findings of small sella turcica, ectopia of the posterior pituitary bright spot, and absence or hypoplasia of the infundibular stalk. Patients present with short stature and other hormonal deficiencies.
- Pituitary duplication is also rare and results in complete duplication of the entire gland, including the infundibulum. It has been associated with midline facial or oral anomalies, particularly facial clefting and hypertelorism.

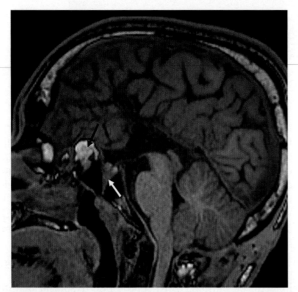

**Fig. 8.12 Persistent craniopharyngeal canal.** Sagittal T1-weighted image shows a persistent craniopharyngeal canal *(white arrow)* extending from the base of the expected location of the sella to the most cranial aspect of the nasopharynx. Note the inferior descent of the pituitary gland along the persistent craniopharyngeal canal. Bonus findings: Complete agenesis of the corpus callosum and the lipoma *(black arrow)* in the anterior cranial fossa.

- Rathke cleft cysts are embryologic remnants of the Rathke pouch, lined with a single layer of cuboidal or columnar epithelial cells and may arise within the sella, the suprasellar region, or both. The cysts can compress normal posterior or anterior pituitary tissue to cause symptoms of hypopituitarism, diabetes insipidus, headache, and visual field deficits, but most patients are asymptomatic. The cysts are well-defined masses that are located between the adenohypophysis and neurohypophysis.
  - Signal characteristics may vary on MRI: high or low signal intensity on T1WI (depending on the amount of proteinaceous contents), high signal intensity on T2WI, and lack of postcontrast enhancement are common (Fig. 8.13). These can appear hypodense on CT. Presence of an intracystic solid nodule is strongly suggestive of a Rathke cleft cyst. The differential diagnosis is craniopharyngioma or cystic pituitary adenoma; first check out the location—if the lesion is between the adeno- and neurohypophysis and lacks calcification, solid component, and enhancement, then favor Rathke cleft cyst. Fluid-fluid levels, septations, and an off-midline location favor a pituitary adenoma.

## CORTICAL MALFORMATIONS

### Proliferation Disorders

#### Primary Microcephaly with Simplified Gyral Pattern.

- These children are microcephalic because of the reduced proliferation of neurons and glia in the germinal zones or increased apoptosis. The head circumference is 3 or more standard deviations below the norm.
- Neuroimaging shows the primary and secondary sulcations; however, it lacks the tertiary sulcations. The primary sulci are shallow grooves on the surface of the brain that become progressively more deeply infolded and that develop side branches, designated *secondary sulci*. Gyration proceeds with the formation of other side branches of the secondary sulci, referred to as *tertiary sulci*. The volume of the white matter in the cerebral hemispheres is reduced.
- This is a heterogenous group of disorders classified under six subgroups of increasing severity of neuroimaging findings. Groups 5 and 6 have the simplest looking gyral pattern and are named *microlissencephaly* (Fig. 8.14).

#### Hemimegalencephaly.

- Hemimegalencephaly is hamartomatous overgrowth of all or part of a cerebral hemisphere with defects in neuronal proliferation, migration, and organization.
- This is a heterogenous disorder that can occur in isolation but is more commonly associated with cutaneous abnormalities and hemihypertrophy. Hemimegalencephaly may occur in a variety of syndromes, including epidermal nevus syndrome, Proteus syndrome, neurofibromatosis type 1 (NF-1), Soto syndrome, tuberous sclerosis (TS), and Klippel-Trénaunay-Weber syndrome, or CLOVES (congenital lipomatous overgrowth, vascular malformations, epidermal nevi, and scoliosis) to name a few. These children are typically macrocephalic at birth. Patients have seizures,

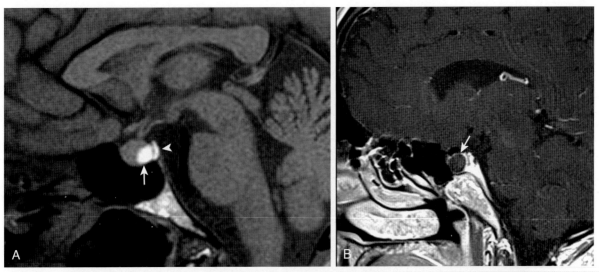

**Fig. 8.13 Rathke cleft cyst.** (A) Precontrast sagittal T1-weighted imaging (T1WI) demonstrates hyperintense lesion in the pituitary gland *(arrow)*. Note the normal precontrast bright T1 signal of the dorsum sellae *(arrowhead)*. (B) Postcontrast T1WI in a different patient nicely demonstrates nonenhancing cyst in the sella representing the Rathke cleft cyst *(arrow)*.

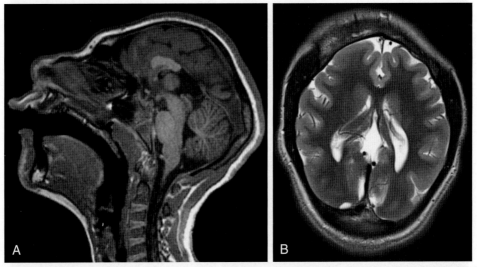

**Fig. 8.14 Microcephaly with simplified gyral pattern.** (A) Sagittal T1-weighted imaging (T1WI) shows the markedly small head size in relation to the face. Note the hypogenesis of the corpus callosum mostly affecting the posterior segment. (B) Note the too few gyri and shallow sulci in this axial T2WI scan.

hemiplegia, developmental delay, and abnormal skull configurations.

---

**TEACHING POINTS**

Hemimegaloencephaly

Neurofibromatosis type 1
Dyke-Davidoff-Masson syndrome/Sturge-Weber association
McCune Albright syndrome
Soto syndrome
Tuberous sclerosis
Klippel-Trénaunay-Weber syndrome
Proteus syndrome
Epidermal nevus syndrome

---

- On MRI and CT, part or all of the affected cerebral hemisphere appears moderately to markedly enlarged. Typically, affected lobes/hemispheres show various degrees of pachygyria and dysplasia of the cortex. White matter volume is increased and usually reveals heterogeneous or high signal, usually attributed to delayed myelination. Characteristically, the ipsilateral ventricle is enlarged, with a dysmorphic pointed appearance of the frontal horn (Fig. 8.15). This unique feature of ventricular dilatation on the side of the enlarged hemisphere separates congenital hemimegalencephaly from other infiltrative lesions. Interestingly, the radiologic appearance may change over time. Patients with hemimegalencephaly of one hemisphere in infancy have been reported to develop atrophy of the affected hemisphere at 1 year of age. Although rare, associated enlargement and

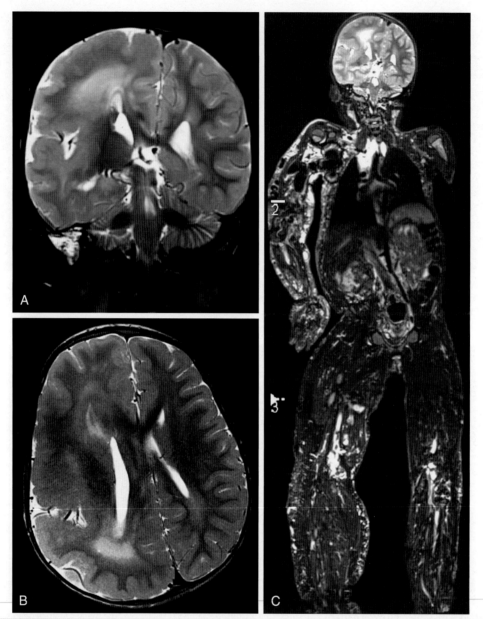

**Fig. 8.15 Unilateral hemimegalencephaly in a patient with congenital lipomatous overgrowth, vascular malformations, and epidermal nevi (CLOVE) syndrome.** (A–B) Coronal T2-and axial T2-weighted imaging demonstrate marked enlargement of the right cerebral hemisphere, diffuse pachygyria of the right cerebral cortex, mild asymmetric enlargement of the right lateral ventricle, and straightening of the right frontal horn. In addition, the T2 signal of the white matter is diffusely abnormal and gray-white matter distinction is fuzzy. (C) Stitched coronal short tau inversion recovery (STIR) sequence of the whole body demonstrates overgrowth in the right upper and lower extremities and torso and, to a lesser degree, in the left lower extremity with extensive venous and lymphatic malformations in this patient with CLOVE syndrome.

dysplasia of the cerebellum and brain stem can be seen, a condition known as *total hemimegalencephaly*.

- Anatomic or functional hemispherectomy may be indicated in cases with intractable seizures if the contralateral hemisphere is normal. Therefore careful evaluation of the contralateral hemisphere is critical in these patients.

## Migrational Disorders

### Lissencephaly

- The term *lissencephaly* means "smooth brain," with paucity of gyral and sulcal development of the surface of the brain.

- Agyria is a global absence of gyri along with thickened cortex and is the same entity as "complete lissencephaly," whereas "pachygyria" refers to partial involvement in a hemisphere.

- Multiple genetic mutations have been identified in lissencephaly, and one of the most well-known is a defect of *LIS1* gene at locus 17p13.3. Miller-Dieker syndrome also has a mutation in chromosome 17 and presents with characteristic facies and lissencephaly on imaging. Mutation in the *DCX* gene (also known as *XLIS*) in chromosome 22 is known as X-linked lissencephaly and accounts for about 75% of lissencephaly mutations. Appendicular and oropharyngeal spasticity develops

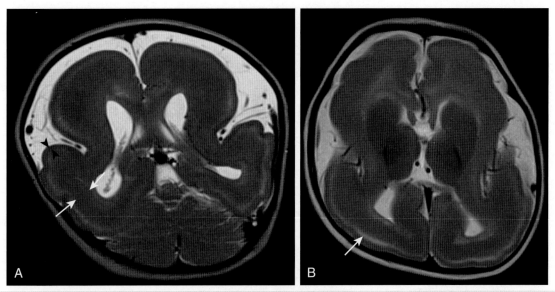

**Fig. 8.16 Lissencephaly.** Note the vertically oriented sylvian fissures giving the brain a figure eight or hour-glass appearance. (A) Coronal T2-weighted imaging shows the thin cortical outer layer *(black arrowheads)* separated from arrested neurons by a normal white matter in the cell sparse zone. The thick layer of arrested neurons is outlined between the two *white arrows*. The thin layer of cortex is outlined by the *black arrowheads*. (B) Very few shallow sulci in the frontal lobes. The T2 bright cell-sparse zone *(arrow)* is quite prominent in the agyric posterior parieto-occipital lobes.

with maturation of the CNS. The X-linked gene *double-cortin (XLIS)* predisposes to lissencephaly in boys and band heterotopia in girls (protected by two X chromosomes). *LIS1* and *DCX* mutations have similar neurologic presentations, namely hypotonia at birth.

- Imaging demonstrates a smooth brain surface, diminished white matter, and shallow/vertically oriented sylvian fissures (thus the figure eight or hourglass appearance on axial images).
  - The thin outer cortex is separated from the thick deeper cortical layers by a zone of white matter, called the *cell-sparse zone.*
  - The trigones and occipital horns of the ventricles are dilated, likely because of underdevelopment of the calcarine sulcus.
  - The brain stem is small, likely secondary to lack of normally formed corticospinal and corticobulbar tracts (Fig. 8.16).

### PACHYGYRIA

- Agyria/pachygyria typically results from abnormal neuronal migration and is considered a subtype of the lissencephaly spectrum of disorders. Patients with congenital cytomegalovirus (CMV) infection have higher incidence of pachygyria.
- Imaging shows thickened gray matter and poor sulcation. Sulci are shallow and few; however, they can be identified neuroanatomically, in contrast to polymicrogyria, where the sulci are abnormal and do not correspond to any normal described sulci in the textbooks (Fig. 8.17). White matter volume is decreased, as opposed to hemimegalencephaly. Abnormal myelination may coexist.

### HETEROTOPIA

- Heterotopia is usually gray matter that is located in the wrong place. Heterotopias form when migration of the neuroblasts from the periventricular region to the pia is

thwarted, possibly because of damage to the radial glial fibers, which orient migrating neurons.
- The heterotopias are named by their morphology and location, such as nodular/focal subcortical, band, or periventricular/subependymal nodular types.

### BAND HETEROTOPIA

- The band heterotopia (double cortex) may present at any age, but it usually forms in childhood with variable degrees of developmental delay and mixed seizure disorders.
- The *DCX* mutation is the most common genetic abnormality, with a strong female preponderance (>90%).
- On imaging, a homogenous band of gray matter is seen between the cortex and white matter, separated from the ventricles and cortex by normal appearing white matter. It may be complete or partial. Partial frontal lobe bands are more common in females, whereas posterior involvement is more common in males. The overlying cortex may be normal or malformed. (Fig. 8.18).

### PERIVENTRICULAR NODULAR (SUBEPENDYMAL) HETEROTOPIA

- Patients with subependymal heterotopias can be divided in two groups: the larger group of patients have symmetric and fewer subependymal heterotopias usually confined to the trigones and temporal/occipital horns (Fig. 8.19). These are rarely familial but can be seen in association with other congenital anomalies such as callosal anomalies, Chiari II malformations, Dandy- Walker malformation, or cephaloceles, to name a few.
- The smaller group of patients may have familial either X-linked or autosomal recessive patterns of inheritance. Mutations in several genes (such as *Filamin*-1 gene on the long arm of the X chromosome) may cause subependymal heterotopias.
- Subependymal heterotopias appear as smooth, ovoid masses that are isointense to gray matter on all imaging

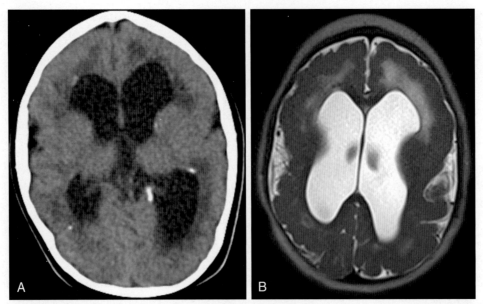

**Fig. 8.17 Bilateral pachygyria in a patient with cytomegalovirus infection.** (A) Axial computed tomography (CT) image shows diffuse thickening of the cortex bilaterally with low density of the white matter. Note the periventricular calcifications. (B) Axial T2-weighted imaging of the brain demonstrate diffuse thickening of the cortex and shallow sylvian fissures. The volume of the white matter is reduced. The increased T2 signal of the white matter corresponds to the decreased density in the CT representing delayed myelination.

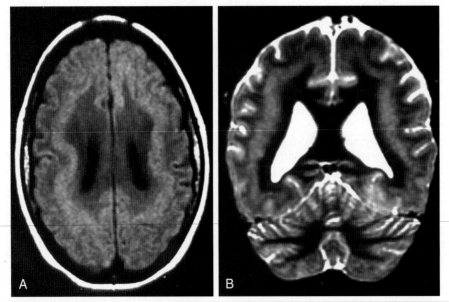

**Fig. 8.18 Band heterotopia.** (A–B) Coronal and axial T1-weighted imaging demonstrate a thin layer of gray matter in the subcortical white matter of bifrontal lobes representing a partial band heterotopia.

sequences (see Fig. 8.19). The long axis of the heterotopias is parallel to the ventricular wall, and the heterotopias do not show evidence of enhancement on postcontrast images, nor do they have perilesional edema. They can grow exophytically, extending into the ventricle, and, if big enough, may have mass effect on the ventricle (see Fig. 8.19). Hyperintensity on T1WI may be because of dystrophic microcalcifications and these may show hyperdensity at CT.

FOCAL SUBCORTICAL HETEROTOPIAS
■ Patients with subcortical heterotopias often have abnormal sulcation patterns superficial to the heterotopia.

The hemisphere ipsilateral to the site of the subcortical heterotopia may be smaller with thinning of the overlying cortex. Subcortical heterotopias may be nodular or curvilinear in shape. The nodular variety of subcortical heterotopias are usually identified in a periventricular or subcortical location, whereas the diffuse (or laminar) heterotopias are seen more commonly in or close to the cortex. Imaging features are similar to that of subependymal heterotopias.

■ Encephaloceles, holoprosencephaly, schizencephaly, Chiari malformations, and agenesis of the corpus callosum may coexist with gray matter heterotopias. If you see one, actively search for other anomalies!

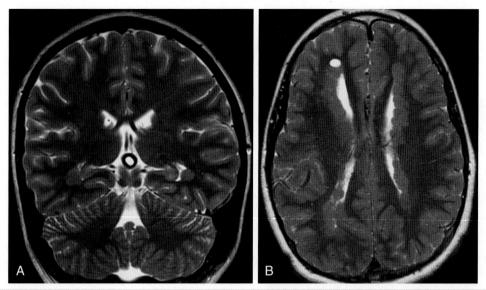

**Fig. 8.19 Examples of nodular heterotopias.** Axial T2-weighted imaging (T2WI) scan shows bilateral extensive nodular masses outlining the lateral ventricles, following the same signal of the cortex.

## Cobblestone Malformations

- Congenital muscular dystrophies (CMD) are included in this group of malformations, characterized by hypotonia at birth, generalized muscle weakness, joint contractures, and other CNS anomalies. Fukuyama type was the first described in this group, an autosomal recessive condition prevalent in Japan. Walker-Warburg syndrome and muscle-eye-brain disease have brain and ocular anomalies.
- There is considerable overlap in pathologic and imaging findings. Walker-Warburg syndrome patients have cobblestone lissencephaly, congenital hydrocephalus, severe congenital eye malformations (microphthalmos, retinal dysplasia, persistent hypoplastic primary vitreous, optic nerve hypoplasia), and may have occipital encephaloceles. The cortex is thick with very few sulci.
- *Cobblestone lissencephaly* refers to the quite distinctively irregular gray-white matter junction possible, reflecting the disorganized neurons interrupting the white matter. More severe cases have pontine hypoplasia with a distinctive kink at the mesencephalic-pontine junction because of cerebellar hypoplasia/dysplasia.
- Fukuyama congenital muscular dystrophy is characterized by frontal polymicrogyria and temporo-occipital cobblestone cortex. In addition, the cerebellum is dysplastic and with subcortical cysts. Muscle-eye-brain disease shows similar features to that of the two previously described entities; however, the severity is somewhat intermediate.

## Focal Cortical Dysplasia

- Cortical dysplasia may be a source of seizures and motor deficits.
- According to the ILAE (International League Against Epilepsy) Task Force classification system, focal cortical dysplasias (FCD) are classified into three major groups: FCD types Ia and Ib; FCD types IIa and IIb; and FCD types IIIa to IIId.

- The signal intensity of the dysplastic cortex and underlying white matter may change with age; therefore, multiple studies may be required to find the FCD in young children. (Table 8.3)

**Table 8.3** The ILAE consensus classification of focal cortical dysplasia (FCD)

| FCD | Histopathology | MR Findings |
|---|---|---|
| Type Ia | abnormal cortical layering, compromising the radial composition of the 6-layered neocortex | Cortex appears normal with normal thickness, however the underlying white matter signal is abnormal. |
| Type Ib | abnormal cortical layering, compromising the tangential composition of the 6-layered neocortex | Cortex appears thin, often within a vascular territory. |
| Type IIa | dysmorphic neurons | Blurring of the gray-white matter junction |
| Type IIb | dysmorphic neurons and balloon cells | Blurring of the gray-white matter junction and abnormal T2 hyperintensity of the subcortical white matter. T2/FLAIR signal abnormality can span the entire cerebral mantle from the cortex to the ventricle, namely "transmantle sign". |
| Type IIIa | cortical dyslamination associated with hippocampal sclerosis | Imaging depends on the associated abnormality. |
| Type IIIb | cortical dyslamination adjacent to glial or glioneuronal tumor | |
| Type IIIc | cortical dyslamination adjacent to vascular malformation | |
| Type IIId | cortical dyslamination adjacent to lesion acquired during early life, e.g. stroke, trauma or infection | |

### FOCAL CORTICAL DYSPLASIA TYPE I (DYSPLASIAS WITH ABNORMAL LAMINATION)

■ Imaging findings may be very subtle, manifested as normal or thinned cortex with underlying abnormal unmyelinated or hypomyelinated white matter (Fig. 8.20). Positron emission tomography (PET) studies show decreased 18-fluorodeoxyglucose (FDG) uptake in the affected region.

### FOCAL CORTICAL DYSPLASIA TYPE II (DYSPLASIAS WITH CORTICAL DYSLAMINATION AND DYSMORPHIC NEURONS WITH OR WITHOUT BALLOON CELLS)

■ This is also called *focal transmantle cortical dysplasia*.
■ Histologically, there is cortex with abnormal lamination, abnormal cells (dysplastic neurons and balloon cells), and glial proliferation and reduced myelination in the affected white matter.
■ Imaging shows focal signal abnormality that extends from the gray-white matter junction to the ventricular surface with hyperintense subcortical white matter on T2WI. The gray-white junction is blurred (Fig. 8.21).
■ Some genetic studies showed alterations within the *TSC1* locus (one of the genes responsible from TS) at higher frequencies in patients with FCD type II compared with the normal population, explaining the striking similarity between FCD type II and cortical tubers associated with TS.

### FOCAL CORTICAL DYSPLASIA TYPE III

■ FCD type III occurs with other lesions such as hippocampal sclerosis (FCD type IIIa), epilepsy associated tumors (FCD type IIIb), vascular malformations (FCD type IIIc), and acquired lesions, such as traumatic or ischemic injury and encephalitis (FCD type IIId). They have no imaging correlate apart from the pathology they are presenting with.

### Hamartomas

■ Hamartomas represent an abnormal nonneoplastic proliferation of disorganized but mature cells, usually a combination of neurons, glia, and blood vessels in an abnormal location.
■ There is a propensity for hamartomatous formation in the hypothalamus typically located between the

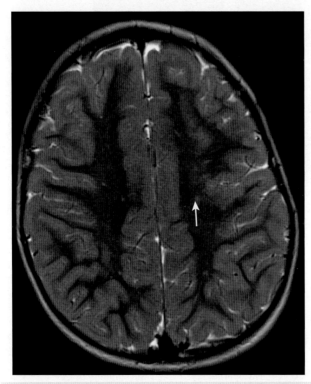

**Fig. 8.20 Cortical dysplasia, type I.** Note the localized blurring of the gray-white matter junction in the posterior left frontal lobe in the medial aspect representing focal cortical dysplasia. In addition, few tiny foci of gray matter signal are seen in the white matter in the vicinity of this focal cortical dysplasia suggesting additional subcortical heterotopias *(arrow)*.

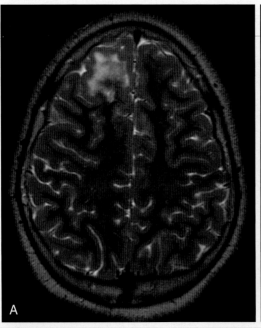
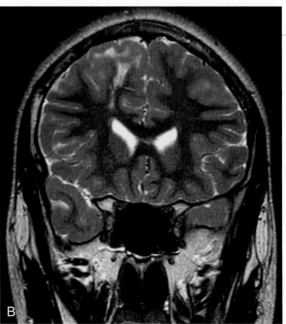

**Fig. 8.21 Cortical dysplasia, type II with balloon cells.** (A) Axial T2-weighted imaging (T2WI) shows a focal area of increased T2 signal in the subcortical white matter of the right frontal lobe radiating to the superolateral margin of the right frontal horn in this coronal T2WI (B).

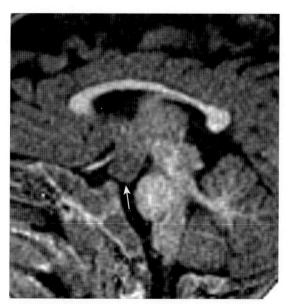

**Fig. 8.22 Hypothalamic hamartoma.** Sagittal T1-weighted imaging shows pedunculated brain tissue extending caudally from tuber cinereum of the hypothalamus.

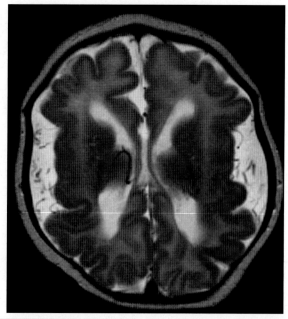

**Fig. 8.23 Polymicrogyria in a patient with bilateral perisylvian syndrome.** Axial T2-weighted imaging shows thick and bumpy insular cortex where gray-white matter differentiation is blurry. The sylvian fissures are open because of abnormal opercularization. Please notice the distinction from pachygyria, in which the normal anatomy of the sulci can be identified.

mammillary bodies and the tuber cinereum of the hypothalamus (Fig. 8.22). Boys are more commonly affected than girls. These patients typically present with precocious puberty (before 2 years of age in boys and slightly later in girls) and gelastic (laughing spells) seizures. However, occasionally, visual disturbances may be present because the hypothalamic hamartoma involves the optic pathways.

- Because a hamartoma is essentially normal brain substance, the hamartoma is isodense with the gray matter on CT and isointense on T1WI on MRI with variable signal on T2WI. The lesion is identified as a bulbous protrusion of the hypothalamic region in the midline. The hamartomas have a normal blood-brain barrier and therefore do not show enhancement on either CT or MR. Occasionally, mass effect may be associated with the hamartoma as evidenced by displacement of the inferior portion of the third ventricle.
- After the hypothalamic region, the next most common location for hamartomas is the cerebral cortex-subcortical region. Occasionally, hamartomas may be seen in a periventricular location. Fetus in fetu refers to duplication of brain structures, usually seen as an extra-axial frontal region mass. The signal intensity approaches that of normal brain. Case studies of ectopic brain in the nasopharynx or pterygopalatine fossa have also been reported.

## Organizational Disorders

### Polymicrogyria

- Polymicrogyria is a malformation of cortical development that results from interruptions in later neuronal migration and neuronal organization. Histologically, there is derangement of the six-layered lamination of the cortex, with an associated derangement of sulcation. Therefore, in polymicrogyria, no normal sulci are seen.
- Patients may present with developmental delay, focal neurologic signs/symptoms, or epilepsy at any age.

- CMV infection, in utero ischemia, or chromosomal mutations can be associated with polymicrogyria.
- It can be focal, multifocal, or diffuse; it can be unilateral or bilateral. Posterior sylvian fissure and frontal lobe are common locations for polymicrogyria.
- On imaging, excessive numbers of small, disorganized cortical convolutions are seen with thickened cortex. The white matter thickness is normal (remember that it is increased in hemimegalencephaly and smaller in agyria). On thin section images, polymicrogyria is "bumpier" compared with pachygyria. Cortex may appear buckled or with an inward folding.
- Another distinguishing feature between pachygyria and polymicrogyria is the possible presence of abnormal deep white matter in the latter. Keep in mind that the degree of myelination affects the imaging appearance. In unmyelinated areas, the polymicrogyria looks thin, whereas in myelinated areas the thickness may reach 5 mm or more with a smoother looking outer cortex.
- The polymicrogyria tends to involve the frontal and parietotemporal lobe. An association with developmental venous anomalies (anomalous venous drainage) is noted with polymicrogyria, as with other dysplastic cortices.
- Congenital bilateral perisylvian (opercular) syndrome is recognized as an entity in which there is polymicrogyria involving the opercular cortex associated with abnormal sylvian fissure sulcation (Fig. 8.23). The inheritance pattern is heterogenous. Patients with congenital bilateral perisylvian syndrome disorder have seizures, congenital pseudobulbar paresis, and developmental delay. The abnormal sylvian fissure may have cortical thickening on either side of it. Schizencephaly may also be present.

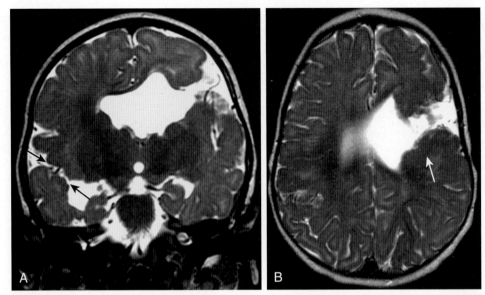

**Fig. 8.24 Schizencephaly.** (A) Coronal T2-weighted imaging (T2WI) shows a cleft extending from the cortical surface of the left frontal lobe to the frontal horn of the left lateral ventricle lined with dysplastic gray matter representing an open lip schizencephaly. Note the additional closed lip schizencephaly in the right temporal lobe *(black arrows)*. Septum pellucidum is absent. (B) Dysplastic gray matter lining of the left frontal open lip schizencephaly is better depicted in the axial T2WI. Note thickened cortex lining the cleft *(arrow)*.

- Bilateral symmetric frontoparietal polymicrogyria syndromes and bilateral medial parieto-occipital polymicrogyria syndromes have also been described.

## Schizencephaly

- Schizencephaly is classified as a malformation of abnormal neuronal organization and is described by gray matter–lined clefts that extend from the pial covering of the cortex to the ependymal lining of the lateral ventricle. Both genetic and acquired causes are considered in the etiology. Non-CNS abnormalities are seen in one third of affected patients, including gastroschisis, bowel atresias, and amniotic band syndromes.
- The abnormality can be unilateral or bilateral, with the lips of the cleft apposed ("closed lipped") or gaping ("open lipped") (Fig. 8.24).
- Bilateral involvement (~40%) is associated with worse prognosis with seizures, worse developmental delay, and developmental dysphasia. Motor dysfunction is more common with frontal lobe schizencephaly, open lipped varieties, and wider gaps in the open lips.
- Schizencephaly occurs most commonly in the frontal (44%), frontoparietal (30%), and occipital (19%) lobes. The gray-white matter junction is irregular along the clefts because of dysplastic gray matter.
- The cleft has a dysplastic gray matter lining with abnormal lamination, most likely polymicrogyria, and is usually seen in the supratentorial space (near the precentral and postcentral gyrus) coursing to the lateral ventricles. Polymicrogyria can also be present in the contralateral hemisphere, especially if there is a unilateral open lip schizencephaly.
- The closed lip variety require attention for indirect findings, such as a dimple at the ventricle-cleft interface. The gyral pattern of the cortex adjacent to the schizencephaly is usually abnormal.
- Schizencephaly is often associated with FCD, gray matter heterotopias, agenesis of the septum pellucidum

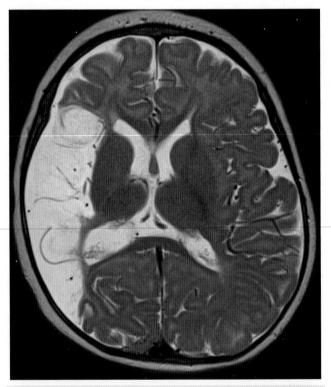

**Fig. 8.25** Intrauterine middle cerebral artery (MCA) infarct in a 7-month-old demonstrates cystic encephalomalacia in the right MCA territory. Note the lack of dysplastic gray matter lining along the borders of the encephalomalacia. In addition, the remaining frontal and occipital lobes demonstrate reduced parenchymal volume, typical of intrauterine territorial infarcts.

(~80%), and pachygyria. If bilateral clefts are present, then the septum pellucidum is almost always absent. Septo-optic dysplasia may therefore coexist. Optic nerve hypoplasia is seen in one third of the patients

- The lining of the cleft with dysmorphic gray matter, best seen on MR, is the distinctive feature and

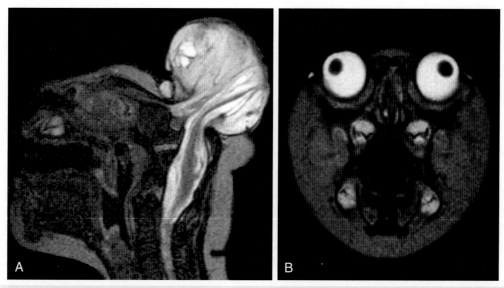

**Fig. 8.26 Anencephaly.** (A) Sagittal T2 and (B) coronal T2-weighted imaging show lack of cranial vault. Tangle of disorganized neuronal elements and glia are noted along with rudimentary brain stem.

distinguishes it from ischemic/encephalomalacic abnormalities, which are usually lined by white matter (Fig. 8.25). Porencephaly, in which there also is a CSF communication to the lateral ventricle (and possibly to the subarachnoid space), is also lined by white matter, not dysplastic gray matter, which distinguishes it from open lip schizencephaly. Prenatal open lip clefts may become closed lip postnatally in 50% of cases.

## Anencephaly

- Anencephaly is failure of anterior neural tube closure (Fig. 8.26), which is a prenatal diagnosis because of early screening in pregnancy for elevated levels of serum alpha-fetoprotein, a marker of neural tube defects.
- The diagnosis by obstetric ultrasound is made when the cranial vault is seen to be small, with only the fetus's face and posterior fossa well seen. Only a nubbin of tissue is seen at the skull base on ultrasound, and amniotic fluid α-fetoprotein levels are elevated.
- These babies die soon after delivery. An association with spinal dysraphism exists.

# Infratentorial Abnormalities

- Inherited (genetic) or acquired (disruptive) causes are identified in congenital abnormalities of the posterior fossa. It is important to differentiate the disruptive causes because the chance of recurrence in other offspring is very limited. Disruptive abnormalities most commonly result from prenatal infections, hemorrhage, and ischemia. If one identifies a unihemispheric abnormality of the cerebellum, disruptive causes should be considered.
- For practical purposes, posterior fossa malformations are classified based on the neuroimaging pattern: (1) predominantly cerebellar, (2) cerebellar and brain stem, (3) predominantly brain stem, and (4) predominantly midbrain. We will focus on the first two in this classification

because they cover the most common malformations of the posterior fossa. Evaluation of vermis is of great importance, so make good use of your midsagittal images! Always pay attention to the size and shape of the fourth ventricle and everything else around it.

## ANOMALIES LIMITED TO THE CEREBELLUM

- The cerebellum consists of the vermis and two cerebellar hemispheres. The cerebellum may be hypoplastic (small volume), dysplastic (abnormal foliation and architecture of the cerebellar white matter), or a combination of both, involving the entire cerebellum, limited to the vermis only, or limited to the cerebellar hemispheres only.

## Dandy-Walker Malformation

- This is the most common malformation of the posterior fossa and is typically sporadic, with a very low risk of recurrence. These days, most cases are prenatally diagnosed. Macrocephaly and symptoms of increased intracranial pressure (ICP) manifest before 1-year-of-age in most patients.
- The key neuroimaging features are (1) hypoplasia of the cerebellar vermis (rarely agenesis), typically involving the inferior portion with the remaining vermis elevated and upwardly rotated, and (2) dilation of the cystic-appearing fourth ventricle, which may fill the entire posterior fossa (Fig. 8.27). The fourth ventricle is enlarged because of vermian hypoplasia. The cerebellar hemispheres display normal morphology, although they are displaced anterolaterally. The posterior fossa is usually enlarged, and the torcular Herophili and transverse sinuses are elevated.
- Additional abnormalities, such as agenesis of the corpus callosum, occipital encephalocele, polymicrogyria, and subependymal/subcortical heterotopias, can be seen in up to 50% of patients. Hydrocephalus is seen in about 90% of patients. Coexisting cardiovascular, urogenital, or skeletal abnormalities also influence the prognosis negatively.

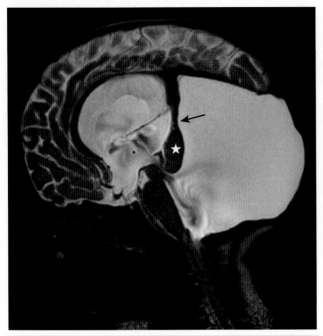

**Fig. 8.27 Dandy-Walker malformation.** Sagittal half-Fourier-acquisition single-shot turbo spin-echo (HASTE) image demonstrates a hypoplastic vermis *(star)* with upward rotation *(arrow)* and cystic dilation of the fourth ventricle enlarging the posterior fossa. Note the elevation of the tentorium, ventral displacement of the brain stem, and supratentorial hydrocephalus. The cerebral aqueduct is patent with cerebrospinal fluid flow artifact through it.

- Neuroradiologists must make the utmost effort not to fall into confusing terminologies such as "Dandy-Walker variant," "Dandy-Walker spectrum," or "Dandy-Walker complex" when they find one or two things wrong with the posterior fossa. Rather, recognize the true Dandy-Walker malformation as previously described and remain with descriptive terminology for the rest of the cases.

## Blake Pouch Cyst

- The Blake pouch is a normal embryologic structure that normally should fenestrate to form the foramen of Magendie. Lack of fenestration in the Blake pouch results in absent communication between the fourth ventricle and subarachnoid space. Foramen of Luschka perforates later in the development by 4 to 5 months, which establishes a new CSF equilibrium. Persistent Blake pouch cyst is the cystic dilatation of the foramen of Magendie and can result in tetraventricular hydrocephalus. The size of the posterior fossa is normal. The cerebellum has normal size and form (Fig. 8.28).
- The typical neuroimaging findings are a retrocerebellar or infraretrocerebellar cyst. The choroid plexus is displaced inferior to the cerebellar vermis. Supratentorial abnormalities other than hydrocephalus are usually absent.

## Mega Cisterna Magna

- Mega cisterna magna refers to an enlarged cisterna magna with a normal intact vermis (measuring >10 mm in mid-sagittal slice). The fourth ventricle is normal in size. The posterior fossa may be enlarged in some patients (Fig. 8.29).
- Normal communication of CSF between the fourth ventricle, cisterna magna, and cervical subarachnoid spaces are seen on CSF flow studies.

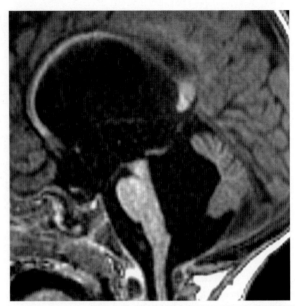

**Fig. 8.28 Blake pouch cyst.** Sagittal T1-weighted image in the midline shows enlargement of the fourth ventricle, which communicates with a cystic infravermian compartment representing the Blake pouch cyst. The vermis is normal. Note the tetraventricular hydrocephalus.

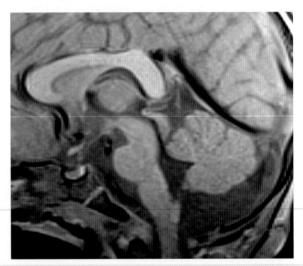

**Fig. 8.29 Mega cisterna magna.** Sagittal T1-weighted imaging in the midline shows mild enlargement of the posterior fossa. Normal vermis, no hydrocephalus.

- This is usually an incidental finding of no clinical consequence. There is no known risk of recurrence in future pregnancies.

## Arachnoid Cyst in the Posterior Fossa

- About 10% of the arachnoid cysts occur in the posterior fossa. The duplication of the arachnoid membrane produces these CSF-filled cysts. They can be retrocerebellar (Fig. 8.30), supravermian, prepontine (Fig. 8.31), or anterior/lateral to the cerebellar hemispheres. No communication is seen with the fourth ventricle.
- Arachnoid cysts occur sporadically without known risk of recurrence. These cysts can be asymptomatic or present with macrocephaly, hydrocephalus, and/or increased ICP, if the CSF flow is obstructed.

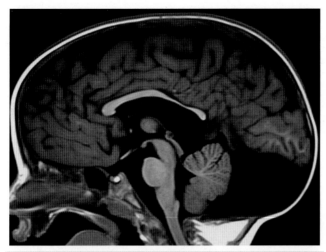

**Fig. 8.30 Retrocerebellar arachnoid cyst.** Sagittal T1-weighted imaging shows a posterior fossa cyst that is isointense to cerebrospinal fluid. Note mass effect on the normally formed vermis, normal fourth ventricle, and scalloping of the occipital bone.

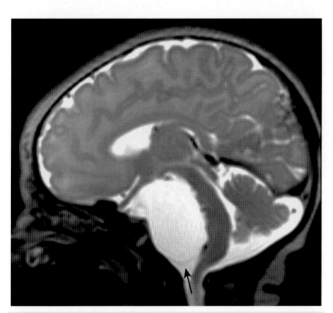

**Fig. 8.31 Prepontine arachnoid cyst.** Sagittal half-Fourier-acquisition single-shot turbo spin-echo (HASTE) shows an extra-axial cyst in the prepontine cistern, displacing cerebral peduncles and pons posteriorly. The inferior cyst wall is nicely delineated in this image *(arrow)*.

- Neuroimaging findings are similar to their supratentorial counterparts, revealing a well-defined, smooth-contoured extra-axial cyst that follows the CSF density/signal on all images. No restricted diffusion is seen. Remodeling/thinning of the adjacent bone can be seen, occurring because of repetitive CSF pulsations. Be cognizant of the association of the arachnoid cyst with acoustic schwannomas in the cerebellopontine angle cistern.
- As opposed to Dandy-Walker malformations, arachnoid cysts do not communicate with an open posterior fourth ventricle and most often do not cause a large posterior fossa. As opposed to a mega cisterna magna, arachnoid cysts may remodel bone, compress cerebellar tissue, and do not have any vessels "floating" within them. As

opposed to Blake pouch cysts, they are rarely below the cerebellum and rarely cause hydrocephalus.

### Isolated Vermian Hypoplasia

- This is a distinct entity not to be confused with Dandy-Walker malformation. Vermian hypoplasia refers to partial absence in the inferior vermis.
- Prenatal diagnosis is most reliable after 18 gestational weeks because incomplete development of the inferior vermis may be physiologic before then.
- More than 75% of these patients have a favorable outcome.

### Distinctions Between Blake Pouch, Mega Cisterna Magna, and Dandy-Walker Malformation

- To summarize the most common cystic lesions in the posterior fossa:
  - The vermis is hypoplastic in Dandy-Walker malformation and inferior vermian hypoplasia.
  - The fourth ventricle is enlarged in Dandy-Walker malformation, inferior vermian hypoplasia, and Blake pouch cysts.
  - Posterior fossa is enlarged in Dandy-Walker malformation and variably in mega cisterna magna.
  - Hydrocephalus is seen in Blake pouch cysts, in most patients with Dandy-Walker, and sometimes in posterior fossa arachnoid cysts.
  - Bony scalloping is seen with posterior fossa arachnoid cysts and may be seen in cases with mega cisterna magna (Table 8.4).

### Rhombencephalosynapsis

- This malformation is characterized by the absence of a vermis with continuity across the midline of the cerebellar white matter and folia, fused dentate nuclei, and superior cerebellar peduncles, resulting in a keyhole-shaped fourth ventricle.
- Coronal T2WI best depicts the continuation of a horizontal folial pattern.
- In some cases, a small and dysplastic vermis may be present, rendering the diagnosis of incomplete or partial rhombencephalosynapsis.
- Ataxia, abnormal eye movement, and delayed motor development are the most common clinical presentations.
- It is sporadic, therefore, risk of recurrence in future pregnancies is low. Most cases are nonsyndromic, except for Gómez-López-Hernández syndrome and in patients with VACTERL (vertebral anomalies, anal atresia, cardiac defects, tracheoesophageal fistula, renal anomalies, and limb anomalies).

## ANOMALIES INVOLVING THE CEREBELLUM AND BRAIN STEM

### Joubert Syndrome

- Joubert syndrome is clinically characterized by hypotonia, ataxia, oculomotor apraxia, neonatal breathing dysregulation, and variable degree of intellectual disability. Autosomal recessive inheritance is seen in all cases apart from *OFD1* mutation where inheritance is X-linked.

**Table 8.4**   Cystic Malformations of the Posterior Fossa

| Feature | Dandy-Walker Malformation | Inferior Vermian Hypoplasia | Blake Pouch Cyst | Mega Cisterna Magna | Arachnoid Cyst |
|---|---|---|---|---|---|
| Vermis hypoplasia | Yes | Yes, inferior portion | No | No | No |
| Enlarged fourth ventricle | Yes | Yes | Yes | No | No, can even be reduced |
| Enlarged posterior fossa | Yes | No | No | Variable | No |
| Hydrocephalus | Yes | No | Yes | No | Sometimes |
| Occipital bone scalloping | No | No | No | Sometimes | Yes |

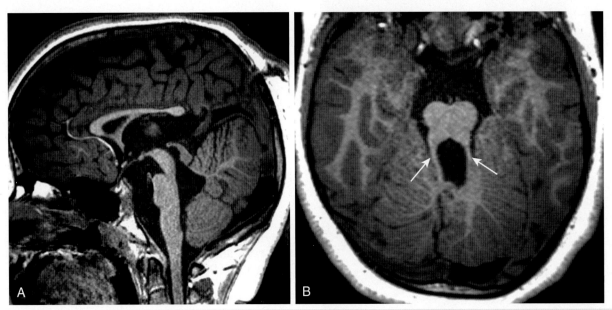

**Fig. 8.32  Joubert syndrome.** (A) Sagittal T1-weighted imaging (T1WI) shows hypoplastic vermis, upward and posterior displacement of the fastigium, mild enlargement of the fourth ventricle, and the narrow pontomesencephalic isthmus. Note the atretic parietal encephalocele *(arrow)*. (B) Axial T1WI scan shows the molar tooth sign, with elongated parallel superior cerebellar peduncles *(arrows)*.

- The classic neuroimaging finding is the "molar tooth sign," which consists of elongated and thickened superior cerebellar peduncles, a deep interpeduncular fossa, and vermian hypoplasia (Fig. 8.32). DTI can show the absence of decussation of superior cerebellar peduncles, which may imply an underlying defect in axonal guidance. Other additional abnormalities can be seen, such as dysmorphic tectum and midbrain, thickening and elongation of the midbrain, and a small pons.
- Additional supratentorial abnormalities are seen in 30% of cases showing callosal agenesis, cephaloceles, hippocampal malrotation, neuronal migrational disorders, and ventriculomegaly. Renal (nephronophthisis), liver (congenital hepatic fibrosis), ocular (coloboma), and skeletal (polydactyly) abnormalities can also be seen. Renal and liver involvement leads to a poorer prognosis.
- The molar tooth sign can also be seen in oro-facial-digital syndrome type VI. Presence of a hypothalamic hamartoma allows for differentiation of oro-facial-digital syndrome type VI from Joubert syndrome.

### Pontocerebellar Dysplasia

- This is a group of autosomal recessive neurodegenerative disorders with prenatal onset. The disease is characterized by hypoplasia of the cerebellum and pons. In cases with prenatal onset, there is progressive atrophy of the already hypoplastic cerebellum. Ten subtypes have been identified.
- On coronal images the appearance of the cerebellum resembles a "dragonfly" with small volume/flattened cerebellar hemispheres and the relatively preserved vermis representing the body. This morphologic appearance is not specific for pontocerebellar hypoplasia and can be seen in the setting of insults (such as those seen in extreme prematurity) and neurometabolic diseases.

### Pontine Tegmental Cap Dysplasia

- *Pontine tegmental cap dysplasia* is characterized by flattened ventral pons, partial absence of the middle cerebellar peduncles, vermian hypoplasia, a molar-tooth-like pontomesencephalic junction, and absent inferior olivary prominence. The combination of a flattened hypoplastic ventral pons and a caplike dorsal pontine protrusion is pathognomonic of pontine tegmental cap dysplasia. *Horizontal gaze palsy with progressive scoliosis* is a rare autosomal recessive disease, characterized by butterfly-shaped medulla and prominent inferior olivary nuclei. The pons is hypoplastic with a dorsal midline cleft.

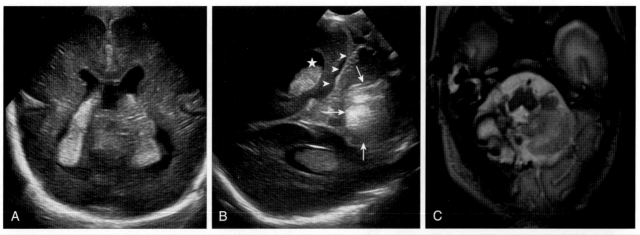

**Fig. 8.33 Cerebellar hemorrhage in a 26-gestational-week premature infant.** (A) Coronal image through the anterior fontanelle demonstrates a simple gyral pattern that is age appropriate. Prominent size of choroid is normal for age. (B) Transtemporal view demonstrates hemorrhage in the fourth ventricle and cerebellar parenchyma occipital horn *(star): arrowheads* outline the tentorium blood-filled fourth ventricle *(white arrows)*. (C) Term equivalent age magnetic resonance imaging of the brain showing marked volume loss and hemosiderin staining in the right cerebellar hemisphere representing disruptive cerebellar injury secondary to hemorrhage.

## Cerebellar Disruptions

- Cerebellar maturation and development are complex, starting in the midst of the first trimester and ending at about 2 years of age. There is rapid growth (30-fold increase in the surface area of the cerebellar cortex) of the cerebellum between 28 gestational weeks and term. This rapid growth is dependent on high levels of energy supply resulting in increased vulnerability, especially between 24 and 32 gestational weeks (Fig. 8.33).
- The cerebellum is vulnerable to metabolic, toxic, and infectious insults, as well as hemorrhage and ischemia; however, in the immediate prenatal, perinatal, and postnatal period, it is resilient to hypoxic ischemic injury. Cerebellar injury occurs in 20% of preterm infants born at less than 32 gestational weeks. Hemorrhage and ischemia may result in parenchymal volume loss.

## CHIARI MALFORMATIONS

Chiari malformations were initially described by Chiari in 1891 as three major malformations of the hindbrain.

### Chiari I Deformity

- Chiari I deformity is classically diagnosed when there is caudal cerebellar tonsillar ectopia with peglike morphology, measuring 5 mm or more below the level of foramen magnum (on the sagittal midslice of the brain, draw a horizontal line between the tip of the basion and opisthion and measure the craniocaudal length of the cerebellar ectopia perpendicular to that line).
- Chiari I deformity may result from multiple different processes. In some cases, there is underdevelopment of the posterior fossa from para-axial mesoderm that forms the occipital somites, resulting in a cranial base dysplasia. The posterior fossa may be relatively small with a short/flattened clivus (Fig. 8.34). There may be basilar invagination or a missing odontoid tip.
- The symptoms are similar in either form ranging from asymptomatic to suboccipital headaches, retro-orbital

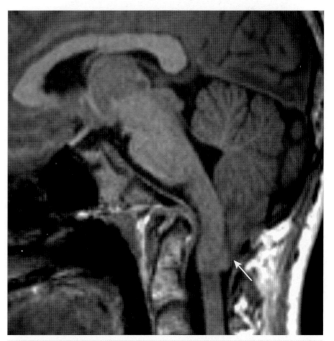

**Fig. 8.34 Chiari I malformation.** Sagittal T1-weighted imaging shows inferior descent of the cerebellar tonsils below the level of the foramen magnum *(arrow)*. The cerebellar tonsils have a peg-like shape. Note the short clivus, posterior tilt of the odontoid process of C2, and kinking at the craniocervical junction.

pressure or pain, clumsiness, dizziness, vertigo, tinnitus, paresthesias, muscle weakness, and lower cranial nerve symptoms (i.e., dysphagia, dysarthria, sleep apnea, and tremors, especially in children younger than 3 years of age). Some patients with tonsillar descent less than 5 mm may be symptomatic in the presence of peg-like morphology of the cerebellar tonsils with associated crowding at the foramen magnum. Conversely, some patients with tonsillar descent of 5 to 10 mm can be completely asymptomatic. Often there is a precipitating event (head trauma or infection) that leads to the onset of symptoms attributable to the Chiari I abnormality.

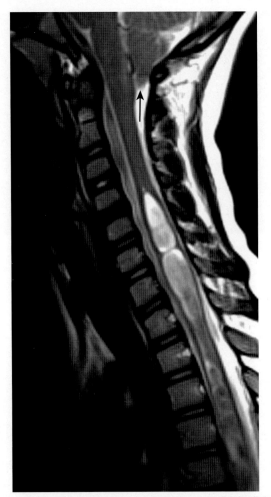

**Fig. 8.35 Chiari I malformation with syrinx.** Sagittal T2-weighted imaging shows segmented syrinx in the distal cervical and upper thoracic spinal cord. Note the cerebrospinal fluid flow artifact in the syrinx. The cerebellar tonsils are low-lying *(arrow)*.

- Syringohydromyelia can be seen in 12% to 23% of the patients with Chiari I deformity (Fig. 8.35), which warrants spine imaging in these patients. It could be absent in children younger than 5 years of age and could develop in late childhood. Posterior indentation of the dens is associated with higher incidence of syringohydromyelia.
- Although anatomic MRI evaluation and clinical presentation is sufficient in most cases, CSF flow studies are useful where the measurements are borderline or when a mismatch is seen between symptoms and measurements. Patients with symptoms almost always have abnormal CSF flow studies. Foramen magnum obstruction may lead to increased systolic spinal cord motion, impaired spinal cord recoil, and impaired diastolic CSF motion anteriorly at the C2 to C3 level and anteriorly and posteriorly in the posterior fossa. Impaired systolic and unimpaired diastolic flow may also be seen just below the foramen magnum. In general, abnormal CSF flow posterior to the tonsils at the opisthion is the most common dynamics abnormality seen in Chiari I.
- Some neurosurgeons perform suboccipital decompression procedures on patients with a variety of clinical symptoms including headaches, vertigo, weakness, and

fibromyalgia who have imaging findings of abnormal CSF motion with tonsillar ectopia.

## Chiari II Malformation

- Chiari II malformation is a complex malformation that involves abnormal development of the hindbrain, spine, and skull base. Chiari II (the original Arnold-Chiari malformation) anomalies occur in 0.02% of births and affect girls twice as often as boys.
- The majority of cases are diagnosed prenatally with ultrasonography and amniocentesis (elevated alpha fetoproteins). The cerebellar tonsils, vermis, fourth ventricle, and brain stem are herniated through the foramen magnum, and the egress from the fourth ventricle is obstructed. A kink may be present at the cervicomedullary junction.

---

**TEACHING POINTS**

Findings in Chiari II Malformation

### Infratentorial Findings

Myelomeningocele
Small posterior fossa
Tonsils and medulla below foramen magnum
Beaking of tectum
Caudal displacement of medulla
Cerebellum wrapped around brain-stem
Petrous bone scalloping
Fourth ventricle compressed, elongated, trapped, and low
Syringohydromyelia
Cervicomedullary kinking
Low torcular
Dysplastic tentorium
Scalloping of clivus posteriorly
Absent hypoplastic arch of C1

### Supratentorial Findings

Hydrocephalus
Callosal hypogenesis
Lückenschädel skull
Falx hypoplasia
Interdigitation of gyri along widened interhemispheric fissure
Fused, enlarged massa intermedia
Colpocephaly
Malformations of cortical development
Caudate hypertrophy, bat-wing lateral ventricles
Biconcave third ventricle

---

- Ultrasound features prenatally include the banana and lemon signs. Banana sign refers to an abnormal shape of the flattened cerebellum that is inferiorly displaced and wraps around the brain-stem. Lemon sign is the abnormal inward scalloping of the frontal bones, seen on transverse images of the fetal skull.
- Virtually all patients have myelomeningoceles. The hindbrain findings of Chiari II are best explained by the theory of McLone and Knepper. In this theory, the hindbrain abnormality results from a small posterior fossa with low tentorial attachment in the setting of a rostral-caudal pressure gradient (secondary to the myelomeningocele). The anchoring of the distal portion of the craniospinal

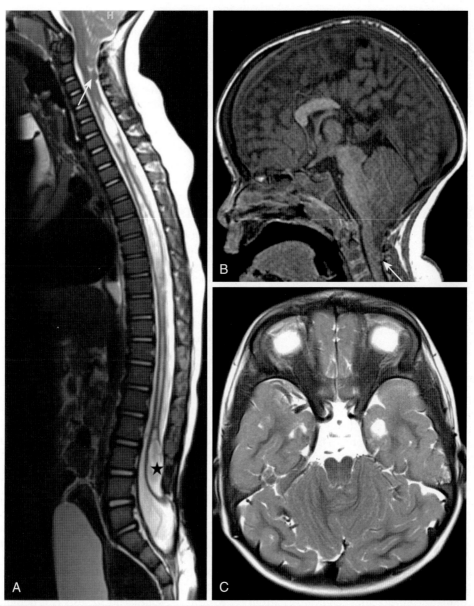

**Fig. 8.36 Chiari II malformation.** (A) Sagittal T2-weighted imaging (T2WI) shows cord tethering in this patient status post myelomeningocele repair. Note the segmented syringohydromyelia and dilated ventriculus terminalis *(black star)*. (B) Sagittal T1-weighted imaging (T1WI) scan shows small posterior fossa, effacement and inferior displacement of the fourth ventricle, beaking of the tectal plate, enlargement of the massa intermedia, and inferior descent of the cerebellar tonsils reaching the level of C3 *(arrow, as also seen on A)*. Note the shortened anteroposterior diameter of the corpus callosum in this patient with agenesis of the posterior segment of the corpus callosum. (C) Axial T2WI scan shows towering of the cerebellum.

axis may account for the downward herniation of intracranial contents in this disorder. Rarely, the tonsils may necrose secondary to compression of critical vessels at the foramen magnum.

- Hydrocephalus may occur prenatally and usually improves after closure of the myelomeningocele. The frontal horns of the lateral ventricles are squared off, the fourth ventricle is compressed, and the aqueduct is stretched inferiorly. The tectum of the midbrain is beaked. The massa intermedia and the caudate heads are abnormally enlarged. The superior cerebellum towers superiorly through a widened tentorial incisura because the posterior fossa is too small. The rest of the cerebellum may literally wrap around the brain stem. Abnormalities of the corpus callosum are seen in 70% to

90% of the cases, predominantly affecting the splenium (Fig. 8.36). Falx cerebri is usually fenestrated, resulting in interdigitation of the sulci.
- Other supratentorial malformations are common, like neuronal migrational disorders such as heterotopias. Abnormal gyral pattern can be seen usually in the medial occipital lobes, having the appearance of multiple small gyri, not to be confused with polymicrogyria, because the cortical thickness is not increased. This appearance is called *stenogyria*.
- Plain radiography or CT of the skull shows irregularity of the surfaces of the inner and outer table of the skull called the *lacunar skull* or *Lückenschädel* appearance (Fig. 8.37).

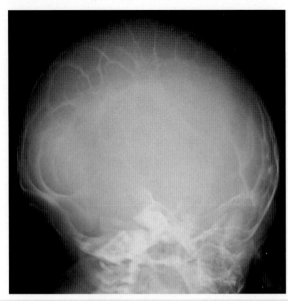

**Fig. 8.37 Lückenschädel skull.** Lateral radiography of the skull in a 1-day-old infant with Chiari II malformation with lacunar skull appearance, secondary to dysplasia of membranous skull vault. Note areas of apparent thinning in the calvarium.

### Chiari III Malformation

■ Chiari III malformations are extremely rare and associated with herniation of posterior fossa contents through a posterior spina bifida defect at the C1 to C2 level. Nearly all Chiari III encephaloceles contain brain tissue, usually the cerebellum, although even the brain stem can herniate through the defect.
■ Common associations include heterotopias, agenesis of the corpus callosum, anomalies of venous drainage, and syringohydromyelia.
■ Meningoencephaloceles in the occipital and high cervical regions are most commonly seen with Chiari III malformations (Fig. 8.38).
■ Symptoms include developmental delay, ataxia, vertical nystagmus, headache, cranial nerve VI through XII findings, and, occasionally, central canal syndromes caused by syringohydromyelia. The prognosis is poor.

## Other Congenital Malformations

### MENINGOENCEPHALOCELES

■ In the United States, parietal (10%) and frontal (9%) meningoencephaloceles are the next most common locations after the occipital region. The majority of parietal cephaloceles are atretic cephaloceles. Vietnamese and Southeast Asian patients have a propensity for nasofrontal (Fig. 8.39) or sphenoethmoidal meningoencephaloceles.
■ Chiari 0 malformation is described as the presence of syringohydromyelia without tonsillar descent. Even though tonsillar descent was absent, "physical barriers" disrupting the CSF flow were found intraoperatively in those patients. Nevertheless, there is no clear imaging criteria to distinguish Chiari 0 from idiopathic syringohydromyelia.
■ Chiari 1.5 malformation has been defined as the presence of brainstem descent in combination with Chiari 1 malformation. However, this entity remains controversial

and treatment decision relies on each patient's presentation and symptomatology.

### CONGENITAL HYDROCEPHALUS

■ Among the congenital malformations of the brain, Chiari II malformation and Dandy-Walker malformation are the most common causes of hydrocephalus.
■ Chiari II malformation accounts for 40% of congenital hydrocephalus in children.
■ Seventy to eighty percent of children with Dandy-Walker malformation have hydrocephalus.

### AQUEDUCTAL STENOSIS

■ Aqueductal stenosis causes lateral and third ventricular enlargement without fourth ventricular dilatation.
■ It can be developmental or acquired (synechiae, bands, clots, fibrotic), seen in around 20% of cases with hydrocephalus.
■ During the normal maturation of CNS, the aqueductal size gradually decreases until birth, reaching a mean cross-sectional diameter of $0.5 \text{ mm}^2$ at birth. Aqueductal stenosis is focal, usually at the level of the superior colliculi or intercollicular sulcus.
■ It can be associated with a tumor (intrinsic or extrinsic compression) such as tectal/tegmental gliomas, which appear as T2/FLAIR hyperintense, nonenhancing, and focal round/oval masses centered at the level of the aqueduct. Pineal region masses often obstruct the aqueduct.
■ Acquired causes of aqueductal stenosis are numerous and include clots adhesions from subarachnoid or intraventricular hemorrhage or fibrosis after infections. Posthemorrhagic hydrocephalus in preterm infants in the setting of germinal matrix spectrum hemorrhages has been extensively studied. In those cases, isolated (trapped) fourth ventricle dilatation can also be seen.
■ The congenital causes may be because of webs, septa, or membranes. The aqueductal web is a thin membrane in the distal aqueduct (Fig. 8.40).
■ *X-linked aqueductal stenosis* is a hereditary-type stenosis with variable symptoms such as intellectual disability, aqueductal stenosis, spasticity of lower extremities, and clasped adducted thumbs. Pathologic studies showed malformations of cortical development in addition to hydrocephalus. Few MRI reports showed fusion of the thalami, small brain stem, and diffuse hypoplasia of cerebellar white matter.

### ARACHNOID CYST

■ Arachnoid cyst is the most common congenital cystic abnormality in the brain. It is typically a serendipitous finding and is usually asymptomatic. It consists of a CSF collection within layers of the arachnoid. The cyst may distort the normal brain parenchyma (Fig. 8.41).
■ The most common supratentorial locations for an arachnoid cyst are (in decreasing order of frequency) (1) the middle cranial fossa, (2) perisellar cisterns, and (3) the subarachnoid space over the convexities. Infratentorially, arachnoid cysts commonly occur in the (1) retrocerebellar cisterns (see Figs. 8.30), (2) cerebellopontine angle cistern, and (3) quadrigeminal plate cistern. Intraventricular cysts are rare but favor lateral and third ventricles (Fig. 8.42).

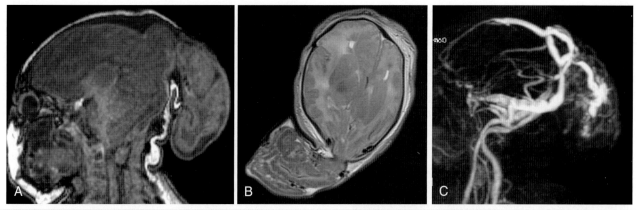

**Fig. 8.38 Chiari III malformation.** (A) Sagittal T1-weighted imaging (T1WI) shows a large calvarial defect with protrusion of occipital and posterior parietal brain through the defect. Note the retraction of the brain stem and posterior fossa toward the encephalocele. (B) Axial T2-weighted imaging (T2WI) scan shows that the calvarial defect is to the left of midline, and the encephalocele contains dysplastic brain tissue. Maldevelopment of most of the visualized cortices and subependymal heterotopias noted. (C) Three-dimensional reconstruction of postcontrast magnetic resonance venography shows aberrant deep draining veins and ectopic venous sinuses, critical information for the neurosurgeons. Hypogenesis of the corpus callosum noted.

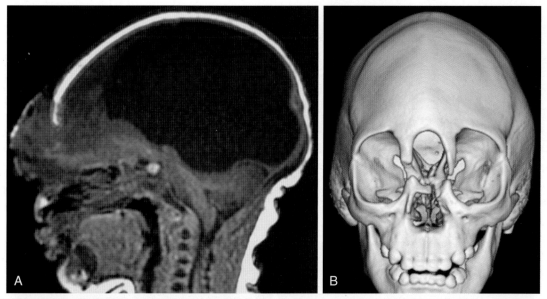

**Fig. 8.39 Frontonasal encephalocele.** (A) One-day-old infant with a large defect in the frontonasal region with extension of the dysplastic brain tissue. Note the ventriculomegaly and dysplastic brain stem. (B) Three-dimensional surface-rendered image of head computed tomography at 15 months of age demonstrates the large bone defect in the frontonasal region.

- CT demonstrates a nonenhancing CSF density mass that typically effaces the adjacent sulci and may remodel bone. The density of the mass measures from 0 to 20 HU (fluid density of CSF).
- In those difficult cases where an arachnoid cyst and a dilated subarachnoid space must be distinguished, MRI, especially high-resolution T2WI (such as CISS/fast imaging employing steady-state acquisition cycled phases [FIESTA] sequence) can be very helpful in delineating the cyst walls.
  - On MRI, the most common appearance is that of an extra-axial mass that has signal intensity identical to CSF on all pulse sequences. Occasionally, the signal intensity may be greater than that of CSF on proton density–weighted imaging (PDWI) scans because of the stasis of fluid within the cyst as opposed to the pulsatile CSF of the ventricular system and subarachnoid

space. FLAIR and diffusion-weighted imaging (DWI) scans usually show a dark mass similar in intensity to CSF (again, pulsation effects may cause some higher intensity). Rarely, the fluid within the arachnoid cyst may be of higher protein content than that of the CSF, accounting for the difference in the signal intensity.

- The differential diagnosis of an arachnoid cyst is limited and generally revolves around three other diagnoses: a subdural hygroma, dilatation of normal subarachnoid space secondary to underlying atrophy or encephalomalacia, and epidermoid.
  - Although subdural hygromas have been thought to be because of chronic CSF leaks through traumatized leptomeninges, in most cases the trauma results in sufficient blood deposited within the "hygroma" so that the signal intensity on T1WI and FLAIR is different from that of

CSF. In addition, subdural hygromas are typically crescentic in shape, whereas arachnoid cysts tend to have convex borders. Both efface sulci and show mass effect.

■ In contradistinction, dilatation of the subarachnoid space secondary to underlying encephalomalacia does not demonstrate mass effect, and the adjacent sulci are enlarged. Another distinguishing feature is the fact that the cerebral veins in the subarachnoid space are seen to course through the CSF in the case of underlying

encephalomalacia (see Fig. 8.25), as opposed to the subdural hygroma and arachnoid cyst, where the veins are displaced toward the surface of the brain.

■ An epidermoid may simulate an arachnoid cyst on CT and T2WI; however, FLAIR and DWI should show higher signal intensity than CSF because of elevated protein content. In fact, T1WI will often also be brighter than CSF.

■ A feature often seen in association with arachnoid cysts that may suggest the diagnosis is bony scalloping. The bone may be thinned or remodeled, probably because of transmitted pulsations and/or slow growth. This would not be seen with hygromatous collections or atrophy. However, the finding may be seen occasionally in epidermoids, in mega cisterna magna, or with porencephaly, where the ventricular pulsations may be transmitted through the porencephalic cavity to the inner table of the skull. The underlying brain parenchyma may appear hypoplastic, yet with normal function. Absence of soft-tissue intensity or density, calcification, or fat distinguishes arachnoid cysts from those of the dermoid-epidermoid line.

## Congenital Infections

■ With respect to in utero infections, the age of the fetus at the time of the insult plays a critical role in prognosis. The infections in the first and second trimester result in congenital malformations, whereas the third trimester infections result in destructive lesions.

■ Another unique feature of prenatal infection is the altered biological response of the fetal brain to injury; the immature brain does not respond to injury by astroglial reaction. The transmission of the infection is either ascending from the cervix (bacterial infections) or transplacental (TORCH: toxoplasmosis, other infections

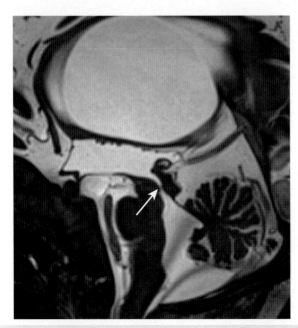

**Fig. 8.40  Aqueductal stenosis.** Sagittal constructive interference steady state (CISS) demonstrates a thin web *(arrow)* in the distal cerebral aqueduct. Supratentorial hydrocephalus is noted. The anterior and inferior recesses of the third ventricle are dilated.

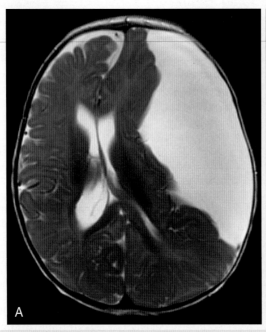
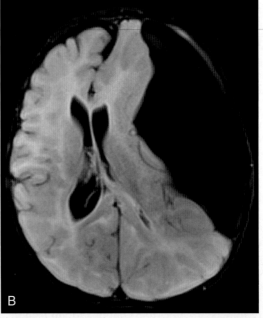

**Fig. 8.41  Arachnoid cyst.** Large extra-axial cystic lesion following the same signal as cerebrospinal fluid on axial T2-weighted (A) and fluid-attenuated inversion recovery (FLAIR) (B) images. Note the midline shift, bowing of the falx, effacement of the left lateral ventricle, and hypoplastic appearance of the left cerebral hemisphere.

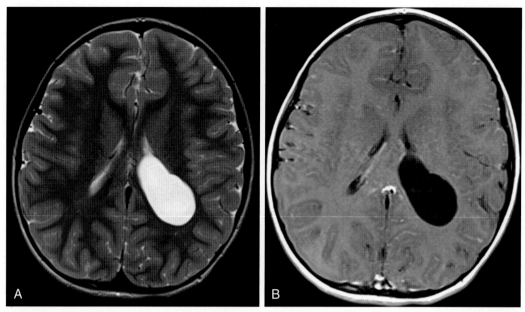

**Fig. 8.42 Intraventricular arachnoid cyst.** Axial T2-weighted imaging (T2WI) (A) and postcontrast T1WI (B) scans demonstrate a cyst in the left lateral ventricle.

such as syphilis and HIV, rubella, CMV, herpes simplex). In many instances, these infections lead to in utero death. Other infants may present with failure to thrive, hydrocephalus, and/or seizures in the perinatal period (Table 8.4). The transmission may be at the time of passage through the vaginal canal during delivery.

■ The neuroimaging findings are variable depending on the timing and severity of injury. Microcephaly, intracranial calcifications, pachygyria/agyria, polymicrogyria, neuronal migrational anomalies, white matter abnormalities/delayed myelination, and cysts can be seen.

■ Intracranial calcifications are not specific for congenital infections, and ischemic/metabolic diseases may result in dystrophic calcifications. Linear branching hyperechogenicities can be seen in the basal ganglia and thalami with transfontanellar head ultrasound, representing lenticulostriatal and thalamostriatal arterial wall calcifications. This entity is called *mineralizing vasculopathy* and can be seen in congenital infections, trisomies, prenatal drug exposure, congenital heart disease, and a variety of anoxic/toxic injuries, as well as a normal variant (far more commonly). Therefore, mineralizing vasculopathy is a nonspecific finding, and unless additional abnormalities are seen in the brain, congenital infection should not be strongly considered.

■ *CMV* is the most common viral infection, seen in approximately 1% of all births in the United States (see Fig. 8.17). Hepatosplenomegaly and petechiae can be the first signs of disease. Lissencephaly, delayed myelination, marked ventriculomegaly, and significant periventricular calcifications are presumed to be a result of early first trimester CMV infections, whereas those infected in the middle of the second trimester typically have polymicrogyria, less pronounced ventriculomegaly, and less pronounced cerebellar hypoplasia. Microcephaly caused by atrophy can also be seen with CMV infections (27%). White matter damage (with increased water content)

can be seen at any gestational age. Periventricular cysts, usually around the occipital poles, may also be present.

■ *Toxoplasmosis* is caused by a protozoan *toxoplasma gondii* and is approximately 10 times less common than CMV. The principal CNS findings are chorioretinitis, hydrocephalus, and seizures. The inflammatory infiltration of the meninges is seen with granulomatous lesions in the brain, thus leading to obstructive hydrocephalus. Unlike CMV, malformations of cortical development are uncommon. Toxoplasmosis calcifies most frequently of the congenital infections (71% of the time in one series). With treatment of congenital toxoplasmosis, 75% of cases show diminution or resolution of the intracranial calcifications by 1 year of age. If treatment does not occur, is delayed, or is inadequate, the intracranial calcifications may increase. The status of the calcifications often mirrors neurologic function. On MR, periventricular and subcortical white matter injury is seen as high signal intensity on T2WI.

■ *Herpes simplex infection* (HSV2) may be acquired as the child passes through the birth canal. The imaging may have a similar appearance to CMV, but microcephaly and microphthalmia are more prevalent. Neuroimaging shows diffusely increased echogenicity or high T2 signal on head ultrasound or MRI, respectively, reflecting diffuse cerebral edema (Fig. 8.43). DWI is the sequence that demonstrates injury the earliest, with areas of restricted diffusion. Contrast enhancement is usually in a leptomeningeal pattern. Progression to chronic encephalomalacic changes (usually cystic) is very rapid within a few weeks. Hemorrhagic foci may be present in the basal ganglia, and cortical laminar necrosis may be seen as high signal on T1WI.

■ *Rubella infection* is extremely rare in Western countries because of maternal screening during pregnancy. It may lead to cataracts, chorioretinitis, glaucoma, and cardiac myopathies. Deafness caused by sensorineural injury is

**Table 8.5**    In Utero Infections

| Characteristic | Rubella | HSV (Type 2 >1) | Toxoplasmosis | CMV | HIV |
|---|---|---|---|---|---|
| Frequency | 0.0001% of neonates | 0.02% of neonates | 0.05% of neonates | Most common; 1% of neonates | Growing exponentially |
| Clinical manifestations | Hearing loss, intellectual disability, autism, speech defects | Skin lesions | Usually fetal death; developmental delay, seizures | Hearing loss, psychomotor retardation, visual defects, seizures, optic atrophy | Asymptomatic at birth, later presentation, developmental delay, late spastic paraparesis, ataxia |
| Ocular changes | Cataracts, glaucoma, pigmentary retinopathy | Chorioretinitis, microphthalmos | Chorioretinitis | Chorioretinitis | conjunctivitis, retinal vasculitis |
| Neuronal migrational anomaly | Rare | None | None | Frequent (polymicrogyria, heterotopia, hydranencephaly, lissencephaly, pachygyria), cerebellar hypoplasia | none |
| Head size | Microcephaly | Microcephaly unless hydrocephalus | Microcephaly | Microcephaly | occasional microcephaly |
| Parenchymal changes | Necrotic foci, delayed myelination | Hydranencephaly; patchy areas of low density in cortex, white matter; vast encephalomalacia; cortical laminar necrosis, no predilection for temporal lobe | Hydrocephalus from aqueductal stenosis, intracranial calcifications | Hemorrhage especially at germinal matrix; loss of white matter, delayed myelination, cortex, subependymal cysts around occipital horns, cerebellar hypoplasia, atrophy | Glial, microglial nodules in basal ganglia, brain stem, white matter; demyelination, atrophy, corticospinal tract degeneration |
| Vessels | Vasculopathy | Can infect endothelial cells | Infarctions | Vasculopathy, vasculitis with calcifications | arteritis, fusiform aneurysms, dilated circle of willis |
| Calcifications | Basal ganglia, cortex | Frequent (71%) of neonates, periventricular, basal ganglia, parenchyma | Frequent (40%), periventricular, can have cortical calcifications | Perivascular in basal ganglia, cerebellum | Basal ganglia |
| Non central nervous system | Patent ductus arteriosus, pulmonic stenosis, rash, hepatosplenomegaly | Hepatosplenomegaly rash | Hepatosplenomegaly | Neck adenopathy, oral candidiasis | adenopathy |

*CMV*, Cytomegalovirus; *HIV*, human immunodeficiency virus; *HSV*, herpes simplex virus.

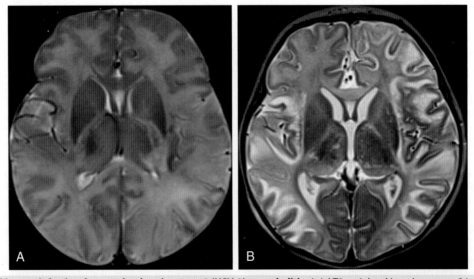

**Fig. 8.43  Neonatal herpes infection: herpes simplex virus type 2 (HSV-2) encephalitis.** Axial T2-weighted imaging at age 24 days (A) and 33 days of life (B). (A) Diffuse marked increase in T2 signal of the entire supratentorial white matter and cortex with relative sparing of the bifrontal cortices. The thalami are swollen with markedly increased T2 signal. (B) Within 7 days, rapid subacute-chronic changes in the brain parenchyma with volume loss and laminar necrosis, in the previously described regions.

very common. Microcephaly and seizures may lead to medical attention. Calcifications in the periventricular white matter and basal ganglia are usually seen as a sequela to the ischemia from vasculopathy.

- *Congenital HIV infection* is a significant health care problem. Transmission of disease to the fetus is about 30% in untreated mothers. Maternal treatment and cesarean section can reduce transmission to fetus to less than 2%. Neuroimaging of congenital HIV shows meningoencephalitis, atrophy, and calcific vasculopathy. Diffuse calcification is seen throughout the brain, not limited to the periventricular region or the basal ganglia. Microcephaly may develop. Congenital HIV infection is also associated with arteritis, fusiform aneurysms, and arterial sclerosis with vascular occlusion. One can see diffuse dilatation of circle of Willis vessels in these children.

- Patients with *congenital acquired immunodeficiency syndrome (AIDS)* rarely present with neurologic symptoms in the neonatal period. Ninety percent of HIV-infected infants get AIDS within the second year of life and thus may develop AIDS encephalitis, infections, and lymphoma at an early age. AIDS encephalitis is characterized by atrophy, diffuse white matter hyperintensity on T2WI, and basal ganglia vascular calcification. Progressive multifocal leukoencephalopathy (PML), toxoplasmosis, and tuberculosis are rare in children with AIDS.

- *Congenital syphilis* leads to seizures and cranial nerve palsies in infancy. Radiologic manifestations include optic atrophy, tabes dorsalis, meningitis, and vasculitis with enhancing meninges and perivascular spaces. Vasculitis may lead to infarctions.

# Phakomatoses

- The phakomatoses refer to a group of congenital malformations mainly affecting the structures of ectodermal origin, the nervous system, skin (thus the neurocutaneous disorders), retina, globe, and its contents. The visceral organs can be involved to a lesser degree.
- The most common and classic ones will be discussed in this chapter including NF, TS, von Hippel-Lindau disease (VHL), and Sturge-Weber syndrome (SWS).
- The quintessential lesion is the nerve sheath tumor, the tuber, the hemangioblastoma, and the angioma.
- Hereditary hemorrhagic telangiectasia, ataxia-telangiectasia, neurocutaneous melanosis, basal cell nevus syndrome, Wyburn-Mason syndrome, and Parry-Romberg syndrome are also classified as phakomatoses.

## NEUROFIBROMATOSIS TYPE 1

- NF type 1 (von Recklinghausen disease; Table 8.6) is an autosomal dominant disease with an incidence of approximately 1 in 3000 to 5000 people in the general population.
- The NF-1 gene is transmitted on the long arm of chromosome 17 (17q11) and is a tumor suppressor gene that is inactivated in patients with this disease.
- The phenotypic appearance is quite variable, both clinically and radiologically. The diagnosis is made if there are two or more of the following findings: (1) six or more

**TABLE 8.6**  Neurofibromatosis Type 1 Versus Neurofibromatosis Type 2

| Feature | NF-1 | NF-2 |
|---|---|---|
| Chromosome involved | 17 | 22 |
| Optic gliomas | Yes | No |
| Acoustic schwannomas | No | Yes |
| Meningiomas | No | Yes |
| UBOs in deep gray matter, cerebellum | Yes | No |
| Incidence | 1/4,000 | 1/50,000 |
| Skin findings | Many | Few |
| Spinal gliomas | Astrocytoma | Ependymoma |
| Skeletal dysplasias | Yes | No |
| Lisch nodules (iris hamartomas) | Yes | No, but sublenticular cataracts |
| Dural ectasia | Yes | No |
| Age at presentation (years) | <10 | 10–30 |
| Vascular stenoses | Yes | No |
| Plexiform neurofibromas | Yes | No |
| Malignant change | Yes | No |
| Sphenoid wing absence | Yes | No |
| Hydrocephalus | Yes, obstructed/ stenotic aqueduct | No |
| CNS hamartomas | Yes | No |
| Paraspinal neurofibromas | Yes | Yes |
| Meningocele | Yes, lateral thoracic | No |

*CNS,* Central nervous system; *NF-1,* neurofibromatosis type 1; *NF-2,* neurofibromatosis type 2; *UBOs,* unidentified bright objects.

café-au-lait spots, (2) two or more Lisch nodules (hamartomas) of the iris, (3) two or more neurofibromas or one or more plexiform neurofibromas, (4) axillary/inguinal freckling, (5) one or more bone dysplasias or pseudarthrosis of a long bone, (6) optic pathway glioma, or (7) a first-degree relative with the diagnosis of NF-1.

- The following features are common characteristics of the disease: gliomas of the optic pathway, kyphoscoliosis, sphenoid wing dysplasia, vascular dysplasias (ectasia, stenosis, occlusions, moyamoya disease or fusiform aneurysms), nerve sheath tumors, macrocephaly, and cognitive impairment (wide range of learning disabilities). Additional findings include spinal dural ectasia (posterior vertebral body scalloping), lateral thoracic meningoceles, aqueductal stenosis, and syringomyelia.

- The most important brain abnormality in NF-1 is the *optic pathway glioma,* typically of the low-grade pilocytic variety. These optic gliomas present in childhood but may have little effect on vision until they are large. Fifteen percent of patients with NF-1 have optic pathway gliomas and only half of the affected patients are symptomatic. Optic gliomas can be confined to the optic nerve (unilateral or bilateral), the optic chiasm, or rarely the optic radiations (Fig. 8.44). Involvement of the optic chiasm

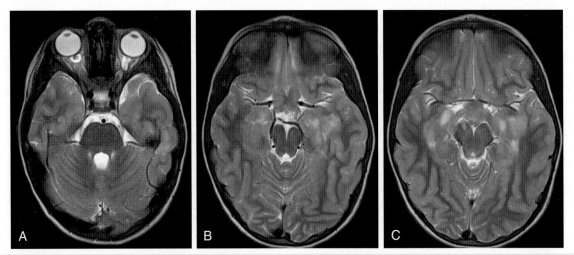

**Fig. 8.44 Neurofibromatosis type 1.** Optic pathway gliomas. Axial T2-weighted imaging demonstrates thickening and tortuosity of bilateral intraorbital optic nerves (A), thickening of prechiasmatic optic nerves and optic chiasm (B), and bilateral optic tracts (C).

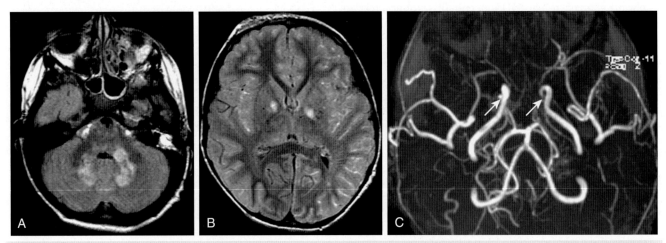

**Fig. 8.45 Neurofibromatosis type 1.** Axial fluid-attenuated inversion recovery (FLAIR) images (A), and (B) demonstrates FLAIR signal hyperintensities in bilateral dentate nuclei and globus pallidi, the most common places for unidentified bright objects. (C) Three-dimensional reconstruction from magnetic resonance angiography demonstrates occlusion of distal internal carotid arteries (paraclinoid Internal Carotid Artery [ICAs] are indicated with *arrows*), bilateral middle cerebral arteries, and anterior cerebral arteries in this patient with moyamoya. The collaterals are not well displayed in this image.

and optic radiations indicates a poorer prognosis. Optic chiasm and hypothalamic involvement may be associated with precocious puberty. On imaging, one may see enlargement of the optic nerves or chiasm. Enhancement is variable. These tumors are generally low-grade pilocytic astrocytomas, are slow growing, and are usually watched; treatment is withheld until the patients become progressively symptomatic.

■ Cerebellar, brain stem, hypothalamic, and cerebral astrocytomas are also seen with NF-1. Patients with NF-1 also have increased incidence of astrocytomas of the spinal cord.

■ White matter volume is increased, which also manifests as an abnormally thick corpus callosum.

■ In addition, the patients have multiple high signal intensity foci on T2WI or FLAIR scans that appear in the cerebellar peduncles or deep gray matter of the cerebellum, the brain stem (especially the pons), the basal ganglia (especially the globus pallidus), the thalamus, and the internal capsule

(Fig. 8.45), likely representing areas of myelin vacuolation. Centrum semiovale and subcortical white matter are typically uninvolved. Typically, these lesions do not enhance and demonstrate normal or near normal proton MR spectroscopy (H1 MRS) findings to those of normal brain, with lack of mass effect/edema. The basal ganglia foci may also be bright on T1WI. These high-intensity foci in NF-1 decrease in size and number with age. When these high-intensity foci enhance or grow larger over time, the possibility of neoplasm must be raised. Short-term follow-up scans are indicated.

■ The presence of a plexiform neurofibroma strongly suggests NF-1. A plexiform neurofibroma consists of sheets of collagen and Schwann cells that spread in an aggressive manner, insinuating themselves in a cylindrical fashion around a nerve (Fig. 8.46). These lesions tend to involve the scalp, neck, mediastinum, retroperitoneum, cranial nerve V, and orbit. The lesions are soft and elastic and probably account for the elephantiasis of NF.

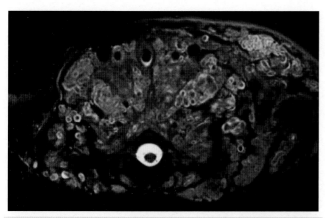

**Fig. 8.46 Plexiform neurofibromas in neurofibromatosis type 1.** Axial T2-weighted imaging: large, infiltrative neurofibromas infiltrating the entire neck, to a point where normal soft tissues cannot be identified. Note the target sign in the neurofibromas.

■ Sarcomatous degeneration of neurofibromas occurs in about 5% of patients with peripheral nerve sheath neural tumors (malignant peripheral nerve sheath tumors [MPNST]). The more neurofibromas one has, the higher the likelihood of malignant degeneration, usually occurring in midadulthood. Plexiform neurofibromas have a higher rate of malignant change, much more so than schwannomas.

## NEUROFIBROMATOSIS TYPE 2

■ NF-2 is an autosomal dominant disease transmitted on chromosome 22q12 and is approximately one tenth as common as NF-1. This is a different entity than NF-1. The patients have fewer skin lesions compared with NF-1, and the pathognomonic imaging sign of NF-2 is bilateral vestibular schwannomas (Fig. 8.47).

■ A definitive diagnosis is made if the patient has one of the following features: (1) bilateral vestibular schwannomas; (2) a first-degree relative with NF-2 and a unilateral vestibular schwannoma or any two of the following: schwannomas, neurofibromas, meningiomas, glioma, juvenile cataract, or retinal abnormality. Cranial nerve V is the second most common site of schwannomas in NF-2. Sensory roots are affected more commonly than motor roots. The patients also have increased incidence of meningiomas and rarely have other glial tumors (ependymomas). A posterior sublenticular capsular cataract in a young patient is also typical of this disorder.

■ Bilateral vestibular schwannomas are usually asymptomatic until adulthood; therefore, hearing loss is an uncommon presentation in childhood. Instead, seizures and facial nerve palsy are more common.

■ On MRI, vestibular schwannomas are slightly T2 hyperintense and enhancing masses located in and around the cerebellopontine angle and/or extending into the internal auditory canal. Arachnoid cysts may accompany the vestibular schwannomas. In addition, meningiomas may occur at this location, although the parasagittal regions predominate. Meningiomas can be seen anywhere else, including the cerebral and cerebellar convexities, or within the ventricles.

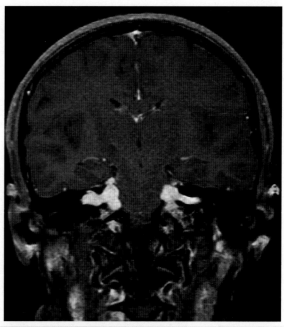

**Fig. 8.47 Neurofibromatosis type 2.** Coronal postcontrast T1-weighted image shows bilateral symmetric enhancing vestibular schwannomas expanding the internal auditory canals and extending into the cerebellopontine angle cisterns.

■ The characteristic spinal manifestations of NF-2, multiple paraspinal nerve sheath tumors, intraspinal meningiomas, and intramedullary ependymomas can be seen in 63% to 90% of cases. In one report, 53% of patients had intramedullary lesions, 55% intradural extramedullary tumors (88% were nerve sheath tumors and 12% meningiomas), and 45% both intramedullary and extramedullary masses (Fig. 8.48). Of those with intramedullary masses, over half had multiple ones. Multiple nerve sheath tumors (both schwannomas [75%] and neurofibromas [25%]) are seen in the cauda equina and may be intradural and/or extradural. Of the intramedullary tumors, ependymomas predominate, but astrocytomas and intramedullary schwannomas may occur. Syringohydromyelia can be seen, secondary to the altered CSF dynamics in the setting of either intramedullary spinal cord tumors or extramedullary masses.

■ See Table 8.5 for a summary of the differences between NF-1 and NF-2. Schwannomatosis is characterized by multiple schwannomas in the absence of vestibular schwannomas, where schwannomas mostly affect the spinal and peripheral nerves. NF-2 and LZTR1 and SMARCB-1 related schwannomatosis can be associated because there are phenotypic overlaps.

## TUBEROUS SCLEROSIS

■ TS (Bourneville disease) is an autosomal dominant disorder that involves multiple organ systems. The *TSC1* gene, localized on the long arm of chromosome 9 (9q34), and the *TSC2* gene, localized to chromosome 16 (16p13), have been identified in patients with TS. It arises in 1 in 6000 to 15,000 live births.

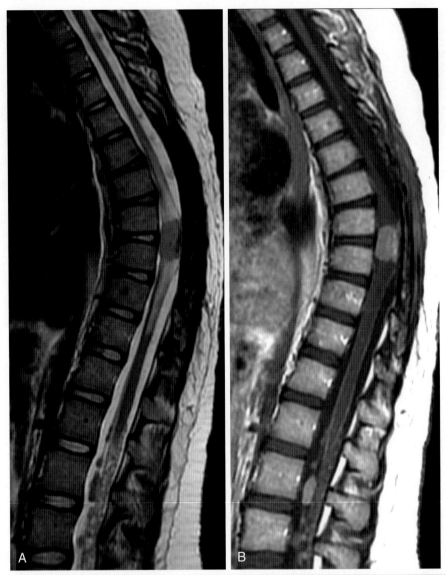

**Fig. 8.48 Neurofibromatosis type 2, ependymomas.** (A) Sagittal T2-weighted imaging (T2WI) demonstrates an expansile intramedullary mass in the mid thoracic spinal cord representing an ependymoma. Note additional multifocal nodular masses along the cauda equina representing schwannomas. (B) Postcontrast T1-weighted imaging (T1WI) scan shows enhancement in all the lesions.

**TEACHING POINTS**

Tuberous Sclerosis Findings

**Clinical**

Adenoma sebaceum
Ash-leaf spot
Café-au-lait spots
Intellectual disability
Retinal hamartomas
Retinal phakoma
Seizures
Shagreen patches
Subungual fibromas

**Central Nervous System Imaging Findings**

Atrophy
Calcified optic nerve head drusen
Cortical tubers

Subependymal giant cell astrocytomas (SEGA)
Intracranial calcifications
Subependymal nodules
Radial glial fiber hyperintensity/myelination disorder

**Non–central Nervous System Imaging Findings**

Angiomyolipomas of kidneys
Aortic aneurysm
Hepatic adenomas
Pulmonary lymphangiomyomatosis
Rhabdomyomas of heart
Renal cell carcinoma
Renal cysts
Skeletal cysts, sclerotic densities, periosteal thickening
Upper lobe interstitial fibrosis, blebs, pneumothorax, chylothorax
Vascular stenosis

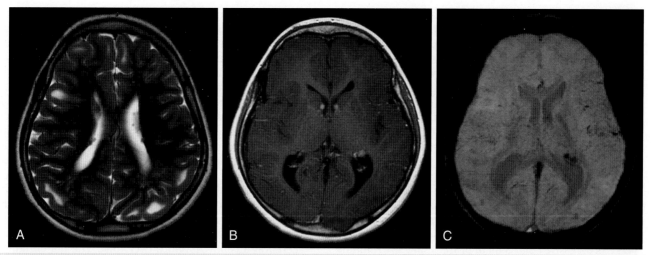

**Fig. 8.49 Tuberous sclerosis (TS).** (A) Axial T2-weighted imaging (T2WI) shows multifocal areas of increased T2 signal in the subcortical white matter representing cortical tubers, the most characteristic lesion in TS. Note the T2 dark subependymal nodules. (B) Postcontrast T1-weighted imaging (T1WI) scan shows enhancing subependymal nodules in the region of the foramen of Monro and also in the left occipital ependyma. (C) Note the signal drop in susceptibility-weighted imaging associated with the left occipital subependymal nodule representing calcification.

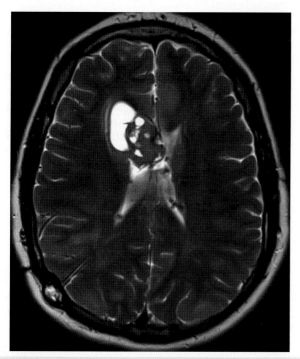

**Fig. 8.50 Tuberous sclerosis, subependymal giant cell astrocytomas.** Axial T2-weighted imaging shows a subependymal giant cell astrocytoma (>12) with solid and cystic components. Note smaller T2 dark subependymal nodules. Patient is shunted.

- The characteristic findings with TS are adenoma sebaceum (60%–90% of cases), intellectual disability (50%), and seizures (60%–80%). All three findings occur in only one third of cases. Patients also may have retinal hamartomas (50%), shagreen patches (20%–40%), ungual fibromas (20%–30%), rhabdomyomas of the heart (25%–50%), angiomyolipomas of the kidney (50%–90%), cystic skeletal lesions, and the intracranial manifestations.

- The intracranial manifestations include supratentorial periventricular subependymal hamartomas/nodules

(the most common lesion, seen in virtually all cases), cortical and subcortical peripheral tubers (the most characteristic lesion, seen in 94% of patients on MR), white matter hamartomatous lesions (Fig. 8.49), and subependymal giant cell astrocytomas (SEGA)(6%–16%) (Fig. 8.50). Cerebellar lesions such as cortical tubers or subependymal hamartomas have been reported in 10% of patients. Patients may have cortical heterotopias and ventriculomegaly as well. Eighty-eight percent of periventricular subependymal nodules are calcified (increasing with age), whereas only 50% of the parenchymal hamartomas are calcified. The frequency of cortical tubers and white matter lesions is highest in the frontal lobes followed by the parietal, occipital, temporal, and cerebellar regions. Tubers may expand gyri or show central umbilication and are bright on long TR sequences.

- Patients with cerebellar tubers are older than those with cerebral tubers, have more extensive disease, and may have focal cerebellar volume loss associated with these tubers.

- White matter lesions may appear on MR as curvilinear or straight thin bands radiating from the ventricles (88%), wedge-shaped lesions with apices near the ventricle (31%), or tumefactive foci of abnormal intensity (14%). Subependymal nodules (31%), cortical tubers (3%), and white matter lesions (12%) may show enhancement on MR. FLAIR imaging is particularly good at spotting subcortical small tubers, even more so than T2WI scans. The number, size, and location of tubers seem to be unrelated to the neurologic symptoms in adults. A greater number of tubers occur in children with infantile spasms, seizures before 1 year of age, and mental disability. The pathogenesis of the various lesions of tuberous sclerosis is thought to be because of the abnormal radial-glial migration of dysgenetic giant cells that are capable of astrocytic or neuronal differentiation.

- In neonates, head ultrasound can identify the subependymal hamartomas. In infants, the subependymal hamartomas are hyperintense on T1WI and hypointense on T2WI (because of unmyelinated white matter), the opposite of what is seen in adults. They are NOT gray matter; therefore, they are not isointense to gray matter and should not be confused with subependymal nodular heterotopias. White matter anomalies are more visible in infants. However, cortical tubers are more difficult to identify in infants.

- TS has an association with subependymal giant cell astrocytomas (SGCA, or SEGA, lesions) that generally occur around the foramina of Monro (see Fig. 8.50). As opposed to subependymal tubers, these lesions enhance commonly and uniformly, are large, grow with time, cause obstructive hydrocephalus, and have a lower rate of calcification. It is believed that these tumors arise from subependymal nodules. The size criteria for SEGA are still being debated, and a size greater than 12 mm has been proposed for SEGA diagnosis. Given the ongoing controversy, progressive enlargement of the lesion size remains the most reliable finding for diagnosis. They occur in approximately 5% to 10% of patients with TS. The risk of malignant degeneration is low.
- SWI should be part of the MRI protocol in patients with TS because calcification can be seen in the most common and characteristic lesions (see Fig. 8.49C).

## STURGE-WEBER SYNDROME

- SWS (encephalotrigeminal angiomatosis) is a sporadic disease with equal occurrence in males and females, affecting the face, choroid of the eye, and leptomeninges.

---

**TEACHING POINTS**

Findings in Sturge-Weber Syndrome

**Clinical**

Accelerated myelination
Choroidal angioma
Glaucoma-buphthalmos
Hemiparesis, hemiplegia
Intellectual disability
Scleral telangiectasia
Seizures
Trigeminal angioma (capillary telangiectasia); port wine stain in cranial nerve V-1 distribution
Visceral angioma

**Central Nervous System Imaging Findings**

Anomalous venous drainage to deep veins
Choroid plexus angioma or hypertrophy ipsilateral to angiomatosis
Dyke-Davidoff-Masson syndrome
Elevated petrous ridge, sphenoid wing
Enlarged frontal sinuses
Hemihypertrophied skull
Hemiatrophy
Intracranial calcification (tram-tracks)
Pial angioma

---

- It typically presents with a facial port wine stain (PWS), ocular choroidal hemangiomas, and cerebral pial angiomatosis.

- Clinical presentation includes seizures, developmental delay, hemiplegia, glaucoma and buphthalmos, choroidal or scleral hemangiomas, and intellectual disability.
- The PWS in the face is a capillary malformation and is usually in the V-1 distribution. As the patient ages, thickening of the capillary malformation is not uncommon.
- The main pathophysiologic abnormality in SWS is venous dysplasia resulting in focal venous hypertension and restricted cortical venous drainage. This leads to dilatation of the deep medullary veins on the affected side. The choroid plexus is commonly enlarged likely because of shunting of blood by the deep medullary veins, which drain into the lateral ventricles. The enlargement of the choroid plexus is known as "angiomatous malformations of the choroid." With elevated venous pressure, the perfusion to the affected cerebral hemisphere decreases and cerebral atrophy develops over time. The pia enhances dramatically on postcontrast T1WI, giving a true demonstration of the degree of the vascular abnormality. Abnormally low signal intensity within the white matter on T2WI is probably related to abnormal myelination from ischemia.
- SWI readily demonstrates cortical calcifications (tramline) in the ipsilateral occipital, parietal, or temporal lobe underlying the leptomeningeal angiomatosis (Fig. 8.51). This can be bilateral in 20% of the cases. Calcification, however, is not seen until about the second year of life.
- Angiography shows similar findings with increased number and size of the medullary veins with decreased cortical veins (anomalous venous drainage) and a capillary stain, usually seen in the parietal and occipital lobes. There is slow cerebral blood flow, and the ipsilateral cerebral arteries are generally small.
- In nearly 50% of patients with SWS, you will find abnormal ocular enhancement, be it because of choroidal hemangiomas or inflammation from glaucoma. Visualization of ocular hemangiomata is increased with bilateral intracranial disease, extensive facial nevi, and ocular glaucoma.
- The Wyburn-Mason syndrome may be a forme fruste of SWS. Patients have a facial vascular nevus in nerve V distribution, retinal angiomas, and a midbrain arteriovenous malformation (AVM). Some have postulated that SWS with involvement of the viscera and extremities is called Klippel-Trénaunay-Weber syndrome (hemihypertrophy, cutaneous angiomas, slow-flow vascular malformations, varices, and/or anomalous venous drainage).

## VON HIPPEL-LINDAU DISEASE

- VHL disease is an autosomal dominant disease with incomplete penetrance and caused by a germ-line mutation of a tumor suppressor gene, namely the VHL gene, on chromosome 3p25.
- VHL disease is characterized by CNS, spinal cord or retinal hemangioblastomas, cysts of the kidney, pancreas, and liver, renal cell carcinomas, islet cell tumors and adenomas.
- Diagnosis is based on a hemangioblastoma of the CNS or retina and the presence of one VHL associated tumor or a previous family history. Pheochromocytomas of the adrenal gland may also be present, linking the

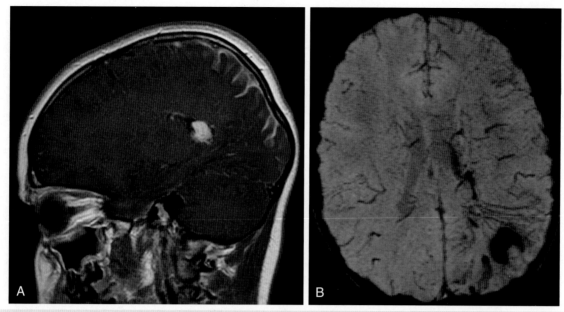

**Fig. 8.51 Sturge Weber.** (A) Sagittal postcontrast T1-weighted imaging shows thickening and enhancement of the parieto-occipital leptomeninges secondary to leptomeningeal angiomatosis. (B) Axial susceptibility-weighted imaging shows signal drop in the subcortical white matter representing calcification. In addition, note the dilated deep intramedullary veins. Overall, left cerebral hemisphere is smaller compared with the right, secondary to atrophy.

multiple endocrine neoplasia syndromes with VHL. Endolymphatic sac tumors (ELST) have also been described with this entity in 15% to 20% of VHL cases. Bilateral ELST suggests VHL.

- Multiple CNS hemangioblastomas are the sine qua non of this syndrome, and they may arise in the cerebellum (most commonly), the medulla, the spinal cord, or less commonly, supratentorially. The lesions may be cystic, solid, or combined. The classic description is a highly vascular, enhancing mural nodule associated with a predominantly cystic mass in the lateral cerebellum. Twenty percent of patients with cerebellar hemangioblastomas have VHL. Cerebellar hemangioblastomas ultimately develop in 83% of patients with VHL.

- Spinal hemangioblastomas represent about 3% of spinal cord tumors. One third are associated with VHL. Of all spinal hemangioblastomas, 80% are single, 20% multiple (almost all associated with VHL), 60% intramedullary, 11% intramedullary and extramedullary, 21% intradural but purely extramedullary, and 8% extradural. Their location is usually characterized by the surgeons as "subpial." They are more commonly found in the thoracic cord than the cervical cord. Most hemangioblastomas seen with VHL are 10 mm or less in size and may be intramedullary or along the dorsal nerve roots. It is extremely rare to see flow voids on MR in hemangioblastomas smaller than 15 mm. A syrinx may be present in 40% to 60% of cases (often out of proportion to the small size of the tumor).

## HEREDITARY HEMORRHAGIC TELANGIECTASIA

- Hereditary hemorrhagic telangiectasia (also known as HHT or Osler-Weber-Rendu syndrome) is an entity consisting of mucocutaneous telangiectasias and visceral AVM.

- One of the many presenting symptoms may be epistaxis secondary to sinonasal mucocutaneous telangiectasias. However, 5% of patients with HHT have a cerebral arteriovenous malformation (AVM) and 2% of AVMs are associated with HHT. When a patient with HHT has one cerebral AVM, there is a 50% chance of a second AVM in the brain elsewhere. There can be additional AVMs in the lungs, liver, spine, gastrointestinal tracts, and pancreas.

## NEUROCUTANEOUS MELANOSIS

- Neurocutaneous melanosis is a sporadic disease discovered in children because of hydrocephalus from gummed up arachnoid villi.

- Melanoblasts from neural crest cells are present in the globes, skin, inner ear, sinonasal cavity, and leptomeninges and are the source of this disorder. It is characterized by cutaneous nevi and melanotic thickening of the meninges. Multiple cranial neuropathies may develop.

- Diffuse enhancement of the meninges of the brain and spine (20%) is seen; the melanin may (Fig. 8.52) or may not be detected on noncontrast T1WI but if so, presents as high signal intensity. Hydrocephalus, cranial neuropathies, and syringohydromyelia may develop.

- Although malignant degeneration of the skin lesions is very uncommon, malignant transformation of CNS melanosis occurs in up to 50% of cases. When this occurs, parenchymal or intramedullary infiltration is the hallmark.

## PHACES SYNDROME

- Presence of hemangiomas in the head and neck with intracranial pathologies qualifies PHACES syndrome (posterior fossa malformations, hemangiomas, arterial anomalies, cardiac anomalies and aortic coarctation,

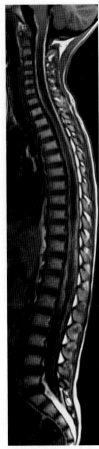

Fig. 8.52 **Neurocutaneous melanosis.** Noncontrast sagittal T1-weighted imaging shows T1 shortening and thickening of the leptomeninges covering the spinal cord and cauda equina secondary to melanin deposition.

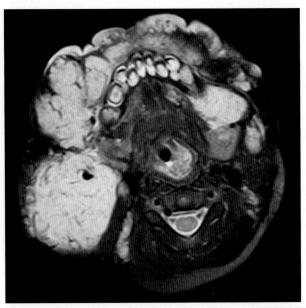

Fig. 8.53 **PHACES (posterior fossa malformations, hemangiomas, arterial anomalies, cardiac anomalies and aortic coarctation, eye anomalies, and sternal clefting and/or supraumbilical raphe).** Large multifocal T2 bright solid masses infiltrating the lower chin and right parotid gland represent infantile hemangiomas. Note smaller ones on the left side.

eye anomalies, and sternal clefting and/or supraumbilical raphe) under the category of phakomatosis.

- The vascular anomaly of the soft tissues in the head and neck is large (>5 cm) and called segmental infantile hemangioma (previously known as *capillary hemangioma* or *strawberry hemangioma*).
- The cerebellar anomalies are the most common structural brain abnormality. Dandy-Walker malformation, cerebellar hypoplasia, and cortical dysplasias can be seen.
- The most common anomalies identified on neuroimaging are vascular in origin such as persistence of the trigeminal artery, and aplasia/hypoplasia of internal or external carotid arteries, vertebral arteries, or posterior cerebral arteries (Fig. 8.53).

# Congenital Spinal Anomalies

Development of the spinal canal and its contents follow four distinct and somewhat overlapping processes: (1) gastrulation and development of the notochord, (2) primary neurulation, (3) segmentation with formation of the somites, and (4) secondary neurulation (caudal cell mass). We will discuss the most common congenital spinal anomalies based on these processes.

## DISORDERS OF PRIMARY NEURULATION

- Separation of the neural tube from the overlying ectoderm during closure of the neural tube is a process called *disjunction*. After disjunction, the ectoderm closes in the midline, dorsal to the closed neural tube. The perineural mesenchyma migrates into the space between the closed neural tube and ectoderm inducing the formation of meninges, bony spinal column, and paraspinous musculature.

### Open Spinal Dysraphism

- Open spinal dysraphism refers to the exposed abnormal neural tissue with leakage of the CSF. The skin, muscle, and bone are deficient with variable degree of severity.
- Complete/segmental nondisjunction of the cutaneous ectoderm from neural ectoderm results in the formation of myeloceles and myelomeningoceles. Many of these disorders are detected prenatally by serologic or amniocentesis tests (elevated alpha-fetoprotein level) and ultrasound. The clinical and neurologic symptoms are believed to arise from two major issues: the neural placode being less functional because of deranged neuroarchitecture and long-lasting intrauterine exposure of the neural tissue to the amniotic fluid.
- A myelocele refers to herniation of the neural placode (a flat plate of neural tissue) through the bony defect such that it lies flush with the surface of the skin of the back. Very little CSF is evident, which is continuous with the subarachnoid space, and only a layer of arachnoid is present at the ventral surface of the myelocele. Both the ventral and dorsal nerve roots arise from the neural placode. A myelomeningocele is identical to a myelocele except for expansion of the ventral subarachnoid space

Grading of Sacrococcygeal Teratoma by Extent

I:   Protrudes predominantly externally with or without presacral component

II:  Protrudes externally and internally with intrapelvic mass

III: Protrudes internally with pelvic and abdominal mass, minimal external component

IV:  Protrudes only internally in presacral space

- Usually, it is seen on imaging as a mixed solid and cystic mass; however, purely cystic forms are seen as well. The deeper the sacrococcygeal teratoma in the pelvis, the worse the prognosis.

## ANOMALIES OF NOTOCORD DEVELOPMENT

### Diastematomyelia

- Diastematomyelia (split cord malformation) refers to a complete or incomplete (anterior only or posterior only) longitudinal split in the cord. The hemicords may be symmetric or asymmetric; however, each involves a central canal and a ventral and dorsal horn. The split may also involve the dura so that there may be two dural sacs; however, more commonly, two hemicords within one enlarged sac is seen.

- It usually occurs in the lower thoracic-upper lumbar region and is associated with bony abnormalities 85% of the time, including spina bifida, widened interpediculate distances, hemivertebrae, and scoliosis. Hairy skin patches occur in 75% of cases. The separation of the spinal cord into two hemicords may be because of a bony spur, cartilaginous separation, or fibrous bands (Fig. 8.60). When this occurs, generally the cord reunites below the cleft. There often is some asymmetry in the size of the hemicords. A bony spur causing the diastematomyelia is more commonly associated with two separate dural sacs than a fibrous split.

- Associated tethering of the conus medullaris, myelomeningoceles (31%–46%), and hydrosyringomyelia can be seen. Almost all cases have some form of formation/segmentation anomaly of the spinal column.

- All these neural tube defects are best evaluated with MR in conjunction with CT. Although CT is useful in detecting the bony canal abnormalities and the bony

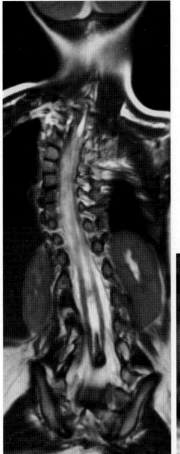
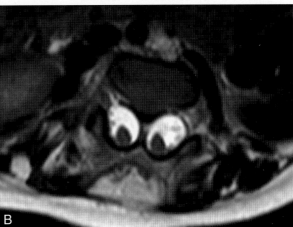

**Fig. 8.60 Diastematomyelia.** (A) Coronal T2-weighted imaging (T2WI) shows scoliosis. Note the two hemicords in the distal thoracolumbar region. The T2 dark bony spur is seen at the lumbosacral junction. (B) Axial T2WI scan shows the bony spur extending between the two hemicords.

spur between the diastematomyelia, MR is superior in locating the distal portion of the conus medullaris and identifying the thickening of the filum terminale, the fatty component to the dysraphic state, and the presence of hemicords. Obviously, the presence or absence of a hydromyelia within the spinal cord is better identified with MR than with CT.

- A full examination of the patient who has spinal dysraphism should include an imaging evaluation of the skull base to assess for a spinal dysraphism and the spine to detect hydromyelia, assess the position of the conus medullaris, identify the structures protruding through the bony defect, and evaluate for block-vertebrae or hemivertebrae.
- Diplomyelia, which is also a split cord malformation, is the complete duplication of the spinal cord, with each cord containing two sets of ventral and dorsal nerve roots, whereas in diastometamyelia, the two hemicords contain only a single set of dorsal and ventral nerve roots.

## NEUROENTERIC CYSTS

- These are usually unilocular, single, smooth cysts most commonly seen in the cervical and thoracic regions. In most cases, the signal intensity follows that of the CSF; however, milky, xanthochromic content may alter the signal intensities on MR. Typically, enteric cysts are located in the ventral or ventrolateral aspect of the cord in an intradural, extramedullary location; however, 10% to 15% of the cases may have an intramedullary component.
- Enteric cysts may be extraspinal, within the mediastinum or abdomen. Dorsal enteric diverticulum refers to an anomaly where the intra-abdominal contents extend through a diastematomyelia and/or malformed vertebral bodies.
- Neuroenteric cysts arise from failure of cleavage between the endodermic bronchial or gastrointestinal tract and the spinal system. The persistent connection (via the canal of Kovalevsky) may be manifest as an intradural extramedullary cyst in the spinal canal (most commonly), but in some cases (<20%), there can be a coexistent thoracic bronchoenteric cyst.
- Over 50% have vertebral segmentation anomalies, including but not limited to hemivertebrae, block vertebral bodies, Klippel-Feil syndrome, butterfly vertebrae, and fused vertebrae. Bony remodeling from the longstanding cyst may be present.

## FORMATION AND SEGMENTATION ANOMALIES OF THE SPINAL COLUMN

- Development of the vertebral column involves three major stages: membranous development, chondrification, and ossification.
- From a practical standpoint, these anomalies refer to either abnormally formed vertebra (such as butterfly or hemivertebrae) or abnormally unsegmented vertebra (such as block vertebra; Fig. 8.61).
- These can be solitary findings or can be seen in other syndromes, such as in VACTERL and OEIS.

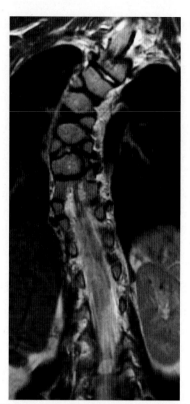

**Fig. 8.61 Formation and segmentation anomalies.** Coronal T2-weighted imaging shows multilevel hemivertebrae with lack of proper segmentation (no visible disc space).

- Although scoliosis is idiopathic in the majority of cases (>90%), the reason for imaging is to exclude or identify formation/segmentation anomalies of the spine. Kidney anomalies are more common in these patients, so take a peek at the kidneys as you review the spine!
- The Klippel-Feil anomaly refers to incomplete segmentation of multiple cervical spine bodies. It may be associated with the Chiari malformations and syringohydromyelia. The C2 to C3 and C5 to C6 levels are the most common sites of segmentation anomalies.

### Other Bony Disorders

Many bony disorders are associated with spinal anomalies. Hypoplasia and/or incomplete development of the C1 arch and/or odontoid process is a common occurrence and is usually asymptomatic. However, occipitalization of the C1 vertebral body may be associated with atlantoaxial instability.

## DURAL ECTASIA

- Dural ectasias can be seen in Marfan syndrome, Loey-Dietz syndrome, and NF-1. If you measure the diameter of the dural sac and correct for vertebral body diameters, you will find that the dural sac ratios in these patients are increased compared with controls, particularly at L3 and S1.
- Associated findings of dural ectasia include widening of the canal, thinning of adjacent bone, enlargement of neural foramina, increased interpediculate distance,

scalloping of the posterior vertebral body, and meningocele formation. The posterior vertebral body is not unique to dural ectasia, because it is also seen in patients with achondroplasia where the spinal canal is narrowed from reduced interpediculate distance.

- Dural ectasia, after excluding NF as a cause, is considered a principal criterion for Marfan syndrome. Genetic mutations associated with Marfan syndrome have been mapped to chromosome 15's long arm (*fibrillin-1* gene). Other manifestations of Marfan's syndrome include aortic dilatation, dissection, coarctation, lens dislocation (up and out), arachnodactyly, pectus excavatum, tall stature, osteopenia, dolichocephaly, pes planus, scoliosis, ligamentous laxity, glaucoma, mitral valve regurgitation, pulmonary cysts, and blue sclera.

## OTHER SPINAL ANOMALIES

### Syringohydromyelia

- Hydromyelia refers to central canal dilatation, whereas a cavity eccentric to the central canal represents a syrinx. On detailed radiologic and pathologic exam, most cases are found to have both, thus the term *syringohydromyelia* is the most commonly used terminology among neuroradiologists.
- Most hydromyelic cavities are associated with congenital spinal and hindbrain anomalies such as Chiari malformations and myelomeningoceles. Most syringes are also congenital but may arise as a result of spinal cord trauma, ischemia, adhesions, or neoplasms.

### Ventriculus Terminalis

- During the development of the spinal cord, the central canal is widest at the conus, which is referred to as *ventriculus terminalis*. This may persist into infancy and even into adulthood. Typically, this is an incidental finding without associated clinical deficits. This appears as an ovoid, non-enhancing, smooth dilation of the central canal with the signal intensity of CSF on all pulse sequences.

### Lateral Meningoceles

- Thoracic and lumbar lateral meningoceles are CSF-filled protrusions of the meninges extending from enlarged neural foramina.
- Thoracic lateral meningoceles are most commonly seen with NF-1 but can be seen in Marfan syndrome. Lehman syndrome includes wormian bones, hypoplastic atlas, and malar hypoplasia with lateral meningoceles. Ehlers-Danlos can also be associated with lateral meningoceles.
- Lumbar lateral meningocele also most commonly occur in the setting of NF-1 or Marfan syndrome.

# Skull Anomalies

## CRANIOSTENOSIS

- *Craniostenosis*, or *craniosynostosis*, refers to abnormal early fusion of one or more of the sutures of the skull (Table 8.7). In 75% of cases, only one suture or part of a

**Table 8.7** Craniostenosis

| Type | Suture Involved | Head Shape |
| --- | --- | --- |
| Dolichocephaly | Sagittal | Long and thin |
| Brachycephaly | Coronal | Round and foreshortened |
| Turricephaly | Lambdoid | High-riding top |
| Plagiocephaly | Any unilateral suture | Asymmetric |
| Trigonocephaly | Metopic | Anteriorly pointed head |
| "Harlequin eye" | Unilateral coronal | One eye points upward |

suture is fused; in 25% of cases, more than one suture is affected. This leads to abnormal head shapes and a palpable ridge at the site of fusion. Males are affected much more often than females. These disorders, if severe and early in development, can cause abnormal growth of the brain. Microcephaly may occur.

- Syndromes associated with early sutural closure include Crouzon syndrome, Apert syndrome, hypophosphatasia, and Carpenter syndrome. Endocrinologic abnormalities, including rickets, hyperthyroidism, and hypophosphatasia, can cause craniosynostosis.
- Premature closure of the sagittal suture, the most common variety (1 in 4200 births), produces a head that cannot grow side to side, so the head looks long and thin, or *scaphocephalic*, also termed *dolichocephalic* (Fig. 8.62).
- If the coronal suture fuses early, the head is short and fat, or brachycephalic (Fig. 8.63). In unilateral coronal synostosis, the ipsilateral forehead appears flattened while there is frontal bossing on the contralateral side, resulting in anterior *plagiocephaly*. There is elevation of the lateral wall and roof of the ipsilateral orbit ("Harlequin eye").
- Lambdoid suture closure can lead to turricephaly, with a high-riding vertex. Unilateral lambdoid suture fusion results in a posterior flattened plagiocephaly.
- Metopic sutural closure causes trigonocephaly with a ridge that runs down the forehead like a triceratops. Communicating hydrocephalus and tonsillar herniation are seen in some patients with complex craniosynostosis.
- Surgery is attempted for cosmetic reasons or when ICP elevation is dangerous secondary to the growth of the brain against the noncompliant calvarium. The elevated ICP may lead to reduction in brain perfusion. If brain growth is stunted because of craniostenosis, operative intervention is also indicated.

## OSTEOPETROSIS

- Osteopetrosis (OP) may be inherited as an autosomal dominant or recessive condition, with at least five types of the disease having been described.
- Imaging abnormalities are more common and severe in autosomal recessive OP.
- Calvarial involvement is frequent in both autosomal dominant and recessive types, with clinical manifestations mostly relating to involvement of skull base foramina. Therefore cranial nerve palsies, optic atrophy, and stenoses of the carotid and jugular vessels may be present.

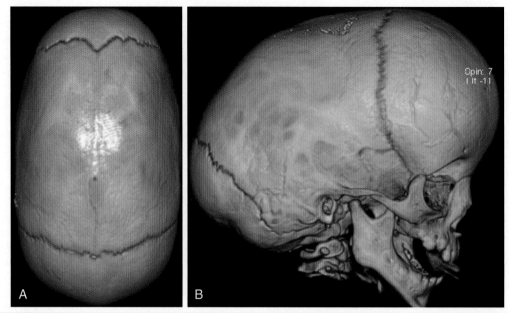

**Fig. 8.62 Scaphocephaly on three-dimensional surface rendered computed tomographic images.** (A) Superoanterior view shows narrow head with reduced biparietal diameter. (B) Lateral view shows elongated head with relatively increased anteroposterior diameter, secondary to early closure of the sagittal suture.

- Diffuse bone thickening and increased marrow density is seen on CT, which corresponds to low signal on T1WI and T2WI. MR may depict optic nerve sheath dilation, tonsillar herniation, ventriculomegaly, or cephaloceles.

## ACHONDROPLASIA

- Achondroplasia is the most common skeletal dysplasia and cause of rhizomelic dwarfism and is characterized by a small foramen magnum but a large head.
- The macrocephaly/megalencephaly may be present with or without hydrocephalus. Megalencephaly (enlarged brain with normal size or slightly enlarged ventricles) may be because of venous outflow obstruction at the jugular foramen or the narrowed foramen magnum level, leading to elevated venous pressure and reduced flow in the superior sagittal sinus. Hydrocephalus likely develops secondary to CSF flow obstruction in the posterior fossa and basal cisterns because of skull base and craniocervical junction abnormalities. The chronic increased venous pressure contributes to hydrocephalus. The end result is increased ICP, maintenance of widened calvarial sutures, and an enlarged head.
- Other craniofacial features of achondroplasia include small foramen magnum, short clivus, platybasia, J-shaped sella, and midface hypoplasia.
- Spinal manifestations include a progressive decrease in the interpedicular distance craniocaudally; small, short bullet-shaped vertebral bodies with posterior scalloping (rounded shape anteriorly); thoracolumbar kyphosis; exaggerated lumbar lordosis; short pedicles; and severe spinal stenosis (Fig. 8.64).

## WORMIAN BONES

- Wormian bones (secondary ossification centers within sutural lines) are seen in osteogenesis imperfecta,

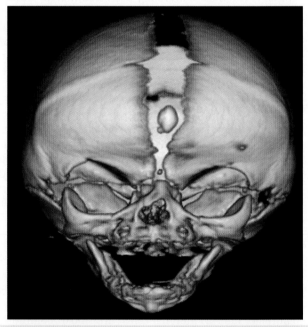

**Fig. 8.63 Brachycephaly.** Three-dimensional surface rendered image; anterior view shows early closure of bilateral coronal sutures in this young infant. Note the bony ridge along the early closed coronal sutures. The anterior fontanelle and sagittal suture are still open. Note the elliptical orbits, known as the "harlequin eye" deformity.

cleidocranial dysplasia, cretinism, pyknodysostosis, Down syndrome, hypothyroidism, progeria, and hypophosphatasia.
- Wormian bones can also be seen as an incidental finding in normal healthy individuals.

## BASILAR INVAGINATION

- Basilar invagination (BI) refers to a developmental anomaly causing upward protrusion of the odontoid process

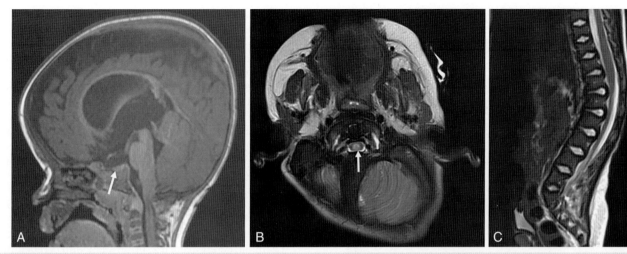

**Fig. 8.64 Achondroplasia** (A) Sagittal T1-weighted image (T1WI) shows frontal bossing, short clivus, j-shaped sella *(white arrow)*, supratentorial ventriculomegaly, and narrowing at the craniocervical junction. (B) Axial T2-weighted imaging (T2WI) shows reduced anteroposterior (AP) diameter of the spinal canal at the craniocervical junction. Abnormal central cord signal is seen likely related to myelomalacia *(white arrow)*. (C) Sagittal T2WI shows a kyphotic deformity in the thoracolumbar junction, scalloping in the posterior vertebral bodies most prominent in the lumbar spine and exaggerated lumbar lordosis.

though the foramen magnum and can cause compression of the ventral brain stem or upper cervical cord.

- Assessment can be made with different methods:
  - Chamberlain's line: from the hard palate to the opisthion (the midportion of the posterior margin of the foramen magnum).
  - McGregor's line: a modification of the Chamberlain's line. Used when the opisthion cannot be identified on a plain radiograph. Connects the posterior margin of the hard palate to the undersurface of the occiput.
  - If the dens extends more than 5 mm (or half its height) above these lines, basilar invagination is present.
- Achondroplasia, Klippel-Feil anomaly, osteogenesis imperfecta, cleidocranial dysplasia, and Morquio syndrome are some conditions associated with this abnormality.
- *Basilar impression* is the term sometimes used when the finding is found secondary to bone-softening diseases, which include Paget disease, rickets, fibrous dysplasia, hyperparathyroidism, and osteomalacia.

## PLATYBASIA

- *Platybasia* means "flattening of the base of the skull" and is diagnosed when the basal angle formed by intersecting lines from the nasion to the tuberculum sellae and from the tuberculum along the clivus to the anterior aspect of the foramen magnum (basion) is greater than 143 degrees.
- Platybasia often occurs with basilar invagination and is seen with Klippel-Feil anomalies, cleidocranial dysplasia, and achondroplasia.

# Perinatal Injury

Although not congenital malformations, there are a few entities that should be included in this chapter. We will briefly touch base on germinal matrix-intraventricular hemorrhage in the preterm infant and hypoxic ischemic encephalopathy in the term infant. Additionally, the topic of temporal lobe seizures and mesial temporal sclerosis will be discussed here.

## IMAGING BRAIN INJURY IN PREMATURE NEONATES

- Several patterns of specific brain injury are seen in premature neonates: Germinal matrix hemorrhage (GMH), intraventricular hemorrhage (IVH), periventricular venous hemorrhagic infarction (PVHI), white matter injury, cerebellar hemorrhage, and atrophy.
- *GMH-IVH:*
  - The capillary bed in the germinal matrix is rich with arterial blood receiving supply from anterior and middle cerebral arteries and internal carotid artery (through the anterior choroidal artery). The venous system drains blood from cerebral white matter (intramedullary veins), choroid plexus (choroidal veins), and thalamus (thalamastriate veins) all coming to a confluence at the caudothalamic notch to form the terminal vein. Finally, the end drainage is into the vein of Galen.
  - The site of origin for germinal matrix hemorrhage is the subependymal germinal matrix, which is the source of cerebral neuronal precursors; this provides glial precursors that become cerebral oligodendroglia and astrocytes.
  - The pathogenesis of GM-IVH is multifactorial, including fluctuating cerebral blood flow, rapid volume expansion, decreased hemoglobin, decreased blood glucose, increased cerebral venous pressure, respiratory disturbances, tenuous vascular supply, vulnerability to hypoxic injury, and deficient extravascular support.
  - Head ultrasound is the best image neuroimaging modality for evaluation of GM-IVH given lack of radiation and bedside serial imaging capability over time.

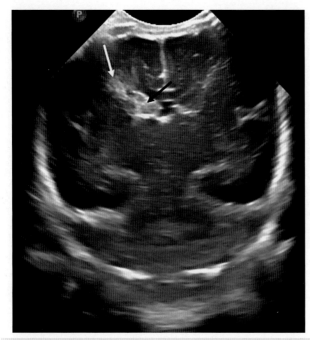

**Fig. 8.65 Germinal matrix hemorrhage (GMH).** Coronally acquired ultrasound image shows focal hyperechogenicity centered in the right caudothalamic notch *(black arrow)* and involving the ganglionic eminence of the germinative epithelium (grade 1 GMH). Note the additional hyperechogenicity *(white arrow)* in the right frontal periventricular white matter representing periventricular hemorrhagic infarction (PVHI). This case illustrates that PVHI is not a continuum of grade 3 GMH. This patient does not have intraventricular hemorrhage or ventriculomegaly.

- GMH-IVH severity can be graded (see Table 8.6):
  - Grade 1 GMH-IVH is hemorrhage limited to the germinal matrix with little to no extension to the ventricular system (Fig. 8.65).
  - Grade 2 GMH-IVH is intraventricular hemorrhage without enlargement of the ventricular system.
  - Grade 3 GMH-IVH is intraventricular hemorrhage with enlargement of the ventricular system.
- *Periventricular venous hemorrhagic infarction (PVHI)* (previously named grade 4) is not an extension of intraventricular hemorrhage. Although it is causally related to GMH-IVH, the pathogenesis is primarily obstruction of flow to the terminal vein typically ipsilateral to the GM, indicating that the primary injury is venous ischemia secondary to venous obstruction, which later develops hemorrhagic conversion. Typically, PVHI is either unilateral (67%) or asymmetric (33%). Approximately 80% of the cases are associated with large IVH (see Fig. 8.65).
- *Cerebellar hemorrhage* can also occur in the germinal zones of the cerebellum, which manifests as peripheral parenchymal hemorrhages (see Fig. 8.33). Cerebellar volume is reduced in preterm infants because rapid growth of the cerebellum occurs in late gestation and premature birth impedes that.
- *White matter injury of prematurity* (often referred as periventricular leukomalacia [PVL]) is usually bilateral and symmetric, nonhemorrhagic, and ischemic or inflammatory injury to the white matter.
  - PVL is an injury to cerebral white matter, classically with two forms: focal and diffuse.

- The focal form is defined as distinguishable cystic focal lesions in the white matter, consisting of localized necrosis deep in the periventricular white matter.
- In diffuse PVL, more commonly seen than focal PVL, focal necroses are microscopic in size and not readily seen by neuroimaging. This form of PVL, which accounts for the vast majority of cases, is termed noncystic PVL.
- The diffuse/noncystic form of PVL is characterized by marked astrogliosis and microgliosis. The decrease in premyelinating oligodendrocytes results in hypomyelination with ventriculomegaly as later sequelae result.
- Neuronal/axonal disease is an important counterpart of PVL. Affected regions include the cerebral white matter (axons and subplate neurons), thalamus, basal ganglia, cerebral cortex, brain stem, and cerebellum.
- On imaging, decreased volume of neuronal structures, such as the thalamus, basal ganglia, cerebral cortex, and cerebellum, is seen as early as term-equivalent age, as well as later in childhood, adolescence, and adulthood.

## HYPOXIC-ISCHEMIC ENCEPHALOPATHY

- Hypoxic-ischemic encephalopathy (HIE) is the leading cause of disability and death in the newborn despite neuroprotective therapeutic treatment options such as cooling.
- HIE is characterized by a deficit in oxygen supply either because of hypoxemia (diminished oxygen in blood supply) or ischemia (diminished amount of blood perfusing the brain) in the neonate. Hypoxemia usually results in impaired cerebral autoregulation, leading to ischemia. Severity and duration of ischemia/hypoxia and the gestational age of the infant are principal factors of the final neuropathology.
- The etiology may be antepartum, intrapartum, or postpartum insults.
- Most common intrapartum events leading to HIE are disturbances to the placenta or cord such as acute placental abruption or cord prolapse, uterine rupture, prolonged labor with transverse arrest, and difficult forceps extractions.
- Postnatal factors such as severe persistent fetal circulation, severe apneic spells, and congenital heart disease make up only 10% of the cases and affect preterm infants more commonly. Apgar scores are diminished at birth with profound metabolic acidosis, hypotonia, lethargy, seizures, coma, and other system involvement (kidneys, liver, etc.).
- Areas of involvement have been described as cerebral (cortex and subcortical white matter usually parasagittal/watershed distribution), deep nuclear (thalamus and basal ganglia especially putamen), brain stem (inferior colliculus and tegmentum), and cerebral white matter (periventricular and central white matter).
- In severe prolonged injury, cerebral, deep nuclear, and brain stem involvement is seen. In severe brief injury, brain stem and deep nuclear involvement is seen.
- In moderate prolonged or intermittent injury, cerebral and/or deep nuclear involvement is seen.

- Mild/moderate, prolonged injury involves the cerebral white matter.
- These findings are usually bilateral and symmetric.
- Head ultrasound shows hyperechogenic generalized brain edema in the white matter and/or basal ganglia reduced resistive indices in the circle of Willis in the first few days of life (Fig. 8.66).
- MRI shows areas of restricted diffusion in the acute phase (first 6 days of life), in the previously described regions with variable degree of increased T2 signal (Fig. 8.67). The findings of diffusion restriction may be present up to 8 to 10 days in those neonates who had cooling treatment because there is delayed pseudonormalization of ADC attributed to cooling.

- Recognition of injury on head CT can be very challenging in the watery neonatal brain, not to mention the disadvantage of the radiation.
- Progression of injury to chronic stages happens much faster in the neonate compared with adults (Fig. 8.68).

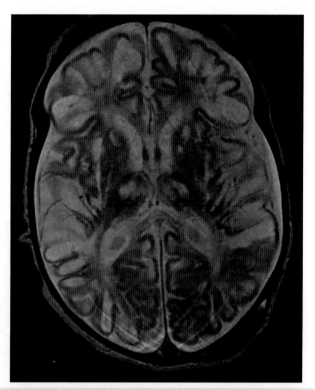

**Fig. 8.68 Same patient as in Fig.** 8.67, follow-up magnetic resonance image (MRI) at day 19 of life. The axial T2-weighted image shows generalized supratentorial volume loss and abnormal white matter hyperintensity, as well as cystic changes in the subcortical white matter, caudate nuclei, putamen, and thalami. This image illustrates the fast progression to chronic stage of ischemic changes in severe hypoxic ischemic encephalopathy (HIE) in neonates.

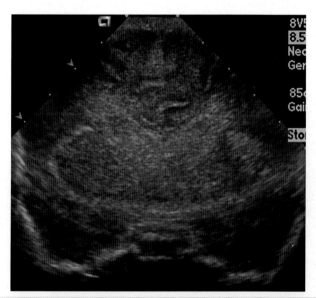

**Fig. 8.66 Hypoxic ischemic encephalopathy (HIE) on head ultrasound.** Coronal ultrasound images show diffuse increased echogenicity of the white matter and deep gray nuclei with increased gray-white matter differentiation.

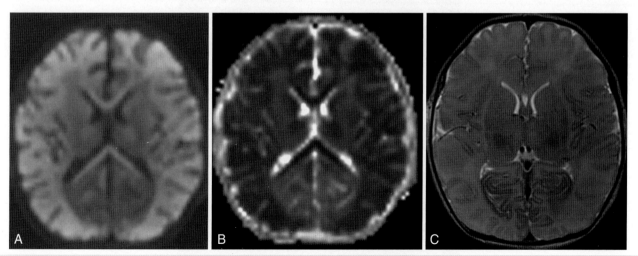

**Fig. 8.67 Hypoxic ischemic encephalopathy (HIE).** (A) Axial diffusion-weighted image and (B) corresponding apparent diffusion coefficient (ADC) map from magnetic resonance imaging (MRI) on day 3 of life on a full-term infant born via C-section after attempted home delivery shows diffusion restriction in the entire supratentorial brain with partial sparing of the mesial occipital lobes. (C) Axial T2-weighted image shows diffuse edema in the affected regions.

- Age of the neonate is quite critical. Hint: The lack of dark T2 signal in the posterior limb of the internal capsule in a 34-gestational-week born preterm should not be regarded as injury because it has not myelinated yet!

## TEMPORAL LOBE SEIZURES AND MESIAL TEMPORAL SCLEROSIS

- Temporal lobe seizures are usually partial (that is, there is no loss of consciousness), as opposed to generalized seizures (where there is loss of consciousness). The causes of temporal lobe seizures are manifold.

---

**TEACHING POINTS**

Causes of Temporal Lobe Epilepsy

Mesial temporal sclerosis (hippocampal sclerosis)
Ganglioglioma
Astrocytomas of all types
Oligodendroglioma

---

Cortical dysplasia
Heterotopia
Vascular malformations
Ischemia
Trauma

---

- Sources of seizure foci in the young patient include tumors, vascular malformations, gliotic abnormalities, FCD, heterotopias, hamartomas, migrational anomalies, and ischemic or traumatic injury.
- Thirty percent of temporal lobe seizures are idiopathic, with no cause, 40% have an underlying visible cause (symptomatic), and 30% are cryptogenic, where the cause may be unknown, but a lesion probably exists. Although 60% of all seizure disorders are well managed with medications, some causes, including mesial temporal sclerosis (MTS), often require surgical intervention. MTS accounts for as many as 50% of subjects undergoing temporal lobe surgery.

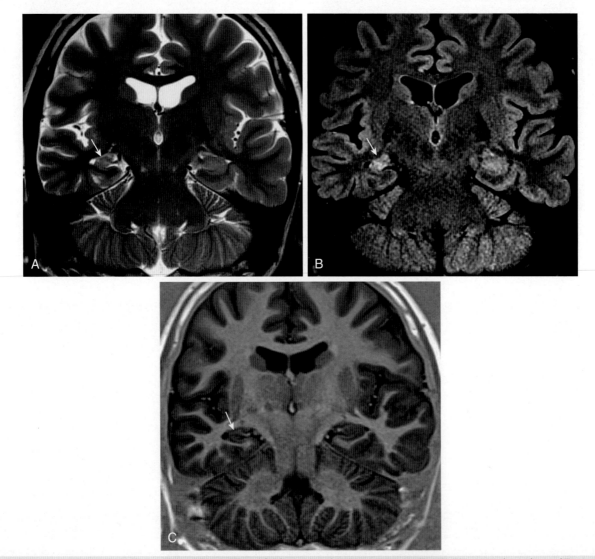

**Fig. 8.69  Mesial temporal sclerosis.** Coronal oblique T2 (A) and fluid-attenuated inversion recovery (FLAIR) (B) images show elevated T2 signal and diminished volume of the right hippocampus compared with the left. To keep things in perspective, this case is *very* obvious, so you can imagine the challenge of making the diagnosis in more subtle cases.

- MTS, also known as hippocampal atrophy, is a common source for poorly controlled seizures in adolescents and young adults. Although most cases present in or after adolescence, the roots of MTS are controversial, with possible association with febrile seizures in infancy. The mechanism for congenital, nonfebrile development of MTS is mysterious but may be because of a perinatal ischemic event because of compression of arteries during delivery, intrauterine hypoxia, hypoxia secondary to status epilepticus, neurotoxic effects of excessive glutamate production, or hypoglycemia. Nonetheless, MTS is considered a progressive disease and the imaging findings of selective atrophy may progress with age. Histopathologically, one sees neuronal loss and gliosis in affected patients.
- On MRI, hippocampal volume loss is the salient feature of MTS. Atrophy of the mesial temporal lobe may affect the amygdala (12%), hippocampal head (51%), hippocampal body (88%), and hippocampal tail (61%). Hyperintense signal on FLAIR/T2WI scans may involve the amygdala (4%), hippocampal head (39%), hippocampal body (81%), and hippocampal tail (49%) or the entire hippocampus (44%). Coronal oblique FLAIR or T2WI through the temporal lobes can show signal intensity changes and inversion recovery T1WI scans (phase-sensitive inversion recovery) can show hippocampal atrophy; these sequences will tell you which temporal lobe is abnormal in the vast majority of cases (Fig. 8.69).
- The imaging findings are more often subtle than glaringly obvious. Keep in mind that there is a normal asymmetry with respect to hippocampal volumes: the left hippocampus is typically 5% to 8% smaller than the right. Also be forewarned that bilateral involvement occurs in approximately 20% of cases, which can make a tricky diagnosis even trickier.
- Another finding in the spectrum of MTS is the loss of the normal cortical interdigitations of the hippocampal head. The sensitivity of this finding is approximately 90%; it may be present even when atrophy and signal intensity changes are absent in the medial temporal lobe.
- Additionally, the fornix and mammillary body ipsilateral to the side of MTS may be atrophic secondary to the decreased input to crossing fibers and limbic contributions (but these findings may also be present in cases of temporal lobe resections, strokes, and tumors).
- In those patients with ipsilateral hippocampal atrophy, surgical removal of MTS is 90% effective in eliminating seizures. Twenty percent of cases show normal MR structural scans, which just goes to show that the diagnosis of this condition should not be based on imaging alone.
- One potential obstacle associated with the work-up for seizures should be recognized. If you image the patient immediately after a seizure or even during status epilepticus that is unapparent to the clinicians, you may see meningeal enhancement and high DWI/FLAIR signal intensity in the seizing temporal lobe. This may imply a more diffuse process than is actually there (encephalitis or gliomatosis) and, in fact, this "abnormality" may resolve completely on MR in a few days. This is probably because of the increased blood flow to the seizing temporal lobe; that is, a perfusion effect.
- Perfuse on this! You completed the *Congenital Anomalies* chapter … and you thought your ex-utero life was complicated!

# PART II

# HEAD AND NECK

# 9 *Orbit*

JARUNEE INTRAPIROMKUL

## Relevant Anatomy

### BONY ORBIT

- The orbit is a cone-shaped structure made up of seven bones (lacrimal, ethmoid, palatine, maxillary, zygomatic, sphenoid, and frontal) (Fig. 9.1). The orbit is bordered superiorly by the anterior cranial fossa, medially by the ethmoid sinus, inferiorly by the maxillary sinus, posteriorly by the middle cranial fossa, and laterally by the temporal fossa.

> **TEACHING POINTS**
>
> The Bones That Make Up the Orbital Walls

- **Roof:** orbital plate of the frontal bone (anterior)
  lesser wing of the sphenoid bone (posterior)
- **Lateral wall:** orbital process of the frontal bone (anterosuperior)
  orbital process of the zygomatic bone (anteroinferior)
  greater wing of the sphenoid (posterior)
- **Floor:** orbital process of the maxillary bone, zygoma (anterolateral)
  orbital process of the palatine bone (posterior)
- **Medial wall:** lamina papyracea and lacrimal bone (anterior)
  lesser wing of sphenoid (posterior)

### GLOBE

- The globe usually approaches a sphere in shape with a diameter of approximately 2.5 cm, containing three enveloping layers: (1) sclera, (2) uvea (including choroid circumferentially), and (3) retina (Fig. 9.2). The outermost collagen-elastic layer is made up of the sclera and cornea. Covering the sclera anteriorly is the conjunctiva, a clear mucous membrane. The middle layer is the vascular pigmented layer termed the *uveal tract*, composed of the choroid, ciliary body, and the iris. The innermost layer of the globe is the retina, which is continuous with the optic nerve. The retina can be further separated into two layers: the outer retinal pigment epithelium, which is attached to the basal lamina of the choroid (Bruch membrane); and, the inner sensory layer, which is responsible for visual perception.
- The globe is divided by the lens into two segments, anterior and posterior. The anterior segment contains the anterior and posterior chambers as well as cornea, lens, iris, and ciliary body. Posterior to the lens is the posterior segment filled with the jelly-like vitreous body (humor), also containing the retina, choroid and sclera.
- The iris separates the anterior chamber from the posterior chamber. The ciliary body lies between the iris

and choroid, contains muscles attached to the lens by the suspensory ligament that control the curvature of the lens, and secretes the aqueous humor, which flows between both chambers.

### ORBITAL SEPTUM

- The orbital septum is a fibrous tissue attached to the outer bony orbital periphery continuous with the orbital periosteum that acts as a barrier to the spread of infection and can be seen on high-resolution magnetic resonance (MR). The superior aspect can be observed descending from the superior orbital rim and fusing with the levator aponeurosis before reaching the superior aspect of the tarsus. The inferior aspect of the septum ascends from the inferior orbital rim toward the lower lid tarsus. It divides the orbit into the superficial anterior preseptal space and the deep postseptal space.

### FORAMINA

- Three major foramina are in the orbit: (1) the optic canal, (2) the superior orbital fissure, and (3) the inferior orbital fissure (Table 9.1; see Fig. 9.1).
- Additionally, the anterior and posterior ethmoidal foramina transmit the anterior and posterior ethmoidal arteries. Supraorbital and infraorbital foramina transmit supraorbital and infraorbital nerve and vessels, respectively. They transmit sensory nerve branches of the trigeminal nerve as well. These are sources of perineural spread from cutaneous cancers back to the cranial nerve (CN) V ganglia.
- The nasolacrimal duct, located in the inferomedial surface of the orbit, communicates with the inferior meatus and can serve as a pathway for nasal tumors to extend directly into the orbit.

### EXTRAOCULAR MUSCLES

- Superior, medial, lateral, and inferior rectus muscles originate from the annulus of Zinn at the optic foramen and insert on the globe. Superior oblique and inferior oblique muscles originate from superomedial to the optic foramen and orbital plate of the maxilla, respectively. The levator palpebrae superioris muscle arises above the superior rectus and inserts into the upper lid.
- The four rectus muscles are classically thought to be connected by an intramuscular fibrous membrane creating the so-called *intraconal space* (Fig. 9.3). For radiologic purposes this boundary serves as a useful landmark in categorizing and diagnosing orbital lesions. Thus, intraconal lesions are associated with the optic nerve and sheath, its vessels, cranial nerves III,IV, and VI, and

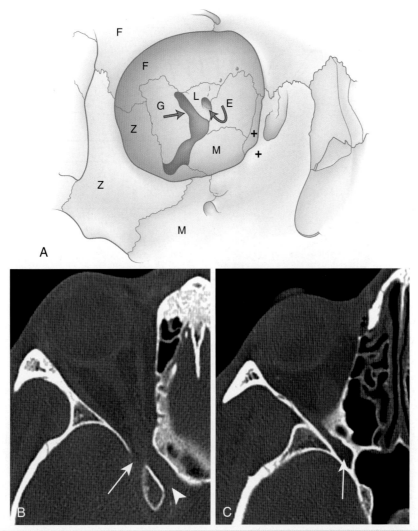

**Fig. 9.1 The bones of the orbit.** (A) A diagram of the bony orbit as seen from the front. The bones of the medial wall are the lacrimal (+), ethmoid (*E:* lamina papyracea), and sphenoid (*L:* lesser wing). The orbital roof is formed by the orbital plate of the frontal bone *(F)* anteriorly and the lesser wing *(L)* of the sphenoid bone posteriorly. The lateral wall of the orbit is composed of the zygomatic bone *(Z)* anteriorly and the greater wing of the sphenoid *(G)* posteriorly. The orbital floor consists primarily of the orbital plate of the maxillary bone *(M)*; however, the zygoma *(Z)* forms part of the anterolateral floor while the palatine bone (not seen) is at the most posterior aspect of the floor. The superior orbital fissure is identified *(straight arrow)*, as well as the optic canal *(curved arrow)*. (B) Axial computed tomography (CT) image shows the superior orbital fissure *(arrow)* and optic canal *(arrowhead)* from the imaging perspective. (C) Axial CT shows the inferior orbital fissure *(arrow)*.

orbital fat; conal lesions involve the muscles; and extraconal disease includes the bony orbit, peripheral fat, nerves and extraorbital structures like the paranasal sinuses, skull, or brain.

**TEACHING POINTS**

Facts on Fat

- The orbit is lined with adipose tissue that is well organized and divided by fibrovascular septae.
- This fat functions as a shock absorber and produces contrast, enabling orbital structures to stand out on magnetic resonance (MR) or computed tomography (CT), and, of course, decreases the conspicuity of enhancing lesions on MR unless fat-saturation MR techniques are used.

## OPTIC NERVE

- The optic nerve is a white matter tract that is sheathed by the leptomeninges and dura mater. The subarachnoid space of the optic nerve sheath is continuous with the intracranial subarachnoid space (see Fig. 9.3) providing a pathway for spread of infection, inflammation, tumors, or hemorrhage. This explains the finding of papilledema in instances of increased intracranial pressure.
- The intraorbital optic nerve has a sinuous course in both horizontal and vertical planes. After the optic nerves leave the canals, they ascend at an angle of approximately 45 degrees as prechiasmatic nerves, meet to form the chiasm beneath the floor of the third ventricle, and proceed posterolaterally to enter the brain as the postchiasmatic optic tracts.

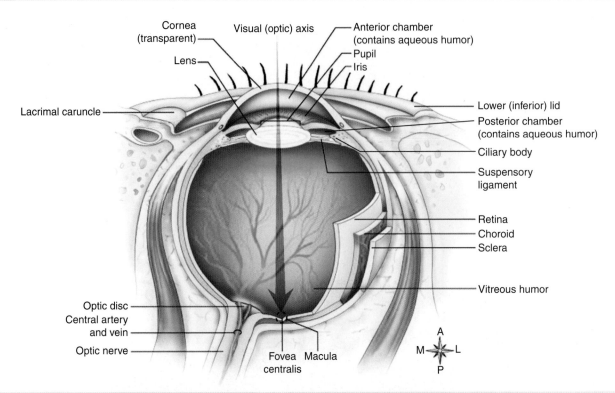

**Fig. 9.2** Cross-section through the left eyeball, viewed from above. (From Thibodeau GA, Patton KT. *Anatomy and Physiology*. 7th ed. St. Louis: Mosby; 2009:515.)

| Table 9.1 | Contents of Major Orbital Foramina | |
|---|---|---|
| **Orbital Foramen** | **Contents** | **Anatomic Considerations** |
| Optic canal | Optic nerve, sympathetic fibers, ophthalmic artery | Formed by the lesser wing of the sphenoid bone, closely approximating the anterior clinoid process. |
| | | Often is bordered by ethmoid or sphenoid sinus aerated cells, which puts the nerve at risk for dehiscence during functional endoscopic sinus surgery. |
| Superior orbital fissure | Cranial nerves (CN) III, IV, first division of CN V, and CN VI; superior ophthalmic vein; sympathetic fibers; orbital branch of middle meningeal artery | Formed from the greater and lesser wings of the sphenoid. |
| | | Separated from the optic canal by a thin strip of bone, the optic strut. |
| Inferior orbital fissure | Second division of CN V, infra-orbital artery and vein, inferior ophthalmic vein | Lies between the orbital plate of the maxilla and palatine bones, and the greater wing of the sphenoid. |
| | | Communicates with the pterygopalatine fossa. |

## VASCULAR STRUCTURES

### Ophthalmic Artery

▪ The ophthalmic artery usually arises from the internal carotid artery just after emerging from the cavernous sinus. On entering the orbit usually via the optic canal, the ophthalmic artery is initially inferolateral to the nerve. The main trunk of the ophthalmic artery divides into two relatively independent systems: the retinal vascular system (central retinal artery), which supplies the optic nerve and inner aspect of the sensory retina, and the ciliary vascular system.

**TEACHING POINTS**

Ophthalmic Artery and Vascular Disease

• The ophthalmic artery constitutes a major anastomotic pathway between the internal and external carotid artery. These anastomoses are listed in Box 9.1 and are particularly important in extracranial occlusive vascular disease.
• The choroid layer of the eye, supplied by the short posterior ciliary arteries, is seen on the lateral conventional catheter arteriogram as a thin crescent with an anterior concavity. A delay in appearance of the choroidal blush suggests hemodynamically significant disease of the internal carotid artery.

▪ Anatomic variations of the ophthalmic artery are important when embolizations and carotid surgery are planned to avoid inadvertent vessel occlusion and blindness. The ophthalmic artery can originate from the middle meningeal artery (meningolacrimal artery), or branches of the meningeal artery may connect with the ophthalmic artery (Box 9.1). Rarely the ophthalmic artery can arise more inferiorly from the cavernous internal carotid artery (ICA) and can enter the orbit through the superior orbital fissure.

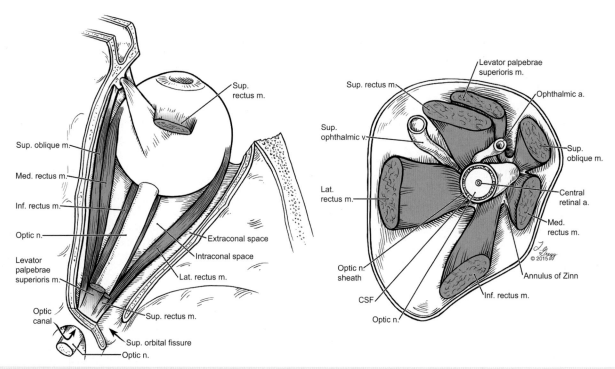

**Fig. 9.3** This diagram shows the classic separation of the sites of pathology in the orbit into ocular disease (the globe), intraconal, conal, and extraconal spaces including the lacrimal sac and gland. *a*, Artery; *CSF*, cerebrospinal fluid; *inf*, inferior; *lat*, lateral; *m*, muscle; *med.*, medial; *n*, nerve; *sup*, superior. (Courtesy Lydia Gregg.)

---

### Box 9.1  External Carotid-Ophthalmic Artery Anastomoses

**Superficial Temporal Artery Branches**

Supratrochlear artery
Supraorbital artery
Internal palpebral artery

**Internal Maxillary Branches**

Anterior deep temporal artery
Middle meningeal artery (anterior division)
Infraorbital artery
Sphenopalatine artery

**Facial Artery Branches**

Angular artery
Lateral nasal artery

---

## Ophthalmic Vein

- The superior ophthalmic vein is formed by the angular, nasofrontal, and supraorbital veins, which converge at the superolateral aspect of the nose. The superior ophthalmic vein (1.5–3 mm in diameter on MR) runs under the orbital roof and through the superior orbital fissure to drain into the cavernous sinus.
- The inferior ophthalmic vein starts as a plexus of small veins beneath the globe and courses posteriorly above the inferior rectus muscle to join the superior ophthalmic vein or to enter the cavernous sinus directly. Inferiorly, a second branch passes through the inferior orbital fissure to drain into the pterygoid venous plexus.
- A medial ophthalmic vein, observed in about 40% of cases, runs in the nasal extraconal space and joins the superior ophthalmic vein near the superior orbital fissure.

## Lacrimal System

- The lacrimal gland is a tear-producing, almond-shaped structure in the anterosuperolateral portion of the orbit lying in the lacrimal fossa at the level of the zygomatic process of the frontal bone.
- Tears produced by the lacrimal glands track medially and flow through the lacrimal puncta in each lid margin. Nasolacrimal drainage follows superior and inferior canaliculi, which are situated along the medial part of the lids and drain via the sinus of Maier into the lacrimal sac (Fig. 9.4). The lacrimal sac is a membranous tissue situated in the medial inferior wall of the orbit (lacrimal fossa) and drains via the valve of Krause into the nasolacrimal duct and through the valve of Hasner into the nasal cavity beneath the inferior turbinate.

---

**TEACHING POINTS**

Consequences of obstructed lacrimal drainage system

Obstruction of the lacrimal drainage system can result in:

- Dacryocystoceles in children
- Epiphora (excessive tearing)
- Dacryocystitis (infection of the nasolacrimal sac) or dacryoadenitis (lacrimal gland inflammation)

---

# Imaging Techniques/Protocols

## COMPUTED TOMOGRAPHY

- Computed tomography (CT) is the modality of choice for orbital trauma in part because of its speed, which is needed because of routine globe movement. Holding one's gaze

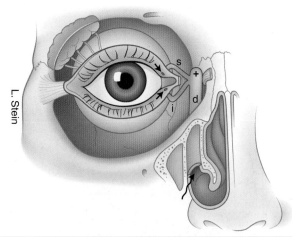

L. Stein

**Fig. 9.4 Interior of the lacrimal system.** The lacrimal puncta in the medial aspect of the lid margin *(small arrows)* drains via the superior *(s)* and inferior *(i)* canaliculi into the lacrimal sac *(+)* via the sinus of Maier. The lacrimal sac lies in the medial inferior wall of the orbit (lacrimal fossa) and drains via the valve of Krause into the nasolacrimal duct *(d)* through the valve of Hasner into the nasal cavity beneath the inferior turbinate *(squiggly arrow).*

steady for 3 to 4 minutes during an MR scan is challenging. Fractures are easier to detect with CT, and bone lesions are usually better visualized with CT. Furthermore, orbital metallic foreign bodies are a contraindication to MR in most cases. One of the most important attributes of CT is its ability to detect calcification and foreign bodies. Widened orbital foramina in the setting of perineural disease extension can also be appreciated by CT.

- Because of the natural soft-tissue contrast between orbital fat and other orbital structures, in most cases dedicated CT of the orbits can be typically performed without intravenous (IV) contrast unless infection or tumor is suspected. Scans currently employ submillimeter slice thickness through the orbits allowing excellent quality coronal and sagittal reconstructions.

## MAGNETIC RESONANCE IMAGING

- Magnetic resonance imaging (MR) has superior soft-tissue contrast compared with CT. It is recommended for characterizing orbital masses arising from the orbit or from direct spread from adjacent compartments, and for evaluation of demyelinating or ischemic optic nerve lesions.

---

**PHYSICS PEARLS**

Magnetic Resonance Imaging of the Orbits

---

- The use of coronally acquired fast spin echo or constructive interference in steady state (CISS) techniques with increased matrix size (512×512) can provide beautiful T2-weighted imaging (T2WI) of the optic nerve, enabling differentiation of the nerve and sheath.
- The major challenge with magnetic resonance (MR) in contrast to computed tomography (CT) is related to the longer scan duration and concomitant image degradation from motion, which in most cases is unavoidable.

- Axial and coronal T1 precontrast and postcontrast images through the orbits at 2- to 3-mm-slice thickness or less are essential. T1 precontrast images should be performed without fat suppression to take advantage of the soft-tissue contrast of orbital fat and other orbital soft tissues. Postcontrast images must be performed with fat suppression to distinguish enhancing pathology from intrinsically hyperintense normal orbital fat.
- Coronal (+/- axial) T2 images with fat suppression at 2- to 3-mm-slice thickness through the orbits are critical for evaluation of the optic nerve signal and caliber. Additional fluid suppression techniques can be employed to further suppress cerebrospinal fluid (CSF) signal within the optic nerve sheath, but with this comes loss of signal to noise ratio. Some combined fat and fluid-suppression techniques include SPIR (spectral inversion recovery) and STIR FLAIR (short tau inversion recovery fluid attenuation inversion recovery).

## ULTRASOUND

- More often used by ophthalmologists than radiologists, ultrasound is used to assess intraocular lesions, including the integrity of the globe after trauma, to look for retained foreign bodies, to demonstrate choroidal rupture, retinal detachment, flow dynamics of vessels in the orbit, some ocular tumors, collections under the ocular membranes, and in the work up of cavernous carotid fistulas.

# Pathology

## OCULAR CALCIFICATIONS

- CT is exquisitely sensitive to ocular calcification. There are various causes of ocular calcification that are listed in Box 9.2. Senescent calcifications of the globe (limbus

---

**Box 9.2   Causes of Ocular Calcification**

**Degenerative**

Cataracts
Optic nerve drusen
Senile calcification of insertion of muscle tendons in the globe

**Chronic/Post-insult**

Phthisis bulbi
Retinal detachment
Retrolental fibroplasia

**Neoplastic**

Astrocytic hamartoma
Neurofibromatosis
Tuberous sclerosis
von Hippel-Lindau syndrome
Retinoblastoma

**Infectious**

Cytomegalovirus
Herpes simplex
Rubella
Syphilis
Toxoplasmosis
Tuberculosis

calcifications, scleral plaques) are usually found at the insertion sites on the globe of the medial and lateral rectus muscles. Trochlear calcifications are seen at the tendon site of the superior oblique muscle. Optic drusen reflects benign calcification, which appears as a punctate calcification located at the optic nerve insertion at the globe, involving the optic disc, and sometimes leading to an appearance ophthalmoscopically as papilledema. Phthisis bulbi is the end stage of globe injury, be it from infection, inflammation, trauma, or autoimmune disease; the globe is non-functional and small, and it eventually calcifies (Fig. 9.5).

## PEDIATRIC OCULAR DISEASES

### Retinoblastoma

- Retinoblastoma (Rb) is the most common intraocular tumor of childhood. Most lesions occur as sporadic mutations (90%), whereas approximately 10% are familial. It is caused by a mutation in both copies of Rb gene *RB1* (the tumor suppressor gene at 13q14.2 location). Heritable Rb is an autosomal dominant trait, with high penetrance and a propensity for bilaterality and multifocality.
- There is a high incidence of nonocular tumors in the hereditary form (including midline, primitive neuroectodermal, pineal tumors, osteogenic sarcoma, soft-tissue sarcoma, malignant melanoma, basal cell carcinoma, and rhabdomyosarcoma). Trilateral Rb is bilateral Rb with associated pineoblastoma. Trilateral Rb plus parasellar or suprasellar neuroendocrine tumor is termed *quadrilateral Rb*.
- Patients with retinoblastoma usually present before the age of 3 years with leukocoria, strabismus, decreased

---

**TEACHING POINTS**

Causes of Leukocoria (White Pupil)

- Leukocoria caused by any opaque tissue that interferes with the passage of light through the globe. Leukocoria has many causes.
  Retinoblastoma
  Congenital cataract
  Retinopathy of prematurity
  Choroidal hemangioma
  Retinal astrocytoma
  Persistent hyperplastic primary vitreous
  Coats disease
  *Toxocara canis* infection

---

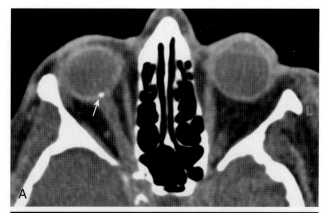
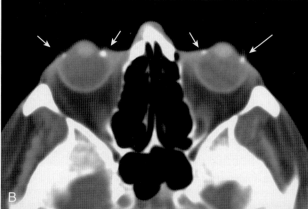
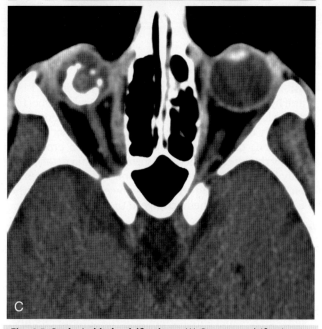

**Fig. 9.5 Ocular/orbital calcifications.** (A) Punctate calcification on computed tomography (CT) at the junction of the head of the optic nerve and right globe *(arrow)*. This is a drusen (body). (B) CT with senescent calcifications in insertions of medial and lateral rectus tendon sheaths *(arrows)*. (C) In this case, phthisis bulbi occurred from trauma to the eye resulting in shrunken globe with calcification.

---

vision, retinal detachment, glaucoma, ocular pain, or signs of ocular inflammation.
- Rb may spread directly into the subarachnoid space via the optic nerve, hematogenously, or via lymphatics and has a propensity to hemorrhage. Metastases from Rb occur within the first 2 years after treatment.
- On CT, homogeneous or irregular calcifications in the posterior portion of the globe are seen in 95% of patients (Fig. 9.6). In children younger than 3 years of age, ocular calcification is highly suggestive of Rb; conversely, its absence

in this same group makes the diagnosis of Rb highly unlikely. These lesions minimally enhance on CT, obscured by the ocular calcification; however, contrast is useful to appreciate the intracranial extension (better assessed with MR).

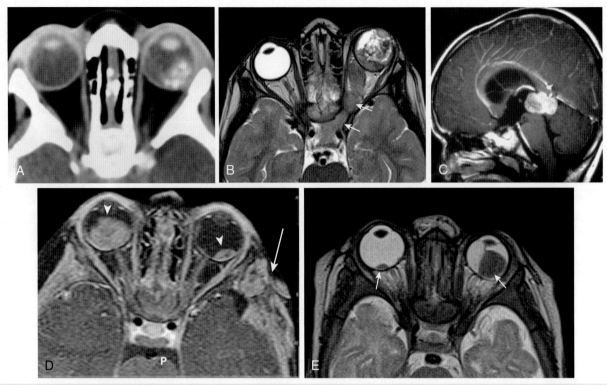

**Fig. 9.6 Retinoblastoma.** (A) On computed tomography, retinoblastoma calcifications are noted extending from the posterior retina into the vitreous on the left. (B) T2-weighted imaging (T2WI) shows retinoblastoma that has spread along the optic nerve *(arrows)* through the optic canal into the intracranial space. (C) Postcontrast T1WI shows enhancing mass at the region of the pineal gland representing pineoblastoma in a patient with bilateral retinoblastoma (the pineal tumor now makes it trilateral). (D) This patient with bilateral retinoblastomas *(arrowheads)* also has a soft-tissue sarcoma *(arrow)* in the left temporalis muscle seen on postgadolinium-enhanced fat-suppressed T1-weighted image. (E) Bilateral retinoblastomas *(arrows)*, larger on the left, are well seen on T2-weighted imaging.

- MR findings in Rb include mildly high intensity on T1WI and hypointensity on T2WI, with the noncalcified portion of the lesion less hypointense than the calcification. High intensity on T1WI may be caused by calcium or by some coexistent paramagnetic substance, tumor protein, or hemorrhagic component. Associated retinal detachment may be high intensity on T1WI and of variable intensity on T2WI, depending on the protein content and whether there is associated hemorrhage in the subretinal fluid.

### Persistent Hyperplastic Primary Vitreous

- Persistent hyperplastic primary vitreous (PHPV) is caused by persistence of various portions of the primary vitreous (embryonic hyaloid vascular system) with hyperplasia of the associated embryonic connective tissue.
- The globe is usually small (microphthalmia), and the lens can be small with flattening of the anterior chamber. Initially, a funnel-shaped (martini glass–shaped) mass of fibrovascular tissue (including the hyaloid artery) is present in the retrolental space and runs in the "Cloquet canal" (between the back of the lens and the head of the optic nerve). PHPV is vascular, and the globe is prone to repeated hemorrhages.
- CT demonstrates generalized increased density in the globe and enhancement of the intravitreal tissue after IV contrast. Unlike Rb, PHPV does not calcify (this is key!). Both can cause retinal detachments.
- CT and MR reveal the retrolental funnel-shaped tissue (between the lens and head of the optic nerve) (Fig. 9.7),

which will enhance after contrast administration. Retinal detachment and blood-vitreous layer may be seen (because of posterior hyaloid detachment). On MR, vitreal intensity is variable.

### Coats Disease

- Coats disease (exudative retinitis/retinopathy) is a vascular anomaly of the retina that may be clinically difficult to distinguish from Rb. This lesion is usually unilateral. These telangiectatic vessels leak serum and lipid into the retina (lipoproteinaceous effusion) and subretinal space, resulting in retinal detachment.
- Patients are usually seen when retinal detachment occurs in the first 2 years of life, although the age at discovery may be as late as 6 to 8 years with approximately two thirds of cases in males.
- The CT appearance is of high density in the vitreous related to the exudate with small eye. Calcification is rare. On MR, the exudate is hyperintense on T1WI and T2WI. There may be contrast enhancement of the detached retina, and it may rarely have mass-like appearance.

### Ocular Toxocariasis

- Toxocariasis occurs because of ingestion of soil contaminated with dog feces containing the ova of the nematode *Toxocara canis* (in dog) or *Toxocara cati* (in cat). The ova hatch in the gastrointestinal (GI) tract and then migrate throughout the body. When larvae of *T. canis* within the eye die, it produces a hypersensitivity response and

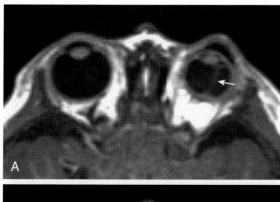

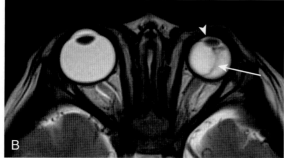

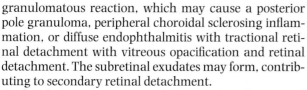

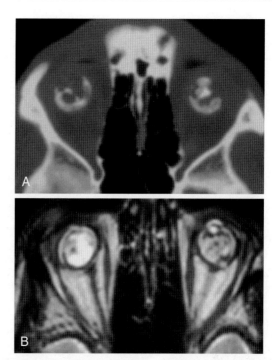

**Fig. 9.7 Persistent hyperplastic primary vitreous.** (A) In this patient with persistent hyperplastic primary vitreous (PHPV), note the presence of Cloquet canal in the left globe *(arrow)*. (B) The T2-weighted imaging scan best shows the persistent canal *(arrow)* and the associated dysmorphic lens *(arrowhead)* in this somewhat small globe.

**Fig. 9.8 Retinopathy of prematurity may present with small dense eyes, sometimes with calcifications.** (A) Bilateral shrunken calcified globes are seen in this patient. They also are abnormally in signal intensity on T2-weighted imaging (B) from the calcification and chronic retinal detachments.

granulomatous reaction, which may cause a posterior pole granuloma, peripheral choroidal sclerosing inflammation, or diffuse endophthalmitis with tractional retinal detachment with vitreous opacification and retinal detachment. The subretinal exudates may form, contributing to secondary retinal detachment.

- Ocular lesions occur months to years after initial infection. The patients may present with decreased visual acuity, leukocoria, vitritis, ocular injection, and strabismus.
- Imaging findings are nonspecific. On CT, diffuse high density may be identified within the globe without calcification. MRI may reveal the posterior granulomas, which are isointense to vitreous on T1-weighted images (T1WI), hyperintense on T2-weighted images (T2WI), and moderately to markedly enhance with IV contrast injection. Subretinal exudate with variable signal intensity and retinal detachment can be observed.

## Retinopathy of Prematurity

- Retinopathy of prematurity (ROP) is the result of abnormal vascular development of the retina. Risk factors are low birth weight (<1 kg) and low gestational age, indicators of prematurity, but episodes of hyperoxia, sepsis, blood transfusions, and hypercarbia can contribute to its occurrence. Prolonged oxygen therapy in premature infants is a major risk factor. It can present as bilateral leukocoria because of traction retinal detachments.
- CT findings are increased density in the posterior portion of the globe with calcification and microphthalmia (Fig. 9.8; Box 9.3). Occasionally, retinal detachment can be identified.

---

### Box 9.3   Big Eye, Small Eye: Causes of Macrophthalmia and Microphthalmia

**Macrophthalmia**

Aniridia
Axial myopia (most common cause of enlarged globe)
Buphthalmos
Congenital glaucoma
Ehlers-Danlos
Homocystinuria
Intraocular masses
Marfan
Neurofibromatosis 1
Proteus
Staphyloma
Sturge-Weber

**Microphthalmia**
PHPV
Trisomy 13 (Patau syndrome)
Surgery
Fetal rubella, varicella, herpes simplex, infection
Holoprosencephaly
Phthisis bulbi
Retinopathy of prematurity
Radiation
CHARGE syndrome
Infant of diabetic mother
Fetal alcohol syndrome
Pseudohypoparathyroidism

*CHARGE,* Coloboma, heart defects, atresia of the choana, retarded growth and development, and ear anomalies; *PHPV,* persistent hyperplastic primary vitreous.

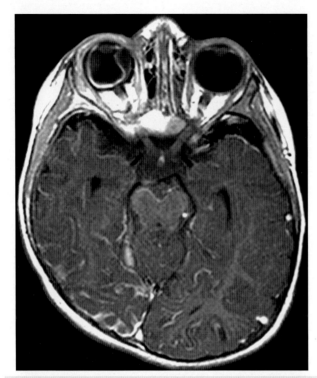

**Fig. 9.9** Choroidal angioma of the right globe in patient with Sturge-Weber syndrome. Note abnormal enhancement of the choroid along with choroidal detachment. Leptomeningeal angiomatosis is present over the right hemisphere and left occipital lobe, with volume loss of the right cerebral hemisphere compared with the left, typical of this syndrome.

## Ocular Manifestation of Neurocutaneous Syndromes

- Retinal astrocytic (glial) hamartomas are observed in cases of tuberous sclerosis and neurofibromatosis 1. A hallmark of von Hippel-Lindau disease is retinal angiomatosis. Hemangioblastomas of the retina and retrobulbar optic nerve and orbit have also been reported in von Hippel-Lindau disease. Choroidal angiomas are reported in Sturge-Weber syndrome (tomato ketchup retina) (Fig. 9.9). Lisch nodules (uveal melanocytic nevi) of the iris are common in neurofibromatosis type 1 (NF-1) but are not appreciable by imaging. The globe may be enlarged and oblong (buphthalmos) in NF-1 and there may be glaucoma on exam. Also remember the potential for sphenoid wing dysplasia in NF-1 with pulsatile exophthalmos clinically.

## ADULT OCULAR DISEASES

### Melanoma

- Uveal melanomas are the most common intraocular malignancy in adults, arising from the melanocytes in the uveal tract (choroid, iris, and ciliary body). They commonly involve the posterior choroid (85% of the cases). Conditions predisposing to uveal melanoma include congenital melanosis, nevus of Ota, blue nevi, ocular melanocytosis, oculodermal melanocytosis, and uveal nevi. They are rare in African Americans, but when they occur tend to be larger, more pigmented, and more necrotic.

- On MRI, melanotic melanomas are hyperintense on T1WI and hypointense on T2WI (Fig. 9.10). The T1 and T2 shortening is a result of paramagnetic effects from free radicals and metal scavenging effects of the melanin. Amelanotic melanomas have MR characteristics similar to those of other tumors (hypointense on T1WI and hyperintense on proton density–weighted imaging [PDWI]/T2WI). There may be associated retinal detachments with subretinal fluid of variable signal intensity.
- On CT, uveal melanomas are high density on noncontrast images and enhance following contrast administration.
- Extraocular invasion is associated with a poorer prognosis and has different therapeutic implications. Choroidal melanoma has a propensity for metastasis to the liver and lung.

### Ocular Metastases

- Metastatic breast, lung, GI, and skin cancers, as well as lymphoma and leukemia are the most common nonmelanoma ocular malignancies seen in adults. Many metastatic neoplasms to the globe affect the uveal tract (most commonly the choroid) and may be clinically asymptomatic.
- On CT and MRI, they appear as eccentric thickening of the uveoscleral rim, usually a broad-based flat lesion (Fig. 9.11). Certain types of choroidal metastases can have similar signal intensity pattern as uveal melanoma (T1 hyperintensity and T2 hypointensity), such as mucin-producing adenocarcinoma and hemorrhagic metastases. Choroidal lymphoma and leukemia can appear on MR to be like uveal amelanotic melanoma, may cause retinal detachment, and may be bilateral (rare for melanoma).

### Chorioretinitis

- Cytomegalovirus (CMV) is the most common opportunistic infection of the retina and choroid. Up to one fourth of patients with acquired immunodeficiency syndrome (AIDS) have CMV. The chorioretinitis may be hemorrhagic and can produce high density on CT or various MR appearances depending on the stage of blood and the retinal enhancement that can be seen (Fig. 9.12). Other infectious pathogens affecting the retina in AIDS include toxoplasmosis, herpes simplex, and herpes zoster.

### Endophthalmitis

- Endophthalmitis is an acute suppurative infection of the aqueous or vitreous humor, acquired either by direct inoculation (e.g., trauma, foreign body, or iatrogenic) or hematogenously from other infected sources (e.g., cardiac). Panophthalmitis is present when infection extends beyond the sclera. Aggressive treatment is warranted to prevent the possibility of permanent blindness. The end-stage appearance is phthisis bulbi.
- On CT, heterogeneous or diffuse increased attenuation within the affected globe can be seen, along with thickening and enhancement of the sclera. Proteinaceous content within the globe can show elevated signal on T1- and T2-weighted images on MRI.

### Scleritis

- Scleritis/episcleritis can be infectious (bacterial, fungal, or viral) or autoimmune (collagen vascular diseases) in origin. It is separated into acute and chronic categories.

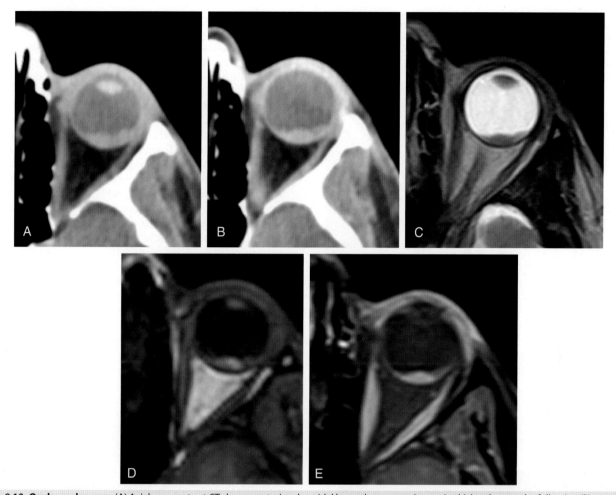

**Fig. 9.10 Ocular melanoma.** (A) Axial non contrast CT shows posterior choroidal hyperdense mass *(arrows)*, which enhances the following (B) contrast administration *(arrows)*. (C) Axial T2-weighted imaging (T2WI) in the same patient shows low signal and precontrast T1-weighted imaging (T1WI). (D) Shows high intensity of the tumor (paramagnetic effect of melanin). Just as on CT, the mass enhances on post contrast fat-suppressed T1WI.

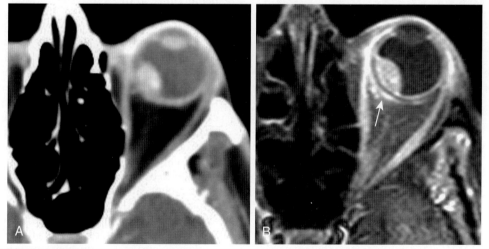

**Fig. 9.11 Choroidal metastasis.** (A) Axial computed tomography (CT) image shows unsuspected choroidal metastasis in a patient with known metastatic colon cancer. (B) Axial postcontrast T1-weighted image shows the postscleral extension of this metastasis *(arrow)* to better advantage compared with CT. Fat suppression is key.

- Findings include nodular/diffuse thickening and enhancement of the posterior sclera and uveal layers. The nodular variety can be mistaken for melanoma; the diffuse type can mimic lymphoma.

## Uveitis

- Inflammation of the uveal tract, which consists of the choroid, ciliary body, and iris, is targeted selectively also by sarcoidosis, ankylosing spondylitis, and inflammatory

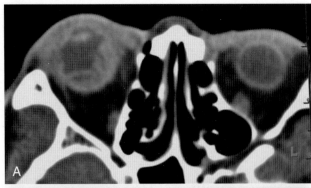

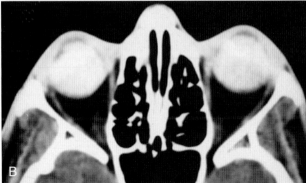

**Fig. 9.12 Cytomegalovirus (CMV).** (A) The patient with acquired immunodeficiency syndrome (AIDS) has a retinal detachment associated with the CMV infection of the chorioretinal membranes. (B) Hemorrhagic CMV. Computed tomography reveals bilateral vitreous hemorrhages in a patient with AIDS.

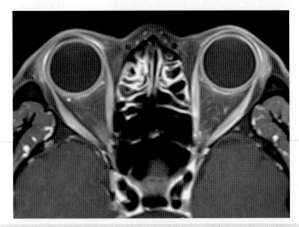

**Fig. 9.13 Visible inflection affecting vision.** Axial fat-suppressed T1WI shows smooth prominent enhancement of the ocular membranes bilaterally, including uveal and scleral layers in this patient with Vogt-Koyanagi-Harada syndrome, a conditional characterized clinically by anterior uveitis, alopecia, poliosis, vitiligo, and cerebrospinal fluid pleocytosis.

bowel disorders. Uveitis can occur secondary to infection as well. On MRI, you can see greater than expected enhancement of affected components on fat-suppressed T1-weighted images (Fig. 9.13).

## Ocular Hemorrhages and Detachments

- Table 9.2 compares the various ocular detachments radiologists commonly encounter, which arise within potential spaces within the globe. The space between hyaloid base and the retina is the posterior hyaloid space (Fig. 9.14). The potential spaces between the layers of

the retina (neurosensory retina and retinal pigment epithelium) are the subretinal spaces, and between the choroid and the sclera is the suprachoroidal space. When the posterior hyaloid membrane separates from the sensory retina, it is termed a *posterior vitreous detachment*; it is curvilinear in shape and anterior to the retina and separate from the optic disc.

- Retinal hemorrhage occurs in 18% to 41% of adults with subarachnoid hemorrhage and may be as high as 70% in children. Retinal hemorrhage in a child should raise a concern for possible nonaccidental trauma. Fundal hemorrhage is believed to be caused by a sudden rise in intracranial pressure (ICP) transmitted into the distal optic nerve sheath. This pressure may compress the central retinal vein and cause the intraocular hemorrhage. Retinal detachments (and vitreous hemorrhages) can be seen as complications of diabetic retinopathy.

- Hemorrhagic choroidal detachment may be observed after penetrating injury or intraocular surgery and has a lenticular morphology. It means there has been rupture of a choroidal vessel, which has an associated poor prognosis. Hemorrhagic choroidal effusions are high density on CT and do not change with position. MR is beneficial in distinguishing hemorrhagic choroidal detachment from serous choroidal detachments. On MR, hemorrhagic choroidal detachment can display a variety of intensity patterns related to the age of the hemorrhage. Serous choroidal detachment has high intensity on T1WI and T2WI.

- Sub-Tenon space is located between the sclera and the fibrous membrane (Tenon capsule) adjacent to the orbital fat extending from the ciliary body to the optic nerve. Hemorrhages in this space, most often from trauma, conform to the curvilinear shape of the eyeball.

- *Terson syndrome* was originally described as vitreous hemorrhage associated with subarachnoid hemorrhage but now has been expanded to any type of intraocular hemorrhage in the settings of intracranial hemorrhage or traumatic brain injury.

### Ocular Injury

Although direct ocular injury can be demonstrated on physical exam, imaging is often required because periorbital swelling can limit direct visual assessment of the eye.

- Ocular hypotony is defined as low tension in the globe and can be seen in the setting of acute traumatic injury. Injury confined to the anterior segment results in a shallow anteroposterior (AP) diameter of the anterior segment, which can be very subtle. Hemorrhage in the anterior chamber is termed a *hyphema*. Injury involving the posterior segment can also be subtle, evidenced by slight dorsal displacement of the lens. If the lens is traumatized, it may show an acute cataract (seen as a lower density disrupted lens), subluxation, or frank dislocation. Presence of intraocular air and/or foreign body material indicates globe rupture, even if there is no obvious globe deformity.

- More often, ocular injury is more dramatic on imaging, evidenced by distorted configuration of the globe, with the "flat tire" sign of the vitreous (Fig. 9.15). Hemorrhage can accumulate within the vitreous segment of the globe and is usually amorphous and hyperdense on CT. Direct injury to the lens or lens displacements can be seen in the setting of trauma but can also be seen in collagen-vascular disease processes.

**Table 9.2**  Types of Ocular Detachments

| Detachment | Separated Layers | Shape | Extent | Association |
|---|---|---|---|---|
| Retinal | Sensory retina from retinal pigment epithelium—subretinal space | V-shaped with apex at optic disc (total) | To ora serrata | Retinoblastoma, Coats disease, *Toxocara* endophthalmitis, diabetes, melanoma, choroidal hemangiomas, after trauma, senile macular degeneration, or persistent hyperplastic primary vitreous (PHPV) |
| Choroidal | Between choroid and sclera—suprachoroidal space | Linear, crescentic, or ring-shaped–serous convex-hemorrhagic | Leaves do not extend to the optic disc because the posterior choroid is anchored by short posterior ciliary arteries and nerves | Ocular hypotony, trauma, surgery, inflammatory choroidal lesions, melanoma |
| Posterior hyaloid space | Between posterior hyaloid membrane and sensory retina | Thin, semilunar, gravitational layering | Variable | Macular degeneration, PHPV, posterior vitreous detachment (PVD) |

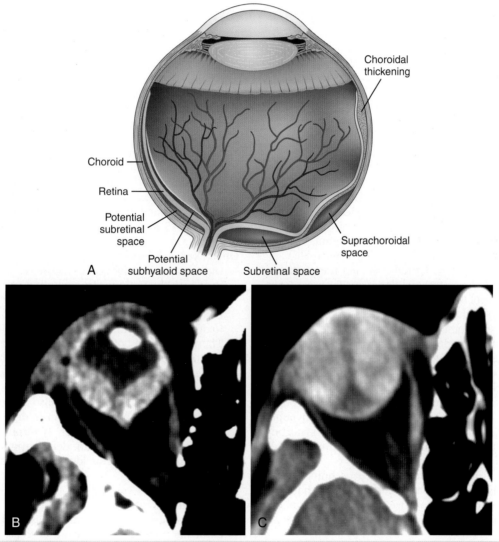

**Fig. 9.14 Ocular collections.** (A) Schematic representation of the various potential spaces for fluid/hemorrhage accumulation in setting of ocular detachments. (B) Axial computed tomography (CT) image shows typical V-shaped appearance of retinal detachment with the apex at the optic nerve head and anterior extent to the level of the ora serrata (at 10 and 2 o'clock). (C) Axial CT image shows typical configuration of choroidal detachment. The margin of the detached choroid extends to the expected location of the vortex veins.

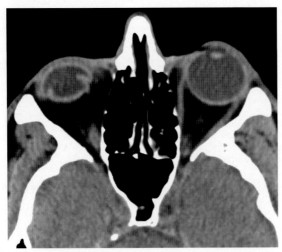

**Fig. 9.15 Deflate-Gate: Ocular hypotony.** Computed tomography after perforation of the right globe. The globe has the appearance of a flat tire compared with the left, which is characteristic of this condition.

**TEACHING POINTS**

Conditions Associated with Lens Dislocations

Marfan: Up and out
Homocystinuria: Down and in
Ehlers-Danlos
Trauma

## Coloboma

- A coloboma of the eye is a congenital defect in any ocular structure caused by incomplete closure of the choroidal fissure. Other structures including the retina, choroid, iris, and lens can be affected. The sclera is normal.
- Colobomas usually arise sporadically and are unilateral, although rarely an autosomal dominant form can exist, with about 60% of those affected having bilateral coloboma.
- It can be seen in the setting of clinical syndromes, such as CHARGE syndrome (coloboma, heart defects, atresia of the choana, retarded growth and development, and ear anomalies), trisomy 13, and Goldenhar syndrome. It may be associated with orbital cysts, midline craniocerebrofacial clefting, including sphenoidal encephalocele, agenesis of the corpus callosum, and olfactory hypoplasia, as well as cardiac abnormalities, genital hypoplasia, and ear anomalies. Patients with Aicardi syndrome may have ocular colobomas and chorioretinal lacunae, microphthalmia, and microcephaly.
- On imaging, there is a cone-shaped or notch-shaped deformity, usually of the posterior globe, that may involve the optic nerve head insertion, with eversion of a portion of the posterior globe (Fig. 9.16).

## Staphyloma

- Staphylomas are acquired defects in the sclera or cornea. They are lined with uveal tissue. Posterior staphyloma is associated with increasing globe size in patients with axial myopia and is usually on the temporal side of the optic disc. It can be a cause of proptosis. On CT and MRI, outward

bulging of the temporal aspect of the posterior portion of the globe with uveoscleral thinning and lack of enhancement can be seen (Fig. 9.17). Although axial myopia is the most common cause, infections (episcleritis), trauma, and surgical complications may lead to this entity.

## RETROBULBAR LESIONS

- Retrobulbar lesions may be conveniently divided into intraconal (lesions associated with the optic nerve, its vessels, and orbital fat), conal (lesions involving extraocular muscles), and extraconal (lesions centered in the bony orbit or extending into the orbit from the paranasal sinuses, skull, or brain).

### Intraconal Lesions

#### Enlarged Cerebrospinal Fluid Space

- An enlarged perioptic subarachnoid space is easily detected by MR and may occur congenitally, because of optic atrophy, or in situations where raised ICP exists (such as idiopathic intracranial hypertension, also known as *pseudotumor cerebri*). Rarely, one may see dural ectasia of the optic nerve sheath associated with NF-1.
- In cases of raised ICP, the globe at its junction with the optic nerve can be indented (reverse cupping) by the transmitted raised ICP, providing imaging evidence of papilledema (Fig. 9.18).
- Marked enhancement of the optic nerve heads has also been observed and thought to be secondary to breakdown of the blood retinal barrier after sudden rise in intracranial cerebrospinal fluid (CSF) pressure. This may be seen in papillitis and acute ICP elevations. There may even be restricted diffusion at the optic nerve head.

#### Optic Nerve Atrophy

- Optic nerve atrophy occurs as the result of a variety of insults to the optic nerve, including compression (such as from pituitary macroadenomas), infections, demyelination, trauma, glaucoma, ischemic optic neuropathy, toxin exposure, and nutritional deficiencies.
- The nerve loses both function and its pink color from loss of vascular supply (optic nerve pallor). On MR, the nerve looks atrophic with volume loss, with or without increased T2 signal (Fig. 9.19).
- Congenital optic atrophy can also be seen. When you see optic nerve hypoplasia in children, think "septo-optic dysplasia" (de Morsier syndrome): optic nerve hypoplasia, midline brain defects (including dysgenesis of the septum pellucidum), and pituitary hormone abnormalities.

#### Optic Neuritis

- Optic neuritis is an inflammatory lesion of the optic nerve clinically associated with pain, decreased visual acuity, abnormal color vision, and afferent pupillary defect.
- Optic neuritis is seen in up to 80% of patients with multiple sclerosis (MS) and may be the first clinical manifestation of MS. In patients with their first attack of optic neuritis, up to 65% have asymptomatic white matter abnormalities in the brain on MR and 50% in 5 years are diagnosed with MS (Fig. 9.20).

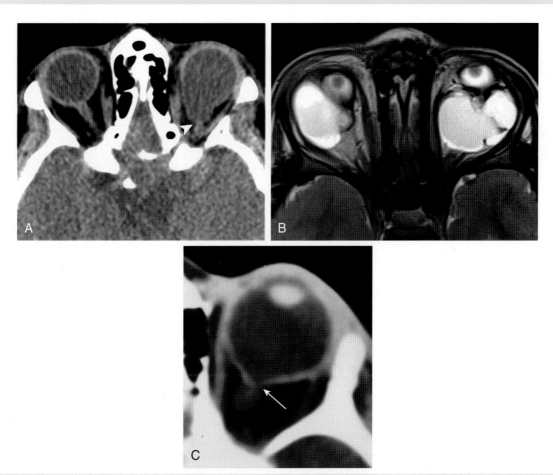

**Fig. 9.16 Coloboma.** (A) Left-sided cone-shaped deformity at the junction of the optic nerve head and globe *(arrowhead)*. (B) Bilateral orbital cysts on axial T2-weighted imaging in a patient with colobomas. (C) Classic in-cupping of the cyst *(arrow)* to the optic nerve insertion of this coloboma.

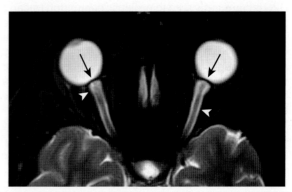

**Fig. 9.18 Increased intracranial pressure.** T2-weighted imaging shows reverse cupping of the optic nerve insertion to the globe *(black arrows)* and prominence to the optic nerve sheath complex *(white arrowheads)* indicative of elevated intracranial pressure and clinically appreciated papilledema.

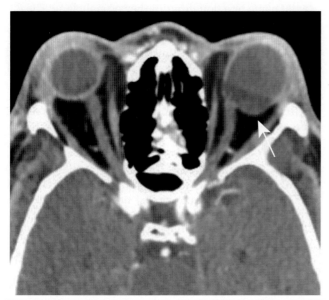

**Fig. 9.17 Computed tomography of posterior staphyloma.** Notice the uveoscleral thinning in the posterior lateral margin of the left globe *(arrow)*.

- Neuromyelitis optica spectrum disorder (a.k.a. NMOSD or Devic disease) is characterized by demyelination in the optic nerves and/or chiasm and long-segment lesions in the spinal cord. Most of the patients have specific immunoglobulin G (IgG) antibodies to the aquaporin 4 water channel on astrocytic foot processes.
- Other less common causes of optic neuritis include ischemia, vasculitis, sarcoid, systemic lupus erythematosus, infection (e.g., syphilis, Lyme disease, toxoplasmosis,

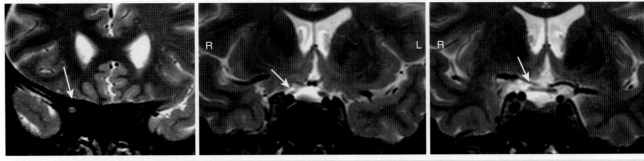

**Fig. 9.19 Optic nerve atrophy on the right.** Serial coronal T2-weighted imaging shows high signal and small volume of the right optic nerve *(arrows)* compared with the left as far back as the chiasm. *L,* Left; *R,* right.

tuberculosis), chemotherapy, myelin oligodendrocyte glycoprotein (MOG) antibody-associated disease, and radiation therapy.
- MRI findings of acute optic neuritis are high T2 signal intensity, enlargement, and enhancement of the optic nerve (best visualized on fat-suppressed postcontrast-enhanced images). In chronic optic neuritis, the nerve shows diminished caliber, although increased T2 signal can persist and does not enhance.

### Optic Pathway Glioma
- Optic pathway glioma (OPG) represents about two thirds of all primary optic nerve tumors, 1.5% to 3% of all orbital tumors, and up to 1.5% of all intracranial tumors. They can occur at any point along the optic pathway. In 10% to 38% of cases (25% average), there is an association with NF-1 (von Recklinghausen disease). OPG is commonly seen in pediatric population (mean age at presentation of 8.5 years; 5 years-old in NF-1 and 12 years-old in the absence of neurofibromatosis, and more than 80% occurring before 20 years of age). Optic nerve gliomas tend to occur more often in females, whereas chiasmal tumors are present equally in males and females; 33% to 60% of chiasmatic gliomas extend into the hypothalamus or third ventricle.
- World Health Organization (WHO) grade I pilocytic astrocytoma is the most frequently seen histopathology and has a favorable prognosis. Malignant glioma is rarely seen, mostly occurring in adults with poor prognosis.
- Patients may be asymptomatic or have variable symptoms (strabismus, visual loss, afferent pupillary defect, and proptosis). Decreased visual acuity occurs late in the course of OPG.
- MR is the imaging modality of choice. A tortuous enlarged nerve usually appears isointense on T1WI and iso to hyperintense on T2WI. OPGs may have cystic components associated with them (as a result of ischemia, radiation therapy, or mucin deposition). The nerve-tumor complex may display kinks or buckling, and perineural axial growth. These lesions demonstrate variable enhancement (Fig. 9.21).
- CT reveals an enlarged optic nerve sheath and canal (if the lesion extends through the optic canal). Enhancement is variable, and calcification is rare unless the patient has been previously treated with radiation.

### Optic Nerve Sheath Meningioma
- Orbital optic nerve sheath meningiomas present with the insidious onset of visual loss, optic atrophy, mild proptosis, and opticociliary shunts (dilated veins from the optic nerve head, observed in 32% of cases). These lesions have a predominance for middle-aged females but may also be seen in children with NF-1 or NF-2 in adults (possibly bilaterally).
- CT findings include a high-density mass that demonstrates enhancement (Fig. 9.22). Calcification is seen in 20% to 50% of the cases (as opposed to optic nerve gliomas, which do not calcify). The "tram-track" sign is a term for the CT appearance of enhancement or calcification of the sheath surrounding of the optic nerve. Bony changes may be present in the region of the optic nerve canal with bone erosion and occasionally hyperostosis.
- MR reveals isointensity or slight hypointensity on T1WI and intermediate intensity on T2WI (see Fig. 9.22). Optic nerve sheath meningiomas enhance (particularly evident with fat-saturation techniques). The enhancement on axial MR has been analogized to "tram-tracks" in the axial plane or a doughnut in the coronal plane. The differential diagnoses include pseudotumor, sarcoid, metastatic disease, lymphoma, and leukemia.
- Perioptic cysts can sometimes be seen on MR, evidenced by dilated subarachnoid space between the distal edge of the optic nerve sheath meningioma and the globe.
- MR is useful for orbital apex and intracanalicular lesions, whereas detection on CT might be difficult in this region because of the high density of adjacent bone.

### Vascular Lesions
- **Infantile hemangiomas** are the most common orbital tumors in infancy. They favor girls and premature infants and present at a mean age just under 1 year old. They may appear in the skin, the subcutaneous tissues, and the extraconal (more often than the intraconal) orbit (Fig. 9.23).
  - They do not present at birth but are seen during the first few weeks to months of life. Infantile hemangiomas have an initial proliferative phase (where they undergo rapid growth), followed by an involutional phase. As they involute between ages 2 and 8, they may undergo fibrofatty change.

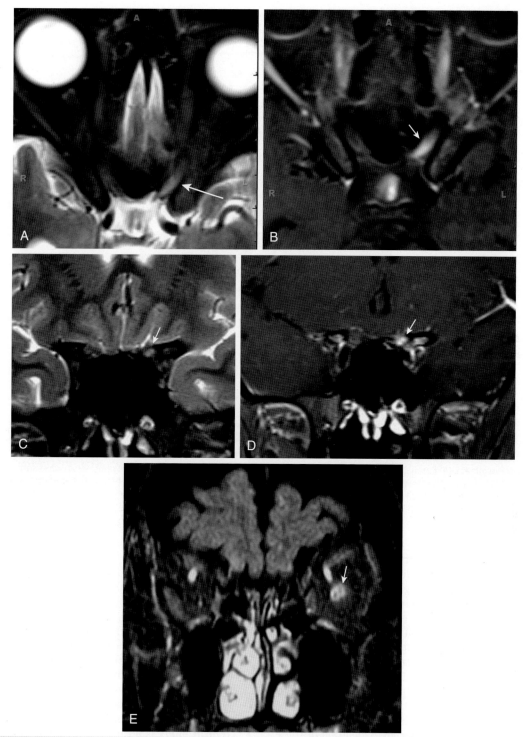

**Fig. 9.20 Optic neuritis.** (A) Axial T2-weighted imaging (T2WI) *(arrows)*, (B) postcontrast T1 *(arrows)*, (C) coronal T2WI *(arrows)*, and (D) postcontrast T1-weighted imaging (T1WI) show abnormal signal and enhancement in the left optic nerve. (E) If you do fluid attenuation coupled with fat suppression, as in this case, you can see the bright left optic neuritis *(arrows)* really well.

- These tumors express glucose transporter 1 (GLUT-1) on immunohistochemical testing. They may be associated with PHACE syndrome (posterior fossa malformations, hemangiomas, arterial anomalies, cardiac defects, eye and endocrine abnormalities, and sternal defects).
- These lesions are typically T2 hyperintense and show homogeneous contrast enhancement. The lesions often show an artery feeding it and are opacified in the arterial phase of a dynamic MR enhanced scan. Flow voids, fibrous tissue, and calcification can be seen in the lesion.
- **Congenital hemangiomas** are less commonly seen. They are fully developed at birth and do not grow. The congenital hemangiomas may demonstrate a rapidly involuting congenital hemangioma (RICH) or

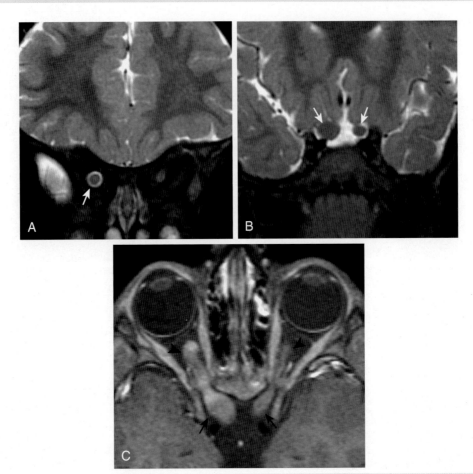

**Fig. 9.21 Optic nerve glioma.** (A) Coronal T2-weighted image (T2WI) shows marked enlargement of the right optic nerve *(white arrow)* compared with the left. Often the T2WI signal of the nerve is normal and, because of the low grade, the tumors may not enhance. (B) More posteriorly at the level of the suprasellar cistern, coronal T2WI shows both optic nerves are markedly enlarged *(white arrows)*, right more than left. (C) Postcontrast T1WI shows enhancement along the involved optic nerve segments within the orbit *(black arrowheads)* and in the suprasellar cistern *(black arrows)*.

noninvoluting congenital hemangioma (NICH) progression. These are difficult to distinguish from infantile hemangiomas based on imaging alone.

- **Venous vascular malformations** (VVMs), previously called *cavernous hemangiomas* (but no longer because they are not tumors like hemangiomas are!), are slow-flow vascular malformation, consisting of dilated endothelial lined vascular channels encompassed by a fibrous pseudocapsule.
  - VVMs are the most common primary orbital vascular mass in adults, presenting in the second to fifth decade of life. They occur in females more commonly than males. There has been a reported association of these lesions with intracranial vascular malformations, blue rubber bleb nevus syndrome, and Maffucci syndrome.
  - Patients typically present with the slow onset of painless proptosis and may have visual disturbance. Growth can be exceedingly slow and may stop after a certain time; however, rapid growth has been observed during pregnancy.
  - CT shows smoothly marginated high-density round or oval intraconal mass that densely enhances with or without phleboliths (that do not occur in infantile hemangioma). Rarely they may be extraconal. Orbital bone expansion may be present.

- On MR, the lesion appears as smoothly marginated, intraconal mass that has no flow voids and demonstrates marked enhancement. VVMs are isointense to muscle and hypointense to fat on T1WI and high intensity on T2WI (Fig. 9.24). On early postcontrast images, they enhance in a patchy fashion with progressive enhancement on delayed images (totally fill in within 30 minutes). They opacify in the later venous phase of the dynamic MR angiography (MRA). There may be combined venolymphatic malformations of the orbit, which have both venous (enhancing) and lymphatic (nonenhancing) components.

- **Orbital varix** is a rare venous malformation. It can be divided into primary, which is idiopathic and most likely congenital, and secondary, which is acquired and associated with carotid-cavernous fistula, dural arteriovenous fistulas, or intracranial arteriovenous malformations and venous vascular malformations (these are discussed in Chapter 3). The spectrum can range from a single dilated venous structure to multiple varicosities.
  - Patients can present with intermittent proptosis in conjunction with Valsalva maneuvers, such as straining or coughing, that increase venous pressure and retrobulbar pain.
  - CT reveals a soft-tissue density lesion of variable shape (such as tubular, tortuous) or may appear as mass-like

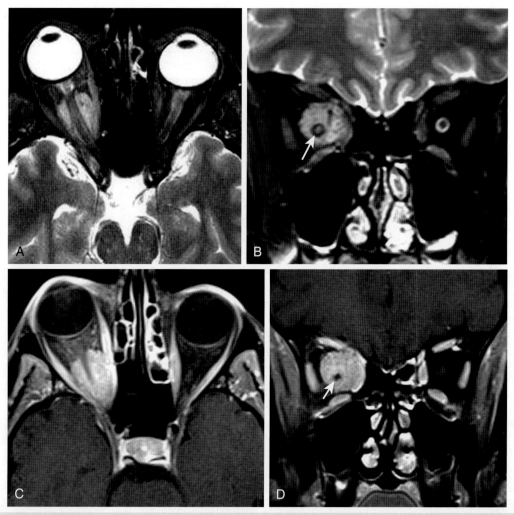

**Fig. 9.22 Optic nerve meningiomas.** (A) Axial and (B) coronal T2-weighted images show hyperintense mass circumferentially investing the right optic nerve *(white arrow)*. There is proptosis of the right globe as a result. Note the elevated T2 signal within the nerve because of the compressive effect by the mass. (C) Axial and (D) coronal postcontrast T1-weighted images show homogeneous contrast enhancement of the mass. (D) Note the nonenhancing optic nerve encased by the tumor *(white arrow)*.

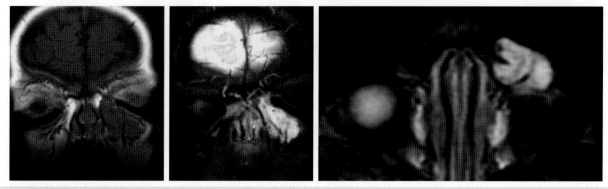

**Fig. 9.23 Rapidly involuting congenital hemangioma (RICH).** This child had a raised red lesion along the left lower eyelid that extended into the orbit that was present at birth. Fortunately, over months it involuted, hence a RICH.

lesion with intense enhancement on enhanced CT. If thrombosis occurs, it appears as high attenuation on noncontrast CT. Varices will increase in size with provocative maneuver that increases venous pressure, such as Valsalva maneuver or prone position (Fig. 9.25).

■ On MR, the venous varices may have complex signal intensity and variable appearance because of clot or hemorrhage. MR may demonstrate turbulent flow in the varix detected as a flow void within the lesion.

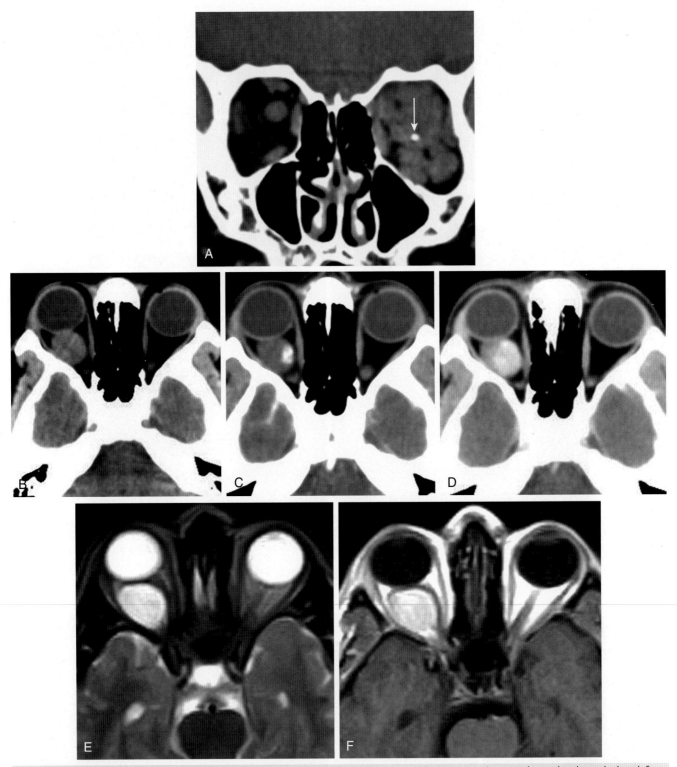

**Fig. 9.24 Venous vascular malformation (VVM).** (A) Note the calcification *(arrow)* among the numerous intraconal vascular channels that define this as a venous vascular malformation. (B) A more classic VVM in a different patient on noncontrast, followed by (C) early and (D) delayed contrast-enhanced computed tomographic images seen as a well-defined intraconal enhancing mass that accrues contrast over time. The same lesion is bright on T2 (E) and shows avid enhancement on postcontrast T1 (F) images.

- **Venolymphatic malformations** (VLM), formerly known as *lymphangiomas*, are congenital no-flow or low-flow vascular malformations, consisting of dysplastic lymphatic and venous channels (lymphatic or venous). They arise from the pluripotent venous anlage. They may be categorized into microcystic and macrocystic (formerly *cystic hygromas*) lymphatic malformations based on cysts greater than or less than 2 cm.
  - VLM may be evident at birth but usually present in childhood. They tend to hemorrhage with the acute onset of symptoms.

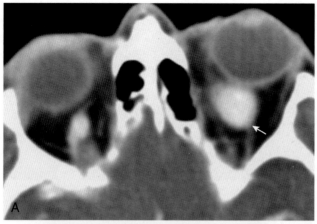

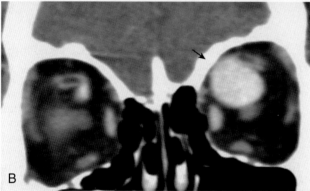

**Fig. 9.25 Venous varix.** (A) Note both the mild left proptosis and the enlarged vascular structure in the left eye *(white arrow)*. (B) On the coronal view one can see that this vessel represents the enlarged superior ophthalmic vein in a venous varix *(black arrow)*. The normal-sized right vein can be seen in comparison.

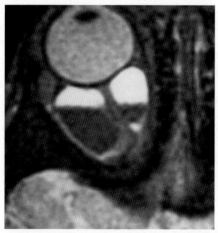

**Fig. 9.26 Venolymphatic malformation.** Axial proton density–weighted imaging in a young patient who had acute proptosis demonstrates hemorrhagic fluid levels as is typically seen with these lesions.

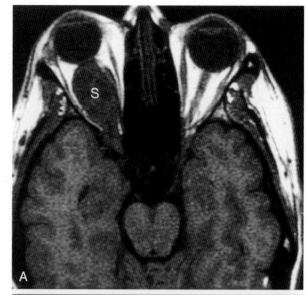

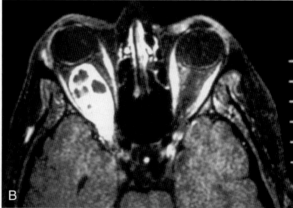

**Fig. 9.27 Schwannoma of the orbit (nerve unknown).** (A) Unenhanced T1-weighted image (T1WI) shows intraconal mass in the right orbit *(S)* causing proptosis. (B) Postcontrast T1WI shows inhomogeneous contrast enhancement of the lesion because of the presence of cystic components that don't enhance.

- VLMs are not well encapsulated and can be multicompartmental, involving both intraconal and extraconal spaces.
- CT demonstrates irregular mass crossing anatomic boundaries and increased density on unenhanced CT scan with variable enhancement after contrast administration. Peripheral enhancement can be demonstrated in cystic regions of the lesion. There may be bony expansion of the orbit. Phleboliths may present in the venous component of the lesion.
- MR reveals multiple or single cysts with variable signal intensity from different ages of blood product and "fluid-fluid levels" (Fig. 9.26).

### Other Neoplasms

- Neurogenic tumors can arise from orbital branches of CN III, IV, V, VI, sympathetic and parasympathetic nerves, and the ciliary ganglion. They include schwannomas, neurofibromas, and amputation neuromas.
- Schwannomas appear similar to those in other locations with cystic and solid components and a propensity to enhance (Fig. 9.27). Neurofibromas may be localized, diffuse, or plexiform, all three associated with neurofibromatosis, with plexiform being pathognomonic.
- Metastases and lymphoma can involve any part of the orbit, presenting as intraconal, conal, or extraconal lesions.

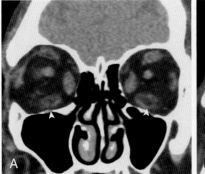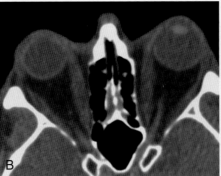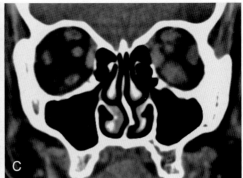

**Fig. 9.28  Thyroid ophthalmopathy.** (A) Thyroid eye disease (TED) manifests proptosis and enlargement of extraocular muscles. Sometimes there is fatty infiltration of the muscles, as seen in these enlarged inferior recti muscles *(arrowheads)*. In this case, the medial recti are also large and the disease is bilateral. (B) Classic medial rectus involvement. (C) Yes, even for unilateral proptosis, TED is the most common diagnosis. TED gets around.

- Metastatic scirrhous breast carcinoma and neuroblastoma in children have a propensity for the extraconal space and enophthalmos and are discussed in the extraconal lesion section.

## Conal Lesions

- **Thyroid eye disease** (Graves orbitopathy, thyroid eye disease, thyroid orbitopathy) leading to proptosis can be present in euthyroid or hyperthyroid persons. Females have a 4 to 1 predominance over males. It may occur before, during, or after treatment and has a subacute onset, extending for months.
  - Signs and symptoms of Graves orbitopathy, including lid lag, diplopia, limited extraocular muscle movements, proptosis, and optic nerve compression result from the periorbital fibrosis that develops when the inflammation resolves. In patients with clinical thyroid ophthalmopathy, 85% have bilateral involvement, 5% have unilateral involvement, and 10% have normal muscles.
  - CT exhibits extraocular muscle enlargement and exophthalmos (greater than two thirds of the globes project anterior to a line connecting lateral orbital wall anterior-most borders [interzygomatic line]). There is fusiform enlargement of the muscle belly with sparing of the muscle insertion, and protrusion of the orbital fat. Coronal scanning is the method of choice for assessing muscle thickness. The most frequently affected muscles are the inferior and medial recti, although the most common single pattern is enlargement of all muscles. The lateral rectus muscle is rarely, if ever, involved alone and is the last to be affected when all muscles are involved (Fig. 9.28). Try this mnemonic for remembering the frequency of muscle involvement—**I'm slo**(w)—inferior, medial, superior, lateral, oblique muscle involvement.
  - Other findings include increased orbital fat (also has been reported to be caused by exogenous steroids and Cushing disease), fatty infiltration of extraocular muscles, swollen lacrimal glands and eyelids, and dilatation of the superior ophthalmic vein.
  - MR may not add much more useful information than CT. Increased T2 signal intensity of the extraocular muscles has been reported, most likely inflammatory changes (increased water content). T2 signal intensity is decreased in those with fibrosis.
  - Multiplanar MR or CT is important in assessing the degree of optic nerve compression by the enlarged muscles at the orbital apex, which is best appreciated on a coronal image. In extreme cases where vision is threatened, orbital decompression is performed with partial removal of the floor or medial wall of the orbit.
- **Idiopathic orbital inflammation (IOI)** has many names: nonspecific orbital inflammation, inflammatory pseudotumor, orbital pseudotumor, and orbital inflammatory syndrome.
  - IOI is a diagnosis of exclusion because it mimics a variety of pathologic states so the appropriate history is essential for making the correct diagnosis. The clinical features include restriction of ocular motility, chemosis, lid swelling, and pain. It is a cause of unilateral exophthalmos. These findings usually have a rapid onset and respond to steroids, although there is also a chronic form with progressive fibrosis and a mild or poor response to steroids.
  - The cause of IOI is currently unknown but believed to be immune-related. It may involve any part of the orbit including the lacrimal gland (dacryoadenitis), the extraocular muscles (myositis), the connective tissue surrounding the dura of the optic nerve (perineuritis), the orbital fat, the epibulbar connective tissue and the sclera (episcleritis/scleritis), and the orbital apex. It can also diffusely involve the orbit or has a mass-like appearance.

---

**TEACHING POINTS**

Facts on Idiopathic Orbital Inflammation (IOI)

- Systemic diseases associated with IOI include IGg-4 related disease, granulomatosis with polyangiitis, polyarteritis nodosa, sarcoidosis, and autoimmune conditions such as lupus erythematosus, dermatomyositis, and rheumatoid arthritis.
- Related and associated fibrotic processes include retroperitoneal fibrosis, sclerosing cholangitis, Riedel thyroiditis, and mediastinal fibrosis. The term *multifocal fibrosclerosis* is used as a collective description of these disorders.

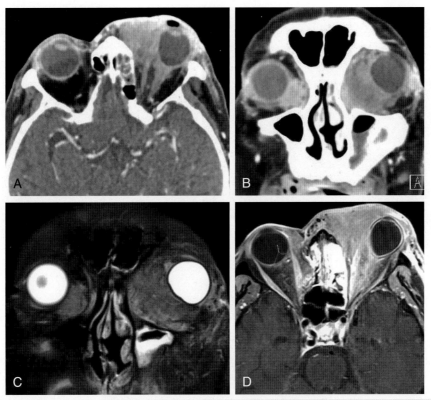

**Fig. 9.29 Idiopathic orbital inflammation.** (A) Axial contrast-enhanced computed tomographic image shows bulky enhancing mass centered in the preseptal tissues/postseptal extraconal medial orbit on the left, distorting the globe and displacing it laterally. (B) On coronal view, there's another mass in the inferomedial orbit on the right. (C) These orbital masses are intermediate signal on T2 and show avid enhancement on postcontrast T1-weighted images (D).

- On imaging, IOI may present as a diffuse, ill-defined retrobulbar enhancing mass obscuring fascial plane, or simply as thickened muscles and/or their tendons and sheaths (Fig. 9.29). Over 70% of cases display proptosis. There may be a subtle increase in the density of orbital fat (dirty fat) or optic nerve thickening.
- The contour of the enlarged muscles may not be smooth, and the tendinous insertions may be affected (in contrast to Graves disease), but not always. At times, IOI may be bilateral and may show intracranial extension.
- On T1WI and T2WI, IOI tends to be low intensity, whereas metastatic lesions have a longer T2.
- **IgG4-related disease** is an inflammatory process of unknown etiology, in which IgG4-positive plasma cells and elevated serum IgG4 are found and can affect any organ system (most commonly the pancreas, hepatobiliary system, salivary glands, orbits, and retroperitoneal space). More recent data suggests that IOI in fact might be part of the disease spectrum of IGg4-lreated diseases. When the orbit is involved, extraocular muscle enlargement is the most common finding but lacrimal gland enlargement, orbital inflammatory soft tissue masses, nerve enlargement, and sinus disease can be seen.
  - MRI characteristics support the densely fibrotic nature of this lesion, including T1 hypointensity, T2 dark signal, and mild contrast enhancement.
- **Tolosa-Hunt syndrome** is an idiopathic inflammatory process within the IOI spectrum that involves the cavernous sinus and orbital apex, classically presenting with painful ophthalmoplegia. Inflammatory tissue can be identified in the orbital apex in the majority of cases.
  - On CT, the low density of orbital fat is replaced by soft tissue. This is a subtle but important finding in lesions of the orbital apex. On MR, soft tissue is isointense to muscle and can be recognized at the orbital apex and/ or the cavernous sinus. This tissue enhances and has signal intensity changes identical to lymphoma, sarcoid, IgG4-related disease, and meningioma, which are in the differential.
- **Sarcoidosis** commonly involves the orbit. Uveitis is the most common manifestation of orbital sarcoidosis, but other sites of involvement include the lacrimal gland, optic nerve/sheath, chiasm, muscles, and retrobulbar tissue producing proptosis (Fig. 9.30). Isolated orbital disease without pulmonary findings is rare; when limited to the orbit, it usually affects the lacrimal glands.
- **Granulomatosis with polyangiitis** (formerly Wegener granulomatosis) is characterized by granulomatous inflammation, tissue necrosis, and vasculitis that involve arteries, veins, and capillaries. It may involve the orbit secondarily from the paranasal sinuses or may present as primary orbital disease. Up to 54% of all patients with the systemic condition have neurologic involvement, and half have disease in the orbit.
  - The most common ocular manifestations are keratitis and scleritis, whereas the orbital involvement produces pain, proptosis, erythematous eyelid edema, and limitation of extraocular movements caused by conal and intraconal spread. The ocular and orbital processes

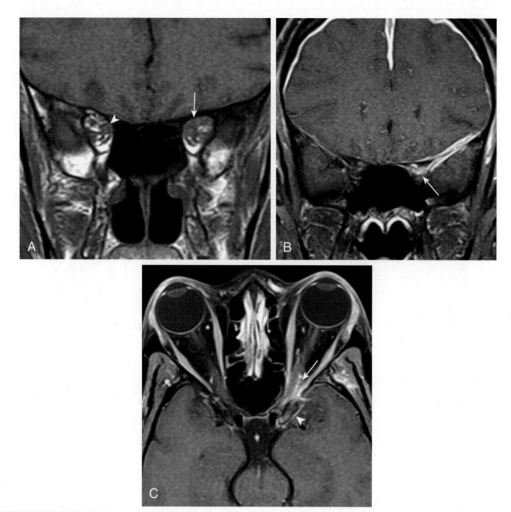

**Fig. 9.30 Orbital sarcoidosis.** (A) Coronal T1-weighted image (T1WI) shows T1 hypointense soft-tissue infiltration at the left orbital apex *(arrow)*. Compare to the normal expected fatty signal surrounding the optic nerve sheath at the apex on the right *(arrowhead)*. (B) Postcontrast T1WI shows abnormal enhancement of this tissue as it invests the optic nerve sheath on the left *(arrow)*. Note extensive dural-based enhancement intracranially. (C) Axial postcontrast T1WI again shows the abnormal enhancement along the optic nerve sheath complex on the left *(arrow)* and adjacent dural enhancement around the left optic strut *(arrowhead)*.

may coexist. Orbital inflammation may cause painful swelling, proptosis, nasal-lacrimal obstruction, or dacryocystitis. Antineutrophil cytoplasmic antibodies are highly sensitive indicators of the disease.

- On MR, this condition has been reported to be hypointense relative to orbital fat on T2WI and enhance homogeneously. The classic lesion is a homogeneously enhancing mass with associated sinus and nasal septal disease and bone destruction (Fig. 9.31). The anterior segment is usually involved more than the posterior segment.

- **Lymphoproliferative disorders** of the orbit are the most commonly primary orbital tumor in adults with the spectrum ranging from benign lymphoid hyperplasia to malignant lymphoma. Lymphoma may occur as a primary orbital tumor or may be associated with systemic lymphoma. In the primary orbital lymphoma, non Hodgkin lymphoma is the most common histology, specifically the mucosa-associated lymphoid tissue (MALT) subtype. Lymphoma is generally seen in older persons presenting with slowly progressive painless periorbital swelling and low-grade proptosis. Most of the cases have unilateral involvement.

- CT reveals a diffuse infiltrative mass that destroys the normal orbital architecture so that anatomic structures cannot be defined. On CT, one may see increased density on the precontrast scan. The lesions can extensively infiltrate muscles and/or the lacrimal gland. Bone destruction is rare (Fig. 9.32).

- On MR, distinguishing lymphoma from orbital IOI on MR is problematic because signal intensities and location are similar, but the latter is painful. Many lymphomas are characterized by very low apparent diffusion coefficient (ADC) values.

### Extraconal Lesions

Orbital infections are among the most common concern prompting imaging of the orbits.

### Periorbital Cellulitis

- The clinical manifestations of preseptal cellulitis are swelling and erythema of the skin and subcutaneous tissues of the eyelids. There is no evidence of proptosis, disturbances of ocular motility, or chemosis. Preseptal periorbital cellulitis is treated medically as an outpatient, and generally imaging is not required.

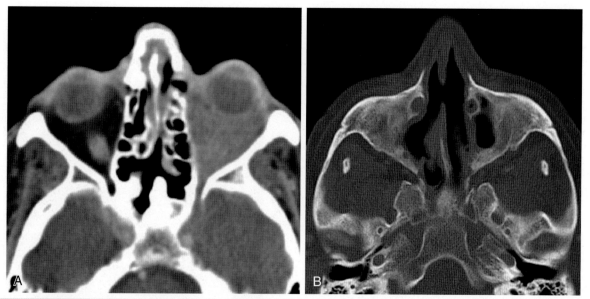

**Fig. 9.31 Granulomatosis with polyangiitis.** (A) On the axial contrast-enhanced computed tomography (CT) image, there is diffuse infiltrative enhancing lesion in left orbit involving intraconal and extraconal spaces. (B) In this same patient, note mucosal thickening and chronic osteitic change of bilateral maxillary sinus walls. Perforation of the nasal septum is also observed.

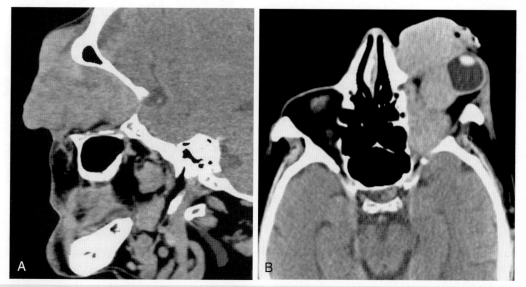

**Fig. 9.32 Lymphoma.** (A) Massive hyperdense tumor in the left orbit on noncontrast computed tomography (CT) without bone destruction favors lymphoma over other cancers. Note tented appearance of the posterior globe margin in (B).

## Orbital Cellulitis and Complications

- The orbital septum is a reflection of orbital periosteum (periorbita) inserting on the tarsal plate of the eyelid. The periorbita is an excellent barrier to neoplastic or inflammatory disease emanating from the sinuses.
- Orbital (postseptal) cellulitis is deep to the orbital septum. It presents with painful ophthalmoplegia, proptosis, chemosis, and decreasing visual acuity. In these cases, imaging is necessary to evaluate the extent of inflammation hiding behind the globe, not directly visible by the examining clinician. Stages of orbital cellulitis are most commonly characterized by the Chandler classification scheme.

**TEACHING POINTS**

Chandler Classification System for Orbital Infections

| Chandler Stage | Features |
|---|---|
| I | Preseptal cellulitis only |
| II | Postseptal orbital fat stranding and edema |
| III | Subperiosteal abscess at lamina papyracea |
| IV | Orbital abscess |
| V | Cavernous sinus thrombosis via superior ophthalmic vein thrombophlebitis |

■ The causes of orbital cellulitis include sinus infection (particularly in the pediatric population, most commonly arising from the ethmoid sinus), bacteremia, skin infection (secondary to trauma, insect bite, and impetigo), or foreign body. Frank abscess may be seen in this setting and can be large enough to cause proptosis and optic nerve sheath stretching, which could portend permanent visual loss. In severe cases, globe tenting (posterior globe with conical configuration) may be seen. If aggressive IV antibiotics are not immediately effective, the abscess may require surgical drainage, often via an endoscopic approach. Orbital abscess is the fourth stage of the Chandler's classification of orbital infection.

### TEACHING POINTS

Nonbacterial Orbital Infections

• Although most cases are bacterial in nature, fungal infection of the orbit can occur, primarily in the immunocompromised individuals, such as those with human immunodeficiency virus (HIV) infection and diabetes.
  • *Aspergillosis* and *Mucormycosis* are the most common fungal orbital infections.
  • The infection usually initiates in the paranasal sinus and extends into the orbit and can result in cavernous sinus inflammation and thrombosis.
  • Think orbital aspergillosis in HIV patients with proptosis, pain, visual loss, and ophthalmoplegia.
• Herpes zoster ophthalmicus, a grouped vesicular eruption, occurs along the dermatomal distribution of first division of cranial nerve V. It is observed in both immunosuppressed and nonimmunosuppressed (usually elderly) individuals. This can be a virulent infection where the virus grows along the optic nerve and vessels producing infarction of the optic nerve and large-vessel vasculitis in the brain.

■ Intracranial complications (including Chandler stage 5 cavernous sinus thrombosis) are associated with a 50% to 80% mortality rate, hence the urgency.
■ CT has an advantage over MR in the diagnosis of orbital cellulitis because of its ability to visualize the air-filled sinuses and demonstrate foreign bodies.
■ CT can distinguish between preseptal cellulitis, orbital cellulitis, and subperiosteal infection (Fig. 9.33).
  ■ *Periorbital cellulitis:* Swelling and obliteration of the preseptal soft tissues without extension deep to the orbital septum.
  ■ *Orbital (postseptal) cellulitis:* Diffuse soft tissue stranding posterior to the orbital septum. The orbital tissue planes are poorly defined, and there may be either an intraconal or an extraconal soft-tissue mass.
■ On MRI, there is stranding of the orbital fat best appreciated on T1WI precontrast. On fat saturated T1WI MR, one can detect enhancement in the preseptal and postseptal tissue, particularly the extraocular muscles or retrobulbar fat.
■ Focal organized collection with ring enhancement suggests discrete abscess on CT and MRI.

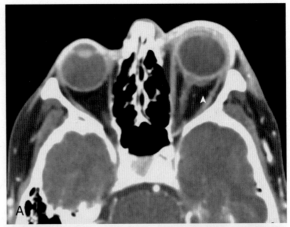

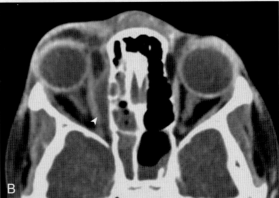

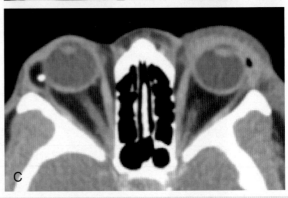

**Fig. 9.33 Manifestations of orbital infection.** (A) Postseptal orbital cellulitis. Computed tomography (CT) shows soft tissue behind the globe *(arrowhead)* and as diffuse thickening over the left globe. Disease behind the orbital septum makes this orbital cellulitis. (B) Subperiosteal abscess. Appreciate the lateral extension of the ethmoid sinusitis into the subperiosteal region fluid collection *(arrowhead)* with lateral displacement of the medial rectus muscle and orbital fat. There is also significant preseptal swelling. (C) Preseptal periorbital cellulitis. There is pronounced left preseptal swelling but no post-septal extension. Note the incidental cute lacrimal fossa dermoid on the right!

■ Subperiosteal abscess is located between the bony wall of the orbit and the periosteum. On CT and MRI, it is characterized as a lentiform rim-enhancing fluid collection along the orbital wall, which demonstrates restricted diffusion and adjacent sinusitis. The most common location of these lesions is in the medial orbit adjacent to the ethmoid air cells. Keep in mind that air-filled sinuses can cause significant distortion on DWI, so don't let the appearance on DWI be your be-all end-all in making this diagnosis.

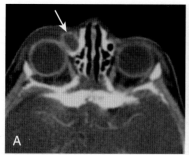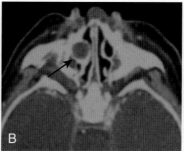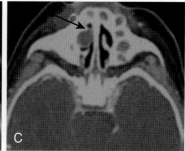

**Fig. 9.34 Dacrocystitis.** (A–C) Peripherally enhancing fluid collection *(arrows)* arising from the nasolacrimal duct canal in this little one indicates infected dacryocystocele. Note associated preseptal soft tissue swelling.

- Orbital infection can produce venous thrombosis of the orbital veins with extension into the cavernous sinus. For this reason, it is important to image the brain in cases of orbital cellulitis complicated by abscess to look for potential intracranial complications, such as frontal epidural abscess, subdural empyema, or an intraparenchymal abscess. Look for absence of enhancement within an asymmetrically enlarged superior ophthalmic vein with possible extension to the cavernous sinus to call venous thrombosis.

### Lacrimal Gland Pathologies

- **Dacryoadenitis** is inflammation/infection of the lacrimal gland. It may be seen in the setting of Mikulicz syndrome (nonspecific swelling of the lacrimal and salivary glands in association with Sjogren syndrome and IgG-related inflammatory disorders). Other conditions such as sarcoid, tuberculosis, IOI, and granulomatosis with polyangiitis can also cause inflammation of the lacrimal gland. Imaging findings of glandular enlargement and hyperenhancement should raise concern for the diagnosis, although precise etiology is determined by the clinical context.
- **Dacryocystitis** is an infection typically caused by obstruction of the lacrimal sac or the nasolacrimal duct and may be acquired as the result of the trauma or congenitally, in the setting of pre-existing dacryocystocele.
  - On imaging, lacrimal sac dilatation is observed on CT or MR, and preseptal swelling and/or cellulitis can be noted in the setting of superimposed infection (Fig. 9.34). Enhancement is seen in the walls of the dilated sac, more pronounced in setting of infection than with dacryocystocele.
- **Neoplasms arising from the lacrimal gland** are histologically similar to the salivary glands. Lymphoid (hyperplasia, lymphoma) and inflammatory lesions make up about one third of lacrimal masses, epithelial tumors represent one half, and the remainder are mesenchymal or metastatic in nature. Malignant disease of the lacrimal gland is rare.
  - The most common tumor is benign mixed tumor (pleomorphic adenoma). Common presentations of patients with lacrimal gland tumors include a palpable lacrimal fossa mass or proptosis. Pleomorphic adenomas have variable appearance on CT and MR depending on the composition and cellularity of the tumors.

They may have cystic degeneration or necrosis and hemorrhage in large tumors. With long-standing lesions, remodeling, lysis, or excavation of bone may be present. Minimal or moderate enhancement can be observed.
- Adenoid cystic carcinoma (most common epithelial malignant tumor) presents with pain, diplopia, and visual loss during a 3- to 6-month period. Bone involvement is common. The overall 5-year survival is 21%, and death is usually secondary to intracranial spread. This tumor has a propensity for perineural spread into the cavernous sinus.
- Mucoepidermoid carcinoma displays high density on plain CT that markedly enhances. Along with sebaceous carcinoma, it may reveal high intensity on T1WI.
- Lymphoid hyperplasia appears as glandular enlargement with a homogeneous density on CT. Generalized contrast enhancement can be seen. A mass lesion in the lacrimal fossa that does not produce bony erosion is most likely lymphoid (lymphoma or lymphoid hyperplasia), whereas epithelial neoplasms generally involve bone. Lymphoma demonstrates diffuse homogeneous involvement of the lacrimal gland that molds to the bony orbit or globe.
- Other malignant tumors include adenocarcinoma, malignant mixed cell tumors, squamous cell carcinoma, undifferentiated (anaplastic carcinoma, sebaceous carcinoma, and metastasis).

### Mucoceles

- Mucoceles are expansile mucus containing cysts typically arising from the sinonasal cavity than can present with extraconal mass effect, diplopia, and proptosis when enlarged. The common locations are the frontal and ethmoidal sinuses. Patients typically have a history of sinusitis, allergy, or trauma.
- CT demonstrates a fluid density smoothly marginated mass (with an enhancing rim) centered in the sinus. Bowing and thinning of the adjacent bony margins of the orbit can be seen.
- On MR, mucoceles have variable intensities depending on the protein concentration and viscosity but commonly are observed to be high intensity on T1WI and T2WI (Fig. 9.35). They demonstrate peripheral enhancement as opposed to neoplasms, which have solid enhancement. These are discussed further in Chapter 12.

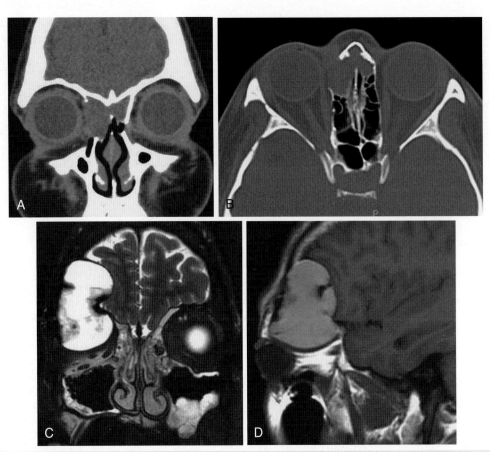

**Fig. 9.35 Mucocele.** (A) Frontoethmoidal mucocele with thinning of the bony wall of the sinus. (B) Note the dehiscent wall of the ethmoid sinus. (C) Different patient with right frontal mucocele demonstrating bright signal on T2-weighted imaging (T2WI) and high signal on T1WI (D) with mass effect on the globe.

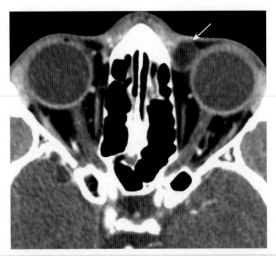

**Fig. 9.36 Computed tomographic image of orbital dermoid: a sight for sore eyes.** There is a smoothly marginated nonenhancing fluid-attenuating mass *(arrow)* abutting the medial left globe. If we saw fat in the lesion, the diagnosis would be a no-brainer. However, identification of fat is not always appreciable on imaging, especially when it's microscopic.

## Dermoids/Epidermoids

- Dermoid and epidermoid cysts (Fig. 9.36) are the most common benign congenital lesion of the orbit (infantile hemangiomas are the most common congenital tumors), accounting for 1% to 2% of all orbital masses. They arise from ectodermal elements trapped in the suture line.
- They usually present in the first decade of life but can be subclinical until adulthood, where they may present by rupturing, inducing granulomatous inflammation, and scar formation.
- The most common location is the superolateral portion of the orbit at the frontozygomatic suture near the lacrimal fossa. These lesions are extraconal and displace the globe medially and inferiorly. They can also arise medially, inferiorly, or posteriorly.
- On CT, you will see a low-density mass and may have either no enhancement or a thin enhancing margin. Dermoid may exhibit fat attenuation and partial marginal calcification. Bony scalloping or remodeling is present. Inflammatory changes of the surrounding tissues can be seen in ruptured dermoid.
- On MR cystic appearance (low signal intensity on T1WI and high signal intensity on T2WI) is expected with epidermoid lesions. Fat component is high signal on T1WI, which suppresses with fat-saturation techniques in the setting of dermoid. Fat may be seen floating in cystic fluid on T1WI with dermoid lesions.

## Orbital Rhabdomyosarcoma

- Orbital rhabdomyosarcoma is the most common primary malignant orbital tumor of childhood as well as the most common site of head and neck rhabdomyosarcomas.

Mean age is 7 to 8 years with 90% occurring before the age of 16 years. Children present with rapidly progressive painless exophthalmos, although about 10% may have headache or periorbital discomfort. On examination, a mass may be palpable and ecchymosis, conjunctival chemosis, and ophthalmoplegia may be present.

- Primary orbital tumor arises from pluripotential mesenchymal cells and may be extraconal or both intra- and extraconal with the superonasal and superior orbit the most typical locations. Secondary involvement can be seen in the nasopharynx, pterygopalatine fossa, infratemporal fossa, or paranasal sinuses (so-called *parameningeal sites*).
- On CT, rhabdomyosarcomas present as an isodense or slightly hyperdense well-defined mass and uniformly enhances. Heterogeneous enhancement is seen in tumor with necrosis and hemorrhage. Bone erosion can be seen in 40% of the cases.
- On MR these lesions are homogeneous, well-defined, moderate-marked enhancing masses, usually isointense on T1WI and hyperintense on T2WI relative to muscle. MR reveals the extent of tumor spread and intracranial extension and this has important prognostic implications.
- Beware that orbital sarcomas of any variety may be seen in the setting of retinoblastoma, be it from the hereditary variety or as a consequence/complication of early age radiation therapy.

## Metastases (Extraocular)

- Metastases account for approximately 10% of orbital neoplasms with an average survival after detection of approximately 9 months. Patients complain of diplopia, ptosis, proptosis, eyelid swelling, pain, and visual loss. Metastasis may be seen involving both soft tissue and bony orbit. Breast and lung cancers account for over 50% of orbital metastases. Bone metastasis to the orbit most commonly involve the greater wing of the sphenoid, affecting the lateral extraconal space. Perineural tumor spread from extraorbital primary tumors can reach the orbit via the superior orbital fissure, inferior orbital fissure, infraorbital nerve canal, and optic canal; some common players include adenoid cystic, squamous cell, and nasopharyngeal carcinomas.
- CT depicts the orbital and cranial soft-tissue components of the lesion. Metastatic lesions are isodense or high density on unenhanced scan and may enhance after contrast administration.
- Infiltrative retrobulbar mass with enophthalmos is characteristic of scirrhous breast carcinoma.
- Metastatic disease may account for 7% of cases of extraocular muscle enlargement found on CT. Isolated enlargement of the lateral rectus should be thought to be secondary to metastasis, idiopathic orbital inflammation or infection, as it does not occur in Graves.
- In childhood, metastatic neuroblastoma is the second most frequent malignant orbital tumor (after rhabdomyosarcoma) with 8% presenting initially with orbital lesions.
  - Metastasis to the bone displaces or elevates the periosteum, producing a smooth extraconal mass

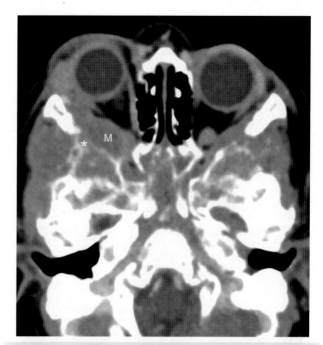

**Fig. 9.37 Neuroblastoma metastases.** Sutural-based metastases centered at the sphenozygomatic suture bilaterally (indicated with *asterisk* on right) are associated with bulky extraosseous soft-tissue tumor extending into the extraconal orbit bilaterally (indicated with *M* on right). There is resulting proptosis on the right. Note extraosseous tumor extension into the masticator space bilaterally and mottled appearance of the central skull base because of additional bony metastases.

(Fig. 9.37). Neuroblastoma metastasis may be found at bony sutures/growth plates.

- These lesions can be high density on CT or display MR characteristics of blood secondary to intratumoral hemorrhage. Neuroblastoma can be distinguished from rhabdomyosarcoma by its high-density values and its lack of preseptal extension (which is much more common in rhabdomyosarcoma).

## Sphenoid Wing Meningioma

- Sphenoid wing meningioma (Fig. 9.38, A and B) presents as a mass associated with hyperostosis displacing extraocular muscles and causing proptosis. It can have a sizable component both in the orbit and intracranially. Proptosis from extraosseous tissue, a blistered appearance to the bone, or purely intraosseous mass can be seen with meningiomas.

## Fibrous Dysplasia

- In fibrous dysplasia, normal bone is replaced by immature bone and osteoid in a cellular fibrous matrix. Pain, swelling, and disfigurement can occur because of its expansile nature. Malignant transformation is rare and is associated with previous radiation.
- Most orbital lesions are monostotic and affect the sphenoid wing (see Fig. 9.38, C) but the disease entity may involve multiple skull bones and cross suture lines. This disease can occur in adults and in adolescents and children.
- On MRI, the appearance is quite variable and can resemble an aggressive bone lesion, with heterogeneous T1 and T2 signal, and heterogeneous contrast enhancement.

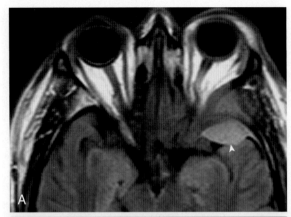
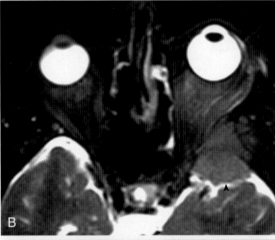
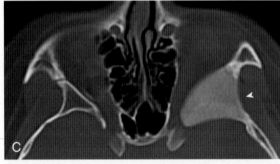

When in doubt, get a CT, which will show the typical confirmatory "ground-glass" appearance.

### Other Primary Bone Lesions

- Primary bone lesions of the orbital walls include eosinophilic granuloma and other fibro-osseous lesions of the orbit, such as osteoma, ossifying fibroma, osteoblastoma, osteosarcoma, osteoclastoma, brown tumor of hyperparathyroidism, aneurysmal bone cyst, and giant cell reparative granuloma.
- Use the clinical information, including the patient's age and presentation, to help guide your differential. Extent of the lesion, zone of transition, presence of extraosseous soft-tissue component, and presence of remodeling versus destruction can help narrow the differential and guide clinical management.

**Fig. 9.38 Sphenoid wing lesions.** Sphenoid wing meningioma *(white arrowhead)* on (A) fluid-attenuated inversion recovery (FLAIR) and (B) T2-weighted imaging shows an intracranial component and an osseous component *(black arrowhead)*. Both meningiomas and fibrous dysplasia (C; *white arrowhead*) can lead to proptosis when the sphenoid wing is affected.

## Relevant Anatomy

### SPHENOID BONE

- Central to the skull base is the sphenoid bone—the main attraction, so to speak. The bone itself has the appearance of a bat with its wings extended (Fig. 10.1) and forms the basis of the anatomic construct of the sella and sphenoid sinus, as well as portions of the orbits and middle cranial fossae.

- The roof of the sphenoid sinus is the planum sphenoidale, which connects the two lesser wings of the sphenoid. Just behind the planum sphenoidale is the sella turcica (Fig. 10.2).

- The pituitary gland sits in the sella turcica, which is bounded anteriorly by the chiasmatic groove (the optic chiasm is not located here; however, the lateral portions of the sulcus lead to the optic canals), the tuberculum sellae, and the anterior clinoid processes (part of the lesser wing of the sphenoid), onto which the tentorium cerebelli attaches. The posterior boundary of the sella is the dorsum sellae, from which arises the posterior clinoid processes, onto which the tentorium and petroclinoid ligaments (from the petrous apex) also insert.

- Inferior to the dorsum sellae is the clivus, which extends inferiorly to the foramen magnum. Anteriorly, the clivus merges with the sphenoid sinus. Its lateral margins are the petro-occipital synchondrosis (also known as the *petrooccipital fissure*, *petroclival synchondrosis*, or *petrooccipital junction*).

- Beneath the sella is the sphenoid sinus, which is usually separated asymmetrically by a vertical bony septum. The sphenoid sinus displays a wide range of normal variations, including asymmetric expansion of its lateral recess into the pterygoid plate or the greater wing of the sphenoid bone. The common wall of the sphenoid sinus and groove for the carotid artery can be quite thin normally.

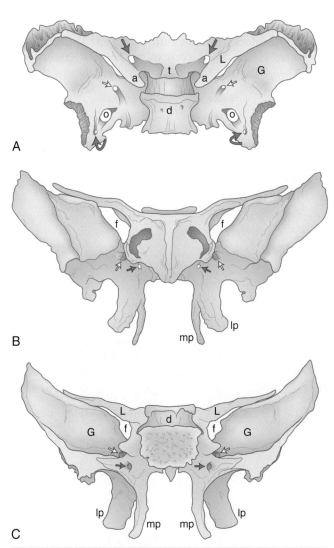

**Fig. 10.1 Diagram of the sphenoid bone.** The feet of the bat are the medial and lateral pterygoid processes, the head being the body of the sphenoid bone, and wings being the greater and lesser wings of the sphenoid. (A) Superior view. (B) Anterior view. (C) Posterior view. Anterior clinoid (a), tuberculum sellae (t), optic canal *(large arrows)*, foramen spinosum *(curved arrows)*, foramen ovale (o), foramen rotundum *(small open arrows)*, dorsum sellae (d), lesser wing of sphenoid (L), greater wing of sphenoid (G), vidian canal *(small closed arrows)*, medial pterygoid plate (mp), lateral pterygoid plate (lp), superior orbital fissure (f).

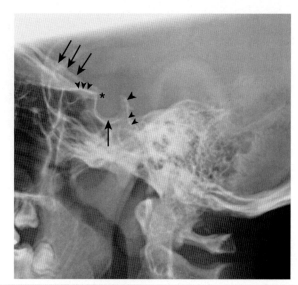

**Fig. 10.2 Lateral radiograph of the sella.** You can appreciate the floor of the anterior cranial fossa *(triple black arrows)*, the planum sphenoidale *(triple black arrowheads)*, the anterior clinoid process *(asterisk)*, the sella turcica *(single black arrow)*, the dorsum sellae *(large single arrowhead)*, and the clivus *(double black arrowheads)*.

## CAVERNOUS SINUS

- On either side of the sella is the cavernous sinus, a trabeculated venous plexus containing cranial nerves III, IV, VI, and the first and second divisions of V (Fig. 10.3). Cranial nerves III, IV, and the first and second divisions of V are in the lateral wall of the cavernous sinus and maintain that order from superior to inferior in the coronal plane. They travel together through the superior orbital fissure into the orbit. Cranial nerve VI is medial in the cavernous sinus but lateral to the cavernous carotid artery.

### TEACHING POINTS
Cavernous Sinus Variations

- The cavernous sinus has many anatomic variations and much controversy about its exact internal venous anatomy.
- It has been reported that the true cavernous sinus (a large venous channel surrounding the internal carotid artery) exists in only 1% of patients.

- In the other instances, the cavernous sinus is formed by numerous small veins including (1) the veins of the lateral wall, (2) the veins of the inferolateral group, (3) the medial vein, and (4) the vein of the carotid sulcus.
- Enhancement within the cavernous sinus can be asymmetric because of these anatomic variations, and this asymmetry alone should not prompt a diagnosis of cavernous sinus thrombosis without other supportive imaging findings.
- Fat in the cavernous sinus is a frequent occurrence.

---

- Many venous connections exist between the cavernous sinuses around the sella. The superior and inferior ophthalmic veins via the superior and inferior orbital fissures respectively drain, along with the superficial middle cerebral vein and sphenoparietal sinus into the cavernous sinus and the cavernous sinus drains into the superior and inferior petrosal sinuses (Fig. 10.4). The basilar venous plexus, the largest intercavernous connection, lies within the dura behind the clivus connecting the two

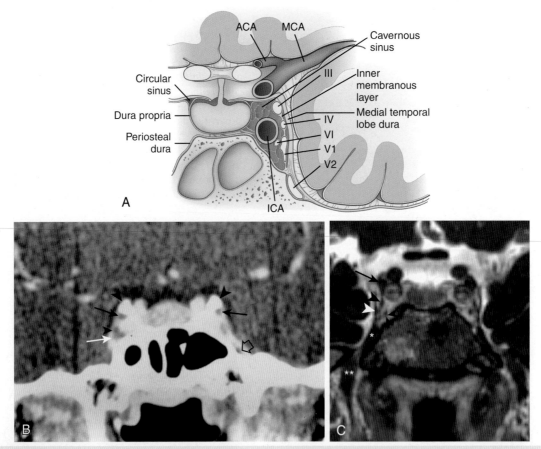

Fig. 10.3 **The low-down on cavernous sinus anatomy.** (A) Rendered diagram in coronal view shows cavernous sinus is in *blue*. Cranial nerves (III, IV, V$_1$, V$_2$, VI). (B) Cranial nerves in cavernous sinus on enhanced computed tomography in coronal plane appear as filling defects within the enhancing cavernous sinuses. Cranial nerve III *(black arrows)* is directly under the anterior clinoid process *(large black arrowheads)*. Also identified on the patient's right side are cranial nerves IV *(small black arrowhead)* and the first division of cranial nerve V *(white arrow)*. On the left side, the second division of cranial nerve (CN) V is marked *(open arrow)*. (C) Coronal contrast-enhanced constructive interference in steady state magnetic resonance image shows the cranial nerves as dark filling defects within the enhancing hyperintense cavernous sinuses. Cranial nerves III *(black arrow)*, IV *(black arrowhead)*, V1 *(white arrowhead)*, and VI *(double black arrowheads)* are indicated. Also seen are V2 headed toward foramen rotundum *(single asterisk)* and V3 *(double asterisk)* extending inferiorly from foramen ovale. *ACA,* Anterior cerebral artery; *ICA,* internal carotid artery; *MCA,* middle cerebral artery

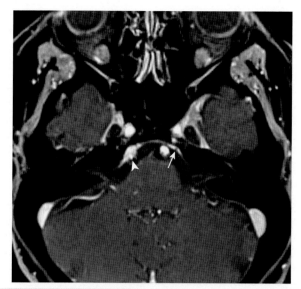

**Fig. 10.4 Inferior petrosal sinus.** On axial T1 fat-suppressed contrast-enhanced magnetic resonance imaging, the sixth cranial nerve can be seen as a "filling defect" *(arrow)* within the enhancing left inferior petrosal sinus as it courses the Dorello canal. There is an enhancing dural-based mass at the level of the Dorello canal on the right *(arrowhead)* felt to represent meningioma, accounting for this patient's clinical presentation of right abducens palsy.

cavernous sinuses and the superior and inferior petrosal sinuses. The coronary sinus is located along the roof of the sphenoid sinus and joins the two cavernous sinuses. There are also venous communications between the cavernous sinus and the pterygoid plexus of veins via emissary veins in the foramen ovale and foramen rotundum and through the inconstant foramen of Vesalius.

## OTHER IMPORTANT NERVES/VESSELS AT THE CENTRAL SKULL BASE

- Cranial nerve V exits the ventral pons as separate motor and sensory roots at the "root entry zone." The roots run forward together through the prepontine cistern and exit through the porus trigeminus of the petrous apex. These roots enter the trigeminal cistern (the space containing cerebrospinal fluid [CSF]), which is in the Meckel cave, a dural invagination at the posterior aspect of the cavernous sinus.

### TEACHING POINTS
Meckel Cave

- The dural layers of the Meckel cave demonstrate thin peripheral enhancement on magnetic resonance imaging (MRI).
- In addition, a discrete semilunar enhancing structure within the inferolateral aspect of the Meckel cave representing the gasserian (or trigeminal) ganglion has been observed to enhance suggesting the lack of a blood-nerve barrier.
- On computed tomography (CT) or MRI, the cerebrospinal fluid in the trigeminal cistern is clearly visualized, and with high-resolution MRI magnetic resonance (MR), the nerve fibers can be seen.

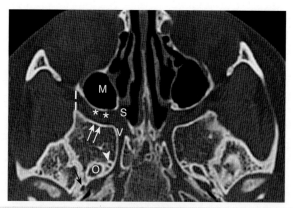

**Fig. 10.5 Anatomy of pterygopalatine fossa (PPF).** Axial computed tomography scan shows the pterygopalatine fossa *(asterisks)* bounded anteriorly by the posterior wall of the maxillary sinus (M) and bounded posteriorly by the base of the pterygoid process *(white arrows)*. The pterygopalatine fossa (PPF) communicates medially with the sphenopalatine foramen (S) and laterally with the masticator space through the pterygomaxillary fissure *(dashed line)*. Also indicated on this image are vidian canal (V), foramen ovale (O), and foramen spinosum *(black arrow)*. The foramen of Vesalius, present in some of us but not all, which carries a sphenoidal emissary vein to the cavernous sinus, is also indicated *(arrowhead)*.

- The three sensory divisions of the trigeminal nerve leave the gasserian ganglion of Meckel cave, with the first and the second divisions running in the lateral wall of the cavernous sinus to exit the superior orbital fissure (along with cranial nerves III, IV, and VI and the superior ophthalmic vein) and foramen rotundum, respectively. The motor root passes under the gasserian ganglion and, after it exits the foramen ovale, combines with its sensory root counterpart to form the mandibular nerve.
- The abducens nerve (cranial nerve VI) exits the pontomedullary sulcus, courses upward through the SAS, enters the Dorello canal, and passes into the cavernous sinus running just lateral to the intracavernous internal carotid artery. Exiting the cavernous sinus, it then enters the orbit through the superior orbital fissure and terminates on the lateral rectus muscle.
- The greater superficial petrosal nerve (GSPN) is a branch of the facial nerve containing sensory and parasympathetic fibers that innervates the lacrimal glands and mucous membranes of the nasal cavity and palate. The GSPN courses anteromedially from the geniculate ganglion and exits the facial hiatus in the petrous bone. It passes under the gasserian ganglion in the Meckel cave and goes forward to the region of the foramen lacerum. Here it merges with the deep petrosal nerve, arising from the sympathetic carotid plexus, and forms the vidian nerve.

### TEACHING POINTS
Introducing Vidian

- The vidian canal connects the pterygopalatine fossa anteriorly to the foramen lacerum posteriorly and transmits the vidian nerve and artery (see Fig. 10.5).
- The vidian nerve runs anteriorly in the vidian canal with the parasympathetic fibers synapsing in the pterygopalatine ganglia and the sensory fibers passing through the ganglion to the nasal cavity and palate.
- The vidian artery, a branch of the maxillary artery, joins the carotid artery in its petrous segment.

## Central Skull Base Foramina

- The major skull base foramina to be aware of and "know by heart" cold are described.

Skull Base Foramina: Survival Guide

| Foramen | Contents |
|---------|----------|
| Superior orbital fissure | Cranial nerves III, IV, first division of V, and VI<br>Orbital branch of middle meningeal artery<br>Sympathetic nerve<br>Recurrent meningeal artery, superior ophthalmic vein<br>Ophthalmic artery (in rare cases) |
| Optic canal | Optic nerve, ophthalmic artery (most often) |
| Inferior orbital fissure | Infraorbital artery, vein, and nerve (branch of second division of cranial nerve V) |
| Foramen rotundum | Second division of cranial nerve V, artery of foramen rotundum, emissary veins |
| Foramen ovale | Third division of cranial nerve V, lesser petrosal nerve, accessory meningeal artery, emissary veins |
| Foramen spinosum | Middle meningeal artery and vein, recurrent branch of third division of cranial nerve V, lesser superficial petrosal nerve |
| Foramen lacerum | Meningeal branch of ascending pharyngeal artery, nerve of pterygoid canal |
| Foramen of Vesalius | Emissary vein from cavernous sinus to pterygoid plexus |
| Vidian canal | Vidian artery and nerve |
| Jugular foramen | Pars nervosa: cranial nerve IX, inferior petrosal sinus<br>Pars vascularis: Cranial nerves X and XI<br>Jugular bulb |
| Hypoglossal canal | Cranial nerve XII, persistent hypoglossal artery (in rare instance when it is present) |
| Pterygopalatine fossa | Pterygopalatine ganglion (V₂)<br>Pterygopalatine plexus |
| Foramen magnum | Medulla oblongata<br>Vertebral artery, anterior spinal artery, posterior spinal artery. |

- The pterygopalatine fossa (PPF) is bounded anteriorly by the maxillary bone, anteromedially by the perpendicular plate of the palatine bone, and posteriorly by the base of the pterygoid process. The PPF is notable because it communicates with other skull base foramina to allow for spread of disease into the orbit (through the inferior orbital fissure), nasal cavity (along the sphenopalatine foramen), infratemporal fossa (via the pterygomaxillary fissure), hard palate (along the greater and lesser palatine nerves), and intracranially (via foramen rotundum and vidian canal) (Fig. 10.5).

## Sellar Structures

- See Fig. 10.6.
- The pituitary gland is surrounded by a dural bag with the medial wall of the cavernous sinus being the lateral extent of the dural bag. The gland is divided into anterior and posterior lobes. The size of the gland varies with sex, age, and physiologic conditions.

Pituitary Gland Size

- In children younger than 12 years of age, the gland should be 6 mm or less, with its upper surface flat or slightly concave. In teenaged females, it may measure up to 10 mm in height, and convex upper margins may be identified. This can be noted in teenaged males but appears to be less striking.
- Convexity has been observed in children with precocious puberty.
- The gland gradually decreases in size after the age of 50 years.
- In females, the maximal height of the pituitary has been reported as 9 mm, whereas in males it is 8 mm.
- The gland changes shape and size during puberty, and pregnancy and lactation up to 12 mm because of physiologic hypertrophy.
- After the first postpartum week, the gland rapidly returns to normal.

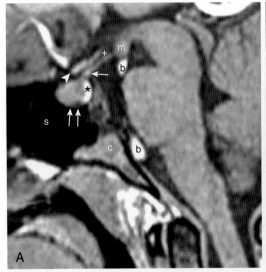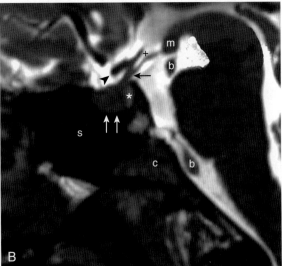

**Fig. 10.6 Normal sellar and suprasellar anatomy.** Sagittal T1-weighted (A) and sagittal T2 constructive interference in the steady state (CISS) (B) images show the posterior pituitary bright spot *(asterisk)*, infundibular recess *(+)*, infundibulum *(arrow)*, chiasm *(arrowhead)*, mammillary body (m), basilar artery (b), clivus (c), floor of sella *(double arrows)*, and sphenoid sinus (s).

- The anterior lobe of the pituitary (adenohypophysis) is divided into the pars tuberalis, pars intermedia, and pars distalis. The pars tuberalis consists of thin anterior pituitary tissue along the median eminence and anterior infundibulum. The pars intermedia lies between the pars distalis and the posterior lobe of the pituitary. It is noted to contain small cysts (pars intermedia cysts, colloid cysts) and may be the origin of Rathke cleft cysts.
- The adenohypophysis secretes prolactin (from lactotrophs), growth hormone (from somatotrophs), thyroid-stimulating hormone (from thyrotrophs), follicle-stimulating hormone and luteinizing hormone (from gonadotrophs), and corticotropin (ACTH) precursor and melanocyte-stimulating hormone (from corticotrophs).
- The neurohypophysis is composed of the posterior lobe, the infundibular stalk, and the median eminence. Besides storing antidiuretic hormone and oxytocin, the neural lobe also contains nonsecreting cells termed *pituicytes*. Their exact role is uncertain.
- The posterior lobe of the pituitary has a direct blood supply from the inferior hypophyseal artery, a branch of the meningohypophyseal trunk arising from the cavernous carotid. The superior hypophyseal arteries, arising from the supraclinoid internal carotid arteries and posterior communicating arteries (usually not visualized on angiography), supply a plexus around the base of the hypophyseal stalk and median eminence and then supply the anterior lobe of the pituitary indirectly through the pituitary portal system.

---

**TEACHING POINTS**

Pituitary Blood Supply Implications

- The implications of this quaint pituitary portal blood supply are that on dynamic imaging, the posterior pituitary and infundibulum enhance immediately because of their direct blood supply, whereas the anterior pituitary is slightly delayed because of the portal system.
- The indirect blood supply to the anterior lobe of the pituitary makes it susceptible to ischemia.

---

- The venous drainage of the pituitary is into the cavernous sinuses.

### Suprasellar Structures

- See Fig. 10.6.
- The diaphragma sellae is the sheet of dura forming a roof over the sella turcica overlying the pituitary gland. The diaphragm has a central hiatus of variable size through which the infundibulum passes. The portion of the hypophysis located just below the diaphragm is concave superiorly like the region just around the stem of an apple and creates the hypophyseal cistern. This cistern is an expansion of the suprasellar cistern and is separated from the interpeduncular and prepontine cisterns by the membrane of Liliequist, located just below the floor of the third ventricle. The basilar artery sits below the membrane and the membrane must be opened to gain access to a basilar artery aneurysm if approached surgically.

- The infundibulum (also called the *pituitary stalk*) arises from the tuber cinereum (a prominence of the inferior portion of the hypothalamus) and courses in an anteroinferior direction toward the pituitary gland.
- The suprasellar cistern is superior to the diaphragma sellae. This cistern contains the circle of Willis with anterior cerebral arteries, anterior and posterior communicating arteries, and the tip of the basilar artery. Anteriorly, the cistern is bounded by the inferior frontal lobes and the interhemispheric fissure, laterally by the medial portions of the temporal lobes, and posteriorly by the prepontine and interpeduncular cisterns. Lying central in the suprasellar cistern is the optic chiasm, which is anterior and superior to the infundibular stalk.
- The hypothalamus forms the ventral and rostral part of the wall of the third ventricle. The chiasmatic and infundibular recesses of the third ventricle project inferiorly into these respective structures (chiasm and infundibulum). Posterior to the infundibular stalk is the anteroinferior third ventricle, as well as the mammillary bodies. The tuber cinereum is the lamina of gray substance from the floor of the third ventricle (hypothalamus) between the mammillary bodies and the optic chiasm.

## Imaging Techniques/Protocols

### MAGNETIC RESONANCE IMAGING

- Sagittal and coronal T1-weighted imaging (T1WI) before and after gadolinium administration with thin sections (<3 mm) are all that is necessary to image the pituitary gland/sella. T2-weighted imaging (T2WI) can occasionally add additional information for the differential diagnosis by providing the intensity characteristics of a particular lesion but is not necessarily essential in typical cases of "rule out adenoma."

---

**TEACHING POINTS**

Expected Imaging of Adult Pituitary Gland

- The anterior lobe of the pituitary gland is isointense to brain on T1-weighted imaging (T1WI) and T2-weighted imaging (T2WI; see Fig. 10.6).
- The posterior pituitary gland is high intensity on the T1WI and of lower intensity on the T2WI (see Fig. 10.6).
- Posterior to this hypointense margin is the hyperintensity of fatty marrow in the clivus.
- After intravenous contrast injection, enhancement is promptly noted on T1WI in the infundibulum with more delayed enhancement at the anterior pituitary. Remember that the posterior pituitary is already high intensity on T1 precontrast.
- The initial enhancement gradually fades in 20 to 30 minutes or more. The pituitary and cavernous sinuses generally enhance to a similar extent.

**Expected Posterior Pituitary Signal Changes**

- The posterior pituitary gland is much more conspicuous in younger people and becomes less conspicuous with increase in age.
- The precise cause of the high T1 signal in the posterior of the pituitary is probably related to the carrier protein (neurophysin) stored in the neurosecretory granules of the posterior pituitary, intracellular lipid in glial cell pituicytes, water interactions with paramagnetic substances, or low molecular weight molecules such as vasopressin or oxytocin.

- Dynamic-enhanced magnetic resonance (MR) after contrast can increase detection of very tiny microadenomas. This consists of rapid imaging at the sella repeated for a short time: 6 to 8 thin sections every 30 seconds, for 3 to 5 minutes, typically in the coronal plane. The dynamic images obtained within the first minute appear to provide the greatest contrast between enhancing normal gland and a pituitary adenoma that does not initially enhance.
- For postsurgical imaging, fat-suppressed postcontrast T1 images should be performed. There is typically considerable fat-packing material present along the transsphenoidal hypophysectomy surgical tract, and fat suppression techniques can help distinguish true enhancing tissue from surgically implanted material and blood products.
- If perineural extension of disease at the skull base is in question, thin section T1 and T2 images in multiple planes without and with contrast through the skull base can be performed.

## COMPUTED TOMOGRAPHY

- Computed tomography (CT) can be performed as a sinus CT exam to evaluate the central skull base region, unless whole brain imaging is required. CT is typically performed without contrast.
- CT is useful in demonstrating calcifications within sellar and parasellar lesions. Bony skull base anatomy, especially the positioning of septa in the sphenoid sinus, is also better visualized on CT, which is important if a transsphenoidal surgical approach is being considered for lesion resection. Widened skull base foramina in the setting of perineural disease extension can also be appreciated by CT.

## VASCULAR IMAGING

- Vascular imaging should be performed by MR angiography/venography (MRA/MRV) or CT angiography/venography (CTA/CTV) when aneurysms, fistulas, and thrombosis or hypervascular masses are suspected or for surgical/treatment planning. CTA and CTV require injection of iodinated contrast material. MRA (time-of-flight) and MRV (time-of-flight or phase contrast (PC) techniques) can be performed without contrast, although contrast-enhanced MRA/MRV can also be performed.

# Pathology

## INTRASELLAR LESIONS

### Congenital Lesions

See Chapter 8.

### Adenoma, a.k.a. Pituitary Neuroendocrine Tumor (pitNET), per 2022 WHO Classification

- Autopsy series indicate that the pituitary gland can be a reservoir for the "incidentaloma," including asymptomatic microadenomas (14%–27% of cases), pars intermedia (Rathke) cysts (13%–22%), and occult metastatic lesions (about 5% of patients with malignancy). This means that clinical input is critical in assessing small lesions of the pituitary because many "normal" patients may have small, insignificant nonsecretory abnormalities visualized on CT or MR.
- In about 75% of cases, microadenomas present because of symptoms from the hormones they secrete. Serum prolactin levels of more than 200 ng/mL are highly specific for prolactin-secreting adenomas. Intermediate levels of prolactin (30–70 ng/mL) may be on the basis of glandular compression from nonprolactinoma lesions. Nonhormonally active lesions become symptomatic because of their size (macroadenomas), producing headache, visual disturbances (classically bitemporal visual defects), cranial nerve palsy, and CSF rhinorrhea.
- Pituitary microadenomas (<10 mm) are generally hypointense compared with the normal gland on T1WI and display a variable intensity on T2WI. The diagnosis of pituitary microadenoma can be made without contrast, but for us mere mortals, microadenomas are more conspicuous with dynamic administration of intravenous (IV) contrast (Fig. 10.7). On postcontrast T1WI, the microadenoma appears hypointense relative to the normally enhancing pituitary gland, especially if dynamic-enhanced MRI is performed. If a delayed scan (20 minutes after the injection of contrast) is performed, the tumor may appear hyperintense relative to the normal glandular tissue or isointense (and hidden).
- Macroadenomas (>10 mm) have roughly the same signal characteristics as microadenomas; however, they have a propensity for hemorrhage and infarction because of their marginal blood supply. Thus these tumors can possess a variable intensity pattern. Cystic regions in macroadenomas produce low intensity on T1WI and high intensity on T2WI.
  - Treatment with bromocriptine increases the likelihood of intratumoral hemorrhages, which may be asymptomatic. Hemorrhage can also be associated with the syndrome of pituitary apoplexy.
- In assessing cavernous sinus invasion, if the pituitary tumor remains medial to a line drawn through the mid diameter of the cavernous carotid artery, cavernous sinus invasion is *not* present. If the tumor extends lateral to a line drawn along the lateral edge of the cavernous carotid artery wall, cavernous sinus invasion *is* present (see Fig. 10.7B). When the tumor is between those lines, all bets are off, but markedly elevated hormonal levels usually mean the cavernous sinus is violated. Alternatively, if one sees encasement of greater than 180 degrees of the

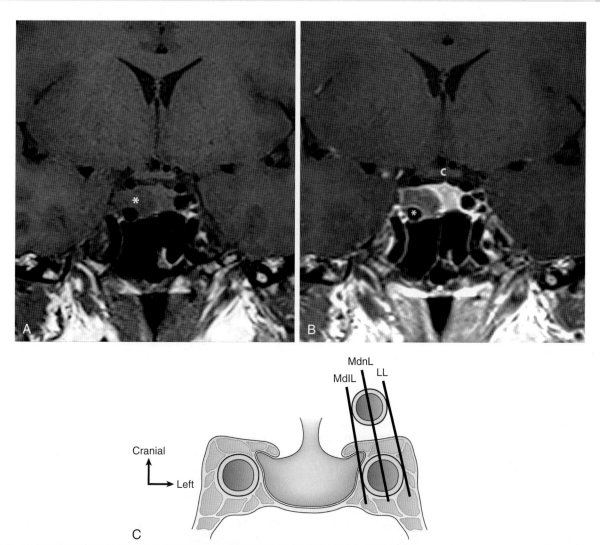

**Fig. 10.7  Magnetic resonance imaging of pituitary adenoma.** (A) On coronal precontrast T1-weighted image, a hypointense nodule relative to the adjacent pituitary parenchyma indicates adenoma in this patient with elevated prolactin level *(asterisk)*. (B) After contrast administration, the adenoma is much more conspicuous because the normal pituitary gland enhances more than the adenoma. Note the cavernous carotid artery flow void *(asterisk)*. In this case, the lateral aspect of the adenoma extends into and through the right cavernous sinus, indicating invasion. No mass effect on the optic chiasm. (C) Coronal schematic rendering through the sella shows the relationships of the intercarotid lateral line (LL), the median line (MdnL) and the medial line (MdIL) of the intracavernous and supracavernous internal carotid artery. Tumor extent between the MDIL and MdnL renders cavernous sinus invasion unlikely, between MdnL and LL possible, just lateral to LL probable, and encasing the ICA, definite. source: Cottier JP, Destrieux C, Brunereau L, et al. Cavernous sinus invasion by pituitary adenoma: MR imaging. *Radiology*. 2000;215(2):463–469. https://doi.org/10.1148/radiology.215.2.r00ap18463.

carotid's circumference, suggest cavernous sinus invasion. If the space inferolateral to the inferior turn of the carotid is invaded (carotid sulcus venous compartment), suggest cavernous sinus invasion.

---

**TEACHING POINTS**

Cavernous Sinus Invasion

- If you see encasement of greater than 180 degrees of the carotid's circumference, suggest cavernous sinus invasion.
- If the space inferolateral to the inferior turn of the carotid is invaded (carotid sulcus venous compartment), suggest cavernous sinus invasion.
- Noninvasion can be assured if (1) there is intervening normal pituitary tissue between the adenoma and cavernous sinus, or (2) less than 25% of the intracavernous carotid artery is encased.

- Pituitary macroadenomas can become very large, to the point that it may be difficult to discern whether the tumor is in fact of pituitary or extrapituitary origin. Such adenomas can result in significant mass effect on the chiasm and adjacent brain parenchyma, resulting in obstructive hydrocephalus and herniation syndromes (Fig. 10.8). If you are unable to distinguish a sellar mass from the (displaced) normal pituitary tissue, assume the lesion is a pituitary adenoma.
- Adenomas have rarely been reported at extrasellar sites not in continuity with the sella, including the sphenoid sinus, nasal cavity, petrous bone, and third ventricle.

## Postoperative Pituitary Imaging

- Imaging is performed after pituitary adenoma resection primarily to assess extent of tumor resection and to serve as baseline for future follow-up imaging. Immediately after surgery, a peripherally enhancing cystic cavity can

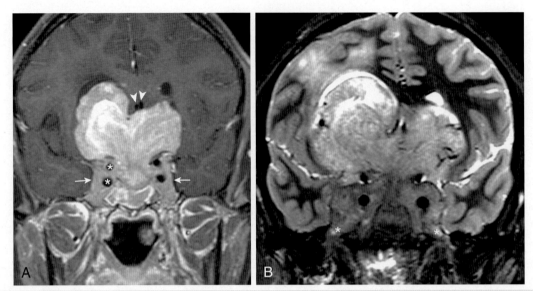

**Fig. 10.8 Giant macroadenoma.** (A) Postcontrast coronal T1-weighted imaging (T1WI) shows enhancing tumor centered within the sella invading the cavernous sinuses bilaterally *(white arrows)*, with preservation of the internal carotid artery flow voids *(asterisks)*. There is significant mass effect upon the inferior frontal lobes. The A2 segments of the anterior cerebral arteries are displaced superiorly by the mass *(arrowheads)*. (B) Coronal T2WI shows edema within the right frontal lobe because of mass effect from this giant macroadenoma. There is leftward midline shift. Note that the tumor has invaded the Meckel cave bilaterally (the normally T2-hyperintense signal within the cave is absent because of tumor invasion, indicated by *asterisks* and is headed into foramen ovale bilaterally.

be seen at the site of previously demonstrated adenoma; although the surgical cavity might show persistent mass effect in the immediate postoperative period, rest assured it will decrease in size over the next few months (Fig. 10.9).

- Additional postoperative changes include fat packing or other surgical material in the sphenoid sinus and persistent enhancement at the operative tract. Recognize that tumors with cavernous sinus invasion are often not completely resected; what one should expect is decompression of the midportion of the tumor where access via the transsphenoidal approach is possible to relieve indentation on the optic chiasm, pituitary stalk, third ventricle, and hypothalamus.

- Remaining normal pituitary tissue is inconstantly identified. It may be difficult to distinguish residual normal pituitary tissue from residual tumor and/or granulation tissue when reviewing the postoperative images. Comparing directly with the preoperative scan can certainly be helpful in this regard; however, identifying these different tissue types is less important than assessing for interval change in tissue bulk in the sella over time and compressive effect on adjacent structures. Hence, serial scanning and hormonal assessment is required in follow-up.

- Occasionally, the optic chiasm and nerves and/or floor of the third ventricle are noted to herniate into the sella. In fact, this results from traction from previous adhesions and from arachnoiditis after surgery. These patients seldom have symptoms.

### Pituitary Apoplexy

- Pituitary apoplexy is a syndrome characterized by acute onset of ophthalmoplegia, headache, visual loss, and/ or vomiting as a consequence of pituitary hemorrhage and/or ischemia, most commonly in the setting of a preexisting pituitary tumor. Sheehan syndrome presents as hypopituitarism as a consequence of pituitary ischemia in the peripartum period.

- Pituitary hemorrhages follow the pattern of intraparenchymal hemorrhages, with acute hemorrhage revealing hypointensity on T2WI and subacute hemorrhages exhibiting high intensity on T1WI (Fig. 10.10). As opposed to most simple intracranial hemorrhages, in which hemosiderin is deposited in the walls of the cavity, pituitary hemorrhage is not associated with hemosiderin deposition. Hemorrhage in a pituitary gland/adenoma can persist for years.

### Abscess

- Abscess can form in the pituitary just as in other parts of the brain. This uncommon lesion can occur after surgery but also in situations that predispose to infection, including sinusitis. The abscess produces compression of surrounding structures. Infection can extend to involve the skull base, leptomeninges, cavernous sinuses, orbits, brain parenchyma, and circle of Willis, so keep your eyes peeled in these situations. Diffusion-weighted imaging (DWI) scans showing restricted diffusion in the sellar region is a giveaway.

### Lymphocytic Infundibuloneurohypophysitis

- This is an uncommon inflammatory disease of the pituitary gland and infundibulum. The condition has also been termed *lymphocytic hypophysitis* (if infundibulum is involved in isolation). It is seen in young females during late pregnancy or in the postpartum period. However, it can also occur in nonpregnant females and males of all ages. Endocrinologic abnormalities can include all anterior pituitary hormonal functions, and when the infundibulum and neurohypophysis are affected, diabetes insipidus can ensue.

- There is enlargement and enhancement of the pituitary gland and thickening of the stalk (Fig. 10.11). The inflammation may extend into the cavernous sinuses. The enlargement may regress spontaneously or with steroids.

### Posterior Pituitary Tumors

- Tumors of the posterior pituitary gland, including pituicytomas and granular cell tumors (choristoma/

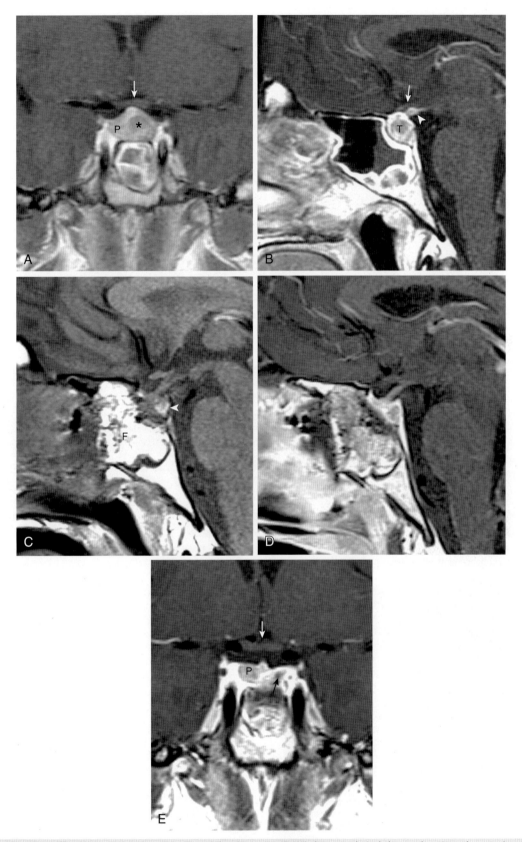

**Fig. 10.9  Postoperative sella.** (A) Coronal postcontrast T1-weighted imaging (T1WI) shows a relatively hypoenhancing adenoma *(asterisk)* in the left aspect of the sella with mass effect upon the inferior margin of the optic chiasm *(arrow)*. Normal pituitary tissue is seen in the right aspect of the sella (P). (B) Sagittal postcontrast T1WI shows the same mass (T), resulting in superior displacement of the infundibulum *(arrowhead)* and chiasm *(arrow)*. (C) After transsphenoidal resection of the adenoma, sagittal T1WI shows fat-packing material in the sphenoid sinus (F) and a small amount of hemorrhage at the site of tumor *(arrowhead)*. Note the more anatomically appropriate positioning of the chiasm and infundibulum on this image, as well as on (D) sagittal postcontrast T1WI. (E) Postcontrast coronal T1WI in the same patient shows surgical cavity at site of resected adenoma *(black arrow)*, residual normal pituitary tissue in the right aspect of the sella (P), and resolution of mass effect upon the chiasm *(white arrow)*.

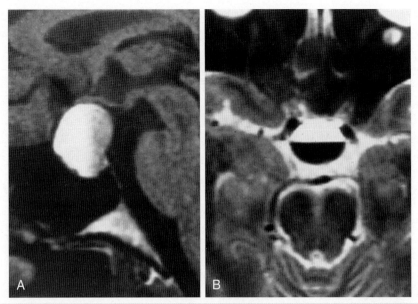

**Fig. 10.10 Pituitary apoplexy.** Sagittal T1-weighted image (T1WI) (A) shows large hemorrhage into a pituitary tumor. There is a fluid level, which is best appreciated on the axial T2-weighted image (T2WI), (B) with the hypointense dependent level containing deoxyhemoglobin. In this case, the patient was acutely symptomatic.

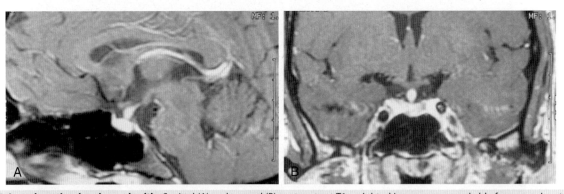

**Fig. 10.11 Lymphocytic adenohypophysitis.** Sagittal (A) and coronal (B) postcontrast T1-weighted images are remarkable for a prominent pituitary gland and vigorous enhancement with enlargement of the stalk. It should not be convex outward.

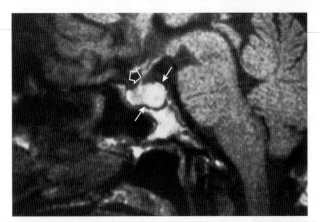

**Fig. 10.12 Pituicytoma.** Sagittal T1-weighted image demonstrates this posterior pituitary tumor *(arrows)*. Observe that the mass is behind the infundibulum *(open arrow)* and thus is located in the posterior pituitary and is high intensity.

myoblastoma), are rare and may produce visual or endocrinologic disturbances (Fig. 10.12).

■ The key to the diagnosis is the sagittal MR, which localizes the lesion to the posterior pituitary. However, these tumors have also been reported in the suprasellar region and third ventricle. They are of variable intensity on T1WI, proton density–weighted images (PDWI), and T2WI, and they enhance.

## Rathke Cleft Cyst

■ Rathke cleft cysts, or *pars intermedia cysts*, arise from a Rathke pouch and may be found in the anterior sellar region (25%), suprasellar region (5%), or both (70%). They are benign lesions lined with cuboidal or columnar epithelium and may contain mucus. Rathke cleft cysts are most commonly asymptomatic, but if large enough, they may cause visual disturbances, pituitary insufficiency, or diabetes insipidus.

■ These lesions have variable intensities on both T1WI and T2WI (Fig. 10.13). Their MR intensity is related to the contents of the cyst (simple versus proteinaceous fluid). An intracystic nodule having high signal intensity on T1WI and low signal intensity on T2WI is seen in three fourths of Rathke cysts. Fluid-fluid levels may also be seen.

■ The principal differential diagnosis of Rathke cleft cyst is craniopharyngioma. Rathke cleft cysts do not calcify, demonstrate smooth contours, and, at most, show rim

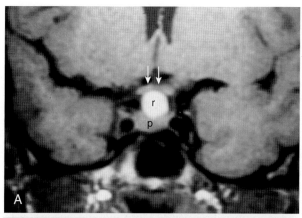

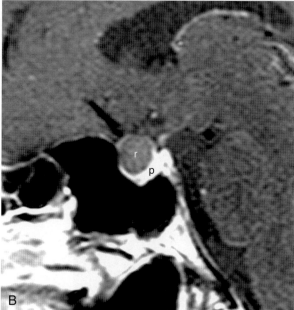

**Fig. 10.13 Rathke cleft cyst.** (A) Coronal T1-weighted image (T1WI) of Rathke cleft cyst (r) in the suprasellar cistern which is high intensity on T1WI. The pituitary (p) and optic chiasm *(arrows)* are identified. (B) Sagittal postcontrast T1WI in a different patient with Rathke cleft cyst shows cystic lesion (r) without enhancing component within the suprasellar cistern, sitting just above normal pituitary tissue (p).

enhancement, whereas the high percentage of craniopharyngiomas have calcifications and demonstrate irregular margins with areas of solid nodular enhancement. Hemorrhagic pituitary microadenoma may also simulate intrasellar Rathke cysts.

### Empty Sella Syndrome

- CSF is easily noted in the empty or partially empty sella because of a patulous diaphragma sella and extension of the suprasellar arachnoid space inferiorly (Fig. 10.14). The sellar floor is often expanded and downwardly displaced. This may be seen with aging and is of doubtful clinical significance. However, the finding may also be seen in pseudotumor cerebri (idiopathic intracranial hypertension). Other findings associated with pseudotumor include an enlarged tortuous optic nerve sheath, bulging of the optic nerve head (papilledema), enlarged Meckel cave, narrowing of the transverse sinuses, prominent arachnoid pits, and meningoceles in other locations. Cases have been reported in which the

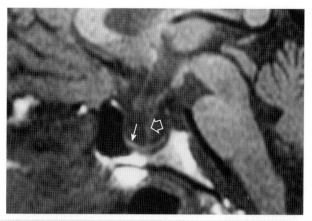

**Fig. 10.14 Partially empty sella.** On this sagittal noncontrast-enhanced T1-weighted image, the sella is expanded without appreciable sellar or suprasellar mass, nor displacement of suprasellar structures from an arachnoid cyst that might otherwise mimic an empty sella appearance (compare with Fig. 10.16). Note the residual pituitary tissue *(solid arrow)* and infundibulum *(open arrow)*.

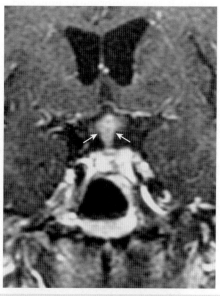

**Fig. 10.15 Sarcoid involving the infundibulum.** Coronal-enhanced T1-weighted image shows an enlarged thickened infundibulum *(arrows)* in a patient with intracranial sarcoid.

appearance of the empty sella was observed to be reversible after treatment of the intracranial hypertension.

### SUPRASELLAR LESIONS

These include pathologies related to the infundibulum (also called the *pituitary stalk*), hypothalamus, optic chiasm, and suprasellar cistern.

#### Infundibular Lesions

- The pituitary adenoma is the most common lesion to affect the infundibulum with displacement, foreshortening, thickening, or effacement of the stalk.
- Diabetes insipidus is a common clinical feature in lesions affecting the stalk and hypothalamus, although there are numerous causes of infundibular thickening and enhancement, including inflammatory, infectious, neoplastic, and drug-induced processes (Fig. 10.15). As such, the clinical context is key in identifying the cause.

**TEACHING POINTS**

Causes of Hypophyseal Thickening and Enhancement

| Inflammatory | Infectious | Neoplastic | Drug-Induced |
|---|---|---|---|
| Autoimmune disorders (e.g., Systemic lupus erythematosus, Sjogren, rheumatoid arthritis, autoimmune thyroiditis, pernicious anemia) | Bacterial | Germinoma | Immune checkpoint inhibitors (often employed with cancer treatment therapies) |
| Systemic processes (e.g., IgG4-related disease, sarcoidosis, granulomatosis with polyangiitis, Langerhans cell histiocytosis) | Viral | Craniopharyngioma | Interferon-alpha (used in treatments for cancer and viral infections) |
| Peripartum/postpartum hypophysitis | Mycobacterial (tuberculosis) | Lymphoma | Ribavirin (antiviral) |
|  | Parasitic | Metastatic disease |  |
|  | Fungal |  |  |

## Arachnoid Cyst

- Approximately 15% of all arachnoid cysts arise in the suprasellar region. Although age at presentation is variable (from childhood to the second or third decade of life), it is hypothesized that they arise developmentally as a result of a lack of perforation of the membrane of Liliequist. If the membrane is imperforate, normal CSF flow anterior to the pons can produce a wind sock, which can subsequently close off and become a true cyst or may remain as an arachnoid pouch. Such a cyst produces mass effect on adjacent structures, including the hypothalamus, chiasm, and brain stem. These cysts can grow and produce hydrocephalus. The density and intensity of these cysts are those of CSF (Fig. 10.16). They are not associated with enhancement or calcification.

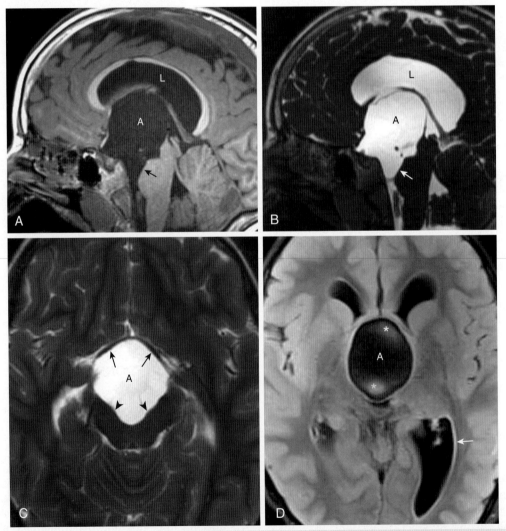

**Fig. 10.16 Arachnoid cyst.** Sagittal T1 (A) and T2 constructive interference in the steady state (CISS) (B) magnetic resonance images through the midline show an extra-axial cerebrospinal fluid (CSF) signal lesion (A) centered within the suprasellar cistern. Note the flattening on the ventral pons because of mass effect *(arrow)* and enlargement of the lateral ventricle (L) because of obstructive hydrocephalus. (C) Axial T2-weighted imaging shows mass effect and lateral displacement of the bilateral A1 segments of the anterior cerebral arteries *(arrows)* and splaying of the bilateral cerebral peduncles *(arrowheads)* by the arachnoid cyst (A). (D) Axial fluid-attenuated inversion recovery (FLAIR) image shows presence of CSF pulsation artifact *(asterisks)* within the arachnoid cyst (A). Note enlarged lateral ventricles and transependymal flow of CSF *(arrow)* because of obstructive hydrocephalus.

- If the arachnoid cyst invaginates into the third ventricle, it can be mistaken for an ependymal cyst (neuroepithelial cyst) of the third ventricle or an enlarged third ventricle. The key here is to determine whether you can separate the third ventricle from the lesion (if you can, it is most likely an arachnoid cyst). High-resolution thin section constructive interference in the steady state (CISS) T2WI can be helpful in distinguishing these lesions. Alternatively, on cisternography, prompt filling with contrast after intrathecal contrast injection indicates a dilated third ventricle as opposed to an arachnoid cyst, which will show delayed contrast filling.

## Craniopharyngioma

- Craniopharyngiomas may be seen in children and adults and make up between 1.2% and 3% of all intracranial tumors. In children, they account for a greater percentage of tumor cases, but more than 50% of craniopharyngiomas occur in adults. Two histopathologic types exist: adamantinomatous and papillary, with different clinical, imaging, and histopathologic/genetic profiles.

**TEACHING POINTS**

Craniopharyngiomas: Adamantinomatous and Papillary

|  | Adamantinomatous | Papillary |
|---|---|---|
| Genetic mutation | Catenin beta 1 (CTNNB1) | BRAF respectively |
| Location | Suprasellar | Intrasellar/suprasellar or intraventricular |
| Age | Children, occasionally adults | Adults |
| Tissue structure | Predominantly cystic | Predominantly solid |
| T1 without contrast | Hyperintense cysts typical | If ever, hypointense cysts |
| Shape | Lobulated | Spherical |
| Encase vessels | Yes | No |
| Tumor recurrence | +++ | + |
| Calcifications | +++ | + |

+, Possible; +++, very likely.

- Craniopharyngiomas are usually centered in the suprasellar (20%), suprasellar and sellar (70%), sellar (10%), or infrasellar regions (<1%), but they can be extensive, including the anterior fossa, middle fossa, posterior fossa, retroclival region, and the third ventricles. Other rare origins include the lateral ventricle, sphenoid bone, nasopharynx, cerebellopontine angle, and pineal gland. A good rule is that if the tumor looks bizarre and has a component at the base of the skull, think craniopharyngioma.
- Three imaging hallmarks of craniopharyngioma have been identified (although an individual lesion may have none or all these characteristics): (1) calcification, (2) cyst formation, and (3) enhancement (solid, nodular) (Fig. 10.17).
  - T1 bright signal intensity, young age, and calcification on CT favor the adamantinomatous over papillary craniopharyngioma. Calcification may be nodular or rim-like, occurring in approximately 80% of cases; for this reason, CT can be a useful adjunct to MRI in

making the diagnosis because calcifications are better appreciated by CT.
  - Cystic regions are observed in about 85% of cases; the cyst can show low density on CT and variable intensity on MR. The intensity on T1WI ranges from hypointense to hyperintense and is usually high intensity on T2WI. The high intensity on T1WI appears to be because of methemoglobin and/or high protein. Some ultra-high protein craniopharyngiomas are low intensity on T1WI. This has been attributed to the increased viscosity associated with such elevated protein levels. The solid portion of the tumor enhances.
- The papillary intraventricular variety of craniopharyngioma is unusual, probably originating from the pars tuberalis that extends to the tuber cinereum in the floor of the third ventricle. These lesions do not extend beneath the floor of the third ventricle (i.e., they are not in the suprasellar space). Other features distinguishing these lesions include higher incidence in adults and male preponderance. Hormonal and visual disturbances are rare, again because of their intraventricular location. There is a lower incidence of calcification or cyst formation, and these lesions show more uniform enhancement. This solid intraventricular lesion has no specific hallmarks, and thus the differential diagnosis includes cavernous malformation of the third ventricle, choroid plexus papilloma, ependymoma, pilocytic astrocytoma, and meningioma.
- Fusiform dilatation (pseudoaneurysm formation) of the supraclinoid carotid artery has been reported postoperatively after craniopharyngioma resection. There is no consensus on the appropriate management of these pseudoaneurysms, however subsequent hemorrhage or cerebrovascular events are unlikely.
- Treatment and retreatment with cyst puncture/drainage and local instillation of antineoplastic drugs for recurrences are common.
- This is a sticky tumor that is hard to get rid of without injury to critical normal structures like the optic apparatus, pituitary stalk, and hypothalamus, making total resection a difficult proposition in many cases.

## Chiasmatic and Hypothalamic Astrocytoma

- Chiasmatic/hypothalamic astrocytomas (gliomas) present as mass lesions in the suprasellar cistern. They are typically isointense to brain on T1WI and high intensity on T2WI (Fig. 10.18). This high intensity may be noted throughout the visual pathway. Enhancement is variable, and calcification in the nonirradiated tumor is rare. At times, a cystic component (fluid attenuation/intensity) is present with the tumor, and they are commonly the grade I pilocytic varieties.
- Hypothalamic gliomas may be difficult to distinguish from chiasmatic lesions; a normal chiasm, with an inhomogeneous mass in the floor of the third ventricle and suprasellar cistern, suggests a hypothalamic as opposed to a chiasmatic astrocytoma. These lesions, because of their location, are rarely resected. Fortunately, they are slow-growing, low-grade tumors so delay, delay, delay until one is forced to radiate and/or operate.
- These tumors may occur in association with neurofibromatosis type 1. Because large optic chiasm low-grade gliomas eventually grow into the hypothalamus,

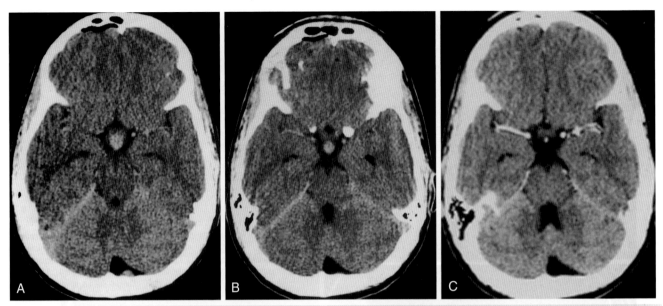

**Fig. 10.20 Germinoma.** (A) Noncontrast computed tomography (CT) demonstrates high density in a suprasellar mass representing a germinoma. (B) Noncontrast CT inferior to (A) shows high density in a markedly enlarged infundibulum containing germinoma. (C) Postcontrast CT after radiation therapy now shows normal appearance of the infundibulum.

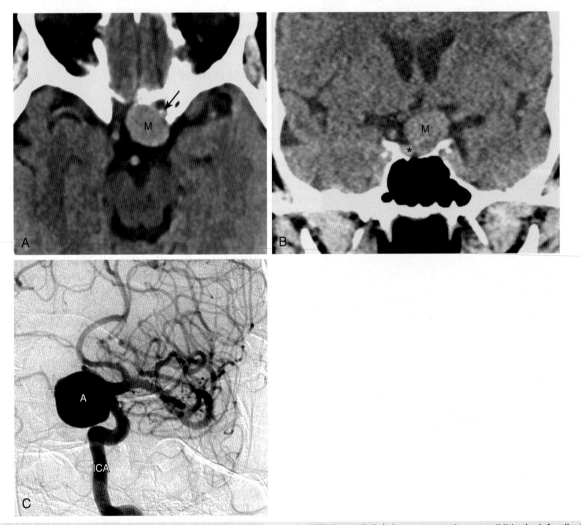

**Fig. 10.21 Intrasellar aneurysm.** (A) Axial noncontrast computed tomography (CT) shows slightly hyperattenuating mass (M) in the left sellar/supra-sellar region, intimately associated with the left cavernous internal carotid artery (ICA; *arrow*). (B) Coronal reconstruction from the same CT confirms left sellar/suprasellar location of the mass (M) and shows its relationship to the pituitary gland *(asterisk)*. (C) Conventional catheter angiography confirms presence of a large aneurysm (A) arising from the cavernous ICA.

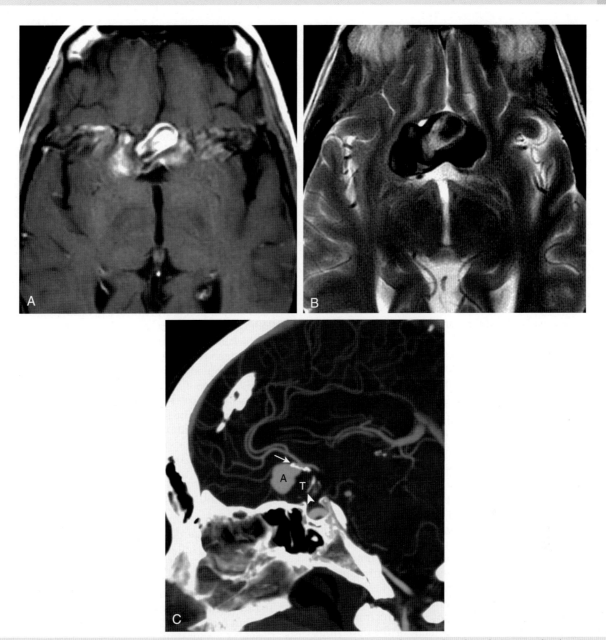

**Fig. 10.22  Giant suprasellar aneurysm.** (A) Axial T1-weighted imaging (T1WI) shows pulsation artifact extending along the image in the phase-encoding direction at the level of a suprasellar mass. (B) Axial T2-weighted imaging (T2WI) shows the suprasellar mass with mixed signal indicating that the lesion is at least partially clotted. Do not biopsy, get a computed tomography angiography (CTA)! (C) Sagittal maximum intensity projection reconstruction from CTA confirms the presence of suprasellar aneurysm (A) arising from the A1-A2 junction. Note the nonenhanced thrombosed component (T) displacing vessels posteriorly *(arrowhead)*. Calcifications are present along the base of the aneurysm *(arrow)*.

- Cavernous ICA aneurysms produce mass effect on the intracavernous cranial nerves. When they rupture, they create carotid-cavernous fistulae as opposed to intradural aneurysms arising more distally from the carotid and its branches, which produce subarachnoid hemorrhage.
- Sometimes the precontrast elevated T1 signal within petrous apex cholesterol granulomas and craniopharyngiomas can mimic a partially thrombosed calcified aneurysm/pseudoaneurysm. Hopefully you can find the normal/displaced ICA flow void nearby to cinch the diagnosis and avoid biopsy!

### Carotid-Cavernous Fistula

- Carotid-cavernous fistula (CCF) occurs as a result of abnormal connection between the cavernous ICA and

cavernous sinus and can be direct/high flow (more common, usually posttraumatic in nature) or indirect/slow flow (spontaneous subacute onset, usually from ruptured cavernous ICA aneurysms). To date, the Barrow classification is the most commonly used system for describing these lesions. Patients with direct CCF typically present with chemosis, pulsatile exophthalmos, and ocular bruit, whereas patients with indirect CCF present with milder chemosis. Treatment options include endovascular ICA stenting and fistula coiling or surgical occlusion with ICA sacrifice. Low-flow CCFs may close spontaneously, although coiling of the cavernous sinus is also an option.
- CTA is the best first test to make the diagnosis, although similar findings can also be demonstrated on MRI.

Barrow Classification of Carotid-Cavernous Fistula

| Type | Features |
| --- | --- |
| A (direct) | Connection between internal carotid artery (ICA) itself and cavernous sinus |
| B (indirect) | Connection between ICA branches and cavernous sinus |
| C (indirect) | Connection between ECA branches and cavernous sinus |
| D (indirect) | Connection between ICA and ECA branches and cavernous sinus |

Associated with an enlarged cavernous sinus is usually an enlarged superior ophthalmic vein or other orbital veins. On CTA obtained in the arterial phase, early or increased venous contrast enhancement isoattenuating to arteries within the affected cavernous sinus relative to the contralateral side can be seen. On time-of-flight MRA, arterialized flow within the affected cavernous sinus can be seen. Occasionally, dilated intercavernous sinus collateral veins can be identified. This can be seen on an angiogram when one internal carotid artery is injected or external carotid artery if supplied by it (Barrow C), and the contralateral cavernous sinus and its tributaries are opacified (see Fig. 3.36).

### Thrombosis of the Cavernous Sinus

- Thrombosis of the cavernous sinus may occur as part of a septic process, tumor extension, spread from invasive fungal sinusitis, extend retrograde from superior ophthalmic vein thrombosis, be associated with spontaneous dural malformations, or result from an interventional or surgical procedure (Fig. 10.23).
- This one is a tricky diagnosis to make, even among the best of us. On MR without enhancement, high intensity may be seen in the subacutely occluded cavernous sinus. However, many times, the sinus may be only partially occluded. Evaluating postcontrast images alone on MR is not very useful because nonthrombosed regions of the sinus enhance, and subacute clot is also high intensity. Absence of gadolinium enhancement of the cavernous sinus without bright signal suggests acute thrombosis. On CT, an irregularly enhancing sinus can be detected with lack of contrast opacification within the thrombosed portion of the sinus. An enlarged superior ophthalmic vein, periorbital swelling, or thickening of the extraocular muscles should send your eyes searching for clot in the cavernous sinus. Be careful not to confuse fat attenuation "filling defects" on CT or high intensity on T1WI in the cavernous sinus with fat seen in normal persons.

### Neurovascular Compression

- Arterial and venous vascular compression upon the cranial nerves as they exit the skull base can be symptomatic, with trigeminal neuralgia being a common presenting complaint. Compression on the trigeminal nerve at the root entry zone can be appreciated on high-resolution T2-weighted MRI (Fig. 10.24). MRA head performed concurrently can aid in diagnosis as well. The most common vessels to compress the trigeminal nerve and require microvascular decompression are (1) the superior cerebellar artery, (2) a vein (perimesencephalic), (3) anterior inferior cerebellar artery, and (4) vertebral artery.

### Perineural Spread of Tumor

- Perineural invasion is a histopathologic diagnosis most commonly made at the primary tumor site, not visibile on imaging, which can portend poorer prognosis. Perineural tumor spread, on the other hand, refers to macroscopic tumor spread away from the primary tumor site, and can be detected by imaging. Head and neck tumors may demonstrate perineural spread through the foramina at the skull base and into the brain. Adenoid cystic carcinoma (ACC), basal cell carcinoma, squamous cell carcinoma, lymphoma, mucoepidermoid carcinoma, melanoma, and malignant nerve sheath tumors all have a propensity for this kind of infiltration (Fig. 10.25). Skin, minor/major salivary glands, and the sinonasal cavity may be the site of origin.
- Enlargement or asymmetry of any basal neural foramina in the appropriate clinical setting should alert you to this possibility of perineural tumor extension (Fig. 10.26). The findings that can be noted with perineural spread include (1) thickening of the nerve; (2) concentric enlargement of the foramen carrying the nerve; (3) enhancement or soft-tissue mass along the course of the nerve; and (4) atrophy, high signal on T2WI, and/or avid enhancement of the denervated muscles supplied by the nerve.
- Always look at the fat in the pterygopalatine fossa (situated behind the maxillary sinus and in front of the pterygoid plates). If asymmetric soft tissue is present there, assume that the branches of V-2 are infiltrated and follow the nerves.

### Cavernous Sinus Infectious and Inflammatory Diseases

- There is a great deal of overlap in imaging features of infectious and inflammatory disorders affecting the cavernous sinuses, including fungal infections, tuberculosis (TB), granulomatous processes like sarcoidosis, granulomatosis with polyangiitis, and IgG-4-related disease. Tolosa-Hunt syndrome resides in this spectrum of disease but remains a diagnosis of exclusion.
- Given cavernous sinus involvement with these conditions, patients can present with deficits in cranial nerves III, IV, VI, or V1; optic nerve; or sympathetic fibers around the cavernous carotid artery. Painful ophthalmoplegia can be present in cases of superior orbital fissure involvement.
- On MR, a spectrum of findings has been observed including infiltrative signal (isointense with muscle on T1WI and iso-dark on T2WI) and/or discrete mass lesion enlarging the cavernous sinus; thrombosis of the cavernous sinus and/or superior ophthalmic vein; and enhancement that can extend into the orbital apex (best identified with fat saturation techniques) and along the floor of the middle cranial fossa (Fig. 10.27).

### Chondrosarcoma

- Chondrosarcoma is a rare neoplasm that is said to arise from embryonal rests, endochondral bone, or cartilage and is located at the skull base, in the meninges, or in the brain. Patients present in their second to fourth decade with long history of headache and cranial nerve problems (particularly cranial nerve VI). To involve the

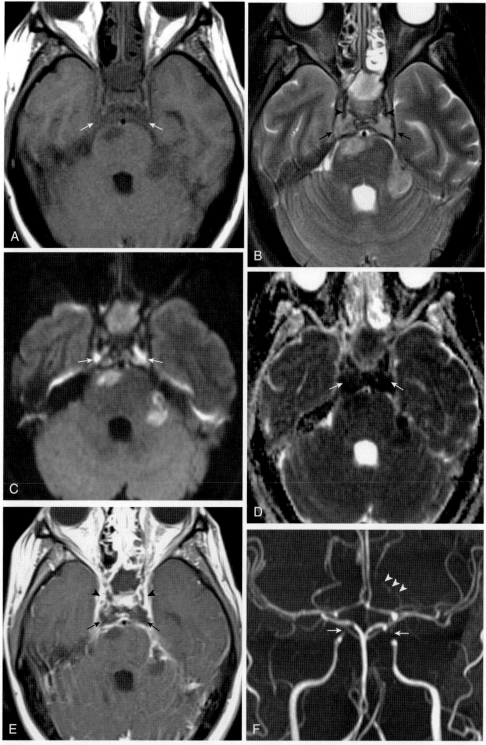

**Fig. 10.23 Cavernous sinus thrombosis in the setting of meningitis.** (A) Axial T1-weighted imaging (T1WI) shows absence of small amount of T1-hyperintense fat signal that can normally be seen in the cavernous sinuses *(arrows)*. (B) Axial T2-weighted imaging (T2WI) shows lateral bulging of the cavernous sinus lateral margins on both sides *(arrows)* and abnormal signal within the posterior aspects of the cavernous sinuses bilaterally. There is also abnormal signal within the right ventral pons and left cerebellopontine angle (CPA) cistern. Note marked narrowing and irregular contours of the cavernous carotid flow voids anteriorly *(arrowheads)* and complete absence of flow voids posteriorly within the cavernous sinuses. Diffusion restriction is seen within the posterior aspects of the cavernous sinuses bilaterally on diffusion-weighted imaging (C; *arrows*), and apparent diffusion coefficient map (D; *arrows*), indicating purulent material. Diffusion restriction is also seen within the right ventral pons and left CPA cistern. (E) Axial postcontrast T1WI shows expansile filling defects within the cavernous sinuses bilaterally *(arrows)* with partially preserved normal enhancement within the cavernous sinuses anteriorly *(arrowheads)*. Note abnormal leptomeningeal enhancement along the pons in this patient with meningitis. Abnormal signal within the pons represents extension of inflammation into the parenchyma, and abnormal signal within the left CPA signal represents loculated meningeal deposit of purulent material. (F) As if that wasn't enough, maximum intensity projection reconstruction from three-dimensional time-of-flight magnetic resonance angiography shows abrupt occlusion of the cavernous internal carotid arteries bilaterally *(arrows)* as well as severe irregularity of the left posterior cerebral artery *(arrowheads)*, indicating arterial vasculitis secondary to meningitis.

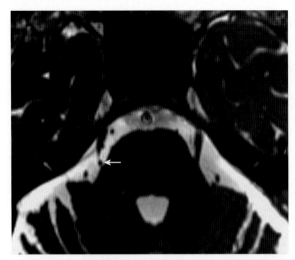

**Fig. 10.24 Neurovascular compression.** In this patient presenting with right-sided trigeminal neuralgia, axial high-resolution T2 constructive interference in steady state (CISS) image shows distal superior cerebellar artery *(arrow)* contacting and laterally displacing the prepontine segment of the right trigeminal nerve at the root entry zone level.

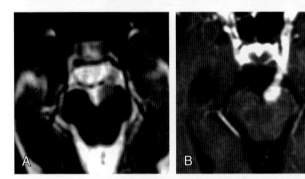

**Fig. 10.25 Lymphoma of cranial nerve III.** Infiltration of the third cranial nerve is best viewed on the postcontrast scan (B), but the enlargement is even evident on the T2-weighted scan (A).

parasellar region, this tumor can arise from the petroclival synchondrosis or petrosphenoid fissure and extend anteriorly toward the cavernous sinus.

- CT is probably more specific for this tumor because of its sensitivity to calcium, demonstrating calcification in more than 60% of cases in a stippled, finely speckled, amorphous, or ring-like configuration. Pure lytic bone destruction may also occur. Contrast-enhanced CT demonstrates enhancing neoplastic tissue.

- MR shows low-to-intermediate intensity on T1WI and classically high intensity on T2WI with heterogeneity. The lesions will enhance, but the degree (and the high intensity on T2WI) is tempered by the amount of calcified matrix, which will not show enhancement (Fig. 10.28). Although chondrosarcomas share T2 hyperintensity with chordomas, parasellar chondrosarcomas are centered "off-midline," in contrast to chordomas, which occur at the midline.

## INFRASELLAR AND BASE OF SKULL LESIONS

These are lesions centered below the sella/central skull base.

### Meningoencephaloceles

- Basal meningoencephaloceles make up approximately 10% of all cephaloceles. These anomalies produce round, smooth erosion in the bone of the particular anatomic region. Their intensity on MR depends on the contents of the cephalocele, which includes meninges, brain which may be dysplastic, and/or CSF.

- At the skull base, you can find sphenopharyngeal (through sphenoid body), spheno-orbital (through superior orbital fissure), spheno-ethmoidal (through sphenoid and ethmoid bones), transethmoidal (through cribriform plate), spheno-maxillary (through maxillary sinus), petrous apex (from Meckel's cave), and mastoid roof meningo(encephalo)celes.

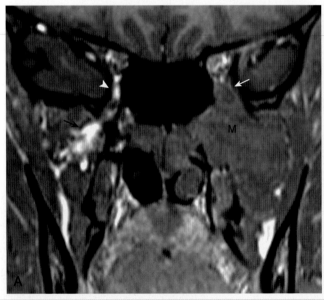

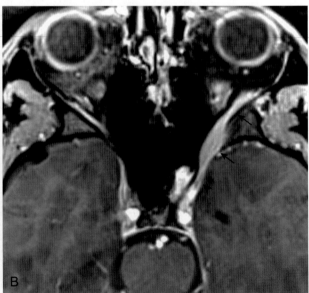

**Fig. 10.26 In diagnosing perineural tumor spread, fat is our friend.** (A) Coronal T1-weighted image (T1WI) shows a tumor mass centered in the left pterygopalatine fossa/masticator space (M) with obliteration of the normal fat in this space as shown on the normal right side *(black arrow)*. There is extension of tumor into the inferior orbital fissure (IOF), which is widened, and normal fat in this space is obliterated by the tumor *(white arrow)*. Compare to the normal IOF on the right *(arrowhead)*. (B) Contrast-enhanced fat-suppressed T1WI shows abnormal enlargement and enhancement within the IOF *(arrows)* with extension along V2 toward the cavernous sinus *(arrowhead)*.

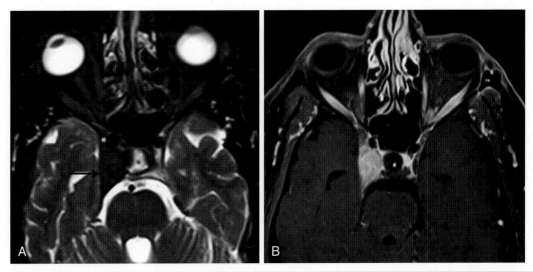

**Fig. 10.27 Inflammatory tissue involving the cavernous sinus.** (A) Axial T2-weighted image shows an impressively T2 dark mass investing the right cavernous sinus *(arrow)* and right parasellar region, strongly suggestive of fibrotic tissue. Some of this tissue is sneaking its way into the right superior orbital fissure *(asterisk)*. (B) On axial fat-suppressed postcontrast T1-weighted image, this tissue shows relatively homogeneous contrast enhancement. This was biopsy proven IgG4-related disease.

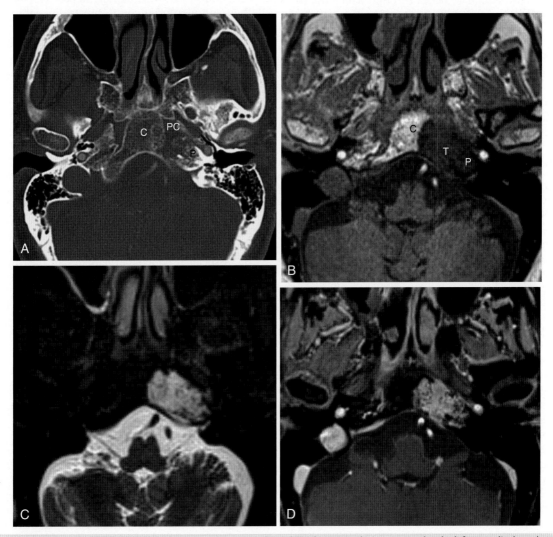

**Fig. 10.28 Chondrosarcoma.** (A) Axial computed tomographic image shows lytic destructive lesion centered at the left petroclival synchondrosis (PC) with lytic change involving the left lateral aspect of the clivus (C) and medial aspect of the left petrous apex (P). (B) Axial T1-weighted imaging (T1WI) shows the tumor (T) again centered in the petroclival synchondrosis with abnormal marrow signal within the left aspect of the adjacent clivus (C) and petrous apex (P). (C) Axial T2-weighted imaging (T2WI) shows characteristic high T2 signal of this lesion. Hypointense foci reflect calcified matrix. (D) The tumor enhances on postcontrast T1W1.

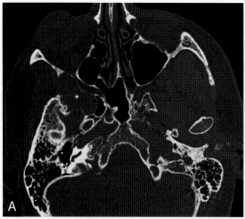
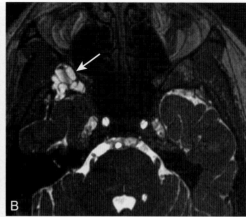
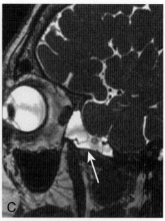

**Fig. 10.29 Meningocele.** (A) Lytic lesion in the sphenoid wing at first, on computed tomography, seems to be a primary bone lesion *(asterisk)*. The axial (B) and sagittal (C) T2-weighted image show the cerebrospinal fluid signal *(arrow)* and communication with the subarachnoid space indicative of a skull base meningocele.

- High-resolution MRI can elegantly show the contents of meningoencephalocele, whereas thin-section CT images can identify the skull base defect through which the tissue herniates (Fig. 10.29). These should be distinguished from physiologic bony excavations from arachnoid granulations, which appear similarly but should not breach the full thickness of the skull.
- Iatrogenic meningoencephaloceles can occur with any type of skull base or endoscopic sinus surgery. The patient may have symptoms of CSF leakage and/or intracranial hypotension with concurrent brain sagging and venous engorgement.

## Chordoma

- Chordomas occur at sites of notochordal remnants and constitute less than 1% of all intracranial tumors. About 35% to 40% of chordomas are cranial, 50% are in the sacrum, and 15% are in the spine. Intracranially, the most common site of origin is the clivus, less commonly the basioccipital and parasellar regions, and rarely the paranasal sinuses. Patients with skull base chordomas present with headache, visual disturbances, and usually cranial nerve VI palsy.
- Although most chordomas are histologically benign, they are locally aggressive, with a poor overall prognosis. Complete surgical removal is rarely possible; thus, partial resection is performed followed by radiation therapy.
- CT and MR are complementary in imaging these lesions (Fig. 10.30). CT demonstrates a midline soft-tissue mass, bone destruction, and calcification. On T1WI, chordomas are isointense to brain parenchyma, although some regions of low intensity (calcification) and high intensity can be identified. On T2WI, high intensity is the rule, and they enhance.
- Chordomas and chondrosarcomas may look identical on MR; however, chondrosarcoma is associated with higher mean ADC values (in the $2000 \times 10^{-6}$ mm²/sec range) than classic ($1500 \times 10^{-6}$ mm²/sec range) and poorly differentiated ($900 \times 10^{-6}$ mm²/sec range) chordomas. Popcorn calcification on CT is a hallmark of chondrosarcoma but is variably present.

## Other Infrasellar Lesions

- *Sellar macroadenomas* typically extend superiorly into the suprasellar region, but occasionally they may be seen extending inferiorly into the infrasellar region, with involvement of the sphenoid sinus, clivus, and even nasopharynx. The imaging appearance is similar to their supratentorial counterparts. Recognition that the lesions arise from the sella can help aid in the diagnosis.
- *Nasopharyngeal carcinoma, sphenoid metastases, and chordomas* arising in the sphenoid sinus can extend to involve the sella in a secondary fashion. Rarely, craniopharyngiomas are found in the upper pharynx.
- *Sphenoid sinus mucoceles* are expansile slow-growing lesions that have a variable intensity pattern but have a tendency for high intensity on T1WI because of proteinaceous contents; these lesions do not enhance centrally, but a thin rim of contrast enhancement can be seen along lesion margins. A thin margin of bone is usually present, best appreciated on CT.
- *Fibrous dysplasia* is a common developmental bone lesion to affect the central skull base. On CT, ground glass density is seen in affected regions, which may be expanded. Lytic changes may be seen within the lesion. When extensive, the associated bone enlargement can narrow skull base foramina and can compress critical soft-tissue structures, such as within the orbit. On MRI, these lesions show a mixed signal intensity on T1WI and T2WI with variable contrast enhancement. These lesions can appear aggressive on MRI, and CT can help specify the diagnosis.

## PANSELLAR LESIONS

These lesions are the sneaky ones that can affect sellar, suprasellar, parasellar, and/or infrasellar regions, sometimes all at once.

## Meningiomas

- Meningiomas at the sella/central skull base region show similar signal characteristics to meningiomas elsewhere in the brain, but in the central skull base region, these lesions have a propensity for extension along skull base foramina with potential for multicompartment involvement. These dural-based tumors can arise from the tuberculum sellae, anterior clinoid processes, diaphragma sellae, planum sphenoidale, tentorial leaflet, and upper clivus.
- Planum sphenoidale meningiomas can infiltrate the sella and optic canals and cause mass effect on the inferior

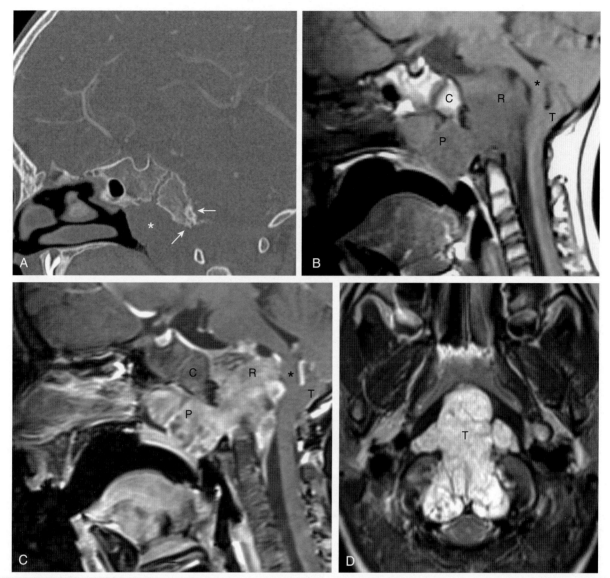

**Fig. 10.30 Clivus chordoma.** (A) Sagittal reconstruction from contrast-enhanced computed tomography shows destructive process centered at the base of the clivus, involving both anterior and posterior margins of the clivus *(arrows)*. Large prevertebral soft-tissue component is appreciated *(asterisk)*, resulting in near complete occlusion of the nasopharyngeal airway. Sagittal precontrast (B) and postcontrast (C) T1-weighted imaging (T1WI) shows the truncated appearance of the clivus (C) because of destructive tumor mass. Prevertebral (P) and retroclival (R) soft-tissue components are shown here. The retroclival component compresses and posteriorly displaces the medulla *(asterisk)* and there is crowding of the cerebellar tonsils (T) because of mass effect. (D) Axial T2-weighted imaging (T2WI) shows characteristic high signal within this lesion (T). Note that the tumor is centered at midline, as opposed to the off-midline chondrosarcoma (compare with Fig. 10.28).

frontal lobes (Fig. 10.31). Paracavernous meningiomas arise from the tentorial leaflet and cause lots of trouble by infiltrating into the orbit via the superior and inferior orbital fissures or optic canal, as well as middle cranial fossa, cavernous sinus, and sella, and can push up into the anterior cranial fossa (Fig. 10.32). In rare cases, they may extend along other neural foramina, such as the foramen ovale with consequent involvement of the masticator space, or along V2 into the pterygopalatine fossa and vidian canal. These lesions may encase and narrow the cavernous ICA (in distinction from pituitary adenomas).

■ CT can reveal hyperostosis adjacent to slightly hyperattenuating mass, occasionally with associated calcifications. On T1WI, meningiomas are isointense to slightly hypointense to brain. On T2WI, they are isointense to slightly hypointense to brain. They enhance avidly and typically demonstrate associated dural tail.

## Epidermoids

■ These are benign congenital lesions resulting from entrapped ectodermal components, which become symptomatic as they enlarge over time because of compression of adjacent structures. Epidermoids may be intradural or extradural, insinuating between and encasing tissues. They can arise in the third ventricle and in the parasellar region around the gasserian ganglion, where they may remodel the petrous apex. They can insinuate throughout the suprasellar region and can grow behind the clivus, thereby pushing the brain stem posteriorly.

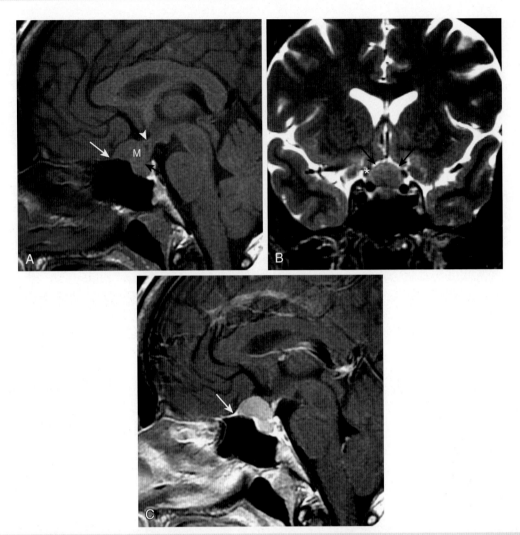

**Fig. 10.31 Planum sphenoidale meningioma.** (A) Unenhanced sagittal T1-weighted imaging (T1WI) shows a mass (M) in the suprasellar region. However, there is a subtle tissue plane present between the mass and pituitary gland *(black arrow)*, indicating that this tumor is not arising from the pituitary gland. There is dural-based attachment on the planum sphenoidale *(white arrow)*, indicating dural origin of this meningioma. The infundibulum is displaced posteriorly *(black arrowhead)*, and the optic chiasm is elevated superiorly *(white arrowhead)* by the mass. (B) Coronal T2WI shows the tumor to be very slightly hyperintense to brain *(arrows)*. Note lateral displacement of the A1 segments of the anterior cerebral arteries *(asterisk)*. (C) After contrast administration, the dural attachment is again seen *(arrow)*, and the tumor is shown to enhance slightly less than the normal pituitary gland.

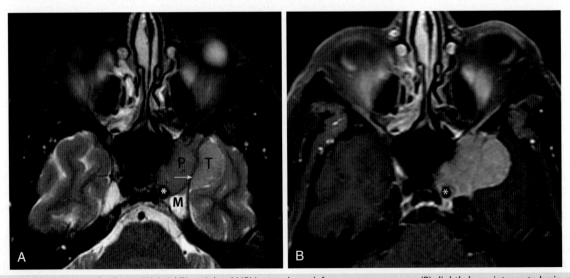

**Fig. 10.32 Paracavernous meningioma.** (A) Axial T2-weighted MRI image shows left paracavernous mass (P) slightly hyperintense to brain, partially encasing the cavernous internal carotid artery (ICA) *(white asterisk)* and invading the ventral aspect of Meckel's cave (indicated by M). Foramen rotundum is obliterated by the mass (compare with normal appearance on the right indicated by *black arrow*), granting tumor access to the inferior orbital fissure *(black asterisk)*. Note middle cranial fossa component (T) on the other side of the tentorial leaflet *(white arrow)*. (B) On fat-suppressed postcontrast T1-weighted image, the mass shows homogeneous contrast enhancement, consistent with meningioma. Note slight narrowing of the left ICA flow void *(asterisk)* compared with the right, a feature which meningiomas can be guilty of.

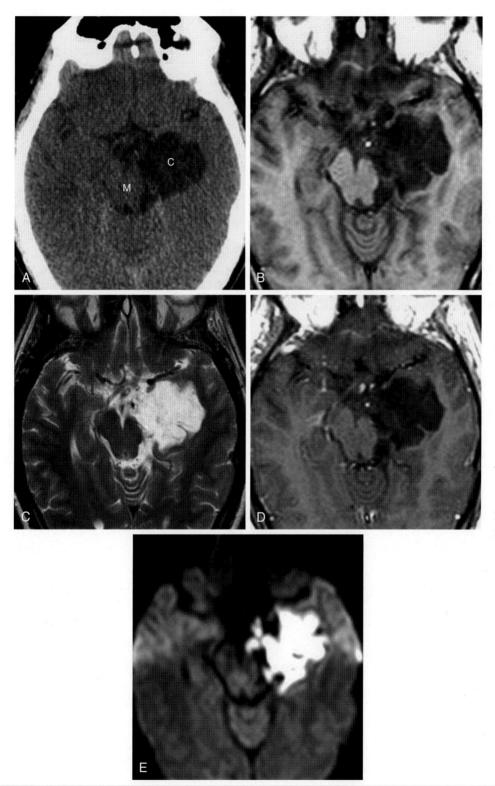

**Fig. 10.33 Epidermoid.** (A) Unenhanced computed tomography (CT) shows lobulated contours of an extraaxial lesion isodense to cerebrospinal fluid (CSF; C) centered in the left middle cranial fossa, with extension into the left parasellar region. Note mass effect upon the left aspect of the midbrain (M). No calcification is seen. (B) Axial T1-weighted imaging (T1WI) and (C) axial T2WI show the lesion to have signal intensity similar to CSF. (D) Postcontrast T1WI shows that the lesion does not enhance. So far this lesion could represent an arachnoid cyst. However, the diffusion-weighted scan (E) nails the diagnosis of an epidermoid.

■ Epidermoids can have the same density and intensity on CT and T1WI and T2WI on MR as CSF. Fortunately, the diagnosis of these lesions has been made rather straightforward with fluid-attenuated inversion recovery (FLAIR) imaging where they are brighter than CSF (Fig. 10.33) and show restricted diffusion because of the highly proteinaceous contents. Occasionally, epidermoids may have rim calcification appreciable on CT. These lesions rarely, if ever, enhance.

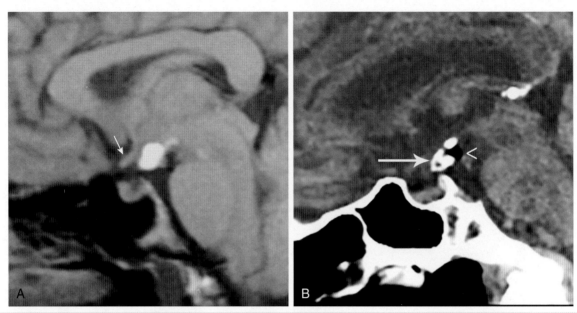

**Fig. 10.34 Incidentally, what is up with that fat?** (A) On this sagittal T1-weighted image, a discrete high intensity mass representing a lipoma is noted in the suprasellar cistern. Optic chiasm *(arrow)* is anterior to the lipoma. (B) Sagittal reconstruction from noncontrast computed tomography (CT) in a different patient shows a suprasellar mass containing calcifications *(white arrow)* and fat density *(arrowhead)* components, compatible with dermoid.

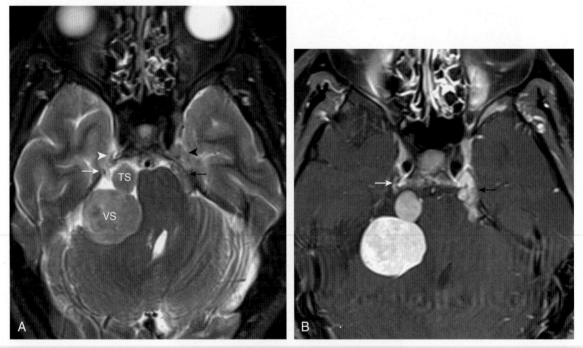

**Fig. 10.35 Bilateral trigeminal schwannomas.** (A) In this patient with neurofibromatosis type 2, axial T2-weighted imaging (T2WI) shows multiple bilateral extra-axial masses hyperintense to brain. On the left, an elongated lobulated mass extends along the prepontine course of the trigeminal nerve *(black arrow)* and into the Meckel cave with effacement of the normal fluid signal present within the cave *(black arrowhead)*, compatible with trigeminal schwannoma. On the right, a rounded trigeminal schwannoma (TS) arising from the proximal segment of the nerve displaces the more distal prepontine segment of the trigeminal nerve laterally *(white arrow)*. An additional lesion along the trigeminal nerve is suspected within right Meckel cave given partial absence of expected fluid signal *(white arrowhead)*. Posterior to this is a large vestibular schwannoma (VS), compressing and displacing the brainstem to the left. (B) These schwannomas enhance homogeneously on postcontrast T1W1. Note the enhancement of schwannomas within left Meckel cave *(black arrow)* and right Meckel cave *(white arrow)*.

## Dermoids, Lipomas, and Teratomas

- Like epidermoid lesion, dermoids, lipomas, and teratomas are developmental lesions and can occur anywhere in the neuroaxis, including the sella/central skull base regions, and can grow to be large, compressing the third ventricle and adjacent structures.

- Dermoids are midline lesions containing fat, squamous epithelium (as do epidermoids), hair follicles, sweat glands, and sebaceous glands. On MR, high intensity on T1WI from fat can be observed in dermoids, lipomas, and teratomas (Fig. 10.34). Lipomas in this region are usually well circumscribed. Teratomas may contain dense calcification or ossification, which has been observed to be in the central portion of the lesion.

### Schwannomas/Neurofibromas

- These are nerve sheath tumors that can arise from peripheral nerves or any of the cranial nerves after they exit the brain stem (except cranial nerve II, of course, where we have "gliomas") (see Chapters 2 and 8). These can be spontaneous or seen among patients with neurofibromatosis types I and II. Symptoms relate to the nerve involved.
- On MR, they are smooth masses, isointense on T1WI and high intensity on T2WI, with avid enhancement (Fig. 10.35). Regions of "cystic" change may be observed in the enhancing mass. They may grow through skull base foramina, producing smooth enlargement.

### Metastases

- Just like everywhere, metastases can affect the sellar/parasellar/infrasellar and central skull base regions. Symptomatology depends on the site and size of the lesion and although there are no specific imaging features, multiplicity favors metastasis.

# 11 Temporal Bone

NAOKO SAITO

## Relevant Anatomy

- At the lateral skull base, the temporal bone helps form the middle and posterior cranial fossae on either side.
- The temporal bone has five bony parts, including the squamous (the thinnest part anteriorly), mastoid (consisting of network of aerated air cells and serves as attachment point for neck muscles as well as houses portions of the facial nerve and venous sinuses), petrous (the most medial part, carrying the internal auditory canal), tympanic (which gives rise the bony external auditory canal) and styloid (linear inferiorly directed bone that serves as attachment point for styloid muscles and ligaments) parts.
- Among its many important roles in the skull, the temporal bone facilitates the transmission of sound that allows us to hear and engage in the world around us.

### TEACHING POINTS
#### Development of the Ear

- The external auditory canal (EAC) is derived from the first branchial groove.
- The cartilaginous EAC and auricle are derived from the first and second branchial arches.
- The first branchial arch forms the bodies of the malleus and incus and the short process of the incus.
- The second branchial arch forms the superstructure (capitulum and crura) of the stapes and long process of the incus, as well as the manubrium of the malleus.
- The first branchial pouch invaginates into the eustachian tube, mesotympanum, and mastoid air cells.

### EXTERNAL AUDITORY CANAL

- The external auditory canal (EAC) is made of fibrocartilage laterally and bone medially.
- The anterior wall of the EAC is the posterior border of the glenoid fossa housing the temporomandibular joint (TMJ). Posterior to the EAC is the mastoid portion of the temporal bone.
- The EAC forms embryologically from branchial grooves, arches, and pouches.

### TEACHING POINTS
#### Tympanic Membrane

- Where the ectodermal external auditory canal (EAC) joins the endoderm of the first branchial pouch is the medial boundary of the EAC, the tympanic membrane.
- The tympanic membrane has a thin anterosuperior portion known as the *pars flaccida* and a tougher posteroinferior pars tensa.

- The umbo is the inward puckering of the tympanic membrane at the attachment of the handle of the malleus.

### THE MIDDLE EAR

- The middle ear, or *tympanic cavity*, is divided into the most superior epitympanum, the mesotympanum at the level of the tympanic membrane, and the hypotympanum lying inferior and medial to the tympanic membrane (Fig. 11.1). It communicates posteriorly with the mastoid antrum via the aditus ad antrum.
- The tympanic membrane and scutum are the lateral border of the middle ear. The medial border of the middle ear is formed by the otic capsule, the dense bone encasing the labyrinthine structures of the inner ear.

### TEACHING POINTS
#### Scutum

- The scutum is a sharp, bony excrescence seen best on coronal images.
- It forms the superomedial margin of the external auditory canal (EAC) (inferolateral attic wall) from which the tympanic membrane descends.
- It protrudes from the roof of the epitympanic cavity, the tegmen tympani.
- The air space between the scutum and the ossicles is called the *Prussak space* and is the first area filled by a pars flaccida cholesteatoma.

- The ossicles are responsible for sound conduction in the middle ear and despite their tiny size, these bones harbor some intricate parts (Fig. 11.2). The epitympanum contains the head of malleus and the body and short process of the incus.
- The rest of the ossicular chain is located in the mesotympanum.

### TEACHING POINTS
#### Ossicular Chain

- The malleus has a head, which articulates with the body of the incus; a neck, an anterior process that attaches by ligaments to the wall of the mesotympanum and to the tensor tympani muscle; a lateral process; and a manubrium, which connects to the tympanic membrane. The tensor tympani muscle attaches to the upper manubrium and neck of the malleus (see Figs. 11.2 and 11.3).
- The incus has a body, short process, and long process. The short process attaches by ligaments to the posterior

tympanic cavity wall, whereas the long process parallels the manubrium posteromedially before bending medially and articulating with the stapes via its lenticular process.

- The stapes has a head (capitulum), which articulates with the lenticular process of the incus, an anterior crus, a posterior crus, and a footplate. The footplate of the stapes covers the oval (vestibular) window. The stapedius muscle arises from the pyramidal eminence and attaches to the head of the stapes. This muscle dampens sound by preventing excessive stapedial vibration. This explains the hyperacusis with seventh nerve palsies because this muscle is innervated by a branch of the facial nerve.

- In the inferoposterior portion of the middle ear cavity, four important structures are visible on axial scans. They are, medially to laterally, the round window niche, the sinus tympani, the pyramidal eminence, and the facial nerve recess (see Fig. 11.1).
  - The sinus tympani and facial nerve recess are indentations in the bone; the pyramidal eminence is a bony hillock separating the two. The stapedius muscle belly and tendon emanate from the pyramidal eminence and attach to the neck of the stapes.

- These recesses are important because disease at these sites can be difficult to see at otoscopy or on direct inspection during middle ear surgery; recognition of disease at these levels on imaging before surgery is key to minimizing residual tissue.
- The middle ear cavity connects via the eustachian tube to the nasopharynx at the torus tubarius.
  - This explains the frequent coexistence of serous otitis media and/or mastoiditis with nasopharyngeal carcinoma or adenoidal hypertrophy. The eustachian tube is a conduit for spread of lesions in both directions (e.g., malignant otitis externa from ear to nasopharynx and carcinoma from nasopharynx to middle ear cavity).

## FACIAL NERVE

- The facial nerve courses through the temporal bone after exiting from the internal auditory canal (IAC) (Box 11.1), giving off important branches on its journey (Fig. 11.3).
- The IAC is separated into superior and inferior sections by the transverse crista falciformis and into anterior and posterior quadrants by the Bill bar (Fig. 11.4). Cranial nerve VII is found in the anterosuperior portion of the IAC ("Seven-Up").

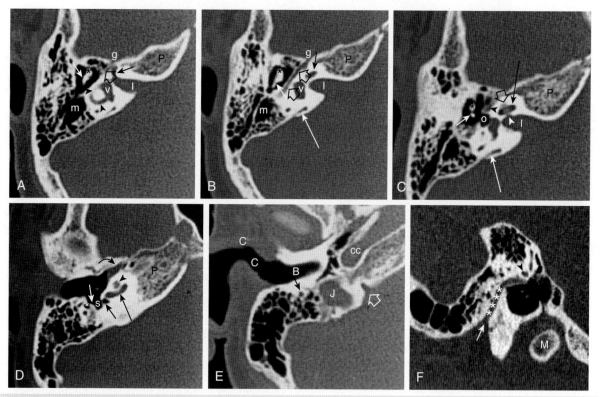

**Fig. 11.1 Computed tomography of the normal anatomy of the middle ear from the superior to the inferior region.** (A) Axial view of labyrinthine portion of the facial nerve *(black arrow)*, geniculate ganglion of facial nerve *(g)*, proximal portion of the horizontal segment of the facial nerve *(open arrow)*, head of malleus *(asterisk)*, and short process of incus *(white arrow)*. Also note vestibule *(v)*, lateral semicircular canal *(black arrowheads)*, mastoid *(m)*, nonpneumatized petrous apex *(P)*, and internal auditory canal (IAC; *l*). (B) Axial view of middle turn of the cochlea *(black arrow)*, geniculate ganglion of facial nerve *(g)*, horizontal segment of the facial nerve *(open arrows)*, head of malleus *(asterisk)*, short process of incus *(small white arrow)*, vestibule *(v)*, mastoid *(m)*, nonpneumatized petrous apex *(P)*, IAC *(l)*, and vestibular aqueduct *(large white arrow)*. (C) Axial view of middle turn of the cochlea *(large black arrow)*, apical turn of the cochlea *(open arrowhead)*, neck of malleus *(asterisk)*, long process of incus *(small white arrow)*, oval window *(o)*, tensor tympani muscle *(small black arrowhead)*, cochlear aperture *(white arrowhead)*, nonpneumatized petrous apex *(P)*, IAC *(l)*, and vestibular aqueduct *(large white arrow)*. (D) Axial view of the hypotympanum. Basal turn of the cochlea *(large black arrow)*, apical turn of the cochlea *(black arrowhead)*, nonpneumatized petrous apex *(P)*, round window niche *(small black arrow)*, superior aspect of the eustachian tube and tensor tympani tendon *(curved black arrow)*, sinus tympani *(s)*, pyramidal eminence *(white arrow)*, and facial nerve recess *(asterisk)*. (E) Axial view of the region inferior to the hypotympanum.

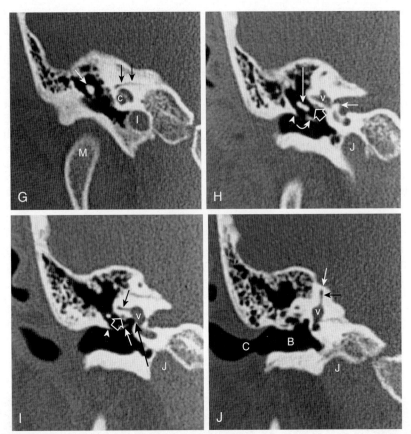

**Fig. 11.1 cont'd.** Cochlear aqueduct *(open arrow)*, cartilaginous portion of external auditory canal (EAC), bony portion of EAC *(B)*, carotid canal *(cc)*, jugular bulb *(J)*, and descending portion of facial nerve *(black arrow)*. (F) Sagittal oblique reconstruction of the right temporal bone shows the descending (mastoid) segment of the facial nerve *(asterisks)* and the stylomastoid foramen *(arrow)*. The tympanic segment of the facial nerve travels just underneath the lateral semicircular canal *(arrowhead)*. Mandibular condyle is noted *(M)*. (G–J) Coronal images from anterior to posterior. (G) Internal carotid artery *(I)*, cochlea *(c)*, facial nerve coursing over cochlea *(black arrows)*, head of malleus *(white arrow)*, and mandibular condyle *(M)*. (H) Crista falciformis of IAC *(small white arrow)*, jugular bulb *(J)*, vestibule *(v)*, head and neck of malleus *(large white arrow)*, tympanic portion of the facial nerve *(open arrow)*, scutum *(arrowhead)*, and incus *(curved arrow)*. (I) Jugular foramen *(J)*, vestibule *(v)*, incudostapedial joint *(white arrow)*, tympanic portion of the facial nerve *(open arrow)*, scutum *(arrowhead)*, oval window *(long black arrow)*, and lateral semicircular canal *(short black arrow)*. (J) Jugular foramen *(J)*, arcuate eminence *(white arrow)*, superior semicircular canal *(black arrow)*, vestibule *(v)*, cartilaginous portion of EAC *(C)*, and bony portion of EAC *(B)*.

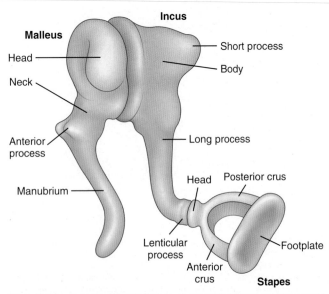

**Fig. 11.2** Schematic shows ossicles including their named parts and articulations.

- The intratemporal segments of the facial nerve as defined by location are: (1) labyrinthine, (2) geniculate ganglion, (3) tympanic or horizontal, and (4) mastoid or descending.
- The labyrinthine segment courses anterosuperiorly and laterally in the fallopian canal from the IAC to the geniculate ganglion.
- The geniculate ganglion is superior to the cochlea and is the fulcrum by which the facial nerve forms its first genu. Here it gives off the greater superficial petrosal nerve anteriorly, which contributes to lacrimation.
- The facial nerve runs posteroinferolaterally on the undersurface of the lateral semicircular canal and above the oval window niche in its horizontal or tympanic segment.
- The facial nerve then makes its second turn (the second genu) to course inferiorly in the mastoid bone in the mastoid or descending segment before exiting at the stylomastoid foramen.
- Along its course it gives innervation to the stapedius muscle and, just above the stylomastoid foramen, to the chorda tympani for taste to the anterior two thirds of the tongue. The chorda tympani doubles back on itself running superiorly and re-enters the mesotympanum before

exiting anteriorly via the petrotympanic fissure to join the lingual nerve.

■ Extracranially, the facial nerve bisects the parotid gland into superficial and deep lobes and branches to innervate muscles of facial expression.

## INNER EAR, PETROUS APEX, AND JUGULAR FORAMEN

■ The petrous apex is the medial most aspect of the temporal bone, a pyramidal shaped portion of the temporal bone that houses the inner ear structures, internal auditory canal (IAC) and portions of the carotid canal (see Fig. 11.1). The petrous apex can consist of solid marrow but can also be pneumatized. The IAC carries the facial nerve as well as the cochlear, superior vestibular and inferior vestibular divisions of cranial nerve VIII (see Fig. 11.4), and delivers them to their respective inner ear structures.

■ The cochlea and semicircular canals make up the principal components of the inner ear (Fig. 11.5). The osseous labyrinth (otic capsule) includes the vestibule, semicircular canals, and cochlea. The membranous labyrinth includes the perilymph (within the scala vestibuli and tympani of the cochlea) and the endolymph (within the cochlear duct, semicircular canals, and vestibular aqueduct).

---

### Box 11.1   Intracranial Segments of Cranial Nerve VII

Cisternal (cerebellopontine angle cistern)
Intracanalicular (internal auditory canal)
Labyrinthine (fallopian canal)
Geniculate ganglion (first genu)
Horizontal (tympanic)
Intramastoid (second genu, descending portion, exits skull base through the stylomastoid foramen)

---

■ The cochlea has apical, middle, and basal turns. The apical turn amplifies low tones, and the basal turn amplifies high tones.

■ The cochlea is filled with perilymph but also has an endolymph channel. The cochlea has a base and a cupula (or *apex*) and is divided by a bony central canal known as the *modiolus*.

■ At the scala vestibuli, perilymph from the vestibule communicates with that of the cochlea. At the end of the scala tympani along the basal turn, the perilymphatic space connects to the round window. The scala tympani and vestibuli join at the helicotrema of the cupula. The cochlear aqueduct is seen on sections below the IAC (see Fig. 11.1E) and extends from the scala tympani posteromedially to drain perilymph into the subarachnoid space of the posterior fossa.

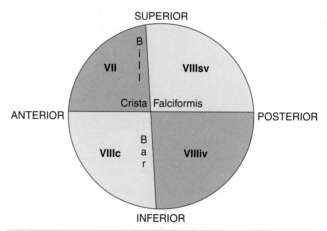

Fig. 11.4 **Internal auditory canal subdivisions.** Diagram demonstrating Bill bar and crista falciformis separating the internal auditory canal (IAC) into four quadrants with cranial nerve VII and cochlear (VIIIc), superior vestibular (VIIIsv), and inferior vestibular (VIIIiv) divisions of cranial nerve VIII.

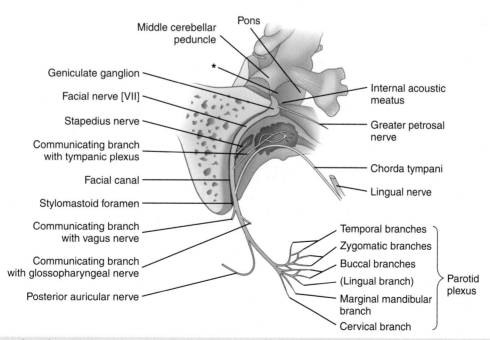

Fig. 11.3 **Facial nerve branches.** Schematic shows branches of the facial nerve, including the greater (superficial) petrosal nerve (for lacrimation and salivation), the stapedius nerve (to dampen sound), the tympanic plexus, the chorda tympani (for taste), and infratemporal branches for facial muscles.
(From Putz R, Pabst R. *Sobotta Atlas of Human Anatomy, Vol. 1: Head, Neck, Upper Limb.* Philadelphia: Lippincott Williams & Wilkins; 2001. Fig. 652, p 370.)

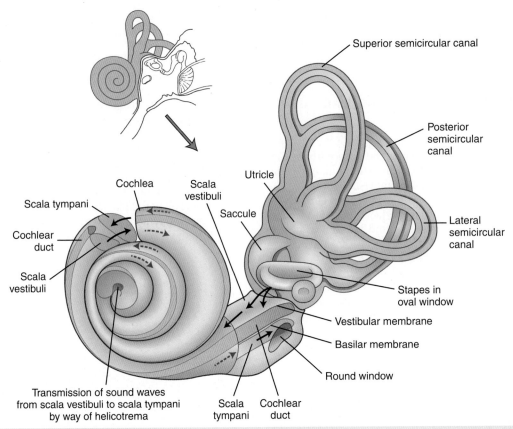

**Fig. 11.5** Schematic shows the vestibulocochlear apparatus and its numerous components.

- The vestibule is the common chamber to which the semicircular canals join. There are lateral, superior, and posterior semicircular canals.
- The superior and posterior semicircular canals share a nonampullated end known as the *crus communis*. The bony ridge over the superior semicircular canal is called the *arcuate eminence*.
- The stapes articulates to the vestibule via the oval window. The vestibule contains the posteriorly located utricle and the round, anterior saccule, the sense organs responsible for balance.
- The endolymphatic sac within the bony vestibular aqueduct courses posterolaterally from the vestibule and dilates into a blind-ending sac (see Fig. 11.1B–C).
- The jugular foramen has two parts divided by a fibrous or bony septum called the *jugular spine*.
  - A pars nervosa is the anteromedial portion of the jugular foramen. It contains cranial nerve IX and the inferior petrosal sinus.
  - A pars vascularis is the posterolateral portion of the jugular foramen. It is larger than a pars nervosa. It contains the internal jugular vein and cranial nerves X and XI.

# Imaging Techniques/Protocols

## COMPUTED TOMOGRAPHY

- Computed tomography (CT) of the temporal bone is performed at high resolution and with a small field of view with thin-slice thickness (about 0.4 mm). CT is typically performed without contrast.

- Axial and coronal images are reconstructed for each side. An oblique reconstruction image (such as Stenver and Pöschl) is useful for detection of the superior canal dehiscence, assessment of the ossicular chain, measurement of vestibular aqueduct, and so on.

## MAGNETIC RESONANCE IMAGING

- High resolution and small field of view with thin-imaging slices (<2 mm) of the temporal bone is essential for detecting tiny lesions in and around the temporal bone.
- Fluid-sensitive, heavily T2-weighted images (T2WI) using steady-state gradient echo (e.g., constructive interference steady state [CISS]) or fast-recovery fast spine-echo (e.g., driven equilibrium [DRIVE]) techniques can provide submillimeter-thickness "cisternogram" type images. These are often used to identify the cochlear nerve in congenital sensorineural hearing loss (SNHL) cases or to detect dehiscence of the superior semicircular canal.
- Precontrast and postcontrast 2-mm-thickness T1-weighted images (T1WI) can assess for potential enhancement of disease processes detected on fluid sensitive sequences.
- Diffusion-weighted imaging (DWI) is useful for diagnosis of a cholesteatoma, being bright on DWI with a diminished apparent diffusion coefficient (ADC). Nonechoplanar imaging (non-EPI) DWI is preferred to echoplanar imaging (EPI) DWI because there is less of a susceptibility artifact.
- A three-dimensional (3D) fluid-attenuated inversion recovery (FLAIR) technique can be performed for detection of hemorrhage or inflammatory exudate in inner ear structures.

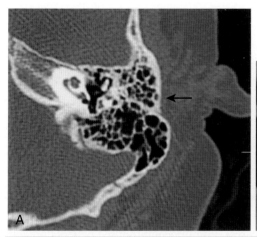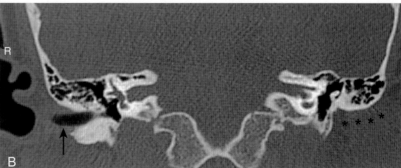

**Fig. 11.6 External auditory canal (EAC) atresia.** (A) Axial computed tomography (CT) demonstrates absence of EAC on the left side *(arrow)*. The ossicles are deformed. (B) The finding is confirmed on the coronal image, where one can see the normal *(R)* right EAC *(arrow)*, the absent EAC *(asterisks)*, and the lateralized ossicles on the left adherent to atretic plate.

---

### Box 11.2   Associations with Microtia

Idiopathic
External auditory canal atresia
Down syndrome
CHARGE syndrome
Crouzon syndrome
Treacher Collins syndrome

---

*CHARGE*, Coloboma, heart defects, choanal atresia, growth and developmental retardation, genitourinary abnormalities, ear abnormalities.

## Pathology

### EXTERNAL AUDITORY CANAL

#### Congenital Anomalies

■ Congenital anomalies of the EAC are rather common, more so than isolated middle ear abnormalities. However, middle ear abnormalities often accompany EAC anomalies. The degree of congenital deformities of the EAC runs the gamut from total atresia to hypoplasia or stenosis of the EAC. Microtia (a small pinna) can be seen in conjunction with EAC atresia or stenosis but can also be seen in association with inner and middle ear anomalies (Fig. 11.6; Box 11.2). Microtia may occur sporadically or as part of a congenital syndrome.

#### External Auditory Canal Atresia/Stenosis

■ With EAC atresia (complete absence of the EAC), there is often concomitant abnormality in the TMJ, with flattening or absence of the glenoid fossa. Dysplasia of the mandibular condyle and defects of the zygomatic arch may be seen. Additionally, atresia of the EAC may be associated with hypoplasia of the malleus, fusion of the malleus and incus, lateral displacement in the epitympanum, or other anomalies of middle ear structures (in more than 50% of cases).

■ In patients with EAC atresia, the horizontal segment of the facial nerve may have an aberrant course in close proximity to the stapes footplate and may be anteriorly located in its descending portion. The facial nerve may also be dehiscent in its tympanic course.

■ With EAC hypoplasia, the slope of the EAC may be more vertically angulated. In addition, keratinous plugs and cholesteatomas may form.

■ Degree of microtia tends to correlate with the extent of stenosis of the EAC.

■ Middle ear malformations also vary with the severity of the auricular anomalies.

---

**TEACHING POINTS**

Middle Ear Malformations in Microtia

• Two thirds of patients with severe microtia or anotia have reduced pneumatization of the middle ear and mastoid.

• In minor microtia (e.g., pocket ear, absence of upper helix, absence of tragus, miniear, clefts), one half of patients have a dysplastic malleus-incus complex, whereas with major microtia, two thirds are dysplastic and one third have absent ossicles altogether.

• The incudostapedial joint is commonly abnormal in both minor and major microtia. Abnormalities of the stapes often coexist.

---

■ It is important to know whether the inner ear structures are normal. Thirteen percent of patients with microtia have dysplastic inner ear structures—usually a hypoplastic lateral semicircular canal.

■ Surgery to correct the EAC is fruitless if the inner ear is nonfunctional. Therefore, assessment of the cochlea to identify a nerve and patency of the cochlear aperture (see later) is required. Surgery for external ear anomalies is difficult because it often requires grafts of bone and cartilage as well as the drilling of new canals. Thus correction just for cosmetic purposes is usually delayed until after adolescence, when growth has slowed down. However, if the ear anomaly leads to learning disabilities (e.g., bilateral hearing loss from EAC atresia), it may be treated before schooling (Table 11.1).

**Table 11.1** Checklist for Evaluating for External Auditory Canal Atresia or Stenosis

| Item | Rationale |
| --- | --- |
| Inner ear structures | No sense fixing the outer and/or middle ear if no sensorineural function |
| Stapes | Implies inner ear anomaly, requires implant |
| Oval and round window | Access to perilymph, endolymph |
| Middle ear space | Need space to place or repair ossicles, transmit sound |
| Facial nerve | Do not want to injure nerve |
| Ossicular anatomy | How many need to be replaced? Are there functioning joints? |
| Carotid artery, jugular vein | Makes for a bloody mess if they are anomalous and in the way |

**Box 11.3    Causes of Calcified External Ear Organs**

Idiopathic
Hyperparathyroidism
Diabetes mellitus
Pseudogout
Gout
Radiation
Frostbite
Relapsing polychondritis
Ochronosis
Acromegaly
Hypoparathyroidism
Addison disease

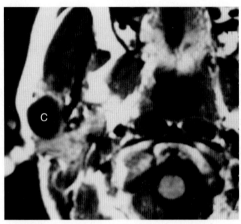

**Fig. 11.7 First branchial cleft cyst.** Axial T1-weighted image shows a cystic (C) mass in the right parotid gland near the external auditory canal. The first branchial cleft anomaly can communicate with the external ear.

## First Branchial Cleft Cyst

- First branchial cleft cysts occur around the ear and/or in the neighboring parotid gland (Fig. 11.7). A fistula from a first branchial cleft anomaly may drain to the EAC at the bone-cartilage interface.
- They typically present in middle age, with recurrent drainage from the EAC.
- On imaging, an organized fluid density/signal mass can be seen in and around the parotid gland. Peripheral rim enhancement can be seen if the cyst becomes infected.

## Calcifications of the External Ear Organs

- Calcifications of the external ear and/or pinna occur in a variety of congenital and acquired lesions. Box 11.3 lists these entities.

## Inflammatory Lesions

### Malignant Otitis Externa

- This is the most severe inflammatory condition affecting the EAC. *Pseudomonas* infection of the EAC is the most common offending pathogen in elderly diabetic patients

(93% of cases). Immunocompromised patients are also at risk. Patients present with pain and purulent discharge from the ear.

- The infection usually begins at the junction of the cartilaginous and bony portion of the EAC along the fissures of Santorini, which lead to the parapharyngeal space.
- The infection can spread to the infratemporal fossa, the nasopharynx, the parapharyngeal space, the adjacent bone leading to osteomyelitis, the TMJ, and the middle and inner ear structures and intracranially in the extradural space. The process may mimic an aggressive neoplasm in many respects and often is difficult to control with antibiotics.
- CT demonstrates soft tissue in the EAC and bony erosion of the EAC walls and skull base.
- Magnetic resonance imaging (MRI) shows edema within the EAC mucosa; the parapharyngeal fat may be obliterated as the infection extends anteriorly and medially, and the tissue planes around the carotid sheath may be infiltrated (Fig. 11.8). Marrow involvement is evidenced by edema (high T2 signal and low T1 signal) and enhancement on MRI, but CT shows later development of bony erosion. Affected cranial nerves can show abnormal enhancement.

### Keratosis Obturans

- This condition, caused by plugs of keratin in the EAC, is very painful (distinguishing it from epidermoid) and is usually seen bilaterally in middle-aged adults with histories of bronchiectasis and/or sinusitis.
- CT shows soft tissue opacifying and expanding the EAC without erosive change. The tissue does not enhance. These plugs can be surgically excised.

### Surfer's Ear

- Patients who swim in cold water are prone to exostoses of the EAC (surfer's ear) (Fig. 11.9). Patients present with conductive hearing loss.
- CT shows smoothly marginated broad-based circumferential sclerosis of the bony EAC resulting in narrowing of the canal. A more pedunculated bony overgrowth at the junction of the cartilaginous and bony EAC can be diagnosed as osteoma. Some authors believe exostoses and osteomas are the same entity.
- These are benign and typically require no treatment, unless hearing loss is severe, in which case resection is warranted.

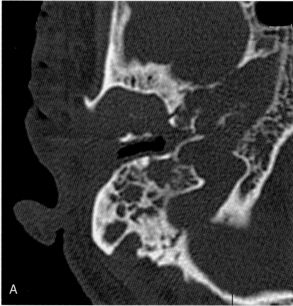

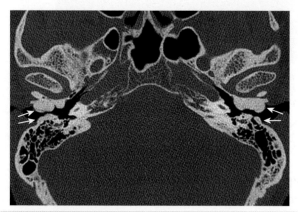

**Fig. 11.8 Malignant otitis externa.** (A) Axial computed tomographic image shows thickening of the external auditory canal (EAC) mucosa, mastoid opacification, and destructive changes at the mastoid and petrous portions of the temporal bone. (B) The fat-suppressed T1-weighted imaging scan shows enhancing tissue in the EAC, mastoid, petrous tip, right side of clivus, right longus colli muscle, and parapharyngeal space.

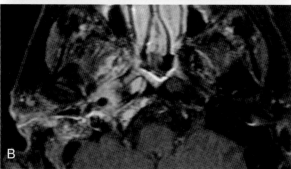

**Fig. 11.9 Exostosis of the external auditory canal (EAC).** Axial computed tomographic image reveals dense EAC exostoses bilaterally *(arrows)*. Note that the hyperostosis is also seen along the posterior margin of the EAC.

## Benign Neoplasms

- Benign masses of the external ear include hemangiomas, nevi, ceruminomas (adenomas of the ceruminous glands), polyps, and salivary gland tumors (Box 11.4).

---

### Box 11.4  Benign and Malignant External Auditory Canal Masses

Cerumen impaction
Foreign body
Exostosis
Hemangioma
Polyp
Basal cell carcinoma
Squamous cell carcinoma
Melanoma
Papilloma
Malignant otitis externa (infection not cancer!)
Keratosis obturans
Epidermoid
Metastasis
Rhabdomyosarcoma
Minor salivary gland neoplasm
Ceruminoma
Chondroid neoplasm
Langerhans cell histiocytosis
Nevi

---

- All of these present on CT and MRI as soft-tissue masses that may expand the EAC without destruction. All may enhance.
- Venous vascular malformations (VVMs), although not true neoplasms, can also occur in the external ear and could be mistaken for hemangioma, a true neoplasm. VVMs may have phleboliths and have more gradual enhancement than hemangiomas on dynamic imaging.

## Malignant Neoplasms

### SQUAMOUS CELL CARCINOMAS

- Squamous cell carcinomas (SCCs) of the EAC are the most common malignant neoplastic processes in this location (see Box 11.4). The lesion may invade the middle ear and temporal bone. Cartilaginous invasion of the external ear or middle ear extension portends poor prognosis and must be treated aggressively. The 5-year prognosis of EAC SCCs without middle ear disease is 59% but is 23% if the cancer extends into the middle ear. Deep lesions in the bony canal have the worst prognosis (Fig. 11.10).
- Pain occurs early because of periosteal spread or extension to the TMJ, where trismus may also arise. Facial nerve involvement also occurs early in the course.
- CT can identify bony erosion and destruction along the osseous margins of the EAC and adjacent TMJ and mastoid air cells. Metastatic adenopathy within the parotid and periparotid nodes that drain the EAC can be seen in conjunction with the primary tumor.
- Although distinguishing the tumor from obstructed opacified air cells can be difficult, on MRI, the tumor tends to be darker on T2WI, whereas obstructed air cells are T2 bright, making MRI a more reliable tool in assessing the margins of the tumor. The tumor enhances solidly. Secretions enhance on the periphery. Intracranial extension is better evaluated by contrast-enhanced MRI.

### Other Primary Malignant Tumors

- Other skin tumors, such as basal cell carcinomas or melanomas, may also affect the external ear in the same

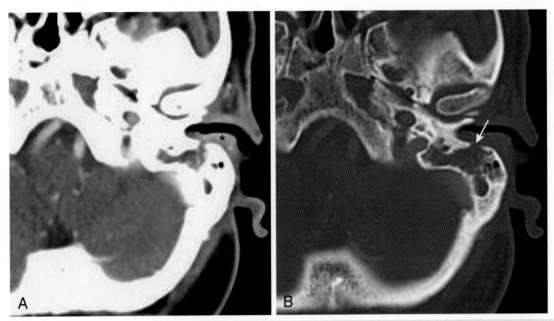

**Fig. 11.10 External auditory canal (EAC) squamous cell cancer.** (A) Axial contrast-enhanced computed tomography (CT) image in soft-tissue windows shows mucosal based thickening along the posterior wall of the EAC *(asterisk)*. (B) Close review of CT in bone windows at the same level shows associated focal bony destruction *(arrow)*, making this lesion suspicious for aggressive process. Biopsy revealed squamous cell carcinoma.

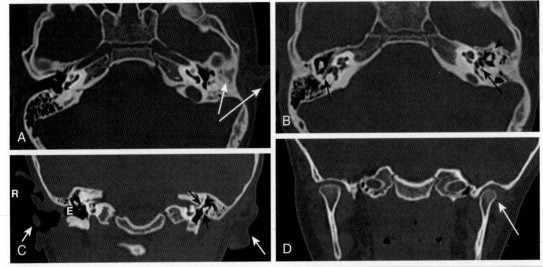

**Fig. 11.11 Left microtia and external auditory canal (EAC) atresia.** (A) Axial computed tomography (CT) scan through the temporal bone shows an absent left EAC and malformed auricle *(arrows)*. (B) The ossicles on the left are fused, and there is no incudomalleolar joint *(arrowhead)*. The position of the facial nerve second genu on the left is anterior to the right *(arrows)*, which puts it in potential danger during the ossicular reconstruction procedure. Note decreased air space of left middle ear. (C) Coronal reconstruction of axial CT images shows the maldeveloped left pinna with microtia (compare *white arrows*), the absence of an EAC on the left (see normal EAC indicated by *E* on the right), with a poorly aerated left middle ear and fused ossicles *(black arrows)*. (D) When the EAC and ossicles are congenitally malformed, the temporomandibular joint *(arrow)* on the same side is also typically maldeveloped as seen on the left: shallow and misoriented.

manner as SCCs. They can demonstrate perineural spread via cranial nerves V and VII.

- Kaposi sarcoma in individuals who are human immunodeficiency virus (HIV) positive can affect the ear.
- In children, rhabdomyosarcomas and lymphomas may present as external ear masses.
- Carcinomas of the parotid gland directly invade the temporal bone and EAC, and perineural growth may occur along cranial nerve VII.
- Metastases rarely affect the EAC portion of the temporal bone.

## THE MIDDLE EAR AND FACIAL NERVE
### Congenital Anomalies

#### Hypoplasia and Fusion

- The middle ear is a site of congenital dysplasia that may be associated with EAC stenosis or atresia or may be isolated to ossicular anomalies (Fig. 11.11).
- Ossicular fusion, hypoplasia, or maldevelopment can occur and may coexist with anomalies of the facial nerve as it runs through the middle ear cavity.
- When isolated middle ear congenital abnormalities occur, the distal incus (especially the long process) and

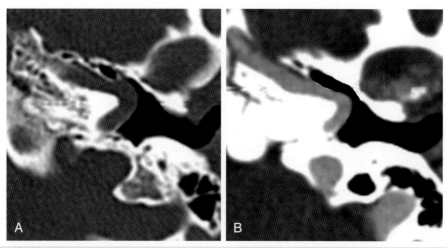

**Fig. 11.12 Aberrant left internal carotid artery.** (A) Axial computed tomography (CT) image in bone windows shows extension of the petrous internal carotid artery (ICA) into the middle ear. (B) If you're not convinced that was the ICA, here's a contrast-enhanced CT showing the expected enhancement in the vessel to alleviate all doubt. Tell your surgeon to resist the temptation to biopsy!

the stapes are most commonly affected in concert, followed by the stapes alone and incus alone. Ossicular anomalies can be associated with dysplasia of the oval and round windows, so be sure to check those structures because surgical repair will need to include window repair if they are indeed dysplastic.

### Variations in Vascular Anatomy

- There are the variations in vascular anatomy that can mimic middle ear tumors and may present similarly on otoscopic examinations as a retrotympanic vascular mass.
- The aberrant internal carotid artery (ICA) passes through the middle ear cavity and runs anteromedially to the horizontal portion of the cavernous carotid canal and is readily diagnosed by MRA and CTA (Fig. 11.12).
- The persistent stapedial artery is rare (<0.5% of patients) and may coexist with an aberrant ICA (60%). Associations with trisomy 13, 15, 21, thalidomide exposure, anencephaly, and neurofibromatosis have been reported.
  - This artery appears transiently in embryologic development as a branch of the hyoid artery (derived itself from the second aortic arch) connecting the external and internal carotid artery. Ultimately, it regresses to form pieces of the caroticotympanic artery. When it persists, it may present as a pulsatile middle ear mass.
  - Imaging findings include absence of the foramen spinosum, a soft-tissue mass along the horizontal portion of the tympanic facial nerve, and an additional branch leading from the petrous carotid artery. It enters the middle ear to create the obturator foramen of the stapes (between the crura) and leaves the middle ear near the geniculate ganglion.
- The jugular bulb wall may be dehiscent or nondehiscent. The nondehiscent jugular bulb has preservation of the bony plate of the top of the jugular foramen, whereas the dehiscent jugular bulb shows no bony margin.
  - High jugular bulbs may extend into the middle ear (Fig. 11.13) or into the petrous bone near the endolymphatic sac. Most people use either the inferior rim of the tympanic annulus or the IAC as the uppermost limit for a normal jugular bulb.

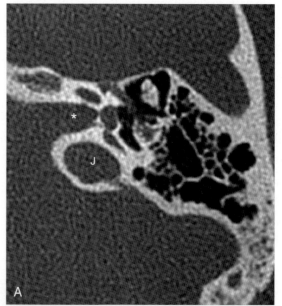

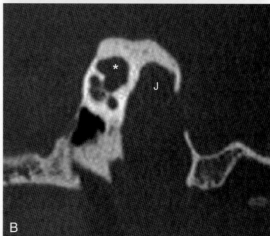

**Fig. 11.13 High-riding jugular bulb.** (A) Axial computed tomography (CT) image shows the jugular bulb (J) at the level of the internal auditory canal (asterisk) in this patient presenting with tinnitus. (B) Sagittal CT reconstruction in the same patient shows that the roof of the jugular bulb (J) approaches that of the internal auditory canal (asterisk).

- Diverticuli of the jugular bulb may also enter the middle ear.
- Sigmoid sinus diverticulum are outpouchings of the sigmoid sinus projecting in the mastoid bone, with or without dehiscence of the sigmoid plate. It is a common cause of pulsatile tinnitus although most times the finding is incidental.

## Epidermoids (Congenital Cholesteatoma)

- Epidermoids are ectodermal/epithelial rests that may arise in a variety of locations within the temporal bone (Box 11.5). To prevent confusion with acquired cholesteatomas, use the term *epidermoids* rather than the older terms congenital cholesteatomas, epidermoidomas, or primary cholesteatomas.
- Patients present with hearing loss, vertigo, or facial nerve palsy. On direct visual inspection, these lesions are pearly white. Treatment is surgical excision.
- On CT, epidermoids appear as noninvasive, low density, expansile, well-circumscribed lesions in the temporal bone with scalloped margins (Fig. 11.14). Although in the middle ear they may be whitish lesions that simulate acquired cholesteatomas, these lesions are not associated with perforation of the tympanic membrane, and patients have no history of antecedent ear infections or previous surgeries. The scutum is usually intact.

---

### Box 11.5 Classic Locations for Epidermoids in the Temporal Bone

Petrous apex
Körner septum (the petrosquamous suture)
Mastoid air cells
Eustachian tube opening
Geniculate ganglion region
Middle ear (including epitympanum junction, incudostapedial joint, sinus tympani, and facial nerve recess)

---

- On MRI, these lesions are nonenhancing, hypointense on T1WI, and hyperintense on T2WI. They are bright on FLAIR scanning and bright on DWI. Epidermoids may be solid or cystic.

## Inflammatory Lesions

### Otitis Media

- Obstruction or impairment of the function of the eustachian tube from nasopharyngeal lymphoid or mucosal hypertrophy caused by upper respiratory tract infections is often responsible for otitis media in children. The most frequent causes of otitis media are *Streptococcus*, *Moraxella catarrhalis*, *Haemophilus influenzae*, and *Pneumococcus*. Otitis media generally responds well to antibiotics.
- Imaging is typically not required in the diagnosis of otitis media unless complications are suspected. The middle ear is filled with fluid density and intensity on CT and MRI, respectively, in uncomplicated otitis media (Fig. 11.15).
- Rarely, ossicular erosions can occur in association with acute otitis media. When they occur, they usually affect the long process of the incus and can lead to conductive hearing loss. The erosions appear on CT as tiny, lytic, punched-out areas in the ossicle.
- Another complication of chronic otitis media is ossicular fixation. This may cause a conductive hearing loss and may be fibrous (soft tissue around the ossicles)
- Finally, tympanosclerosis can also be seen in the setting of chronic otomastoiditis (on CT, calcification around ossicles, ossicular ligaments, and/or tympanic membrane).

### Mastoiditis

- Mastoiditis may occur secondary to otitis media or de novo. Infection may travel from the middle ear via the aditus ad antrum (the narrow channel connecting the middle ear cavity to the mastoid antrum) to the mastoid air cells. Again, routine imaging is not indicated unless complications of mastoiditis are suspected.

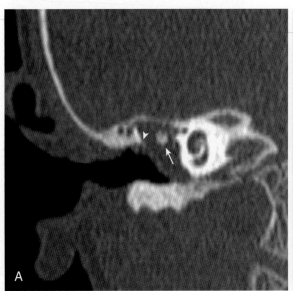
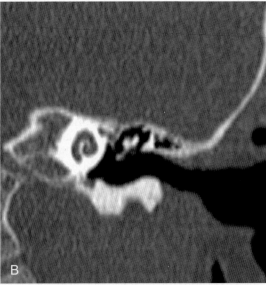

**Fig. 11.14 Epidermoid in middle ear cavity.** (A) Coronal computed tomography (CT) image in 5-year-old child presenting with hearing loss on the right shows expansile tissue in the middle ear, resulting in medialization of the ossicles, demineralization of the malleolar head *(arrow)*, with intact scutum *(arrowhead)*. The tympanic membrane was intact on direct inspection, but there was no question about the presence of the characteristic pearly white mass behind it. (B) Compare these findings with the normal left side.

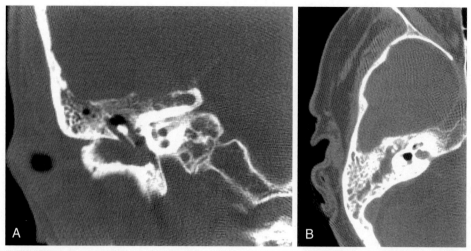

**Fig. 11.15  Acute otomastoiditis.** (A) An air-fluid level is seen in the epitympanic space with complete opacification of the mesotympanum on this coronally acquired computed tomographic image. The mastoid air cells are also opacified. (B) Air in the vestibule and in the cochlea (pneumolabyrinth), seen in this patient with otomastoiditis, implies an open connection between the middle ear and the inner ear.

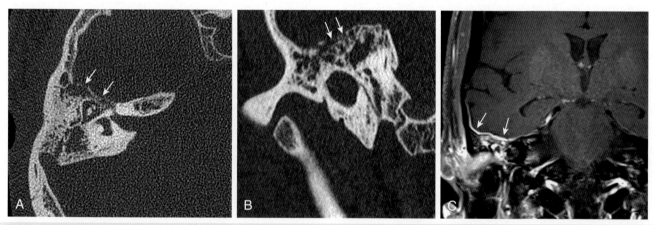

**Fig. 11.16  Coalescent mastoiditis.** (A) Axial and (B) coronal computed tomographic images show destruction of mastoid air cell septations and areas of dehiscence along the anterior and superior walls of the mastoid bone *(arrows)*. (C) Coronal postcontrast T1-weighted image shows abnormal dural-based enhancement along the floor of the middle cranial fossa *(arrows)*, likely reactive, as a consequence of breach of the mastoid roof.

Noninflammatory effusions are common when tubes are placed in the nose or mouth, in association with brain irradiation, or when the eustachian tube is obstructed.

- CT reveals opacification of air cells. The fluid is bright on T2WI and FLAIR even when not infected. Occasionally, air-fluid levels within the small mastoid air cells can be seen. Middle ear and/or petrous apex opacification may coexist.
- Coalescence of mastoiditis portends a poor prognosis because it represents bony infection (osteomyelitis) with destruction (Fig. 11.16).
  - *β-Hemolytic streptococci* and *pneumococci* are the usual pathogens in (coalescent) mastoiditis.
  - CT shows bone destruction involving the mastoid septations and/or overlying cortex associated with the mastoid opacities. These findings may also be seen on malignant otitis externa pseudomonas infection spreading from the EAC to the mastoids.
  - Contrast-enhanced imaging by CT or MRI can provide additional important findings of subperiosteal abscess

within the adjacent scalp, intracranial extension of infection with cerebritis or frank abscess formation, and adjacent venous sinus thrombosis.

- A Bezold abscess is another complication of acute otomastoiditis. It is an inflammatory collection that occurs within the soft tissues inferior to the mastoid tip as the infection spreads from the bone to the adjacent soft tissue (Fig. 11.17). It can spread down the plane of the sternocleidomastoid muscle to the lower neck.

### Acquired Cholesteatomas

- Recurrent otitis media and acquired cholesteatomas are easier to distinguish in textbooks than in real life, where imaging characteristics may overlap (Table 11.2). Acquired cholesteatomas are erosive collections of keratinous debris from an ingrowth of stratified squamous epithelium through a perforated tympanic membrane.
- The diagnosis of cholesteatoma is usually made by the clinician based on clinical presentation, tympanic membrane perforation, and the "pearly white" appearance of the middle ear lesion on otoscopic evaluation.

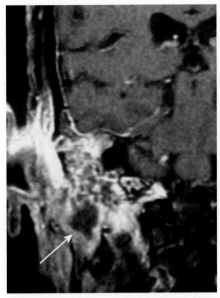

**Fig. 11.17 Bezold abscess.** Coronal postcontrast T1-weighted image shows ring-enhancing abscess *(arrow)* just below the opacified mastoid tip.

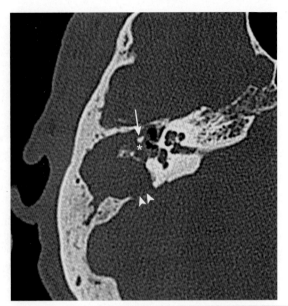

**Fig. 11.18 Acquired cholesteatoma.** This rampant cholesteatoma has eroded the ossicles as well as the posterior wall of the mastoid air cells *(arrowheads)*. Remnants of malleus and incus are present *(arrow)*, and the middle ear cavity *(asterisk)* is opacified.

**Table 11.2**    Cholesteatoma Versus Otitis Media

| Feature | Cholesteatoma | Otitis Media |
|---|---|---|
| Middle ear opacified | Yes | Yes |
| Scutum | Eroded | Normal |
| Ossicular erosion | Yes | Infrequent |
| Ossicular displacement | Yes | No |
| Expansion of aditus ad antrum | Sometimes | No |
| Lateral semicircular canal fistula | Sometimes | No |
| Gadolinium enhancement | Rare | Rare |
| T2-weighted image signal intensity | Intermediate | Bright |
| Tympanic membrane retracted | Yes | No |
| Diffusion-weighted imaging signal | Bright | Low unless really purulent |
| Tegmen tympani erosion | Sometimes | No |
| Facial nerve canal dehiscence | Sometimes | No |

- CT imaging is useful to better understand the full extent of the lesion for surgical planning. The key features in identifying a lesion as a cholesteatoma are the presence of mass effect, bony erosion, and/or expansion (Fig. 11.18).
- MRI is not typically required in the primary diagnosis of cholesteatoma but can be helpful in distinguishing recurrent cholesteatoma from granulation tissue in patients who have undergone surgical resection in the past and have continued symptoms. Cholesteatomas are hypointense on T1WI, intermediate on T2WI, and do not enhance, as opposed to granulation tissue (postoperative), which does enhance. Cholesteatomas will show diffusion restriction; granulation tissue does not (Fig. 11.19). For this reason, DWI is important to include in the workup of suspected recurrent cholesteatoma after resection.

- There are two major types of acquired cholesteatomas: pars flaccida cholesteatomas and pars tensa cholesteatomas. This is a favored location for acquired cholesteatomas because of perforation or a retraction pocket of the pars flaccida and/or pars tensa of the tympanic membrane.

**TEACHING POINTS**

Pars Flaccida Cholesteatomas

- After perforation in the pars flaccida, this cholesteatoma can extend into the Prussak space.
- On computed tomography (CT), a soft-tissue mass causing erosion of the scutum and medial displacement of the malleus and incus is seen. The head of the malleus and body of the incus are the area most susceptible to erosion.
- From the Prussak space, the lesion often spreads through the aditus ad antrum, expanding its waist as the inflammatory process proceeds into the mastoid air cells.

**TEACHING POINTS**

Pars Tensa Cholesteatomas

- Pars tensa cholesteatomas are much less common than pars flaccida cholesteatomas.
- They arise from perforations through the posterosuperior-most portion of the pars tensa, which is the inferior portion of the tympanic membrane. From this location, the sinus tympani, pyramidal eminence, and facial recess may be expanded and/or eroded.
- Pars tensa cholesteatomas present with a mass in the hypotympanum of the middle ear, erosion of the long process of the incus or stapes, epitympanic spread, and ossicular displacement. The scutum is usually intact.

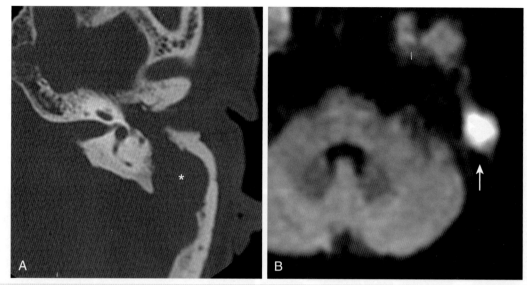

**Fig. 11.19 Recurrent cholesteatoma.** (A) Axial computed tomographic image in a patient with recurrent ear drainage many years after cholesteatoma resection shows expansile opacification within the mastoid bone *(asterisk)* with complete absence of normal mastoid bony architecture (automastoidectomy). Opacification is also present in the middle and external ears. (B) The expansile soft tissue shows diffusion restriction *(arrow)*, indicating recurrent cholesteatoma.

- Complications of cholesteatomas include a perilymphatic fistula from the middle ear into the semicircular canals (4%–25% of cases), with the lateral semicircular canal most commonly affected (Fig. 11.20). This may be identified as a dehiscence in the bony labyrinth with a soft-tissue mass expanding the region of the oval window or lateral margin of the lateral semicircular canal.
- Cholesteatomas may erode the tegmen tympani (the roof of the epitympanic space) and subsequently invade the intracranial compartment or be a source for cerebrospinal fluid (CSF) leak (Fig. 11.21).
- Another area of potential erosion is the lateral or inferior wall of the tympanic portion of the facial nerve. If there is dehiscence or skeletization of the facial nerve canal or sinus tympani, the surgeon must know this preoperatively so that removal of the cholesteatoma is done in a careful manner so as not to injure the underlying structures.

## Other Inflammatory Conditions of the Middle Ear

- Granulomatosis with polyangiitis (formerly *Wegener granulomatosis*) can attack the eustachian tube and from there invade the nasopharynx or skull base.
- Langerhans cell histiocytosis affects the temporal bones of children as eosinophilic granulomas in isolation or as part of the wider spectrum of disease (histiocytosis X, Langerhans granulomatosis) (Fig. 11.22).

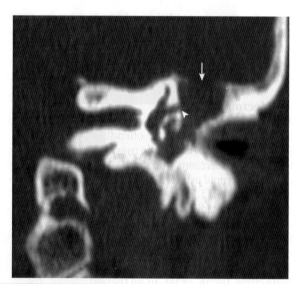

**Fig. 11.20 Lateral semicircular canal dehiscence from cholesteatoma.** Coronal reconstruction of temporal bone computed tomographic image shows cholesteatoma focally eroding the lateral margin of the lateral semicircular canal *(arrowhead)* and the tegmen tympani *(arrow)*.

**TEACHING POINTS**

Eosinophilic Granuloma

- Eosinophilic granuloma has a propensity for involving the mastoid portion of the temporal bone.
- Hearing difficulties without pain may be the initial complaint.
- Computed tomography (CT) shows a well-defined lytic lesion with beveled edges involving the outer table more than the inner table. On magnetic resonance imaging (MRI), the lesion is dark on T1-weighted imaging (T1WI) and bright on T2-weighting imaging (T2WI) and enhances.
- If suspected, be sure to check for other lesions elsewhere in the skull, skull base, and orbits because multiplicity is common (Fig. 11.22).

- Another cause of lysis of the temporal bone is osteoradionecrosis. This has been described most commonly after irradiation for nasopharyngeal carcinoma.

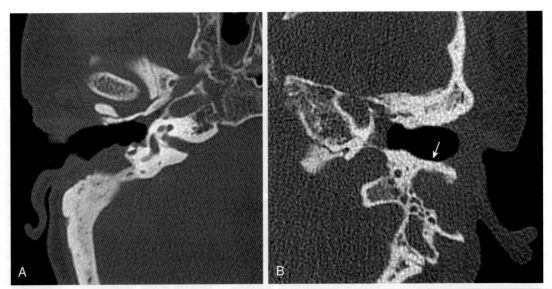

**Fig. 11.23 Up or down?** (A) Axial computed tomography (CT) image shows canal wall down mastoidectomy defect with surgical absence of the posterior wall of the external auditory canal (EAC). There is accumulation of debris/granulation tissue in the mastoidectomy "bowl." (B) Axial CT image shows typical appearance of canal wall up mastoidectomy defect with intact posterior wall of the EAC *(arrow)*.

---

### Box 11.6    Types of Synthetic Ossicular Prostheses

Stapes prosthesis
Incus interposition graft
Applebaum prosthesis (a synthetic prosthesis from long process of incus to capitulum of stapes)
Black oval top synthetic prosthesis (from tympanic membrane to capitulum of stapes or oval window)
Richards synthetic prosthesis (from tympanic membrane to capitulum of stapes or oval window)
Goldenberg prosthesis (from tympanic membrane to capitulum of stapes or oval window, or stapes to malleus or footplate to malleus)

Stone JA, Mukherji SK, Jewett BS, Carrasco VN, Castillo M. CT evaluation of prosthetic ossicular reconstruction procedures: what the otologist needs to know. Radiographics. 2000 May-Jun;20(3):593–605.

unless flow voids are seen. VVMs may occur in the bone in and around the geniculate ganglion, the so-called facial nerve "hemangioma" (see later).

### Dural Vascular Malformations

■ Another entity that may cause tinnitus is a dural vascular malformation. These commonly affect the transverse sinus and, in some cases, may be because of previously thrombosed veins or sinuses, resulting in abnormal collateral flow of arteries and veins around the thrombosis.
■ If no soft-tissue mass in the middle ear or skull base is seen on cross-sectional imaging in patients with objective tinnitus, angiography may be indicated to detect this lesion (Fig. 11.27).

### Facial Schwannomas

■ If the facial nerve canal is widened, a facial nerve schwannoma should be considered. MRI should be performed to assess for an expansile enhancing lesion along the entire course of the nerve (Fig. 11.28).
■ Differential diagnosis includes vestibular schwannomas within the IAC or glomus tumors within the tympanic cavity.

### Facial Nerve Venous Vascular Malformations

■ Facial nerve VVMs (previously called *hemangiomas*) can occur in the IAC, around the geniculate ganglion, and at the posterior genu of the facial nerve canal.
■ These malformations often present with slowly evolving facial paresis and twitching.
■ On CT, bone erosion with a soft-tissue mass is seen and involved marrow space may have a "honeycomb" bony trabecular internal architecture (Fig. 11.29).
■ The borders of a VVM are indistinct compared with the well-demarcated schwannoma. The distinction is important because a schwannoma is rarely resected without sacrificing the nerve, but a VVM can sometimes be separated from the nerve.

### Facial Nerve Enhancement

■ The facial nerve normally may show some enhancement at the geniculate ganglion and in its horizontal and descending portions. Enhancement of the facial nerve in the cerebellopontine angle cistern, IAC, in the labyrinthine portion, and in the parotid gland, by contrast, is always abnormal.
■ The reason for the normal enhancement is the prolific circumneural arteriovenous plexus around the nerve. The plexus is not present in the IAC or intralabyrinthine and extracranial portions of the nerve.
■ There are many causes of facial nerve enhancement (Box 11.10). Bell palsy is thought to account for 80% of facial nerve paralysis. Smooth linear enhancement is seen along the course of the affected facial nerve at the fundus of the IAC or opening to the labyrinthine portion.
■ Parotid malignancies, especially adenoid cystic carcinoma and lymphoma, have a propensity for tracking up the facial nerve. Perineural tumor spread along the facial nerve is seen as enlargement and enhancement of the nerve itself, secondary enlargement of the stylomastoid foramen, or loss of normal fatty tissue surrounding the

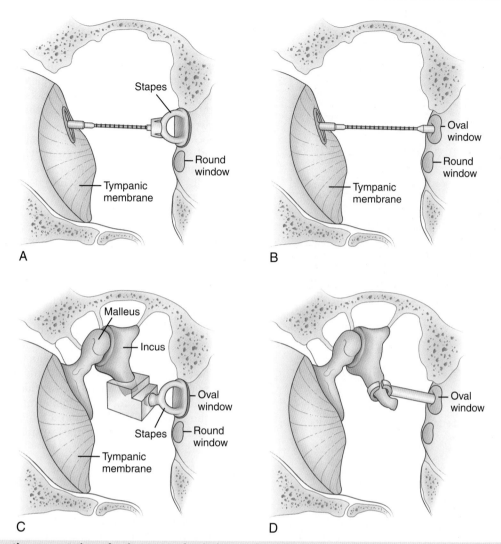

**Fig. 11.24 Schematic representations of various types of ossicular prostheses (by no means all-inclusive!).** (A) Partial ossicular replacement prosthesis (PORP) extends from the tympanic membrane to the stapes capitulum. (B) Total ossicular replacement prosthesis (TORP) extends from the tympanic membrane to the oval window. (C) The L-shaped configuration of the Applebaum prosthesis is depicted, with one end of the prosthesis extending over the partially resected long process of the incus and the other extending over the capitulum of the stapes. (D) In the case of stapedectomy, the stapes is resected, and an implant extends from the incus to the oval window.

---

**Box 11.7    Causes of Ossicular Prostheses Failure**

Recurrent otitis media
Recurrent cholesteatoma
Reparative granulomas (foreign body reactions)
Ossicular subluxation or dislocation, adhesions, fracture of the
  prosthesis
Granulation tissue
Recurrence of otospongiotic bone
Excessive postoperative bony reaction
Extrusion of the prosthesis

---

nerve within the foramen (Fig. 11.30). Enhancement along the nerve can be smooth or nodular.

## Malignant Neoplasms

■ Malignancies of the middle ear are uncommon. Usually, these masses are derived from EAC structures and secondarily invade the middle ear.

■ Primary rhabdomyosarcomas of the middle ear may arise from muscular cells along the eustachian tube opening.

■ Rarely, ectopic salivary gland tissue may be present within the middle ear cavity and neoplasms such as adenocarcinoma or adenoid cystic carcinoma may arise in such ectopic salivary tissue.

■ The most common primary tumors to metastasize to the temporal bone are lung and breast cancer.

## INNER EAR AND PETROUS APEX

### Congenital Anomalies

■ The majority (80%) of congenital hearing loss is caused by membranous pathology involving inner ear hair cells, without detectable morphologic changes on high-resolution CT and MRI. Radiologists can play a useful role in detecting morphologic abnormalities of the inner ear in the remaining 20%. The goal of imaging is to identify

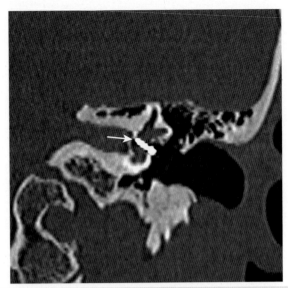

**Fig. 11.25 Subluxed stapes prosthesis.** Coronal computed tomographic image shows a displaced stapes prosthesis extending through the oval window deep into the vestibule *(arrow)*. Ouch! The prosthesis should normally not extend 0.25 mm deep to the oval window.

---

### Box 11.8   Causes of Pulsatile Tinnitus

Sigmoid sinus diverticulum
Idiopathic
Idiopathic intracranial hypertension (pseudotumor cerebri)
Ménière disease
High-grade stenosis of internal carotid artery[a]
High-riding jugular bulb
Paraganglioma (glomus jugulare, glomus tympanicum, glomus jugulotympanicum)
Hemangioma/venous vascular malformation
Cholesterol granuloma
Meningioma
Aberrant carotid artery/persistent stapedial artery
Dural vascular malformations, fistulas
Carotid aneurysms
Otosclerosis
Paget disease

[a] May be "objective tinnitus."

---

the specific morphologic abnormalities present because these findings will play an important role in managing the hearing loss (placement of hearing aid, cochlear implantation, or auditory brain stem implantation) and anticipation of potential surgical risks (facial nerve course) and complications (CSF leaks and meningitis).

■ Although many causes of sensorineural deafness are derived from acquired disorders of the inner ear, several different types of congenital anomalies cause inner ear dysplasias and hearing loss. Underlying causes for these anomalies include thalidomide exposure, congenital rubella or cytomegalovirus infection, and eponymical genetic disorders.

■ The otic capsule structures develop between gestation weeks 3 and 10. Congenital inner ear abnormalities vary in degree of severity, ranging from mild dysplasias to complete aplasia depending on when during embryogenesis the failure of normal development occurred.

■ Although our understanding of inner ear anomalies is ever evolving, the following classification is currently advocated (Table 11.3):

   ■ Labyrinthine aplasia (Michel deformity) consists of absent cochlea, vestibule, semicircular canals, and vestibular and cochlear aqueducts. Otic capsule can be hypoplastic or absent, and only the temporal bone segments of the facial bones are identifiable.

   ■ Rudimentary otocyst is a malformation lying between the spectrum of Michel and common cavity deformity and consists of ovoid otic capsule without internal

---

### Box 11.9   Vascular Intratympanic Masses

High riding/dehiscent jugular bulb or diverticulum
Paraganglioma (glomus jugulare, glomus tympanicum, glomus jugulotympanicum)
Hemangioma/venous vascular malformation
Cholesterol granuloma/chronic hypervascular inflammatory tissue
Meningioma
Aberrant carotid artery/persistent stapedial artery
Petrous carotid aneurysms

---

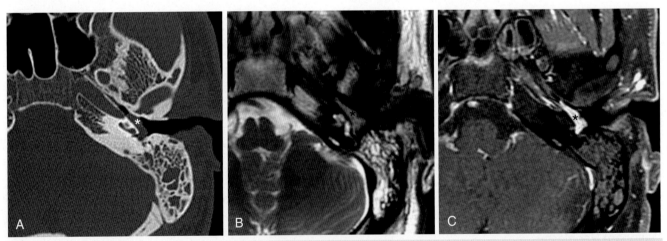

**Fig. 11.26 Glomus tympanicum.** (A) Axial computed tomographic image shows small soft-tissue mass in the middle ear *(asterisk)*. Although nondescript in its appearance, in the setting of pulsatile tinnitus, glomus tympanicum is the major diagnostic consideration. The location, overlying the cochlear promontory *(asterisk)* is perfect for glomus tympanicum. (B) Axial T2-weighted image (T2WI) shows a slightly hyperintense to brain mass in the middle ear *(asterisk)*. Note opacification of mastoid air cells attributable to obstruction of the eustachian tube by the tumor. (C) Postcontrast fat-suppressed T1-weighted imaging (T1WI) shows the mass to be avidly enhancing *(asterisk)*.

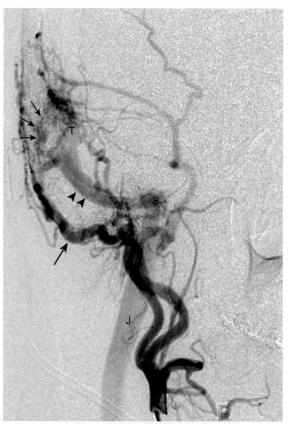

**Fig. 11.27 Dural arteriovenous fistula on conventional catheter angiogram.** In this patient presenting with tinnitus, selective catheterization of the external carotid artery demonstrates an enlarged occipital artery *(large arrow)* and multiple fistulous connections (one of which is indicated by *small arrows*) to the venous drainage system. Note the early enhancement within the torcular *(T)*, transverse sinus *(arrowheads)*, sigmoid sinus *(S)*, and jugular vein *(J)*.

auditory canal. Portions of the semicircular canal may be present.

- Cochlear aplasia (Fig. 11.31) consists of absent cochlea accompanied by anterior displacement of the facial nerve canal with normal positioning of the vestibule and semicircular canals, which can be normal in morphology or dilated. The internal auditory canal is normally positioned, and otic capsule morphology is normal.
- Common cavity deformity (Cock's deformity) consists of a solitary rounded cavity in place of cochlea and vestibule in continuum with the internal auditory canal. Dysmorphic semicircular canals may also be present.
- Incomplete partition (IP) type of the cochlea involves a spectrum of malformations (IP I-III) in which cochlea and vestibule are anatomically separate, but there are specific defects in the modiolus and interscalar septae.
  - In IP-I, the cochlea is normally positioned but maintains cystic configuration because of absent modiolus and interscalar septae and communicates with the labyrinth (cystic cochleovestibular malformation) (Fig. 11.32).
  - In IP-II, the apical portion of the cochlea is malformed with rounded configuration representing combined apical and middle cochlear turns

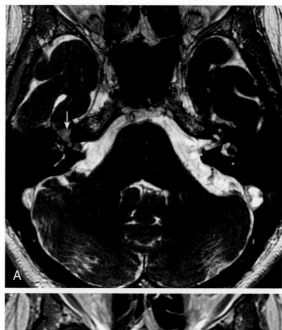

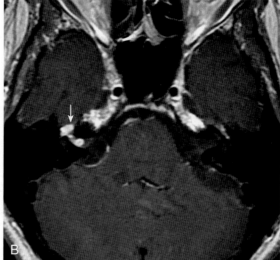

**Fig. 11.28 Facial nerve schwannoma.** (A) Axial T2 constructive interference in steady state (CISS) image shows expansile mass within the lateral aspect of the internal auditory canal extending along the facial nerve canal on the right *(arrow)*. Compare with normal appearance on the left. (B) Postcontrast T1-weighted image shows enhancement of this mass involving the canalicular and labyrinthine segments and genu of the right facial nerve *(arrow)*.

because of defect in modiolus. If vestibular aqueduct and vestibule are concurrently dilated, this can be described as a Mondini malformation.
  - In the very rare IP-III, the modiolus is completely absent, but interscala septae are present. On imaging, the optic capsule is thinned, the internal auditory canal is wide, and labyrinthine segment of facial nerve course is displaced, located superior to the cochlea.
- For information on the enlarged vestibular aqueduct with normal cochlea, see the next section.
- Cochlear aperture abnormalities are characterized by a small or absent cochlear nerve canal (i.e., cochlear fossette), which should normally be greater than 1.4 cm in width. The internal auditory canal may

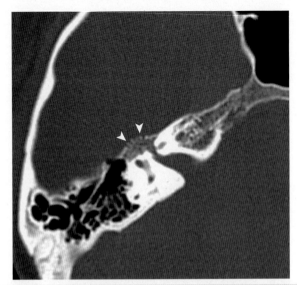

**Fig. 11.29 Venous vascular malformations (VVMs) of the facial nerve.** Axial computed tomography demonstrates an expansile mass *(arrowheads)* with permeative change in the bone surrounding the facial nerve canal. Internal architecture should suggest the diagnosis of VVM.

**Box 11.10   Causes of Abnormal Facial Nerve Enhancement**

Bell palsy
Cholesteatoma
Fracture
Infection (viral, Lyme disease, spread from otitis media or malignant otitis externa)
Schwannoma
Venous vascular malformation
Sarcoidosis or other inflammatory process
Perineural malignant spread
Meningioma

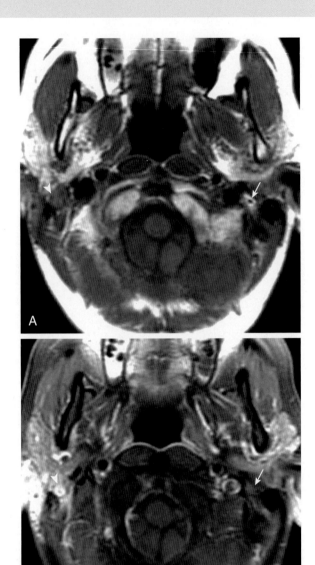

**Fig. 11.30 Perineural tumor spread in a patient with adenoid cystic carcinoma of the right parotid gland.** (A) Axial T1-weighted image (T1WI) shows normal appearance of the facial nerve as it exits the stylomastoid foramen on the left *(arrow)*. Note hypointense nerve surrounded by normal hyperintense fat signal within the foramen. On the right, the fat within the foramen is effaced by infiltrative soft tissue *(arrowhead)*, indicating perineural spread of tumor along the right facial nerve. (B) Axial postcontrast T1WI shows abnormal enhancement in the right stylomastoid foramen *(arrowhead)*, confirming perineural tumor spread. Note normal postcontrast appearance of the stylomastoid foramen on the left *(arrow)*.

be narrowed, and the cochlea can be otherwise normal appearing. MRI can help determine whether the cochlear nerve is normal, hypoplastic, or absent.

■ Cochlear nerve deficiency is a cause of SNHL and consists of diminished caliber of absence of the cochlear nerve. This condition can be congenital or acquired (attributable to atrophy).
   ■ Making this diagnosis is important because cochlear implants are contraindicated.
   ■ On MRI, sagittal reconstructions from high-resolution T2WI can show the small or absent nerve in the anterior inferior aspect of the IAC.
   ■ On CT, the cochlear nerve canal is small in caliber as it enters the basal turn of the cochlea (cochlear aperture stenosis).
■ If the cochlear aqueduct is congenitally enlarged, hearing may be impaired.
   ■ A medial orifice size of greater than 1.5 mm should be considered abnormal, and a midportion diameter of greater than 1.2 mm is suspicious.
   ■ An enlarged cochlear aqueduct, because it represents a communication between the scala tympani and the

subarachnoid space, has been implicated in children with recurrent meningitis and ear infections. This anomaly has also been associated with the poststapedectomy "gusher," so named because CSF and perilymphatic fluid intermingle in spurts.

**Vestibular Aqueduct Abnormalities**

■ Enlarged vestibular aqueducts cause high-frequency hearing loss and may be seen in isolation or in association with abnormal cochlea spiralization (76%), cystic vestibules (31%), or abnormal semicircular canals (23%). It can be seen as part of the IP-II spectrum (Fig. 11.33).

**Table 11.3**   Congenital Inner Ear Anomalies

| Malformation | Features |
|---|---|
| Labyrinthine aplasia (Michel deformity) | Absent cochlea, vestibule, semicircular canals, vestibular and cochlear aqueducts |
| Rudimentary otocyst | Ovoid otic capsule without internal auditory canal |
| Cochlear aplasia | Absent cochlea, anterior displacement of facial nerve canal |
| Common cavity deformity | Cystic cavity without differentiation into cochlea or vestibule |
| Incomplete partition type I | Cochlea lacks entire modiolus, with cystic cochlea and vestibule |
| Incomplete partition type II | Cystic apical and middle turns of cochlea. Add dilated vestibule and vestibular aqueduct and you get Mondini malformation |
| Incomplete partition type III | Absent modiolus, thinned otic capsule, widened internal auditory canal (IAC), displaced labyrinthine segment facial nerve |
| Enlarged vestibular aqueduct | Enlarged vestibular aqueduct with or without abnormal cochlea spiralization or abnormal semicircular canals |
| Cochlear aperture abnormalities | Small or absent cochlear nerve canal |

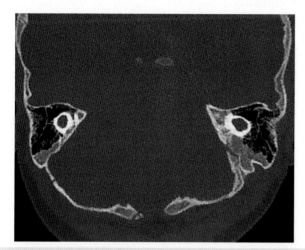

**Fig. 11.31 Cochlear aplasia.** Axial computed tomography shows complete absence of the cochlea with abnormal cystic-appearing vestibule bilaterally.

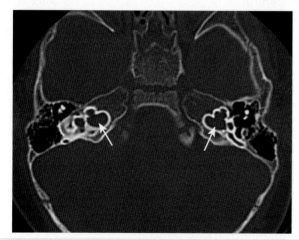

**Fig. 11.32 Incomplete partition type I.** Axial computed tomography shows cystic-appearing cochlea with absent modiolus bilaterally *(arrows)* and cystic-appearing vestibule bilaterally.

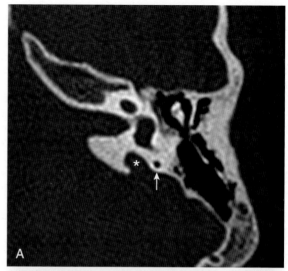

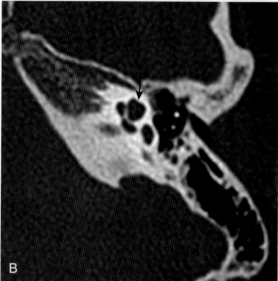

**Fig. 11.33 Large vestibular aqueduct syndrome with incomplete partition type II.** (A) Axial computed tomographic image shows enlargement of the vestibular aqueduct (the bony housing of the endolymphatic sac, *asterisk*). The normal vestibular aqueduct should be similar in diameter to the adjacent posterior limb internal capsule *(arrow)*. (B) In this same patient more superiorly, the cochlea shows abnormal morphology, with cystic appearance of the apical and middle turns *(arrow)*.

- The midpoint of the normal duct should have a transverse diameter equal to or less than 1.5 mm in size or about the same size as the adjacent posterior semicircular canal.
- One may see the dilated endolymphatic sac on MR as brighter than CSF on T1WI as a result of high-protein, hyperosmolar fluid.
- CHARGE syndrome (coloboma, heart defects, choanal atresia, retardation, genitourinary abnormalities, ear abnormalities), Pendred syndrome, and congenital cytomegalovirus infections may predispose to enlarged vestibular aqueducts. A narrowed vestibular aqueduct less than 0.5 mm in diameter may be seen with Ménière disease.

## Semicircular Canal Abnormalities

- If one sees an isolated semicircular canal deformity without cochlear anomalies, it implies that the defect occurred after 8 to 9 weeks of gestation; by that time, the cochlea has completely developed. Aplasia of the semicircular canals can be seen in CHARGE syndrome.
  - Lateral semicircular canal hypoplasia is most often seen because the lateral semicircular canal is the last to form embryologically (superior first, posterior second, lateral last). Hearing loss occurs rather than imbalance.
  - In addition to absence or small caliber of the semicircular canals, compensatory enlargement of the vestibule will occur.
- Superior semicircular canal dehiscence is characterized clinically by sound- and/or pressure-induced vertigo.
  - Oscillopsia (the perception that stationary objects are moving) and vertigo evoked by loud noises are part of the Tullio phenomenon, a frequent clinical finding.
  - Although the defect has been described in congenital and syndromic conditions, there is an increased prevalence of the defect among older age groups, suggesting that this is more commonly an acquired condition.
  - High-resolution CT shows a dehiscence of the bone overlying the superior semicircular canal, unilaterally or bilaterally. Of note, the finding may be seen in patients without the typical clinical presentation and is of doubtful clinical significance in these cases.
  - Surgical exploration of the middle cranial fossa has confirmed the CT findings in selected patients; covering up the gap may lead to symptom relief.

## Congenital Internal Auditory Canal Abnormalities

- IP type III (IP-III) is an X-linked deformity manifested by bulbous dilatation of the IAC laterally along with enlargement of labyrinthine segments of the facial and superior vestibular nerve canals. The bone between the IAC and basal turn of the cochlea can be deficient or absent.
- Atresia or stenosis of the IAC is often associated with absence of cranial nerve VIII and, less commonly, VII, best appreciated on MRI using heavily weighted T2 thinsection images. Often the facial nerve will leave the IAC early or aberrantly while cranial nerve VIII is aplastic or hypoplastic.

## Congenital Syndromes

- Inner ear dysplasias are rather common in patients with Down syndrome with hypoplastic inner ear structures, vestibular malformations, and deficiencies of the lateral semicircular canal reported. Additionally, fusion of the lateral semicircular canal and vestibule, large vestibular aqueduct syndrome, cochlear nerve deficiency, and IAC stenosis or duplication can be seen.
- In patients with achondroplasia, one can see (1) poorly developed mastoid air cells; (2) upward tilting ("towering") of the petrous ridges and IACs; (3) rotation of the cochlea and ossicles; (4) changes of chronic otomastoiditis; and (5) narrowing of the skull base and foramen magnum.

- Additional congenital syndromes associated with inner ear anomalies include (but are not limited to) neurofibromatosis, osteogenesis imperfecta, Apert syndrome, and Treacher Collins syndrome.

## Labyrinthine Disease

### Perilymphatic Fistula

- A perilymphatic fistula is an abnormal connection between the subarachnoid space and the perilymphatic space of the inner ear. The usual sites of the fistula in children are at the oval and round windows, often with associated stapes superstructure malformations.
- Congenital sources include enlarged vestibular aqueducts, Mondini malformations, and Michel anomalies. Acquired causes of perilymphatic fistulas include acquired cholesteatomas, chronic otitis media, and trauma.
- In the trauma setting, the presence of air in the labyrinthine structures on CT can indicate perilymphatic fistula.
- Spread of middle ear infections to the meninges or of meningitis to the inner or middle ear can occur through perilymphatic fistulas.

### Labyrinthitis

- Labyrinthitis may be attributable to viral, bacterial, luetic, or idiopathic causes. Autoimmune labyrinthitis occurs when antibodies to cochlear antigens form; there is often enhancement of the cochlea bilaterally on MRI.
- In the early phase of inflammation, the labyrinthine structures can appear normal on CT but can show some loss of expected fluid signal and/or enhancement within these structures on MRI. Precontrast T1 high signal within the labyrinthine structures can indicate presence of hemorrhage. Abnormal signal on 3D FLAIR or enhancement of the labyrinth on MR in patients with sudden hearing loss and vertigo can be seen in labyrinthine infection (Fig. 11.34).
- Cochlear enhancement or vestibular apparatus enhancement may occur and often correlates with electronystagmogram findings and clinical symptoms. Other causes of labyrinthine enhancement are listed in Box 11.11.

### Labyrinthine Ossification

- Labyrinthitis ossificans (LO) occurs in the later stages after labyrinthitis (see Box 11.11). Fibroblasts in the labyrinth are induced by an inflammatory state to produce fibrosis, and they may differentiate into osteoblasts to form ossific deposits in the cochlea. Patients present with sensorineural hearing loss and vertigo.
- LO is best evaluated with CT, which will show bony replacement of the labyrinthine portion of the inner ear with dense sclerosis (Fig. 11.35). Imaging findings include cochlear stenosis (approximately 40%), cochlear fibro-ossific change (perhaps better seen with high-resolution T2WI MRI because the fibrous obliteration may not be evident on CT), and cochlear ossification (>30%).
- Ligamentous calcification and bony obliteration of semicircular canals can be another manifestation of LO.

### Otospongiosis (Otosclerosis)

- Otospongiosis is a process whereby endochondral bone at the otic capsule is replaced by spongy bone. Otospongiosis

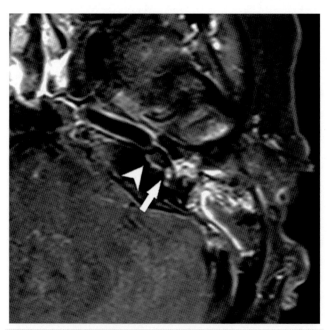

**Fig. 11.34 Labyrinthitis.** Axial T1-weighted postcontrast image shows enhancement in the basal turn of the cochlea *(arrowhead)* and vestibule *(arrow)* in this patient with adjacent otomastoiditis.

## Box 11.11   Causes of Labyrinthine Enhancement and Ossification

| Causes of Labyrinthine Enhancement | Causes of Labyrinthine Ossification |
|---|---|
| Postoperative after schwannoma resection | Chronic labyrinthitis (bacterial) |
| Labyrinthitis (viral, bacterial, luetic, Lyme disease, sarcoidosis, sickle cell disease, hemorrhagic) | Complication of meningitis |
| Posttrauma with hemorrhage into labyrinth | Complication of chronic otitis media |
| Autoimmune labyrinthitis (antibodies to cochlear antigens) | Labyrinthine fistula(infection/ cholesteatoma/trauma) |
| Labyrinthine schwannoma | Trauma/hemorrhage |
| Cogan syndrome (interstitial keratitis, vestibuloauditory abnormality, vasculitis) | Labyrinthectomy |
|  | Otospongiosis |
|  | Paget disease |
|  | Sickle cell disease |

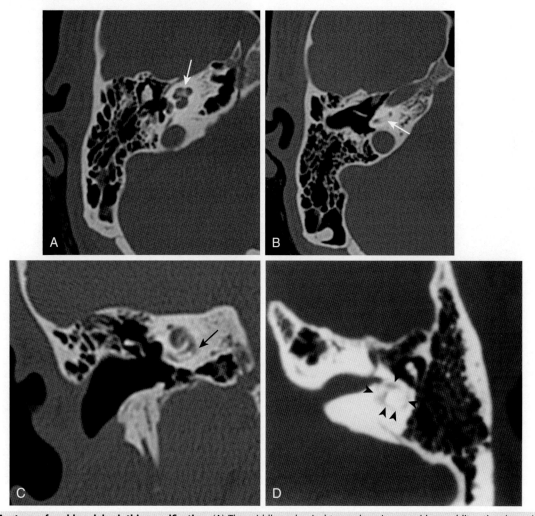

**Fig. 11.35 Montage of cochlear labyrinthine ossification.** (A) The middle and apical turns show increased bony obliteration *(arrow)*. That is too much for a normal modiolus. (B) The basal turn *(arrow)* was also involved. (C) The coronal computed tomography is definitive. The *arrow* is on basal turn ossification. (D) Labyrinthitis ossificans. The vestibule and semicircular canal *(arrowheads)* show the same obliterated appearance resulting from labyrinthitis ossificans.

is usually bilateral and seen most frequently in young to middle-aged females. There are fenestral and cochlear (retrofenestral subtypes). Early on, this process can be seen as demineralization of the involved bone relative to the preserved otic capsule bone density. Later in the course of the disease, the bone becomes sclerotic in appearance, and the pathology is no longer readily detectable.

- Fenestral otospongiosis is more common than cochlear otospongiosis.
  - Fenestral otospongiosis typically involves the fissula ante fenestram, which is found at the oval window border with the anterior crus of the stapes.
  - On CT, there is demineralization at the fissula, and the stapes is essentially glued in position to the oval window, preventing transmission of sound and resulting in conductive hearing loss. The oval window niche is narrowed with fenestral otospongiosis with plaques of bone anteriorly.

- The surgery of choice for fenestral otospongiosis is a small fenestral stapedotomy or total stapedectomy. With a total stapedectomy, a prosthesis must be inserted into the oval window. Metal, Teflon, and wire devices are commonly used.
- In the cochlear (retrofenestral) form of otospongiosis, the middle and basal turns of the cochlea are most frequently involved, showing areas of demineralization marginating these structures (Fig. 11.36).
  - A "double ring" (lucent) sign caused by resorption of bone immediately around the membranous cochlea may be seen as a result of the normal basal turn lucency paralleled by otospongiosis.
  - A cochlear implant may be required in patients with cochlear otospongiosis. This operation is a surgical procedure that consists of inserting multichannel electrodes through the round window into the cochlea with the distal end along the basal membrane

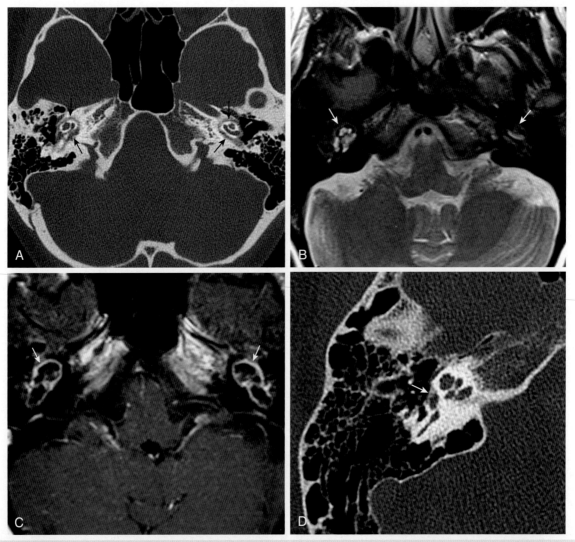

**Fig. 11.36 Otospongiosis.** (A) Axial computed tomographic image shows abnormal lucency in the bone surrounding the cochlea bilaterally in this patient with cochlear otospongiosis *(arrows)*. (B) Axial T2-weighted image (T2WI) shows abnormal hyperintense signal and (C) axial postcontrast T1WI shows abnormal enhancement within the demineralized bone surrounding the cochlea and vestibular structures *(arrows)*. (D) Demineralization at the fissula ante fenestram *(arrow)* is seen with fenestral otospongiosis with identical imaging findings seen in patients with osteogenesis imperfecta (OI). This patient has OI.

of the cochlea where the auditory nerve transmits the sound. A list of what the surgeon needs to know before implantation is given in Box 11.12.

- The differential diagnosis includes osteogenesis imperfecta, otosyphilis, and, rarely, fibrous dysplasia and Paget disease. The normal cochlear cleft of childhood may simulate early otospongiosis because it is in proximity to the fissula but is better defined and resolves with age.

## Ménière Disease

- Ménière disease is a clinical syndrome characterized by episodic vertigo, hearing loss, and tinnitus. The pathogenesis of Ménière disease (endolymphatic hydrops) is characterized by distension of the labyrinthine structures that contain endolymph into spaces that normally contain perilymph, such as the cochlear aqueduct, saccule, utricle, and semicircular ducts.
- On MRI, absence of T2-hyperintense signal on high-resolution T2WI can be seen. More recently, 3D FLAIR imaging at 24 hours after intratympanic (through the tympanic membrane or through the eustachian tube) or at 4 hours after intravenous injection of gadolinium has been shown to demonstrate differential enhancement within endolymph and perilymph with a high sensitivity and specificity.

## Paget Disease

- Paget disease may cause either sensorineural or conductive hearing loss. The increased vascularity of involved temporal bone can also account for the clinical presentation of pulsatile tinnitus.
- In its early phases, you can see a diffuse expansile lytic process with trabecular disorganization (similar to appearance elsewhere in the skeleton) involving the bony labyrinth; however, in the late phases, increased density is seen (Box 11.13). The lytic phase appears to begin medially in the petrous apex and to progress laterally (Fig. 11.37).

## Fibrous Dysplasia

- Fibrous dysplasia may affect the temporal bone, causing increased density in a ground-glass pattern.
- The mastoid portion is affected most commonly, and the involvement may lead to conductive hearing loss.

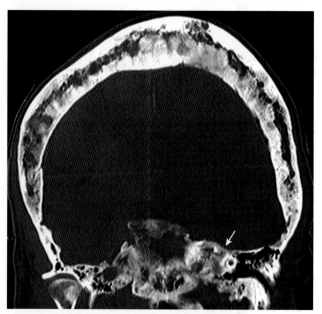

**Fig. 11.37 Paget disease of the temporal bone.** Axial computed tomography reveals diffuse increased bone density with thickening throughout the base of the skull. Note the predominance in the petrous apex *(arrow)* with relative sparing laterally.

## Petrous Apex Lesions

### Petrous Apicitis

- Petrous apicitis is a nondestructive inflammatory condition of the aerated petrous apex (Box 11.14). Pneumatization of the petrous apex is present in 30% to 35% of people; thus petrositis can develop in these persons.

## Benign Neoplasms of the Inner Ear

- Intralabyrinthine schwannomas are rare tumors but enhance markedly on MRI. They are usually situated close to the round window niche. They are an unusual cause of hearing loss, as opposed to the more typical vestibular schwannomas (see Chapter 2, Fig. 2.6). The tumors are associated with neurofibromatosis II.
- Cranial nerve V schwannomas (see Fig. 10.35) may also occur along the petrous apex even to the trigeminal impression of Meckel Cave where the Gasserian ganglion resides. These lesions begin in an extraosseous location but may erode the medial petrous bone near the trigeminal impression. They enhance solidly or heterogeneously.

## Malignant Neoplasms of the Inner Ear

- There are relatively few primary malignant lesions of the inner ear. SCC of the skin is probably the most common malignancy to affect the inner ear by direct extension.
- Hematogenous metastases may occur in the inner ear. Rarely, neurofibrosarcomas, rhabdomyosarcomas, lymphomas, or malignant hemangiopericytomas may occur in this location.
- Perineural spread of malignancies along the facial nerve may lead to destructive processes affecting the inner ear.

## Endolymphatic Sac Tumors

- These tumors of the endolymphatic sac were previously called *adenomatoid papillary tumors*. More recently, their site of origin has been reevaluated, and it currently appears that they need not be of endolymphatic sac origin. Some arise from the top of the jugular bulb, the mucosa of the aerated cells around the jugular bulb, or the mastoid air cells.

- There is a strong association with von Hippel–Lindau disease. Approximately 11% to 16% of patients with von Hippel–Lindau disease have an endolymphatic sac tumor, and of these one third are bilateral.
- The tumors are characterized by aggressive bony destruction and calcified matrix on CT and bright signal on T1WI, possibly from hemorrhage (Fig. 11.39). Tumors larger than 2 cm may have flow voids because of branches of the external carotid artery that supply this hypervascular tumor. The orientation of the tumor, parallel to the posterior margin of the petrous temporal bone, simulates the vestibular aqueduct.

## JUGULAR FORAMEN LESIONS

- Lesions that occur in this location include glomus tumor, neurogenic tumors (neurofibroma or schwannoma), meningioma, superior spread of nasopharyngeal carcinoma, and metastatic disease (Box 11.15; Table 11.4).
  - The glomus tumor, neurofibroma, schwannoma, and metastatic lesions often erode/remodel bone in the jugular foramen. Meningiomas that extend into the jugular foramen usually demonstrate a dural base and an enhancing tail; meningiomas are discussed in detail in Chapter 2.

---

### Box 11.15   Differential Diagnosis of Jugular Foramen Masses

Enlarged jugular bulb/diverticulum
Paraganglioma
Nasopharyngeal carcinoma spread
Schwannoma
Meningioma
Metastasis
Chondroid lesion

---

**Table 11.4**   Differential Diagnosis of Jugular Foramen Masses

| Entity | T2WI Intensity | Enhancement | Calcification/Bone Erosion | Helpful MR Technique | Angiographic Appearance | CT Density |
|---|---|---|---|---|---|---|
| Glomus jugulare | Salt-and-pepper | Marked: downward dip on dynamic enhancement | Erosion | Dynamic enhancement, MR venogram | Hypervascular with arteriovenous shunting, stain | Hyperdense |
| Schwannoma | Hyperintense; may have cystic degeneration | Moderate: upward slope on dynamic scanning | No; bone remodeled | Traditional | Hypovascular | Isodense |
| Metastasis | Hyperintense | Moderate | Erodes bone and infiltrates | Traditional | Most often hypovascular; exceptions include hypervascular metastases such as renal, thyroid | Isodense |
| Enlarged jugular bulb | Flow effects | Varies with technique, turbulence | No | MR venogram | Venous phase | Vascular |
| Nasopharyngeal carcinoma | Hyperintense to intermediate | Moderate | Erodes bone and infiltrates, look for perineural spread | Traditional | Most often hypovascular | Isodense |
| Meningioma | Isointense to slightly hyperintense | Marked | Osteolysis versus hyperostosis | Traditional | Hypervascular; persistent stain on all tests | Slightly hyperdense |

*CT,* Computed tomography; *MR,* magnetic resonance; *T2WI,* T2-weighted image.

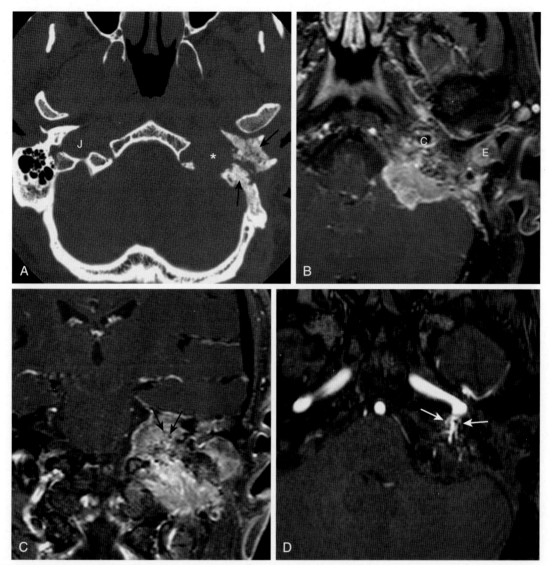

**Fig. 11.40 Glomus jugulare.** (A) Axial computed tomographic image shows marked expansion of the left jugular foramen *(asterisk)*, compared with the normal foramen on the right *(J)*. Note permeative marrow change in the adjacent mastoid bone on the left *(arrows)*, which is very characteristic of glomus jugulare. (B) Axial postcontrast T1-weighted image (T1WI) shows enhancing tumor arising from the expanded jugular foramen with extension into the posterior fossa, encasement of the carotid artery *(C)*, and extension into the external auditory canal *(E)*. (C) Coronal postcontrast T1WI again shows enhancing tumor centered within the jugular foramen with extension below the skull base along the course of the jugular vein. Flow voids are present *(arrows)*, contributing to the characteristic salt-and-pepper appearance of this tumor. (D) Three-dimensional time-of-flight magnetic resonance angiography shows high-flow shunting to the tumor *(arrows)*.

- The glomus jugulare tumor is a paraganglioma arising from the jugular foramen, most commonly from the adventitia of the jugular vein in the jugular foramen, although glomus bodies also accompany the auricular branches of the vagus nerve (Arnold nerve) or the tympanic branch of the glossopharyngeal nerve (Jacobson nerve) presenting as middle ear masses (glomus tympanicum). The glomus jugulare occasionally extends from the skull base superiorly into the middle ear cavity (thereby called a *glomus jugulotympanicum*).
  - A hereditary form of paragangliomatosis is associated with multiple glomus tumors including jugulare, vagal, carotid body, and tympanicum tumors. Overall, multiple paragangliomas occur in 15% of patients with a glomus tumor. Paragangliomas rarely will metastasize.

- The glomus jugulare can occlude the jugular bulb and characteristically grows into the jugular vein (unusual for the other masses in the region). It may grow inferiorly into the jugular vein or may grow from the jugular bulb region into the sigmoid and transverse sinuses. Alternatively, the mass may cause thrombosis of the adjacent venous sinuses.
- On MRI, the glomus jugulare, when large, has a typical MRI salt-and-pepper appearance on T2WI and enhanced T1WI (Fig. 11.40). This is seen as flow voids within the tumor, surrounded by tumor substance. Time-of-flight magnetic resonance angiography (MRA) can show prominent flow-related signal within the mass.
- On conventional angiography, the glomus tumor is evidenced by a hypervascular mass, often supplied by

ascending pharyngeal and occipital branches, with a persistent stain.

## TRAUMA

- Fractures of the temporal bone can range from simple-appearing nondisplaced fractures to very complex injuries.

Secondary Sings of Temporal Bone Fractures

- Occult fractures should be suspected even if a clear fracture plane is not seen when secondary signs of injury are present, including opacification of mastoid air cells, adjacent pneumocephalus, and pneumolabyrinth.
- Temporal bone fractures can be seen with diastatic (widened) sutures.

- Beware of normal sutures, fissures, and vascular channels in the temporal bone that can mimic the appearance of a fracture!

- Fractures can be described as "otic capsule sparing" and "otic capsule violating" injuries with regard to involvement of the cochlea and labyrinth in the setting of temporal bone injury.
- Injury to the facial nerve can occur usually from local effects at the geniculate ganglion rather than transection. Sensorineural hearing loss can also be seen as a complication, and transection of the cochlear nerve can occur at the IAC apex (Fig. 11.41).
- Involvement of the EAC and glenoid fossa of the TMJ is very common.
- When the middle ear is involved, ossicular dislocation can be seen (Fig. 11.42). Ossicular fractures are extremely rare but do occur.

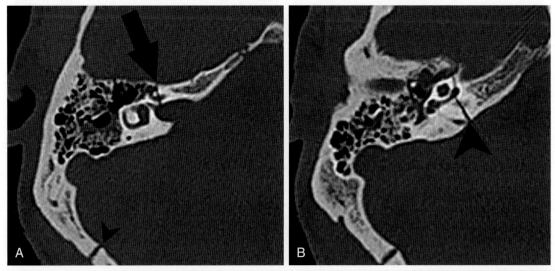

**Fig. 11.41 Temporal bone fracture violating otic capsule.** (A) Linear nondisplaced fracture *(black arrow)* through the otic capsule focally violates the internal auditory canal and the labyrinthine segment of the facial nerve canal. Note diastasis of the occipitomastoid suture as part of the acute bony injury (arrowhead). (B) More inferiorly, the fracture plane *(arrowhead)* just misses the margin of the cochlear aqueduct but does extend right through the basal turn of the cochlea.

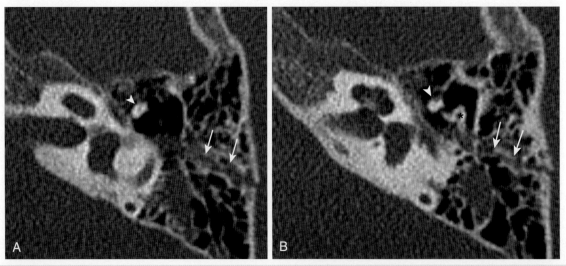

**Fig. 11.42 Ossicular dislocation.** Axial computed tomographic images (A) and (B) show nondisplaced fracture through the temporal bone *(arrows)*. There is associated opacification within the mastoid air cells. Note that the head of the malleus *(arrowhead)* seems to be "falling off" of the short process of the incus *(asterisk)*. This is incudomalleolar dislocation, most often found in the setting of trauma.

**TEACHING POINTS**

Ossicular Chain Dislocations in Trauma

- The incudostapedial joint, being the weakest of the middle ear articulations, is most commonly affected.
- This is detected by seeing a fracture of the long process of the incus with separation of more than 1 mm from the stapes head posterolaterally.
- Incudal dislocations are the source of nearly 80% of the cases of posttraumatic conductive hearing defects. Look for these or you won't find them!

---

- Disruption of other vital structures including adjacent venous sinuses and carotid canal must be reported, followed by recommendation for angiographic evaluation, preferably by CT, to assess for acute arterial and venous injury including dissection, pseudoaneurysm, vasospasm, cavernous-carotid fistula, traumatic occlusion, and thrombosis (Fig. 11.43).

- Be sure to evaluate the intracranial contents for associated extra-axial hemorrhages and parenchymal contusions in the temporal lobe.

- Other complications of temporal bone fractures include otorrhea, meningitis, traumatic meningoencephaloceles, perilymphatic fistula, and CSF leakage. Disruption of the jugular foramen can result in cranial nerve IX, X, and XI palsies, and injury to the petrous apex can cause stretch injury to the abducens nerve as it enters the Dorello canal.

- Beware the normal sutures, fissures, and vascular channels in the temporal bone that can mimic the appearance of a fracture! Knowing your anatomy helps, but when in doubt, look for asymmetry (if it's symmetric, it's probably not a fracture) and expected secondary signs like scalp overlying scalp swelling and adjacent intracranial pneumocephalus to help sort things out.

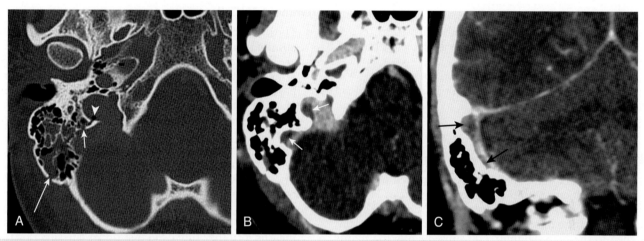

**Fig. 11.43 Temporal bone fracture.** (A) Axial computed tomography (CT) image shows minimally displaced fracture through the mastoid portion of the temporal bone *(large arrow)*, which extends anteromedially to the jugular foramen. There is focal disruption of the bone adjacent to the expected course of the sigmoid sinus *(small arrow)* as well as focus of gas within the jugular foramen *(arrowhead)*. These imaging findings should raise suspicion for acute venous injury and prompt further imaging work-up. (B) Axial and (C) coronal images from subsequently performed CT venogram show nonocclusive filling defects within the sigmoid sinus and jugular vein, indicating acute venous thrombosis *(arrows)*.

# 12 *Sinonasal Disease*

KAREN BUCH

## Relevant Anatomy

### PARANASAL SINUSES

The paranasal sinuses develop in a systematic fashion, with some sinuses present at birth and others developing in childhood.

### The Maxillary Sinus and Its Drainage Pathway

- The maxillary sinuses are the largest paired paranasal sinuses. Mucus within the maxillary sinuses is swept by cilia toward the drainage recesses (Fig. 12.1). This occurs via the maxillary ostium located superolaterally, then to the infundibulum, and subsequently the hiatus semilunaris into the middle meatus, nasal cavity, and ultimately the nasopharynx. Approximately 30% of patients have an accessory ostium present, inferior to the primary opening.
- The infundibulum is located lateral to the uncinate process and medial to inferomedial border of the orbit.
- The uncinate process is a sickle-shaped bony extension of the lateral nasal wall. The uncinate can attach to lamina papyracea (LP) (medial orbital wall), forming a blind pouch called the *recessus terminalis*.
- The middle meatus is a channel between the middle nasal turbinate and the uncinate process.
- The hiatus semilunaris is a slit-like air-filled space, anterior and inferior to the largest ethmoid air cell, known as the *ethmoidal bulla*, and directly *above* the uncinate process.

### The Ostiomeatal Complex

- The ostiomeatal complex (OMC) represents the common drainage pathway of the frontal, maxillary, and anterior ethmoid air cells (Fig. 12.2). The structures of the OMC include: (1) the maxillary sinus ostium, (2) the infundibulum, (3) the uncinate process, (4) the hiatus semilunaris, (5) the ethmoid bulla, and (6) the middle meatus.

### The Frontal Sinuses

- These paired paranasal sinuses are housed within the frontal bone. They are separated from each other by an osseous septum. Drainage from the frontal sinuses can be variable, but generally occurs via the infundibulum within the inferomedial corner of the frontal sinus to a narrow passage known as the *frontal recess*. From the frontal recess, drainage often extends to the ethmoidal infundibulum, through the hiatus semilunaris, and into the medial meatus.

### Ethmoid Air Cells

- These air cells are located within the midline of the ethmoid bone. Anterior and posterior ethmoid sinuses are separated via the *basal lamella*, defined as the lateral attachment of the middle nasal turbinate to the lamina papyracea. The fovea ethmoidalis is a bony extension of the orbital plate, which forms the lateral part of the ethmoid roof and merges medially with cribriform plate.
- The anterior ethmoid air cells drain to the hiatus semilunaris and middle meatus via the ethmoid bulla.
- The posterior ethmoid air cells drain to the superior meatus via the sphenoethmoidal recess (SER). They are located behind the basal lamella of the middle turbinate and drain via the superior meatus, the supreme meatus, or other tiny ostia just under the superior turbinate. They drain along with the sphenoid sinuses into the SER of the nasal cavity and pass secretions into the nasopharynx.
- There are several named ethmoid air cells, which include:
  - *Haller cells*, maxilloethmoidal air cells or infraorbital air cells. These anterior ethmoid air cells are located along the inferior margin of the orbit and protrude into the maxillary sinus. They are seen in 10% to 45% of patients. When Haller cells are enlarged, they may narrow the infundibulum or maxillary sinus ostium (Fig. 12.3).
  - *Agger nasi cells*, the most anterior ethmoid air cells, often located anterior, lateral, and below the frontal recess. They are present in more than 90% of patients (Fig. 12.4).
  - *Ethmoidal bullae*, ethmoid air cells directly above and posterior to infundibulum and hiatus semilunaris. Large ethmoidal bullae can obstruct the infundibulum and hiatus semilunaris and obstruct drainage of the maxillary and anterior ethmoid sinuses.
  - *Frontal cells*, anterior ethmoid air cells that can sometimes be seen along the anterior aspect of the frontal recess. Based on the Kuhn classification, they can be located above the agger nasi cell (single, Kuhn type 1,

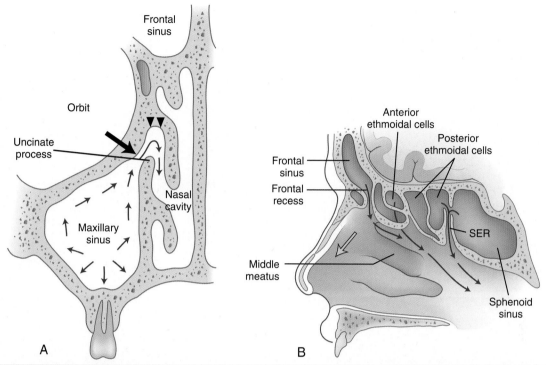

**Fig. 12.1  Major sinonasal drainage pathways.** (A) On this coronal view schematic, mucociliary clearance passes from the antral floor along the walls of the maxillary sinus toward the main maxillary sinus ostium. It then passes lateral to the uncinate process in the infundibulum *(fat black arrow)* into the hiatus semilunaris *(arrowheads)* and then to the middle meatus. (B) Note flow of mucus from frontal, ethmoid and sphenoid sinuses on sagittal view schematic posteriorly (small arrows) and flow anterior to the middle meatus in the forward direction (large arrow). The frontal recess, middle meatus, and sphenoethmoidal recess *(SER)* are the respective egresses from the sinuses. (Modified from Zinreich SJ, Kennedy DW, Rosenbaum AE, et al. Paranasal sinuses: CT imaging requirements for endoscopic surgery. *Radiology.* 1987;163:769–775.)

or multiple type 2) or may extend into (type 3) or be contained within (type 4) the frontal sinus.

- *Onodi cell* (Fig. 12.5), the most posterior ethmoid air cell and that may pneumatize into the sphenoid bone, superior to the sphenoid sinus, often accompanied by pneumatization of the optic strut and anterior clinoid process. If perforated surgically, it may lead to injury intracranially or within the optic canal.
- The sinus lateralis, located between the ethmoidal bulla and basal lamella (the lateral attachment of the middle turbinate to the lamina papyracea of the orbit). The sinus lateralis includes the suprabullar and retrobullar recesses. These may open into the frontal recess or into a space posterior to the bulla: the hiatus semilunaris posterioris.

### Sphenoid Sinuses

- This is the most posterior of the paranasal sinuses located within the central body of the sphenoid bone. Aeration of the sphenoid sinuses is highly variable and can lateralized into the sphenoid wings. Presence of septae can result in multiple compartments within the sphenoid sinuses. The sphenoid sinuses communicate with the roof of the nasal cavity via the SER, located along the anterior wall of the sphenoid sinuses.

### The Nasal Cavity

- The bony housing of the nasal cavity consists of lateral walls (common walls with the medial wall maxillary sinus) and floor (the hard palate) (see Fig. 12.2).

- The nasal cavity contains three sets of nasal turbinates: the superior, middle, and inferior turbinates. Occasionally, a fourth superior-most turbinate can be seen: the supreme turbinate. Paradoxial turns of the nasal turbinates have been described as a reversal in characteristic medially directed curve of middle turbinates.
- *Concha bullosa* is a term referring to an aerated middle turbinate, which usually communicates with the anterior ethmoid air cells. These are seen in approximately 34% to 53% of patients. When the concha bullosa is very large and obstructs drainage pathways, it may predispose to sinusitis.
- The nasal septum is a midline structure between right and left turbinates. There are three parts to the nasal septum including (1) a cartilaginous anteroinferior portion; (2) a bony posteroinferior portion (*vomer*), and (3) a superoposterior bony portion, the perpendicular plate of the ethmoid bone. The nasal septum is rarely aerated.
- The nasolacrimal duct (NLD) is a structure describing the inferior continuation of the lacrimal sac. It is made of an osseous component (within the lacrimal groove descending in the nasolacrimal canal of the maxilla) and a membranous component, which runs in the nasal mucosa and terminates below the inferior nasal meatus as a slit-like opening called the *valve of Hasner*. The NLD courses inferior from the lacrimal sac bordering the medial canthus in close association with agger nasi air cells (Fig. 12.6). Inflammation of agger nasi cells may be associated with epiphora because of this close relationship.

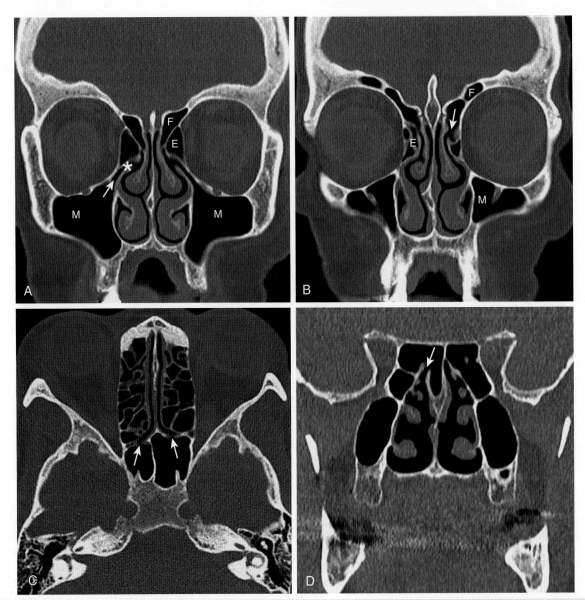

**Fig. 12.2 Nasal cavity and major drainage pathways of the paranasal sinuses.** (A) Coronal computed tomography (CT) reconstruction shows an intact midline nasal septum attaching to the anterior skull base at its superior extent and the hard palate at its inferior extent along with middle and inferior turbinates on either side. Note the lateral wall of the nasal cavity is common with the medial wall of the maxillary sinus. The maxillary sinus ostium *(arrow)* and uncinate process *(asterisk)* facilitate drainage from the maxillary sinus (*M*) into the nasal cavity. Frontal (*F*) and ethmoid (*E*) sinuses are also indicated. (B) More posteriorly in the same patient, the frontal recess is indicated *(arrow)*, facilitating drainage from the frontal sinus (*F*) and ethmoid (*E*) air cells toward the middle meatus. Maxillary sinus (*M*) is indicated. On axial (C) and coronal (D) CT, the sphenoethmoidal recess (SER) *(arrows)* leads from the sphenoid and posterior ethmoid sinus into the nasal cavity.

# Imaging Techniques/Protocols

- Computed tomography (CT) is the workhorse for imaging of the sinonasal cavity, with plain radiographs fallen wayside.
  - 1 to 2 mm axial images through the paranasal sinuses with coronal and sagittal reconstructions in soft tissue and bone algorithms are typically performed.
  - Intravenous (IV) contrast is not necessary unless there is concern for an invasive sinonasal mass or aggressive infectious process with potential for spread of disease to the orbits, intracranial space, or cavernous sinus.
- Magnetic resonance (MR) has an important role when aggressive infections are suspected, for intracranial

complications of sinusitis, and in the imaging workup of sinonasal masses.

**TEACHING POINTS**

Imaging Evaluation of the Paranasal Sinuses on Magnetic Resonance Imaging

- It is not uncommon for a sinonasal mass to cause sinus outlet obstruction. On computed tomography (CT), it can be difficult to distinguish trapped secretions from the mass itself. This is where magnetic resonance imaging (MRI) plays an important role in the evaluation of sinonasal disease.

- Sinonasal secretions are often bright on T2-weighted imaging (T2WI) and dark on T1-weighted imaging (T1WI), but these features are heavily dependent on protein content. High-protein content leads to high T1WI and decreased T2 signal intensity.
- In fungal sinusitis, very low T2 signal intensity is often seen related to paramagnetic effects of iron or manganese metabolized by fungi.
- To distinguish infection from tumor, it is important to remember that inflamed mucosa avidly enhances in a peripheral manner, whereas tumors usually enhance solidly and centrally.
- Subtle extension of disease into the adjacent orbit and intracranial compartment can be more readily apparent on MRI than CT. Look for signal changes in the orbits and subtle dural-based enhancement at the floor of the anterior cranial fossa!

- Typical sequences employed include pre- and fat-suppressed post contrast T1-weighted imaging (T1WI), T2-weighted imaging (T2WI), fat-suppressed T2, and diffusion-weighted imaging (DWI).
- If perineural disease is in question, pre- and postcontrast T2WI and T1WI isotropic three-dimensional (3D) acquisitions (typically using gradient echo or fast spin echo techniques) can allow for high-resolution imaging with multiplanar reconstructions for a more comprehensive assessment of small nerves within their respective neural foramina.

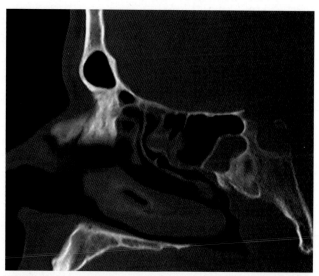

**Fig. 12.5 Onodi cell.** On this sagittal computed tomography (CT) image, there is an aerated posterior ethmoid air cell (Onodi cell) sitting on top of an opacified sphenoid sinus. Perforation of this air cell at surgery could result in violation of the intracranial compartment in this case.

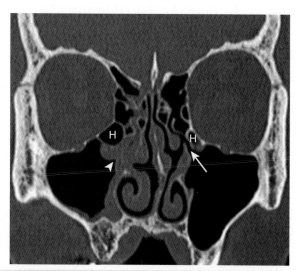

**Fig. 12.3 Haller cell.** Coronal computed tomographic image demonstrates Haller cells (*H*) bilaterally. On the left, the air cell is small enough that it does not narrow the left maxillary sinus ostium (*arrow*). However, on the right side, the ostium is occluded (*arrowhead*) because of the presence of the larger Haller air cell and mucosal thickening.

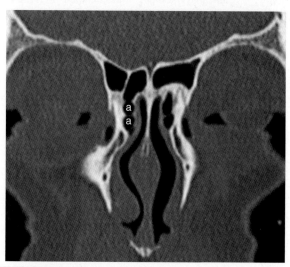

**Fig. 12.4 Agger nasi cells.** Coronal computed tomographic image shows bilateral agger nasi air cells (*a*) on right.

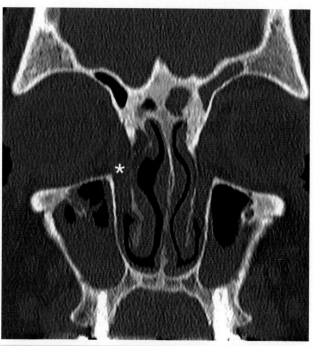

**Fig. 12.6 Nasolacrimal duct.** On this coronal computed tomography (CT) image, the bony housing of the nasolacrimal duct is shown bilaterally (*asterisk*) on the right nasolacrimal duct canal.

# Pathology

## CONGENITAL DISORDERS

- **Piriform aperture stenosis**, is a congenital condition with the piriform aperture being abnormally small in size, with a width measuring less than 11 mm. Piriform aperture stenosis is associated with abnormal dentition and a midline bony inferior palatal ridge. It is a common cause of infantile airway compromise.
- **Choanal atresia** is defined by a posterior choanal opening less than 5 mm in width in neonates and 1 cm in adolescents and can present in a variety of clinical syndromes (Box 12.1). Infants present with respiratory distress, and the clinical team is unable to pass a nasogastric tube. Choanal atresia is also associated with thickening of the vomer (Fig. 12.7).
    - The vomer should measure less than 3 mm in thickness in children younger than 8 years old.
    - Imaging is used to determine whether the obstruction is related to membranous (15%) or bony (85%) structures. Additionally, imaging is used to evaluate for associated congenital central nervous system (CNS) or non-CNS anomalies that can coexist.
- **Congenital sinonasal masses** are a result of aberrations during embryogenesis (Table 12.1). During embryogenesis, the dura contacts the dermis at the nasion region as the neural plate retracts. Normally, the dermal connection regresses, but if this fails, a cerebrospinal fluid (CSF) connection to the intracranial contents may persist (Fig. 12.8). Lesions include:
    - Nasal gliomas, which consist of dysplastic ectopic glial cells, are not neoplasms despite the name. They are more commonly extranasal than intranasal in location (see Fig. 12.8).
    - Meningoencephalocele contains meninges and brain tissue (usually dysplastic) because of a persistent CSF connection between dura and dermal connection (Fig. 12.9).
    - Dermal sinus tract, appearing as a pit in the middle of the nose with a persistent intracranial connection in 25% cases. This may result in the development of meningitis, osteomyelitis, and intracranial abscess because of this persistent connection. This may or may not have fat associated with it (usually not).
    - Epidermoids are slow growing and often painless cystic lesions. These lesions do not have hair, fat, or other dermal elements like their dermoid counterpart.

## INFLAMMATORY LESIONS

### Sinusitis

- Sinusitis is one of the most common afflictions in the United States (affecting over 31 million people in the United States per year). Acute sinusitis is often associated with an antecedent viral upper respiratory tract infection. The mucosal congestion from the viral infection (rhinovirus, respiratory syncytial virus, parainfluenza virus, coronavirus) results in obstruction of drainage. This creates a favorable environment for bacterial superinfection. The ethmoid air cells are most commonly involved. Common bacterial pathogens include *Streptococcus pneumoniae*, *Haemophilus influenzae*, β-hemolytic Streptococcus, and *Moraxella catarrhalis*.

---

**Box 12.1    Entities Associated With Choanal Atresia**

Achondroplasia
Fetal alcohol syndrome
CHARGE syndrome (coloboma, heart defects, choanal atresia, retardation, genitourinary abnormalities, ear abnormalities)
Crouzon syndrome
Apert syndrome
Holoprosencephaly
Treacher Collins syndrome
Amniotic band syndrome
Thalidomide embryopathy

---

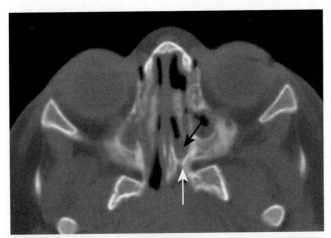

**Fig. 12.7 Membranous and bony choanal atresia.** On the *left*, the nasal passageway narrows and the vomer is thicker, and both bony (posterior; *white arrow*) and soft-tissue (anterior; *black arrow*) plugs are seen. No luck passing the tube on the *left* side.

---

**Table 12.1    Congenital Nasal Lesions**

| Lesion | Imaging Findings | Clinical Examination | Treatment |
|---|---|---|---|
| Nasal glioma | Soft-tissue mass with characteristics of the brain | Intranasal or extranasal mass | Excision |
|  | No connection or fibrous connection to the brain or CSF |  |  |
| Dermoid/epidermoid | Variably cystic/soft-tissue mass | Nasal dimple | Exploration and excision |
|  | ±Sinus tract | Sinus tract |  |
|  | Inflammatory changes |  |  |
| Encephalocele | Connection to CNS with associated defect in skull bone | Pulsatile mass | Patch dura |
|  |  | Dural covering | Reduce brain tissue |
|  | Brain or meninges included |  |  |
|  | Other CNS anomalies |  |  |

*CNS*, Central nervous system; *CSF*, cerebrospinal fluid.

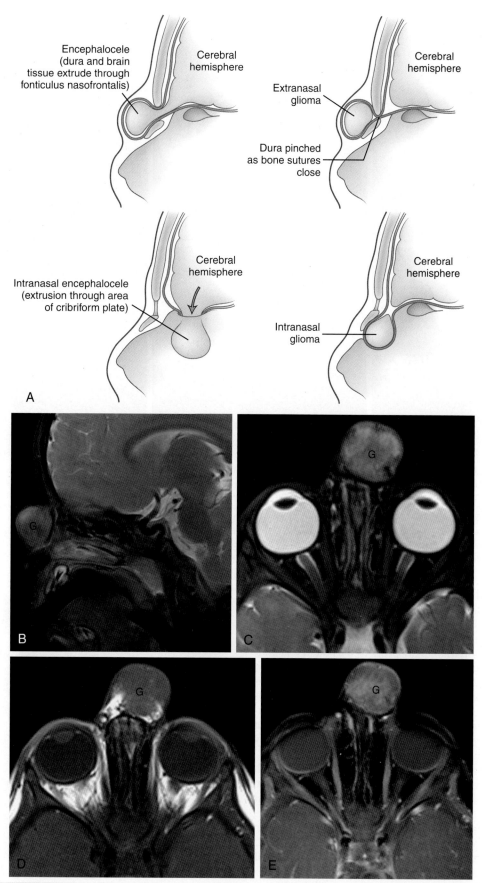

**Fig. 12.8 Congenital nasal lesions.** (A) Sagittal schematic representation of encephaloceles *(left)* and nasal gliomas *(right)*. Sagittal T2 (B), axial T2 (C), and axial precontrast (D) and postcontrast (E) T1-weighted images (T1WI) show an extranasal soft-tissue mass *(G)* looking kind of brainy with mild enhancement; there is no attachment to the intracranial structures. Again, not nasal and not glioma = nasal glioma (go figure!). (A, From Gorenstein A, Kern EB, Facer GW, Laws ER Jr. Nasal gliomas. *Arch Otolaryngol.* 1980;106:536.)

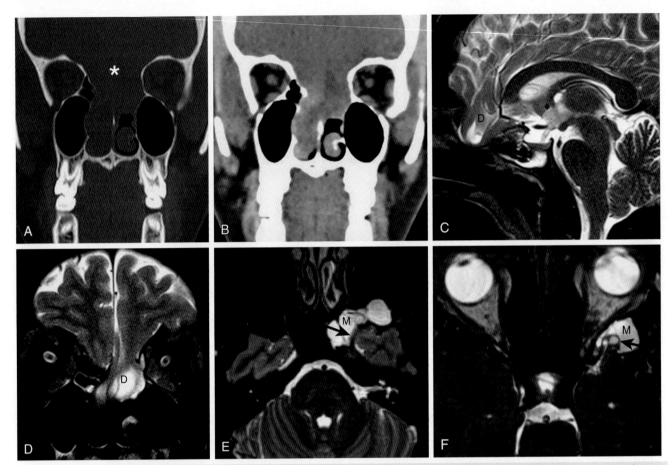

**Fig. 12.9 Meningoencephaloceles galore.** Contrast the previous case with this one. An intranasal meningoencephalocele is seen on coronal computed tomography (CT) in bone (A) and soft-tissue (B) windows. There is a large deficiency at the cribriform plate (A, *asterisk*), allowing for herniation of brain tissue into the nasal cavity. Sagittal imaging (C) and coronal (D) T2-weighted imaging (T2WI) confirm the herniation of brain tissue (D) into the nasal cavity. Note the T2 hyperintensity within the herniated tissue, indicating dysplastic brain. (E) And one more … on this axial T2WI, you might be fooled into calling this a lateralized sphenoid sinus filled with snot but it's not (heh heh). Note the focal deficiency of the middle cranial fossa transmitting a small amount of brain tissue (*arrow*), making this a meningoencephalocele (M). (F) For you nonbelievers out there, slightly more superiorly in this same patient, axial T2 constructive interference in steady state imaging shows another defect along the middle cranial fossa, transmitting clearly dysplastic brain tissue (*arrow*) into the aerated but opacified sphenoid wing, again cinching the diagnosis of meningoencephalocele (M).

- Acute sinusitis is a clinical diagnosis made without imaging! CT imaging is reserved for recurrent sinusitis, atypical sinus infections, or sinusitis complications, with intention of surgical intervention.
- Acute sinusitis on imaging appears as air-fluid levels and/or frothy secretions present in cases of clinically suspected sinusitis (Fig. 12.10). It is important to note that sterile secretions appearing as fluid levels can also be seen in patients performing nasal irrigation, intubated patients, drowning victims, and trauma patients. Mucosal thickening that is new compared with recent prior studies may also imply active inflammation in the appropriate clinical context.
- On the other hand, bone thickening and sclerosis secondary to reactive osteitis from adjacent chronic mucosal inflammation is a hallmark feature of chronic sinusitis (Fig. 12.11).
- Hyperdense paranasal secretions typically occur from inspissated proteinaceous secretions, fungal sinusitis (Fig. 12.12), hemorrhage in the sinus in the setting of trauma, and calcification with various patterns.
- Rarely, chronic sinus inflammation can result in chronic negative pressure in the sinus and ultimately hypoventilation, and over time the sinus can become small in size,

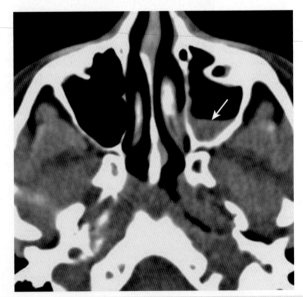

**Fig. 12.10 Acute sinusitis.** An air-fluid level can be seen in a number of clinical scenarios, but if the clinician is concerned about acute sinus inflammation, the air-fluid level would be a salient imaging sign (*arrow*).

sometimes referred to as *sinus atelectasis* or *silent sinus syndrome* (Fig. 12.13). When this phenomenon affects the maxillary sinus, the negative pressure can cause the orbital floor to become depressed, the maxillary walls to retract centrally, and the retromaxillary fat to expand.

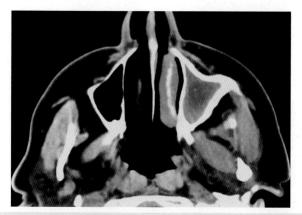

**Fig. 12.11 Chronic sinusitis.** Marked bony thickening and sclerosis around the opacified left maxillary sinus signifies osteitis from chronic sinus disease.

The ocular globe may be displaced inferiorly (hypoglobus) or retract (enophthalmos).

- Additional structures to evaluate on sinus CT include:
  - Teeth: Periodontal disease can incite maxillary sinus infection (odontogenic sinusitis), with dehiscence of maxillary alveolus adjacent to inflamed carious tooth. In such cases, sinus disease will not resolve until the infected tooth is removed.
  - Temporomandibular joint (TMJ): Malocclusion and degenerative changes of the TMJ may result in maxillofacial pain syndrome, which can simulate pain from sinusitis. Look for joint space narrowing, osteophytes, and sclerosis at the joint.
  - Sella: The detection of incidental sellar lesions may mimic opacified paranasal/sphenoid/Onodi sinuses.
  - Nasopharynx: Lesions may extend into paranasal sinuses and mimic opacification from inflammation.

## Mucocele

- Mucoceles result as a complication of sinusitis (Fig. 12.14) wherein trapped secretions from outlet obstruction contribute to slow-growing expansion of the affected sinus. They can involve any of the paranasal

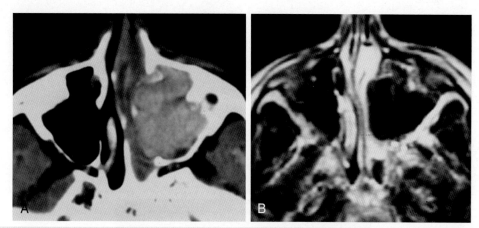

**Fig. 12.12 Fungal sinusitis.** (A) Unenhanced computed tomographic scan shows a hyperdense opacified left maxillary antrum. (B) On T2-weighted imaging (T2WI), the secretions were black, suggesting inspissation, paramagnetic accumulation, or fungal sinusitis; Cultures grew *Drechslera* fungi.

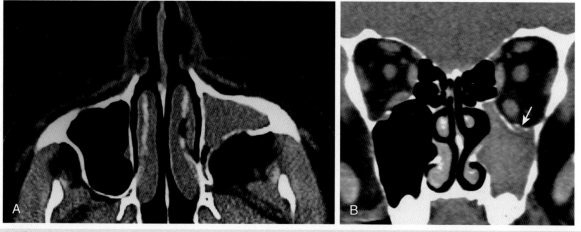

**Fig. 12.13 Silent sinus syndrome.** (A) Note the retracted posterior wall of the *left* maxillary antrum. Fat fills the vacuum. The sinus is nearly completely opacified. (B) On this coronal computed tomographic image in a different patient, the *left* maxillary sinus is completely opacified and smaller than the *right*. Note the slightly thickened walls of the *left* maxillary sinus from chronic inflammation. The orbital floor of the *left* is depressed *(arrow)* compared with the normal *right* side. The sinus has become "atelectatic."

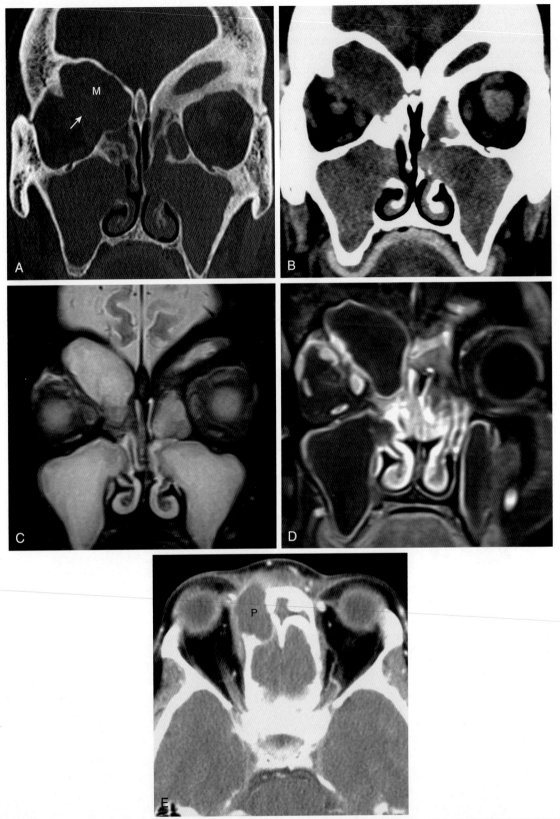

**Fig. 12.14  Mucocele.** (A) Coronal computed tomography (CT) in bone windows shows an expansile lesion within the right frontal sinus *(M)* resulting in dehiscence of the superomedial orbital wall *(arrow)*. There is also complete opacification and osteitis of the included portions of the left frontal, bilateral ethmoid, and bilateral maxillary sinuses. (B) Coronal CT in soft-tissue windows shows the lesion to be near fluid density. Note the displacement of the superior and medial rectus muscles by this lesion. Although very often mucoceles contain proteinaceous contents, in this case (C) coronal T2-weighted imaging (T2WI) and (D) postcontrast T1WI show the lesion to be of fluid signal with only mucosal enhancement present (similar to the other paranasal sinuses). (E) On this axial contrast-enhanced CT of a different patient, a similar lesion shows peripheral contrast enhancement and overlying soft-tissue swelling, consistent with pyomucocele *(P)*. Bonus concomitant chronic inflammation in the left frontal and bilateral maxillary and ethmoid sinuses is included in this case, free of charge.

sinuses but most commonly involve the frontal sinus (65%) followed by the ethmoid air cells (25%) and the maxillary sinus (10%). These require surgical excision, including restoration of sinus drainage to prevent recurrence. If large, the mucocele resection may require extensive facial reconstructive surgery.

- On CT, there is complete sinus opacification, often with bony expansion with thinning or even dehiscence of involved sinus walls. When large enough, expansion of the sinus can lead to involvement and critical mass effect upon orbital and intracranial structures.
- On MRI, signal intensity varies based on protein content with low protein content mucoceles showing T1 dark, T2 bright signal, and higher protein content showing T1 bright and T2 dark signal and inspissated secretions (or calcifications) showing dark signal on both pulse sequences.
- Mucoceles can become superinfected, in which case there can be thick rim enhancement on contrast-enhanced CT and MRI.

### Functional Endoscopic Sinus Surgery Scanning

- For patient with recurrent troublesome symptoms of rhinosinusitis despite maximal medical management, functional endoscopic sinus surgery (FESS) provides surgical options to alleviate symptoms. The goal of FESS is to maintain the normal mucosa of the sinonasal cavity and to preserve the natural pathway of mucociliary clearance, by way of enlarging the natural ostia and passageways of the paranasal sinuses.
- The extent of surgery depends on extent of sinonasal disease and patient factors. More extensive surgery may be required for patients with complicated acute sinusitis and in patients with sinonasal polyposis. Surgery can include uncinectomy, medialization, or partial resection of the middle turbinate, anterior and posterior ethmoidectomy, as well as sphenoid sinusotomy. Frontal sinus drainage surgery can involve anterior ethmoidectomy without instrumentation of the frontal sinus (Draf I), removal of agger nasi and frontal recess air cells (Draf IIa), unilateral drilling of frontal sinus floor (Draf IIb), and drilling of the entire frontal sinus floor and resection of the intersinus septum and upper nasal septum (Draf III).
- CT imaging is necessary preoperatively not just to evaluate extent of sinus disease but to assess bony anatomy

and evaluate for tricky anatomic variations that can complicate the surgical procedure (Fig. 12.15).

- Evaluation of osseous dehiscence for guidance during FESS includes an assessment of the following:
  - The integrity of the cribriform plate (thinned, dehiscent, deep, shallow) to prevent intracranial injury and CSF leak. The lateral lamella is a vulnerable vertical segment of bone that connects the fovea ethmoidalis with the lamina cribrosa upon which the middle turbinate attaches. A longer lateral lamella puts the skull base at risk during turbinectomy or ethmoidectomy compared with a shorter one. Sometimes right and left lateral lamellae are asymmetric in length, putting one side more at risk compared with the other. The Keros classification refers to the length of the lateral lamella, with 1 to 3 mm described as Keros type 1 (one fourth of the population), 4 to 7 mm as Keros type 2 (just under three fourths of the population), and longer than 8 mm as Keros type 3 (super rare)
  - The lamina papyracea to prevent violation of the orbit and intraorbital hematoma
  - The sphenoethmoidal junction to prevent optic nerve injury (look out for that Onodi air cell!)
  - The lateral wall of the sphenoid sinus and insertion of sphenoid sinus septa near or on the common wall of the carotid canal to prevent carotid artery injury or pseudoaneurysm (Fig. 12.16)
  - The ethmoidal notch at the superomedial orbital wall, which transmits the anterior ethmoidal artery; if there is an air cell above the notch (the notch is uncovered), the vessel is at risk for injury during ethmoidectomy, whereas absence of air cell (the notch is covered) poses less of a risk to the vessel
- It is important to be aware of expected postoperative changes, which may occur from FESS. These include:
  - Placement of osteoplastic frontal sinus grafts: These are placed during frontal sinus obliterative procedures when FESS has been unsuccessful in opening the frontal recess. These patients may develop pain secondary to neuromas, mucoceles, or recurrent sinusitis if the sinus is not plugged completely.
  - Fat grafting to obliterate the sinuses: The fat graft has a typical low-density appearance on CT and high T1 signal on T1WI. The amount of fat signal intensity in

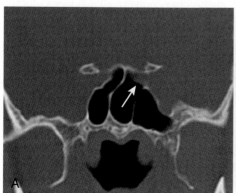
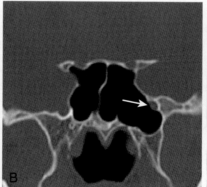
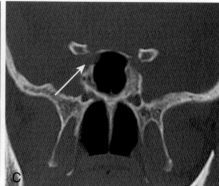

**Fig. 12.15 Potential sites of disaster: Dehiscent areas in the sinuses.** (A) Along the *left* optic canal in the sphenoid sinus *(arrow)*. (B) Along the *left* maxillary nerve *(arrow)*. (C) Along the *right* optic nerve *(arrow)*.

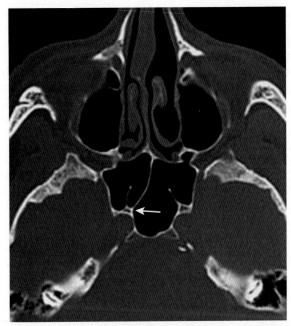

**Fig. 12.16 Sphenoid sinus septum.** On this axial computed tomographic image, the sphenoid sinus septum attaches to the medial wall of the *right* internal carotid artery *(arrow)*. Overvigorous removal during sphenoid sinus surgery can cause a laceration in the carotid wall (ouch!).

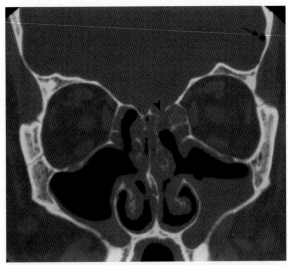

**Fig. 12.17 Postoperative study after uncinectomies and ethmoidectomies.** Despite the surgery to open the ostia and ethmoid sinuses, this patient continued to have acute maxillary sinusitis attacks (note the air-fluid levels on the coronal prone study) and chronic mucosal changes in the ethmoid sinuses. Extra credit: Did you catch the dehiscent area in the *left* fovea ethmoidalis *(arrowhead)*? This may be a manifestation of the disease or the surgery. The dot of intracranial air *(arrow)* is the second edge of the film diagnosis.

obliterated sinus decreases over time as fibrosis occurs. MRI can evaluate adipose tissue, look for mucoceles, and differentiate viable adipose tissue from fat necrosis in the form of oil cysts.

- Absence of anatomic structures like the uncinated process (antrostomy), middle turbinate (turbinectomy), and anterior ethmoid septae (ethmoidectomy), or a widened sphenoethmoidal (sphenoidotomy) or frontal recess (frontal sinusotomy) can indicate prior FESS.
- CT can also be used to evaluate postoperative complications from FESS. Some complications to look out for include:
  - Orbital hematoma, which may occur from transection of an ethmoidal artery at FESS. The hematoma may compress or compromise blood flow of the retinal artery, leading to optic nerve ischemia. On imaging, orbital hematoma will appear as a hyperdense mass on CT with, occasionally, diffuse orbital fat edema. It is important to assess for optic nerve compression or inadvertent transection as well. It is important to alert the clinician to any of these findings for urgent treatment, which will include a decompressive canthotomy to relieve the increased intraorbital pressure and possible evacuation/drainage of the hematoma.
  - Injury to the medial orbital wall, which can occur while removing middle turbinate. A resultant contusion may occur to the medial rectus muscle with fat herniation into the sinus. Intraorbital emphysema may be seen in this setting as well.
  - Trauma to cribriform plate (Fig. 12.17) and damage from overvigorous removal of the superior attachment of the middle turbinate at the fovea ethmoidalis. This

complication may lead to CSF leak, pneumocephalus, postoperative meningitis, and/or epidural abscess.

## LESS COMMON INFLAMMATORY CONDITIONS OF THE PARANASAL SINUSES

- Granulomatous diseases such as sarcoidosis and granulomatosis with polyangiitis can have sinonasal involvement, which can result in nasal septal perforation (Fig. 12.18), although there is a differential diagnosis for septal perforations (Box 12.2). Granulomatous disease processes and nonHodgkin T-cell lymphoma may present with nasal septal perforations, bony/skull-base erosions, and soft-tissue masses in the sinonasal cavity.
- NonHodgkin T-cell lymphoma may present as a soft-tissue mass with osseous erosion involving the medial wall of the maxillary antrum or the hard palate.
- Foreign body granuloma, polyarteritis nodosa, lupus, and hypersensitivity angiitis may also present with destructive sinonasal masses.
- Pseudotumors can also be seen, which may result from inflammatory diseases that can simulate an aggressive sinus process. More recently, these pseudotumors have been classified under IgG4-related disease.

### Complications of Sinusitis

- There are several infectious complications of sinusitis that are important to know. These entities can result in significant morbidity and even mortality for patients. These complications include:
  - The development of meningitis, thrombophlebitis, extra-axial empyemas, and intracranial abscess from perineural and perivascular spread of infection (Fig. 12.19).

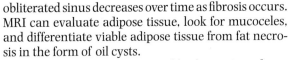

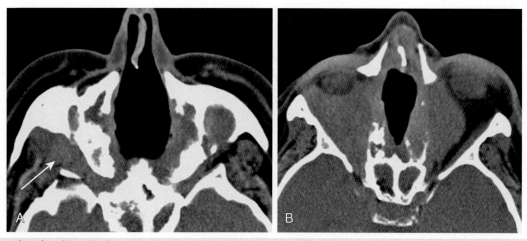

**Fig. 12.18 Septal perforations.** (A) This patient had granulomatosis with polyangiitis. The nasal septum is gone, and the patient had infiltration of the orbits and the soft tissue around the *right* maxillary antra *(arrow)*. (B) Similar findings with septal and lateral nasal wall destruction, as well as orbital soft-tissue extension are seen in this case of sarcoidosis.

### Box 12.2   Causes of Nasal Septal Perforation

Cocaine
Iatrogenic
Foreign body reaction
Sarcoidosis
Granulomatosis with polyangiitis
Lymphoma
Tuberculosis
Syphilis
Rhinoscleroma
Leprosy

- Skull-base osteomyelitis from spread of infection into the adjacent marrow and soft tissues. An entity known as "Potts puffy tumor" (not a tumor!) describes a sinus infection with osteomyelitis of the frontal sinus bone with extraosseous extension/abscess formation into the overlying scalp. There may be concomitant intracranial extension of infection as well, with meningitis, extra-axial abscess, and cerebritis.
- Orbital infections/abscess formation can occur without dehiscence of bone and occurs along vascular channels (Fig. 12.20). This pattern of infection is most commonly seen among children, in which ethmoid sinus infection extends into the adjacent orbit with formation of a subperiosteal abscess along the medial orbital wall. There can be mass effect on the orbital structures by the abscess, proptosis, vision-threatening stretching of the optic nerve, and ophthalmic vein thrombosis—yikes!
- Cavernous sinus thrombophlebitis can be associated with sphenoid sinus inflammation.

### Fungal Sinusitis

- **Fungal mycetoma**, or "fungal ball" in a noninvasive fungal infection; typically affects a solitary sinus, most commonly the maxillary and sphenoid sinuses (Fig. 12.21A).
  - The diagnosis can be made when there is calcification in association with sinus opacification on CT. When

large enough, there can be sinus outlet obstruction leading to changes of chronic sinus inflammation including osteitis (thickening and sclerosis) of the involved sinus walls.
  - On MRI, there is low T1 and T2 signal within the affected sinuses. Mucosal enhancement on postcontrast T1WI is expected.
- **Allergic fungal sinusitis**, A nonvirulent form of the disease often seen in patients with history of asthma/atopy. It is important to note that this entity occurs in immunocompetent hosts. Treatment with steroid therapy and local excision is more effective than antifungal treatment; therefore, recognizing the imaging features of allergic fungal sinus disease is critical in the management of these patients.
  - Imaging appearance typically includes increased attenuation within multiple paranasal sinuses on CT. There is often complete opacification with expansion, erosion, or remodeling and thinning of the sinuses and/or expansion of the ostia as signature features (Fig. 12.22). Findings can be unilateral or bilateral. On MRI, the signal intensity in the sinuses is usually low on T2WI and often bright on T1WI.
- **Acute invasive fungal sinusitis** (see Fig. 12.21B–C), Describes a fulminant disease with high morbidity and mortality most commonly caused by Mucor or Aspergillus. Patients are typically immunocompromised and present acutely with high fevers, facial pain, epistaxis, oculomotor palsy, and loss of sensation in the malar regions. Treatment includes wide local excision with IV antifungal drugs. Additional treatment may include orbital exenteration, hyperbaric oxygen treatment, and radical surgical therapy.
  - The spread of infection from the sinuses to the intracranial compartment may cause vascular insults such as cavernous sinus thrombosis, thrombophlebitis, arteritis, and arterial or venous cerebral infarcts. The prompt detection of this complication can lead to life- or vision-saving therapy.
  - Imaging appearance is notable for mucosal thickening on CT usually at the nasal cavity, with osseous

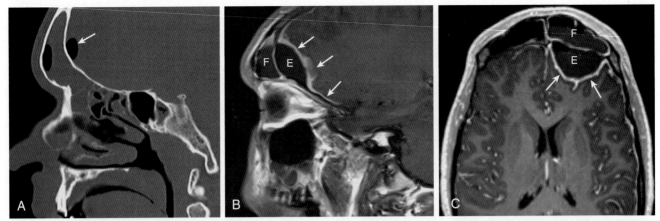

**Fig. 12.19 Epidural abscess associated with sinusitis.** (A) Sagittal computed tomography (CT) shows opacification within the frontal sinus with air-fluid level indicating acute sinusitis. Thickening of the frontal sinus walls indicates element of chronic inflammation. This could be run-of-the-mill acute on chronic frontal sinusitis except for the air bubble intracranially *(arrow)* indicating intracranial extension of infection. (B) Sagittal and (C) axial postcontrast T1-weighted images (T1W1) show the frontal sinus opacification *(F)*, as well as an organized peripherally enhancing fluid collection within the subjacent epidural space *(E)*. Note thickened, enhancing dura *(arrows)*.

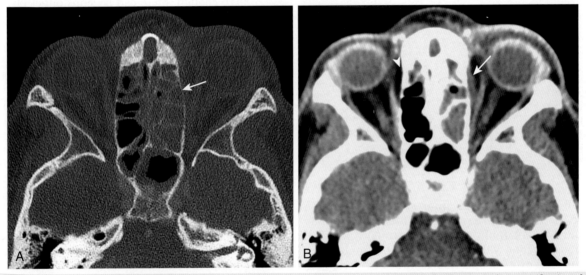

**Fig. 12.20 Orbital inflammation from sinusitis.** (A) Axial bone targeted computed tomographic image shows near complete opacification of the left ethmoid air cells with preservation of the integrity of the lamina papyracea *(arrow)* in this 12-year-old patient. (B) Axial postcontrast image in soft-tissue windows at the same level shows developing subperiosteal phlegmon in the medial left orbit *(arrow)*. Compare this with the normal orbital fat on the other side *(arrowhead)*.

destruction, nasal septal ulceration, and fat stranding involving the antral fat pads, orbital fat pads, and surrounding the nasolacrimal duct. MRI is often used to get a better understanding of the extent of the fungal infection. On MRI, there is typically hypointense signal on T1WI and T2WI within the paranasal sinuses, with absence of mucosal enhancement an important feature because of mucosal necrosis. Lack of enhancement of one or more nasal turbinates in this setting is described as the "black turbinate sign."

- Marrow signal changes and invasion into adjacent compartments including facial soft tissues, orbits, and central skull base.
- **Chronic invasive fungal sinusitis**, on the other hand, is a more indolent infection (on the order of months)

seen among immunocompetent people with or without a history of chronic sinusitis.

- As with its acute counterpart, both intrasinus and extrasinus soft-tissue inflammation can be seen, along with bone destruction and erosion at sites of extrasinus extension of infection.

## Polyposis

- Polyposis is a manifestation of allergic sinusitis but can occur in the absence of allergies. It occurs in 1.3% of the general population and up to 16.2% of patients with chronic sinusitis. In polyposis, there is nonneoplastic hyperplasia of inflamed mucous membranes within the nasal cavity and paranasal sinuses because of obstruction of small seromucinous glands. Polyposis is associated with aspirin intolerance, nickel exposure (4%),

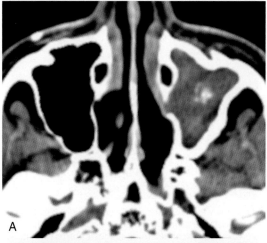

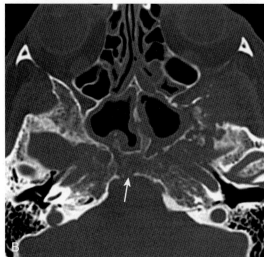

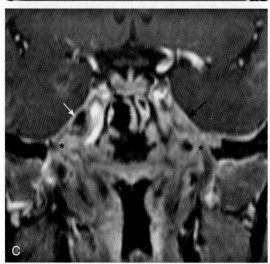

**Fig. 12.21 Fungal sinus disease.** (A) Central calcification in this opacified left maxillary sinus raised possibility of mycetoma, which was confirmed at surgery. Note thickened, maxillary sinus walls indicating osteitis from chronic inflammation. (B) This is not a run-of-the-mill sphenoid sinus mucosal thickening. On closer inspection, there are destructive changes involving sphenoid sinus walls and septum. Destruction and permeative lytic change of the central skull base, sphenoid wings, clivus *(arrow)*, and petrous apices are also present in this patient with invasive fungal sinusitis. (C) Coronal postcontrast T1-weighted imaging (T1WI) in the same patient as (B) shows abnormal enhancement at foramen ovale bilaterally *(asterisks)* resulting from soft-tissue invasion by aspergillosis. Note extension of infection into the left Meckel cave *(black arrow)* compared with the not-yet-violated right Meckel cave *(white arrow)*.

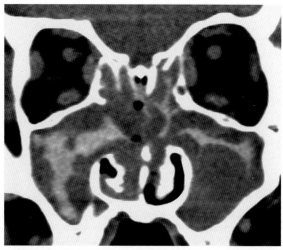

**Fig. 12.22 Allergic fungal sinusitis.** On this unenhanced coronal computed tomographic image, note the expanded paranasal sinuses that are nearly completely opacified with mixed but predominantly hyperattenuating material; a typical appearance for allergic fungal sinusitis.

cystic fibrosis (10%–20%), asthma (30%), allergic rhinitis (25%), and Kartagener syndrome. Steroids can be used for treatment and may decrease the size of polyps and keep the inflammatory process at bay.

- On CT, typically there is enlargement of sinus ostia with rounded masses in nasal cavity, with expanded sinuses or involved portions of the nasal cavity. Sinus contents are usually fluid dense but sometimes can be heterogeneous, reflecting proteinaceous debris or fungal infection (Fig. 12.23). There may be thinning of bony trabeculae and, less commonly, erosive bone changes at anterior aspect of the skull base. Involvement is usually bilateral with nasal cavity involvement in greater than 80% of cases. As with allergic fungal sinusitis, a peripheral rim of hypointense mucosa suggests a nonaggressive chronic polypoid sinusitis.
- On MR, mucosal disease is often bright on T2WI with variable degrees peripheral enhancement related to regions of hypertrophied mucosa. Contrast this with the various etiologies for T2 dark signal on MRI (Box 12.3).
- The **antrochoanal polyp** is a unique inflammatory polyp in that it is usually a solitary lesion felt to arise from prior infection, most commonly seen in the maxillary sinus, but can be seen in any of the paranasal sinuses.
  - Classically, on CT, the polyp presents as an expansile fluid-density mass protruding through an expanded maxillary sinus ostium into the posterior nasal cavity and can bulge into the nasopharynx (Fig. 12.24). Bony remodeling (thinning) can be seen, but destruction should not be present in these cases.

## Cystic Fibrosis

- Cystic fibrosis is an autosomal recessive disease resultant in inhibited mucociliary clearance resulting in thick mucosal secretions. The sinonasal development is often slowed by chronic infections. Paranasal sinus mucosa is often polypoid in appearance with hyperdense sinus contents, and mucocele formation is not infrequent. The

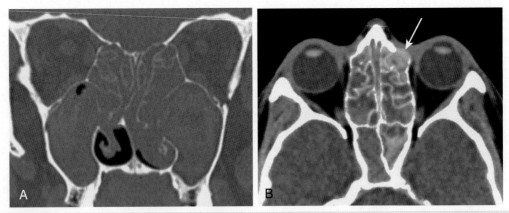

**Fig. 12.23 Sinonasal polyposis.** (A) The coronal computed tomographic image filmed in bone windows belies the extensive high-density secretions seen best in soft-tissue settings. (B) Note the expansion of the sinus walls with a focal area of dehiscence *(arrow)* where the polyp has skeletonized the bone. This type of hyperdensity may characterize fungal infection or inspissated secretions, but the expanded bone suggests polyps (with or without fungus).

---

### Box 12.3    Etiologies for T2 dark signal on MRI

Teeth
Inspissated secretions
Fungus balls
Osteomas
Sinoliths
Hemorrhage
Odontogenic lesions
Chondroid lesions
Amyloidomas
Fibrosis

---

triad of sphenoid and frontal sinus hypoplasia, medial bulging of the lateral nasal wall (indicative of maxillary sinus polyposis), and ethmoid opacification in a child is highly suggestive of cystic fibrosis.

### Meningoencephaloceles and Cerebrospinal Fluid Leaks

- These entities may occur from congenital defects, trauma, or after skull-base surgery (see Figs. 12.9 and 12.17). Rhinorrhea may be present and can result from a dural tear or presence of a postethmoidectomy encephalocele. Repair is necessary to prevent development of meningitis and ensuing complications of intracranial infection. Intracranial hypotension from chronic CSF leakage may be a complication of this process and leads to brain sagging, subdural collections, and meningeal enhancement.
- On CT, a bony defect can be demonstrated in the area of suspected leak. Intrathecal myelographic contrast injection can be used to help localize the site of leak (Fig. 12.25), with presence of contrast in the sinonasal compartment at the site of leak.
- On MR, it is important to evaluate for extension of brain herniation through the osseous defect. This is typically done using heavily T2-weighted thin section MR sequence termed *MR cisternography* (often CISS or FIESTA sequences), which can help identify site of CSF

leaks as well as presence of brain/meningeal tissue extending through the defect (meningoencephalocele) (Fig. 12.26).

### BENIGN NEOPLASMS

- **Inverted papillomas** are benign sinonasal lesions and account for 4% of all tumors of the nasal cavity. Inverted papillomas are associated with squamous cell carcinoma (SCC) in approximately 15% of cases. These lesions can demonstrate aggressive bone destruction pattern and may cross the cribriform plate into the anterior cranial fossa. They typically arise from the lateral nasal wall, nasal septum, or medial maxillary sinus. Treatment is resection with recurrent rates reported at 22% to 40%.
  - Imaging appearance on CT is not terribly specific but can show an expansile enhancing soft-tissue mass in the nasal cavity, which can often but not always contain stippled calcification. If you see focal hyperostosis in the lesion, this can indicate the point of origin and can have implications for surgical approach. Bone destruction suggests malignant transformation to SCC.
  - On MR, these lesions classically show a convoluted "cerebriform" appearance on T2WI and postcontrast sequences, a feature that is unique to this entity (Fig. 12.27). Areas of low signal on T2WI are characteristic. As opposed to inflammatory polypoid masses (which show mucosal enhancement peripherally), inverted papillomas enhance solidly. Unfortunately, so do the coexistent cancers. The presence of necrosis may be an indicator of coexistent SCC.
- **Fibrous dysplasia** is one of the most common bone lesions affecting the paranasal sinuses. There is often an expansile appearance to the involved bone with classic ground-glass attenuation on CT (Fig. 12.28). On MR, the appearance can be a little less straightforward, with variable signal intensity and enhancement (although most commonly dark on all pulse sequences). Rarely, large vascular flow channels can be seen. Bony expansion by these lesions can lead to obstruction of the sinus drainage pathways and cause sinusitis and even mucoceles. Orbital and intracranial involvement by fibrous dysplasia can cause a whole host of other problems too, due to mass effect.

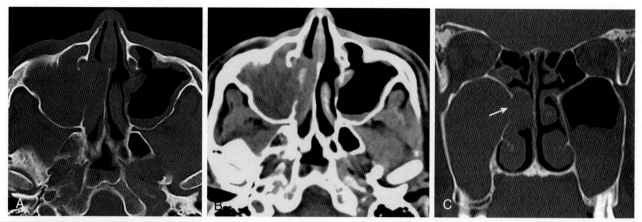

**Fig. 12.24  Antrochoanal polyp.** Axial computed tomography (CT) in bone (A) and soft-tissue (B) windows shows a fluid density expansile lesion opacifying the right maxillary sinus and extending through the ostium into the right nasal cavity. (C) Coronal CT from the same patient shows widening of the right ostium *(arrow)* by this antrochoanal polyp.

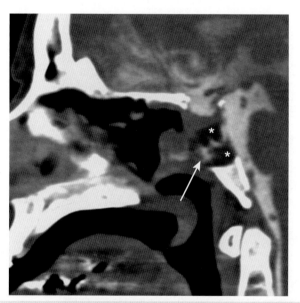

**Fig. 12.25  Cerebrospinal fluid leak.** Sagittal computed tomography (CT) image from CT cisternogram in a patient reporting continuous clear nasal drainage after transsphenoidal resection for pituitary tumor shows clear seepage of contrast *(arrow)* through the fat-packing material *(asterisks)* in the surgical bed into the posterior nasal cavity (sniffle, sniffle).

- **Osteomas** are benign bony masses within any of the paranasal sinuses but most often in the frontal and ethmoid sinuses. Although they are benign, infrequently they may be a source for recurrent headache and/or recurrent sinusitis if large enough and in a position to obstruct sinonasal drainage pathways (Fig. 12.29). These can result in mucocele formation and/or pneumocephalus as the posterior wall of the frontal sinus is breached. The classic presentation of patients with osteomas includes severe sinus pain associated with takeoffs from airplane flights. Osteomas are better evaluated with CT than MRI given their hyperdense calcified composition (simulating sinus aeration on MRI). Gardner syndrome is a syndrome with colonic polyps and osteomas.

## MALIGNANT NEOPLASMS

- When suspecting a sinonasal malignancy, making the correct histopathologic diagnosis is the job of the pathologist. Although it is reasonable to take a stab at making the diagnosis on imaging, the radiologist's role is to help identify the primary tumor focus and search for sites of invasion (e.g., skull base, orbit, brain, and vessels), look for mass effect on critical structures, and check for perineural tumor spread, and lymphadenopathy. These findings will have an important impact on treatment planning.

- Differential considerations for a sinonasal mass with cause intracranial erosion include carcinoma (usually SCC), olfactory neuroblastoma, sarcoma, lymphoma, melanoma, and metastasis. Necrosis, hemorrhage, or calcification in carcinomas, olfactory neuroblastomas, and sarcomas may cause signal heterogeneity on MRI.

- **SCC** makes up approximately 80% of all malignancies affecting the paranasal sinuses, with 80% of SCC occurring in maxillary antrum. Approximately 75% of patients are greater than 50 years of age, with males more commonly affected than females. Risk factors include exposure to human papillomavirus (HPV), occupational exposure to nickel and chrome pigment, use of Bantu snuff and cigarettes.

  - On CT, the hallmark of imaging malignancies of the sinonasal cavity is bony destruction, which is seen in approximately 80% of SCCs at initial presentation. When bone destruction is seen, pay close attention to extension of the tumor mass outside the bony confines of the involved sinus. Look for soft-tissue extension into the facial soft tissue, orbit, and destruction at the anterior skull base, which can signify intracranial tumor involvement. Check the adjacent foramina for evidence of perineural extension of tumor. For example, check the inferior orbital nerve canal at the roof of the maxillary sinus in a maxillary sinus cancer case. From there, tumor can extend into the premaxillary soft tissues of the face anteriorly and/or the pterygopalatine fossa posteriorly. Replacement of pterygopalatine fossa fat by soft tissue is a reliable CT finding of V2 nerve spread.

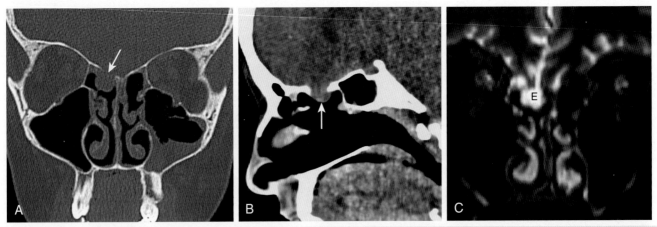

**Fig. 12.26 Postoperative meningocele.** (A) Coronal computed tomography (CT) shows a focal bony defect at the right cribriform plate *(arrow)* after functional endoscopic sinus surgery (FESS). (B) Sagittal CT in soft-tissue windows shows that the tissue herniating through the defect could be fluid or soft tissue, hard to tell *(arrow)*. (C) Heavily T2-weighted coronal magnetic resonance (MR) image demonstrates fluid signal reflecting herniation of the meninges *(E)* through the defect at the cribriform plate.

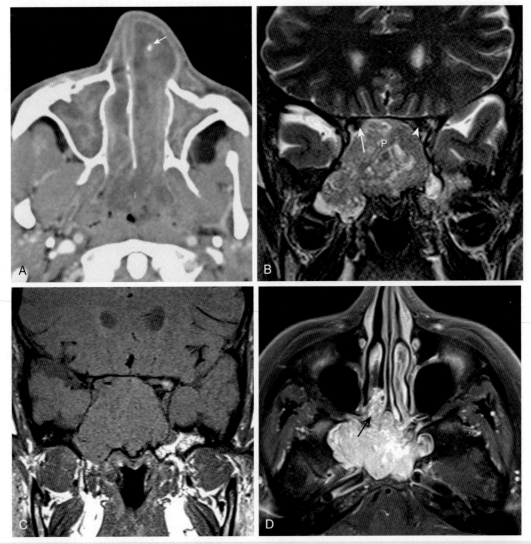

**Fig. 12.27 Inverted papilloma.** (A) On this contrast-enhanced axial computed tomography (CT) image, an expansile mildly enhancing mass occupying the nasal cavity on the *left* bulges anteriorly through the nasal vault and posteriorly to the nasopharynx. There is tiny focus of calcification *(arrow)*, which could lead you to suspect this to be an inverted papilloma. Inspissated hyperdense trapped secretions are present in the bilateral maxillary sinuses. (B) Coronal T2-weighted imaging (T2WI) in another patient shows a mass *(P)* occupying and expanding the sphenoid sinus (a somewhat unusual location for an inverted papilloma). There is a "cerebriform" pattern to the signal intensity of the lesion, which has been described with inverted papillomas. The right optic nerve is slightly compressed because of the expansile nature of this lesion *(arrow)*, compared with the normal optic nerve appearance on the *left (arrowhead)*. (C) On coronal T1-weighted imaging (T1WI), the lesion is isointense to muscle, but with contrast administration (D), the lesion enhances avidly. Note insinuation of the papilloma through the sphenoethmoidal recess (SER) into the posterior nasal cavity *(arrow)*. Based on imaging alone, we cannot readily distinguish this lesion from a sinus cancer. The diagnosis of inverted papilloma was rendered by the pathologist in this case.

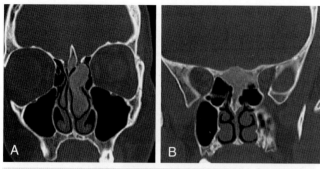

**Fig. 12.28 Polyostotic fibrous dysplasia.** (A) The left, middle turbinate and ethmoid strut is ground-glass in appearance and expansile. (B) There is also involvement of the floor of the anterior cranial fossa and nasal septum.

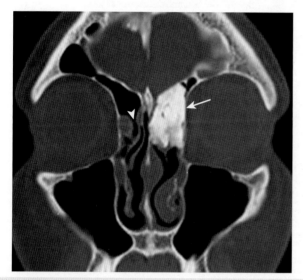

**Fig. 12.29 Osteoma.** Coronal unenhanced computed tomography (CT) shows sclerotic lesion with narrow zone of transition sitting at and occluding the left frontal recess *(arrow)*. Note the patent frontal recess on the right *(arrowhead)* for comparison. This is a characteristic look and location for sinus osteoma and, in this case, is large enough to cause recurrent frontal sinusitis as a result of its obstructive nature.

**TEACHING POINTS**

Imaging Findings of Perineural Tumor Spread on CT and MRI

Enlargement of the affected neural foramina
Eroded bony margins of the affected neural foramina
Enlarged nerves within the affected foramina
Loss of fat signal/density within the affected foramina
Denervation injury of muscles innervated by the affected
  nerve

- On MR, relatively hypointense signal is seen on T2WI, unlike mucosal inflammation that is typically T2 bright (Fig. 12.30). These tumors enhance, but to a lesser degree than that of the mucosa (Fig. 12.31). Contrast-enhanced imaging is helpful to delineate epidural or meningeal invasion of neoplasms through the anterior skull base.

- **Sinonasal undifferentiated carcinoma** (SNUC) is a very aggressive malignancy with a very poor prognosis. It is most commonly encountered in the ethmoid sinus. There is often early bone destruction with involvement of adjacent structures, including the nose, skin, orbit, and calvarium even at the time of presentation. The imaging appearance is similar to SCCs gone wild, often with areas of necrosis and heterogeneous enhancement. Dural metastases occur at a high rate with this neoplasm.

- **Minor salivary gland cancers** represent a wide variety of histologic types, including adenoid cystic carcinoma, mucoepidermoid carcinoma, and adenocarcinoma. Adenoid cystic carcinoma is the most common subtype of these tumors. Adenocarcinoma has a predilection for the ethmoid sinuses and tends to be more common in woodworkers. Adenoid cystic carcinomas have a propensity (50%–60% rate) for perineural tumor spread (Fig. 12.32).
  - Although adenocarcinoma tends to have low signal intensity on T2WI, this is not unique to sinonasal cancers and there are no specific imaging features of salivary gland tumors. Adenoid cystic carcinomas, by virtue of the different histologic varieties, are cancers that may rarely appear bright on T2WI images.

- **Melanoma** is two to three times more common in the nasal cavity compared with paranasal sinuses. It is associated with melanosis, a condition where there is diffuse deposition of melanin along mucosal surface of sinonasal cavity (Fig. 12.33). The nasal septum is the most common site of involvement, followed by the nasal turbinates. Patients may present with epistaxis. Melanoma also has a propensity for perineural tumor spread in addition to hematogenous dissemination.
  - On MR, the paramagnetic effect of the melanin causes T1 and T2 shortening, accounting for high signal intensity on T1WI and low signal intensity on T2WI. Melanin content within these lesions is variable though, and T1 high signal is not always reliably present. Amelanotic melanoma may have low intensity on T1WI and bright signal intensity on T2WI images.

- **Olfactory neuroblastoma** (a.k.a. esthesioneuroblastoma) arises from olfactory epithelium in the nasal vault from cells derived from the neural crest. There is a bimodal peak, with the first peak occurring at 11 to 20 years of age, and the second peak affecting middle-aged adults with a male predilection. Presenting symptoms include nasal obstruction, epistaxis, or anosmia. Lymphatic and hematogenous metastases can be found with rates of recurrence greater than 50%.
  - On CT, olfactory neuroblastoma often appears as a soft-tissue mass in the high nasal cavity or ethmoid vault (Fig. 12.34). Calcifications can be seen occasionally.
  - On MR, these tumors typically have low signal intensity on T2WI, and are associated with tumoral cysts (a virtually pathognomonic feature in an otherwise diverse group of differential diagnoses). There is a propensity for crossing the cribriform plate with intracranial extension in 35% to 40% of cases.

- **Sarcomas** are rare aggressive tumors of the sinonasal cavity. The chondrosarcoma is the most common sarcoma to occur here and typically occurs along the nasal septum (in the cartilaginous portion).

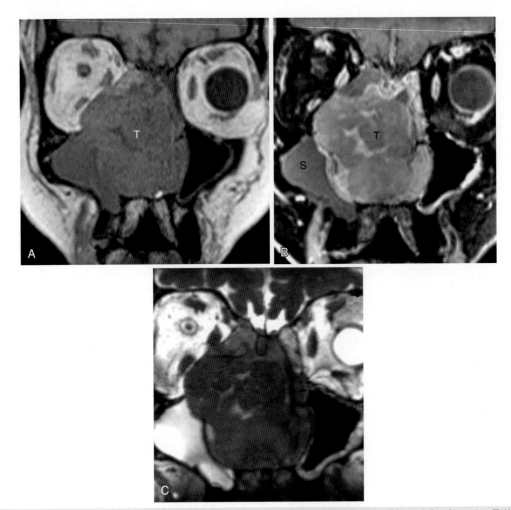

**Fig. 12.30 Differentiation of tumor versus inflammation on magnetic resonance imaging.** (A) Coronal T1-weighted imaging (T1WI) shows a bulky enhancing mass *(T)* within the nasal cavity. The mass is invading the right inferomedial orbit. It is unclear whether the maxillary sinus next door is full of tumor or secretions blocked within the sinus because of obstruction at the ostiomeatal complex. (B) Coronal enhanced fat-suppressed T1WI demonstrates solid enhancement within this neoplasm *(T)*. Note that much of the material within the right maxillary sinus does not enhance, indicating backed-up secretions *(S)*. Thus, with contrast, the border of the tumor is well delineated. (C) In this case, there is also marked signal difference between the tumor and the secretions in the maxillary sinus on coronal T2-weighted imaging (T2WI).

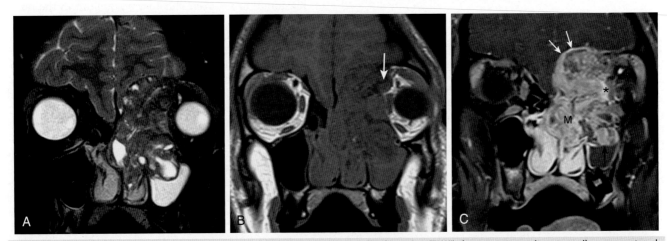

**Fig. 12.31 Poorly differentiated squamous cell carcinoma.** (A) Coronal T2-weighted imaging (T2WI) shows an aggressive, expansile mass centered within the left nasal cavity and maxillary ostium with extension laterally into the orbit and superiorly into the cranial vault. (B) On coronal T1-weighted imaging (T1WI) the mass is isointense to muscle. Infiltration of the orbital fat on the *left* can be seen, with invasion of the superior oblique muscle *(arrow)*, effacement of medial orbital fat, and displacement of other orbital structures laterally. Note the violation of the cribriform plate on the *left*. (C) The mass *(M)* enhances heterogeneously with contrast on this coronal T1WI. Note the thick and slightly nodular dural-based enhancement at the anterior skull base *(white arrows)*, indicating dural invasion. Orbital invasion is again demonstrated *(asterisk)*. The margin of enhancing tumor within the maxillary sinus *(black arrow)* can be distinguished from backed-up fluid within the sinus, which does not enhance.

- On CT, whorl-pattern of calcification (rings and arcs) can be seen in chondrosarcoma.
- On MR, chondrosarcomas tend to demonstrate high signal intensity on T2WI.
- **Lymphoma** can occur in the paranasal sinuses and nasal cavity. Nasal lymphoma often presents with nasal obstruction (80%), nasal discharge (64%), epistaxis (60%), and nasal septal perforations. Most nonHodgkin lymphomas in this location are of T-cell lineage (75%). Advanced age and bulky disease are associated with reduced survival.
  - On CT, these tumors can present as well-defined isolated masses or infiltrating soft tissue. There is soft-tissue obliteration of the involved nasal passages and sinuses (usually the maxillary sinus), with erosion of the bony sinus margins and/or invasion of the adjacent spaces including orbits and nasopharynx. Necrosis and erosion of the nasal septum is common with T-/natural killer (NK) cell lymphomas.
  - Lymphoma appears on MRI as a T2 dark enhancing mass with diffusion restriction with low apparent diffusion coefficient (ADC) values.
  - Perineural tumor involvement is very likely in lymphoma cases, so it is imperative to analyze the skull-base foramina in the vicinity of the soft tissue mass.
  - Patients may also have cervical lymphadenopathy.
- Some rare birds in the sinonasal primary malignancy category include:
  - Neuroendocrine carcinoma (which includes both small- and large-cell carcinomas), which can coexist with squamous cell or adenocarcinomas.
  - The NUT (nuclear protein in testis) carcinoma (also known as *NUT midline carcinoma* [NUTML]), which can affect the mediastinum but also the sinonasal cavity and is more commonly seen in children and young adults. Imaging features are not specific but often shows aggressive sinonasal mass invading orbits and anterior cranial fossa, with regional and distant metastases in half of cases at the time of presentation.
  - HPV-related carcinoma with adenoid cystic-like features, which can very rarely affect the sinonasal compartment.
- **Metastatic disease** to the sinonasal cavity is extremely rare but most commonly results from renal cell carcinoma. Multiple myeloma may affect the walls of the paranasal sinuses, as can plasmacytomas, and is typically associated with lytic lesions with associated soft-tissue components (Fig. 12.35).
  - **Nasopharyngeal carcinoma** (NPC) has a high rate of sinonasal involvement via extrapharyngeal spread. NPC that has spread to the maxillary sinus and orbit portends the worst prognosis.

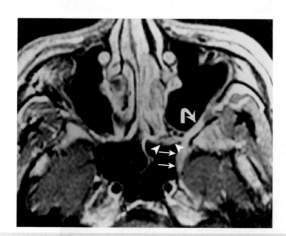

**Fig. 12.32  A tricky case.** In a patient with adenoid cystic carcinoma, follow-up exam including axial-enhanced T1-weighted image (T1WI) demonstrates enhancing tumor traveling along the foramen rotundum on the *left* side *(arrows)* and extending through the pterygopalatine fossa *(arrowheads)* and pterygomaxillary fissure *(curved arrow)*. This is perineural spread of adenoid cystic carcinoma.

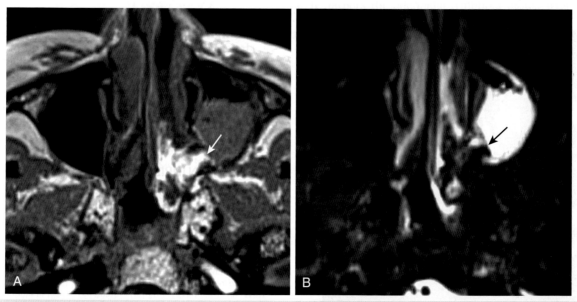

**Fig. 12.33  Sinonasal melanoma.** (A) Bright on T1-weighted imaging (T1WI) and (B) dark on T2-weighted imaging (T2WI), this nasal cavity melanoma *(arrow)* was very well localized. Sinonasal melanomas span the gamut from tiny discolored mucosal lesions identified incidentally for epistaxis to much larger and more aggressive invasive masses. Remember that they need not be bright on T1WI, which is merely a reflection of the quantity of melanin.

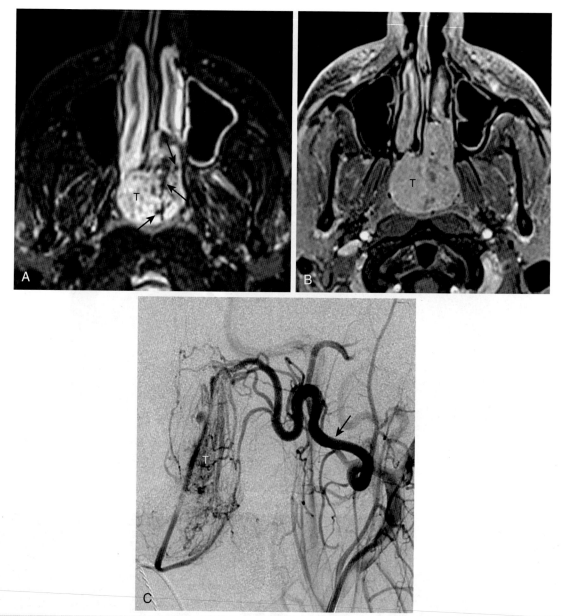

**Fig. 13.20 Juvenile angiofibroma.** (A) Axial T2-weighted imaging (T2WI) in a young male presenting with epistaxis shows a large mass in the nasopharynx extending into the posterior aspect of the left nasal cavity *(T)*. The mass shows numerous serpentine flow voids *(arrows)*. (B) On this postcontrast T1-weighted imaging (T1WI), the mass *(T)* is shown to enhance avidly. (C) Conventional catheter angiogram shows marked enlargement of the maxillary artery *(arrow)*, which provides the major arterial supply to the tumor *(T)*. Preoperative embolization can reduce the morbidity of a surgical excision.

## BENIGN NEOPLASMS OF THE AERODIGESTIVE TRACT

### Juvenile Nasopharyngeal Angiofibroma

- The classic benign nasopharyngeal tumor is the juvenile nasopharyngeal angiofibroma (JNA). It is characterized by its high vascularity and its propensity for bleeding. The typical patient is a male adolescent who has recurrent epistaxis.
- It can extensively involve the sphenopalatine foramen, the pterygopalatine fossa itself, and/or the nasal cavity. Look for enlarged foramina on CT and MRI.
- It may have aggressive growth via the pterygopalatine fossa and its numerous connections to the infratemporal fossa, skull base and orbit. Sixty percent recur after resection.
- On MRI, the salient feature of the angiofibroma is the abundance of flow voids from its high vascularity. This enhancing tumor has a characteristic "salt (tissue) and pepper

(flow voids)" appearance, which is also described with paragangliomas (Fig. 13.20). The salt and pepper may be "served" both on T2WI and contrast-enhanced T1WI.
- On angiography, these tumors are highly vascular and are usually supplied by branches of the ascending pharyngeal artery and the internal maxillary artery. Embolization of the tumor may be useful preoperatively to reduce blood loss.

### Neurogenic Tumors

- As the larynx and pharynx are surrounded by neural networks, schwannomas of the hypoglossal, vagal, or laryngeal nerve can be seen throughout. Although the majority are asymptomatic and seen as incidental, well-defined submucosal masses, there may be consequential atrophy of the muscles they innervate with fatty replacement.

- The aryepiglottic fold and arytenoid region are most commonly involved, presumably because of superior laryngeal nerve course.

### Other Rare Birds

- Other rare benign tumors of the aerodigestive mucosa include tumors of mesenchymal origin (e.g., lipoma, granular cell tumor, leiomyoma, rhabdomyoma). Most extracardiac rhabdomyomas arise from pharyngeal constrictor muscles, the floor of the mouth, and the tongue base. Paragangliomas of neuroendocrine origin may occur in the larynx. The most common benign minor salivary gland tumor of the aerodigestive system is the pleomorphic adenoma.

## MALIGNANT NEOPLASMS/TNM STAGING: SQUAMOUS CELL CARCINOMA

- Head and neck cancer constitutes 3% of all malignancies, and there are approximately 60,000 new cases each year in the United States. Tobacco and alcohol consumption, betel nut chewing, diet, ultraviolet light exposure, and viral infections (human papillomavirus [HPV] and EBV) are risk factors for squamous cell cancer development along the aerodigestive tract regardless of the subsites. For oropharyngeal tumors in particular, the HPV-16 risk factor has become the most common one, outstripping smoking and alcohol consumption.
- The prognosis for oral cavity and oropharyngeal carcinoma for all-comers is about 50% for 5-year survival. Markers for a worse prognosis include expression of mutated tumor suppressor gene *p53*, enhancement of oncogene *cyclin D1*, and high levels of vascular endothelial growth factor. The latter works to increase radioresistance and increase hematogenous metastases and leads to lower survival and disease-free rates. Those with HPV-16 genotype have a far better prognosis and treatment response.
- The TNM staging is crucial for prognosis stratification, treatment planning, and coordinating clinical trials for novel drug development at different treatment centers for the same disease type. T refers to primary Tumor extent, N to regional lymph Nodes, and M to distant Metastases. On the basis of the TNM stage of a tumor, a final disease staging is assigned, and treatment regimens are planned.
- The American Joint Commission on Cancer (AJCC) provides periodic updates on TNM staging. The most recent update became effective January 1, 2018, in the eighth edition of the AJCC Cancer Staging manual.
  - It reflects major changes in T and N staging necessitated by the more accurate and probabilistic individualized outcome prediction models—incorporating additional anatomic and nonanatomic prognostic factors beyond the TNM system, shift in causality from smoking to virus-driven cancer especially in the oropharynx, better locoregional control with radiotherapy leading to dose de-escalation, and from a one-chemotherapy fits all approach to personalized immunotherapy and vaccine developments.
- Currently, AJCC TNM staging depends solely on anatomic cross-sectional imaging, clinical evaluation, and pathologic analysis. The value of metabolic imaging with FDG-PET is well established but has not made its way into the manual yet.
- The eighth edition of AJCC adopted two new pathologic terms: "depth of invasion" in oral cavity T staging and "extranodal extent" in nodal staging of all aerodigestive tract epithelial cancers for prognostic stratification of survival and treatment modulation.
- It also exclusively dedicated T0 disease for virus mediated (hr-HPV or EBV) pharynx cancers presenting with nodal masses but no identifiable primary mass by clinical, endoscopic, or diagnostic imaging modalities.
  - T0: No primary identified
- Tx and Tis are reserved for nonvirus mediated cancers of the pharynx and larynx.
  - Tx: Primary tumor cannot be assessed
  - Tis: Carcinoma in situ
- Carcinoma of unknown origin: These are the cervical nodal squamous cell carcinoma (SCC) metastases in which a primary cannot be found on CT, MRI, FDG PET, or endoscopy. The AJCC recommendation is first to document whether the SCC metastasis is associated with HPV or EBV and stage and treat the patient accordingly:
  - HPV-mediated nodal metastasis: Treat as oropharyngeal primary
  - EBV-mediated nodal metastasis: Treat as nasopharygeal primary

### Nasopharyngeal Carcinoma

- A bimodal distribution appears in the incidence of nasopharyngeal carcinoma.
  - A younger age group (15–25 years old) is seen with nonkeratinizing nasopharyngeal carcinoma in Southeast Asia, where it accounts for 18% of all cancers. Chinese Americans have a sevenfold increased risk of nasopharyngeal carcinoma over non-Chinese counterparts.
  - Westerners who get nasopharyngeal carcinoma are usually older adults (40–60 years old) developing keratinizing carcinomas.
- The AJCC staging guide considers spread of cancer from mucosa to deeper soft tissues such as prevertebral muscles and ultimately intracranial compartment via the skull base. T staging does not include any size measurements but does include local extent evaluation. Although perineural spread exposes a high and direct risk for intracranial extent, it is not a prognostic risk factor identified in the AJCC.
- Epithelial malignancies make up 80% of nasopharyngeal cancer (NPC), followed by lymphoma, minor salivary gland tumors, and rhabdomyosarcoma. The World Health Organization (WHO) recognizes three histologic types of NPC (Table 13.1):
  - Nonkeratinizing (undifferentiated) carcinoma is the most common histologic type of NPC and shows consistent association with EBV (>95%).
  - Keratinizing SCC is associated with EBV in endemic areas but is less commonly EBV positive in nonendemic areas (75%). Compared with nonkeratinizing carcinoma, it is more commonly advanced (76% keratinizing vs. 55% nonkeratinizing), with less common lymph node metastasis (29% keratinizing vs. 70% nonkeratinizing).
  - Basaloid SCC is the rarest form.

**Table 13.1**    Nasopharyngeal Carcinoma and Lymphoma Subtypes

| Feature | Major Risk Factors | Radiation Sensitivity | Frequency | AIDS Association | Survival |
|---|---|---|---|---|---|
| Keratinizing squamous cell carcinoma | Smoking, alcohol, radiation induced, Caucasian | — | 2nd | Yes | Fair |
| Nonkeratinizing squamous cell carcinoma (differentiated and undifferentiated) | Highest Epstein-Barr virus (EBV) risk, Southeast Asian, nitrosamines in salted food, burning incense sticks | Highest | 1st | Yes | Very good |
| Basaloid squamous cell carcinoma | EBV, human papillomavirus (HPV) | — | 3rd | No | Poor |
| Lymphoma<br>– Non-Hodgkin lymphoma (NHL)<br>– B cell<br>– T/NK cell | HIV | — | Rare | Yes | Very good |

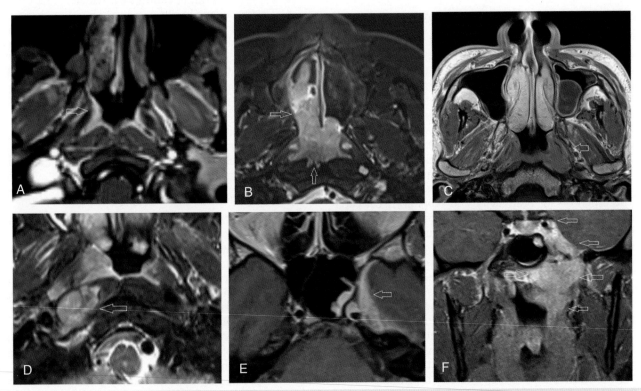

**Fig. 13.21  The many faces of nasopharyngeal cancer (NPC).** (A) Asymmetric mucosal thickening and enhancement of the right demonstrates subtle mucosal-based tumor *(arrow)* on postcontrast T1-weighted imaging (T1WI). (B) Axial short inversion time inversion recovery Short Tau Inversion Recovery (STIR) image in a different patient shows mass arising from nasopharynx extending into the posterior nasal cavity (right more so than left, *horizontal arrow)* and infiltrating the longus coli muscle at its posterior extent *(vertical arrow).* (C) Axial postcontrast T1-weighted imaging (T1WI) shows nasopharyngeal mass effacing the left fossa of Rosenmüller and infiltrating the left parapharyngeal space *(arrow).* (D) Axial STIR image shows right nasopharyngeal mass in conjunction with separate metastatic lateral retropharyngeal node *(arrow)* invading the adjacent longus coli muscle. (E) Axial postcontrast image shows thickening and enhancement of the left V2 in foramen rotundum indicating perineural tumor spread in a patient with NPC *(arrow).* (F) On this postcontrast coronal T1WI, arrows indicate the margins of infiltrative NPC. On the lateral aspect of the tumor from *bottom to top,* arrows indicate the primary tumor, invasion of the masticator space and trigeminal fat pad, enlarged V3, and paracavernous invasion, respectively. Note destruction of the central skull base on the *left.*

■ Endoscopic evaluation of NPC can underestimate extent of disease, and the invasive nature of the primary lesion is best evaluated by cross-sectional imaging techniques (Fig. 13.21). In this case, fat is your friend; loss of fat attenuation or signal on CT and MRI, respectively, between tensor and levator veli palatini muscles or in the parapharyngeal tissue suggests malignancy. Whenever new otitis media or mastoid effusion occurs in an adult, think nasopharyngeal carcinoma and be sure that you scrutinize this area.

■ For T staging, the following structures need to be addressed individually in CT or MRI report:
  ■ Parapharyngeal space
  ■ Skull base
  ■ Retropharyngeal (RP) space
  ■ Carotid space
  ■ Prevertebral, masticator space, nasal cavity, and sphenoid and ethmoid sinus
  ■ Perineural spread through the various skull base foramina to the intracranial space

NPC has no specific features that would differentiate it from lymphoma or minor salivary gland tumors.

- On CT, there is similar density of tumor to that of muscle limiting recognition of early cancer in the setting of minimal symptoms. Look for Rosenmüller fossa and parapharyngeal fat effacement. If in doubt, recommend MRI with contrast.
  - Check the skull base neural foramina size and symmetry. By the time the skull base foramina have enlarged, the tumor spread is likely far advanced.
- On MRI, a STIR hyperintense and enhancing lesion on postcontrast T1 with fat saturation results in loss of nasopharyngeal soft tissue and surrounding fat distinction. Precontrast T1, which may be hiding the primary mass, will show the effacement of parapharyngeal fat very well.
- Keep in mind that normal nasopharyngeal mucosa, the adenoidal tissue, and tumor enhance. Fat saturation on postcontrast T1 MRI is necessary to better evaluate the invasion of skull base foramina and perineural spread.
  - The involvement of cranial nerve V from the pterygopalatine fossa up to the cavernous sinus is much better seen with fat-suppressed postcontrast T1WI scans. If intracranial extension is seen, orbits, cavernous sinuses, and prepontine cisterns must be scrutinized.
  - Skull base involvement through the sinus of Morgagni along the eustachian tube or to the foramen lacerum is also well demonstrated on unenhanced T1WI.
- Treatment of nasopharyngeal carcinoma is primarily nonsurgical, deploying single modality treatment with intensity modulated radiotherapy (IMRT) in early-stage disease and combined IMRT + chemotherapy in locally advanced or metastatic disease. IMRT can deliver doses up to 70 to 80 grays while sparing the vital intracranial and spinal structures. These techniques, with chemotherapy, have rendered nasopharyngeal carcinoma an eminently curable disease at a local level; unfortunately for the patient, the tumor has a relatively high propensity for hematogenous spread. The 5-year survival rates are as follows:
  - Stage I disease is 72% (only 9% of people with NPC are diagnosed at this stage)
  - Stage II disease is 64%, and Stage III disease is 62% (the majority of NPC is diagnosed at these stages)
  - Stage IV NPC is 38%
- T imaging: It is the only pharynx subsite where *size does not matter*, and local extent makes the pillars of the T staging (Table 13.2).
  - Is parapharyngeal fat infiltrated? (T2)
  - Are medial pterygoid, lateral pterygoid, prevertebral muscles infiltrated? (T2)
  - The prevertebral muscle involvement was considered T4 in the seventh edition of AJCC but because of intensity-modulated radiotherapy providing better local control and improve overall survival, these cases were downstaged to T2.
  - Is the bony skull base or paranasal sinuses involved? (T3)
  - Is the mass beyond the lateral margin of lateral pterygoid muscle? (T4)
  - Any intracranial extent is considered T4.
- N imaging (Table 13.3):
  - First echelon nodal spread from nasopharyngeal carcinoma is to RP and high jugular (level II) lymph

**Table 13.2** Nasopharyngeal Carcinoma T staging (AJCC 8th ed.)

| T Category | T Criteria |
| --- | --- |
| TX | Primary tumor cannot be assessed |
| T0 | No tumor identified, but Epstein-Barr virus (EBV)-positive cervical node(s) involvement |
| Tis | Tumor in *situ* |
| T1 | Tumor confined to nasopharynx or extension to oropharynx and/or nasal cavity without parapharyngeal involvement |
| T2 | Tumor with extension to parapharyngeal space and/or adjacent soft-tissue involvement (medial pterygoid, lateral pterygoid, prevertebral muscles) |
| T3 | Tumor with infiltration of bony structures at skull base, cervical vertebra, pterygoid structures, and/or paranasal sinuses |
| T4 | Tumor with intracranial extension, involvement of cranial nerves, hypopharynx, orbit, parotid gland, and/or extensive soft-tissue infiltration beyond the lateral surface of the lateral pterygoid muscle |

*AJCC*, American Joint Commission on Cancer.

(From Amin MB, Greene FL, Edge SB, et al., eds. AJCC Cancer Staging Manual. Springer International Publishing: American Joint Commission on Cancer; 8th ed. New York; 2017.)

**Table 13.3** Nasopharyngeal Carcinoma N staging (AJCC 8th ed.)

| N Category | N Criteria |
| --- | --- |
| NX | Regional lymph nodes cannot be assessed |
| N0 | No regional lymph node metastasis |
| N1 | Unilateral metastasis in cervical lymph node(s) and/or unilateral or bilateral metastasis in retropharyngeal lymph node(s), 6 cm or smaller in greatest dimension, above the caudal border of cricoid cartilage |
| N2 | Bilateral metastasis in cervical lymph node(s), 6 cm or smaller in greatest dimension, above the caudal border of cricoid cartilage |
| N3 | Unilateral or bilateral metastasis in cervical lymph node(s), larger than 6 cm in greatest dimension, and/or extension below the caudal border of cricoid cartilage |

*AJCC*, American Joint Commission on Cancer.

(From Amin MB, Greene FL, Edge SB, et al., eds. AJCC Cancer Staging Manual. Springer International Publishing: American Joint Commission on Cancer; 8th ed. New York; 2017.)

nodes. Nodal spread is so common (80%) that even if not shown by imaging, upper cervical nodes are automatically treated with IMRT.
  - No matter how small the NPC, large volume bilateral nodal disease could be present; that is probably why the T staging of NPC is not based on size criteria, unlike the oral cavity and other pharyngeal cancers.

## Oropharyngeal Squamous Cell Carcinoma

- The eighth edition of AJCC has major changes in oropharyngeal SCC (OPC) T staging because of favorable prognosis in high risk-HPV (hr-HPV)-associated cancer of the oropharynx. hr-HPV will be used to indicate HPV-16 and -18 strains through this chapter. The 5-year overall survival is 82% for patients with hr-HPV-associated OPC and 35% for those with non-HPV-associated disease.

- In hr-HPV-associated OPC, in setting of absence of smoking history and a low nodal status (N0, N1), locoregional control rate can go up to 95% for early-stage and 78% for late-stage HPV-associated OPC at 3 years.
- For non-HPC-associated OPC, the locoregional control rate is only 76% for early-stage disease and 62% for late-stage disease.
- Given survival differences, the AJCC stages hr-HPV-associated OPC separate from non-HPC-associated oropharyngeal cancer. The latter is staged within the general category of non-HPV-associated pharynx cancers along with hypopharynx (Tables 13.4 and 13.5).
- HPV DNA detection is expensive and not widely available in every practice; therefore, p16 immunohistochemistry (IHC) has been introduced as a surrogate marker for HPV infection. Currently, p16 IHC has been endorsed for accurate T staging for any oropharynx cancer. P16 detection is especially important in those with an endophytic component in the base of tongue to accurately identify the origin (oropharynx vs. posterior oral cavity).
- The most common locations for OPC are the palatine tonsils (Fig. 13.22) and the base of the tongue. Luckily, posterior oropharyngeal wall cancers, which have direct access to prevertebral space, are exceedingly uncommon.
- Tonsillar carcinomas have a propensity for invasion into the tongue musculature beyond the circumvallate papillae, thereby spreading across the anatomic boundary between the oropharynx and oral cavity. Tonsillar carcinomas also may spread laterally and superiorly to invade the retromolar trigone and pterygomandibular raphe.
- On CT, because of common dental hardware artifacts, oropharynx evaluation could be quite troublesome unless

**Table 13.4** hr-HPV Mediated (p16+) Oropharyngeal Carcinoma T Staging (AJCC 8th ed.)

| ✓ T Category | T Criteria |
| --- | --- |
| T0 | No primary identified |
| T1 | Tumor 2 cm or smaller in greatest dimension |
| T2 | Tumor larger than 2 cm but not larger than 4 cm in greatest dimension |
| T3 | Tumor larger than 4 cm in greatest dimension or extension to lingual surface of epiglottis |
| T4 | Moderately advanced local disease |
| | Tumor invades the larynx, extrinsic muscle of tongue, medial pterygoid, hard palate, or mandible or beyond* |

*AJCC*, American Joint Commission on Cancer; *hr-HPV*, high-risk human papillomavirus.

(From Amin MB, Greene FL, Edge SB, et al., eds. AJCC Cancer Staging Manual. Springer International Publishing: American Joint Commission on Cancer; 8th ed. New York; 2017.)

*Note: Mucosal extension to lingual surface of epiglottis from primary tumors of the base of the tongue and vallecula does not constitute invasion of the larynx. The specific extrinsic muscles invaded that warrant T4 designation are controversial and inconsistent between AJCC and Union for International Cancer Control.

**Table 13.5** Oropharyngeal (HPV-, p16-) Carcinoma T Staging (AJCC 8th ed.)

| ✓ T Category | T Criteria |
| --- | --- |
| TX | Primary tumor cannot be assessed |
| Tis | Carcinoma in situ |
| T1 | Tumor 2 cm or smaller in greatest dimension |
| T2 | Tumor larger than 2 cm but not larger than 4 cm in greatest dimension |
| T3 | Tumor larger than 4 cm in greatest dimension or extension to lingual surface of epiglottis |
| T4a | Moderately advanced local disease |
| | Tumor invades the larynx, extrinsic muscle of tongue, medial pterygoid, hard palate, or mandible* |
| T4b | Very advanced local disease |
| | Tumor invades lateral pterygoid muscle, pterygoid plates, lateral nasopharynx, or skull base or encases carotid artery |

*AJCC*, American Joint Commission on Cancer; *HPV*, human papillomavirus.

(From Amin MB, Greene FL, Edge SB, et al., eds. AJCC Cancer Staging Manual. Springer International Publishing: American Joint Commission on Cancer; 8th ed. New York; 2017.)

*Note: Mucosal extension to lingual surface of epiglottis from primary tumors of the base of the tongue and vallecula does not constitute invasion of the larynx. The specific extrinsic muscles invaded that warrant T4 designation are controversial and inconsistent between AJCC and Union for International Cancer Control.

the mass is big enough to cause mass effect and efface surrounding tissues. Maneuvers to open the space between maxilla and mandible should be exercised with a mouthpiece or by placing a syringe at the time of imaging. The real size of the oropharynx mass therefore can be underestimated, causing understaging of the tumor mass.
- MR is the preferred modality because of higher soft-tissue resolution. Precontrast T1 and STIR images provide details of parapharyngeal fat, soft palate, and epiglottic infiltration. Postcontrast T1 with fat saturation gives an accurate estimate of the tumor mass size.
- The current preferred treatment modality for oropharyngeal cancers with local and nodal disease is radiotherapy to provide best functional outcome. FDG-PET CT is best suited for systemic staging (Fig. 13.23). In early T stages, carefully selected patients can be offered surgical interventions including minimally invasive robotic removal of the mass.
- T staging pearls include the following:
  - Is it hr-HPV (p16) positive or negative?
  - How big is the mass? The size criteria are the same for oropharynx, oral cavity, and hypopharynx cancers. Numbers to remember are: less than 2 cm, 2 to 4 cm, and greater than 4 cm.
  - Which neighbouring structures are involved within the local infiltrative margins?
  - T3: Limited extension to the lingual surface of epiglottis.
  - T4: Anything beyond lingual surface of epiglottis, including extrinsic tongue muscles, medial pterygoid, hard palate, mandible, and carotid space.
  - Pre-epiglottic fat invasion: Base of tongue cancers have easy access to vallecula and once infiltrated, it is surgically impossible to remove the fat while maintaining

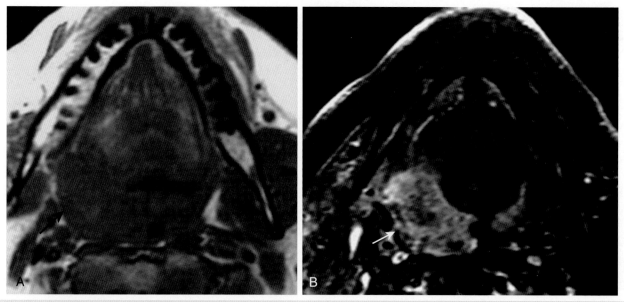

**Fig. 13.22 Tonsillar squamous cell carcinoma.** (A) T1-weighted imaging (T1WI) scan shows a hypointense mass centered in the right palatine tonsil *(arrow)* with partial effacement of the right parapharyngeal fat. These tumors often invade anterolaterally to enter the retromolar trigone, medially to enter the soft palate, and anteriorly to invade the tongue base. (B) Tonsil and tongue cancers are very well-depicted on fat-suppressed T2-weighted imaging (T2WI) *(arrow)*. Immunohistochemical analysis revealed this to be hr-HPV-related oropharyngeal squamous cell carcinoma.

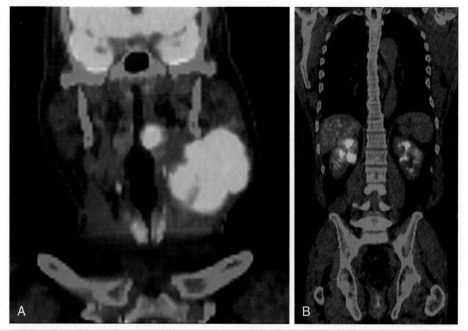

**Fig. 13.23 Systemic staging using fluorodeoxyglucose (FDG) positron emission tomography (PET).** (A) Fused FDG PET-computed tomography (CT) neck image in coronal plane shows marked metabolic activity in the left palatine tonsil, the primary tumor site, as well as a very large nodal conglomerate in the left neck. (B) Fused FDG PET-CT body image in the coronal plane shows no evident metastatic disease elsewhere in the body.

the integrity of the epiglottis's petiole (inferior stem). Sagittal CT or T1 (pre- or fat-saturated postcontrast images) should be routinely checked for that purpose.

- Mandibular invasion: T1 showing loss of the hypointense cortex, fat-suppressed T2 showing high signal infiltration, and postcontrast fat-suppressed T1 showing enhancement of the involved bone can indicate marrow invasion. Infiltration of the bone marrow of the mandible or the maxilla is better appreciated with

MRI, appearing as low signal on T1WI infiltrating the normally high-intensity fatty marrow in an adult.

- If tumor abuts the mandible but is not fixed to the periosteum or mandible, the periosteum is resected as the margin.
- For tumor fixed to or superficially invading the periosteum and/or cortex, inner cortex resection (marginal mandibulectomy) can be performed. Once the cortex has been violated or marrow has been

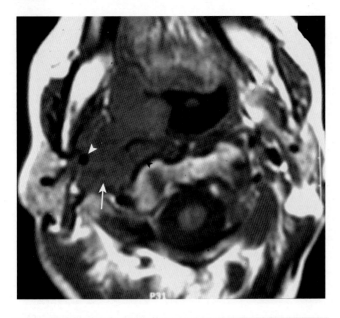

**Fig. 13.24 Spread of oropharyngeal cancer.** This tumor has spread posterolaterally to the prevertebral musculature *(black arrowhead)*, to the carotid artery where the mass *(arrow)* encases the medial 180 degrees of the carotid *(white arrowhead)*. It is also in the parapharyngeal tissues.

infiltrated, local control is achieved with segmental mandibulectomy and microvascular osteomusculocutaneous free flaps.

- Prevertebral muscle invasion: If a cancer is fixed to the prevertebral musculature (longus capitus–longus colli complex) the patient is deemed unresectable and there may be issues about curative radiotherapy (Fig. 13.24). STIR images can show intramuscular papillary projections from the mass.
- Perineural spread: High-resolution MR appears to have the advantage in evaluating the nerves over CT, showing abnormal enlargement and enhancement of the involved nerves. Infiltration of the normal fat surrounding nerves can also be a good indicator of perineural tumor spread, readily visualized on T1 precontrast imaging without fat saturation. Foraminal enlargement and bony infiltration is a reliable finding on CT but is uncommonly seen.
- Pterygomandibular raphe invasion: This fibrous structure stretches from the medial pterygoid muscle's insertion on the medial pterygoid plate to the mylohyoid ridge of the mandible. It serves as the origin or insertion of the buccinator muscle and the pharyngeal constrictor muscles.
  - The pterygomandibular raphe is one of the boundaries between the oral cavity and the oropharynx as it effectively divides the anterior tonsillar pillar and the retromolar trigone.
  - The retromolar trigone, a portion of the oral cavity, is the area behind the maxillary teeth but in front of the coronoid process and ascending ramus of the mandible.
  - Tumor can spread along this plane superiorly to the temporalis muscle, medially into the trigeminal fat pad where the lingual and inferior alveolar

**Table 13.6** Oropharyngeal hr-HPV Mediated (p16+) Carcinoma N Staging (AJCC 8th ed.)

| ✓ | Category | Carcinoma N Criteria |
|---|----------|---------------------|
| | NX | Regional lymph nodes cannot be assessed |
| | N0 | No regional lymph node metastasis |
| | N1 | One or more ipsilateral lymph nodes, none larger than 6 cm |
| | N2 | Contralateral or bilateral lymph nodes, none larger than 6 cm |
| | N3 | Lymph node(s) larger than 6 cm |

*AJCC,* American Joint Commission on Cancer; *hr-HPV,* high-risk human papillomavirus.

(From Amin MB, Greene FL, Edge SB, et al., eds. AJCC Cancer Staging Manual. Springer International Publishing: American Joint Commission on Cancer; 8th ed. New York; 2017.)

**Table 13.7** Oropharyngeal (HPV-, p16-) Carcinoma N staging (AJCC 8th ed.)

| ✓ | Category | N Criteria |
|---|----------|-----------|
| | NX | Regional lymph nodes cannot be assessed |
| | N0 | No regional lymph node metastasis |
| | N1 | Metastasis in a single ipsilateral lymph node, 3 cm or smaller in greatest dimension and ENE(-) |
| | N2a | Metastasis in a single ipsilateral node larger than 3 cm but not larger than 6 cm in greatest dimension and ENE(-) |
| | N2b | Metastases in multiple ipsilateral nodes, none larger than 6 cm in greatest dimension and ENE(-) |
| | N2c | Metastases in bilateral or contralateral lymph nodes, none larger than 6 cm in greatest dimension and ENE(-) |
| | N3a | Metastasis in a lymph node larger than 6 cm in greatest dimension and ENE(+) |
| | N3b | Metastasis in any node(s) and clinically overt ENE(+) |

Note: A designation of "U" or "L" may be used for any N category to indicate metastasis above the lower border of the cricoid (U) or below the lower border of the cricoid (L). Similarly, clinical and pathologic ENE should be recorded as ENE(-) or ENE(+).

*AJCC,* American Joint Commission on Cancer; *HPV,* human papillomavirus.

(From Amin MB, Greene FL, Edge SB, et al., eds. AJCC Cancer Staging Manual. Springer International Publishing: American Joint Commission on Cancer; 8th ed. New York; 2017.)

nerves run, or inferiorly into the floor of the mouth. If tumors spread anteriorly from the medial pterygoid plate, they can enter the pterygopalatine fossa and cause even more trouble.
- N staging pearls include the following (Tables 13.6 and 13.7):
  - How many nodes are there?
  - What is the largest size?
  - Ipsilateral or bilateral?

## Oral Cavity Squamous Cell Carcinoma

- The oral cavity consists of the lips, buccal mucosa, gingiva, dentition, anterior two thirds of the oral tongue, the floor of the mouth, and the bony hard palate. The risk factors for oral cavity SCC include smoking, alcohol abuse, HPV exposure, chewing tobacco, and betel nuts. The lower lip is the second most common site of SCC in the head and neck after the skin from sun exposure.

- One of the major AJCC eighth edition changes involved oral cavity SCC with incorporation of the depth of invasion (DOI) on histopathology and removal of extrinsic tongue muscle infiltration from T staging because deeper extent was associated with worse survival outcomes and extrinsic muscle invasion was hard for pathologists to define and lacked specificity. With current diagnostic radiology techniques, the DOI cannot be reliably measured.
- Findings on imaging have direct treatment implications.
  - If only unilateral disease is present, swallowing and phonation can be preserved. Patients who undergo hemiglossectomy can form a bolus and can speak reasonably intelligibly, if not a little garbled. It is important to identify spread of tumor across the fatty lingual septum that defines the midline of the tongue and laterality at the base of tongue.
  - If the midline of the base of the tongue has been violated by cancer, the possibility of having a complete resection with adequate margins while maintaining a functioning tongue is remote. In such cases, large soft-tissue flap reconstructions will be required to maintain swallowing function and in some cases tracheostomy is needed for airway protection.
- Imaging of oral cavity cancers is critical but has its challenges.
  - On CT, dental hardware artifacts can obscure superficial tumors, even with contrast administration. CT is very helpful for findings of bone erosion.
  - Be aware that floor-of-mouth cancers may cause obstruction of the submandibular duct. This causes an enlarged, edematous, painful, submandibular gland that may simulate inflammation caused by calculous disease and lead to delayed diagnosis.
  - On MRI, pulse sequences that are of the greatest use with tongue are the following:
    - T2: Tumors are brighter than the very dark intrinsic musculature of the tongue.
    - Coronal STIR: This sequence can help identify tumor infiltration at the floor of mouth.
    - Postcontrast fat-suppressed T1: This is useful for measurement of the mass.
    - Precontrast T1: This is an important sequence to evaluate for mandibular marrow invasion.
  - Greater and lesser palatine foramina, inferior alveolar canal, and pterygopalatine fossa can be avenues for the possible spread of cancers along VII and VIII division nerves. The foramen rotundum and foramen ovale should be assessed with imaging to ensure that intracranial extension of tumor along the cranial nerves has not occurred.
  - The tongue undergoes predictable changes after it has been denervated (usually as a result of primary tumor resections, neck nodal surgery, radiotherapy, anterior horn cell disease [amyotrophic lateral sclerosis: ALS], and occasionally from primary neoplasms of the hypoglossal nerve). In the first few months, you can see high signal on T2WI in the ipsilateral hemitongue and a relatively normal

**Table 13.8** Oral Cavity Carcinoma T staging (AJCC 8th ed.)

| ✓ T Category | T Criteria |
| --- | --- |
| TX | Primary tumor cannot be assessed |
| Tis | Carcinoma in *situ* |
| T1 | Tumor ≤2 cm with depth of invasion (DOI)* ≤ 5 mm |
| T2 | Tumor ≤2 cm with DOI* >5 mm |
|  | or tumor > 2 cm and ≤4 cm with DOI* ≤10 mm |
| T3 | Tumor > 2 cm and ≤4 cm with DOI* > 10 mm |
|  | *or* tumor > 4 cm with DOI* ≤10 mm |
| T4a | Moderately advanced local disease |
|  | Tumor > 4 cm with DOV > 10 mm |
|  | *or* tumor invades adjacent structures only (e.g., through cortical bone of the mandible or maxilla or involves the maxillary sinus or skin of the face) |
|  | Note: Superficial erosion of bone/tooth socket (alone) by a gingival primary is not sufficient to classify a tumor as T4. |
| T4b | Very advanced local disease |
|  | Tumor invades masticator space, pterygoid plates, or skull base and/or encases the internal carotid artery |

*DOI is depth of invasion and **not** tumor thickness.

(From Amin MB, Greene FL, Edge SB, et al., eds. AJCC Cancer Staging Manual. Springer International Publishing: American Joint Commission on Cancer; 8th ed. New York; 2017.)

T1WI. After about 5 months, fatty infiltration of the tongue, (manifesting as high signal on T1WI and low density on CT) and volume loss may be seen. The same pattern is seen with denervated muscles of mastication.

- T staging pearls include the following (Table 13.8; Fig. 13.25):
  - How big is the mass? The size criteria are the same for oral cavity, oropharynx, and hypopharynx cancers. Numbers to remember: less than 2 cm, 2 to 4 cm, and more than 4 cm.
  - What is the depth of invasion? This is unique to oral cavity cancer and can only be assigned by a pathologist in a biopsy or surgical specimen.
    - DOI ≤5 mm: T1
    - DOI <5 mm and ≤10 mm: T2
    - DOI >10 mm: T3 or T4
  - Which tissues are infiltrated?
    - T4a: Cortical bone of mandible, maxilla, or skin of the face or maxillary sinus
    - T4b: Masticator space, pterygoid plates, skull base, or carotid artery is encased.
- The imaging features that do not necessarily affect T staging but involve surgical management include question of perineural tumor spread.
  - If the tumor is posteriorly located, is there extension into the retromolar trigone and pterygomandibular raphe and maxilla that would provide easy access to the skull base by perineural spread? Don't forget to check pterygopalatine fossa, especially greater and lesser palatine nerves and the foramina.

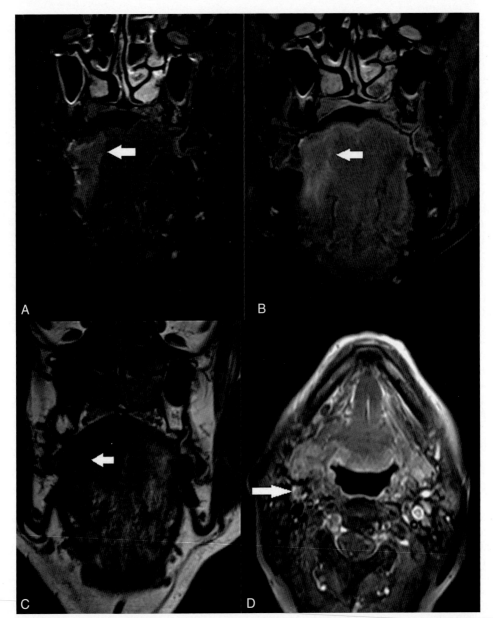

**Fig. 13.25 Oral cancer.** There is a 3 cm (T2) mass at the right lateral oral tongue seen on (A) coronal short inversion time inversion recovery (STIR), (B) coronal postcontrast T1, and (C) coronal precontrast T1 images. The AJCC eighth edition does not count extrinsic tongue infiltration for T staging. However, the postsurgical pathology showed 11 mm depth of invasion, upstaging the mass to T4. (D) Fat-saturated postcontrast T1-weighted imaging (T1WI) shows a right level 2 A metastatic node. The heterogenous enhancement and rounded contour makes the node very suspicious by imaging, despite its small size.

- The N staging pearls include the following (Table 13.9):
  - Nodal disease is less frequent with superficial oral cavity primary cancers than OPC (30% compared to 65%, respectively). Nodal spread impacts significantly on patient outcome (reducing 5-year survival by 50%), emphasizing the importance of identifying pathologic nodes in all patients with cancer.
  - Drainage of the anterior two thirds of the tongue goes to the submandibular lymph nodes and from there to the high internal jugular chain.
  - Because reactive lymph nodes in the submandibular region may grow to more than 1 cm in size, submandibular nodes are not suggested to be neoplastic until they are more than 1.5 cm in diameter. Keep in mind that enhancement characteristics of lymph nodes are more helpful in determining metastatic involvement than size alone.

## Hypopharyngeal Squamous Cell Carcinoma

- Most hypopharyngeal cancers (60%) arise in the pyriform sinus, with the remainder evenly split between postcricoid and posterior pharyngeal locations. The pyriform sinus cancers metastasize early, invade aggressively into the soft tissue of the neck, and present late (because this area is clinically silent; Fig. 13.26).
- The anatomy of the hypopharynx gets somewhat confusing because of the following:

**Table 13.9** Oral Cavity Carcinoma N staging (AJCC 8th ed.)

| ✓ cN Category | cN Criteria |
|---|---|
| NX | Regional lymph nodes cannot be assessed |
| N0 | No regional lymph node metastasis |
| N1 | Metastasis in a single ipsilateral lymph node, 3 cm or smaller in greatest dimension ENE(-) |
| N2a | Metastasis in a single ipsilateral node larger than 3 cm but not larger than 6 cm in greatest dimension, and ENE(-) |
| N2b | Metastases in multiple ipsilateral nodes, none larger than 6 cm in greatest dimension, and ENE(-) |
| N2c | Metastases in bilateral or contralateral lymph nodes, none larger than 6 cm in greatest dimension, and ENE(-) |
| N3a | Metastasis in a lymph node larger than 6 cm in greatest dimension and ENE(-) |
| N3b | Metastasis in any node(s) and clinically overt ENE |

*Note:* A designation of "U or "L" may be used for any N category to indicate metastasis above the lower border of the cricoid (U) or below the lower border of the cricoid (L). Similarly, clinical and pathologic ENE should be recorded as ENE(-) or ENE(+).

*AJCC,* American Joint Commission on Cancer.

(From Amin MB, Greene FL, Edge SB, et al., eds. AJCC Cancer Staging Manual. Springer International Publishing: American Joint Commission on Cancer; 8th ed. New York; 2017.)

- The anteromedial margin of the pyriform sinus is the lateral aspect of the aryepiglottic fold, which is considered a portion of the supraglottic larynx.
- Because tumors in the pyriform sinus often obliterate the space between the lateral/pharyngeal mucosa of the aryepiglottic fold and the mucosa of the pyriform sinus, it is often difficult to determine whether a tumor is supraglottic (arising from the aryepiglottic fold), or hypopharyngeal (arising along the lateral aspect of the pyriform sinus). If the endoscope can pass medial to the tumor, it is a lateral pyriform sinus cancer (hypopharyngeal); if it can pass lateral to the tumor, it is arising from the aryepiglottic fold (supraglottic).
- Pyriform sinus cancers spread through the thyrohyoid membrane or cricothyroid membrane into the neck where they may encircle the carotid arteries and be deemed inoperable.
- As in laryngeal carcinoma, one of the major issues regarding hypopharyngeal tumors is the invasion of cartilage. The superior aspect of the thyroid cartilage is particularly vulnerable to hypopharyngeal cancer.
- MRI has higher sensitivity but lower specificity than CT in the evaluation of early laryngeal cartilage invasion. MRI may be able to detect the more subtle cartilaginous invasion before through-and-through disease is present but also may have false positives with inflammatory reactions. For this indication, T1-enhanced fat-suppressed MRI appears to be a particularly valuable pulse sequence. In the later stages, infiltration of the strap

muscles superficial to the cartilage is seen equally well on MRI and CT.
- T staging pearls include the following (Table 13.10):
  - Number of subsites that are invaded (pyriform sinus, postcricoid region, posterior wall)
  - Size of the lesion (<2 cm, 2-4 cm, >4 cm)
  - Presence or absence of fixation of the hemilarynx
  - If the tumor invades adjacent structures such as the thyroid or cricoid cartilage, hyoid bone, or extends out into the soft tissues of the neck, the lesion is considered a T4a cancer
  - If there is invasion of the prevertebral fascia, encasement of the carotid artery, or involvement of mediastinal structures, it is considered T4b
- N staging pearls include the following (Table 13.11):
  - Nodal disease is frequent, with 65% to 80% at presentation.
  - Level 4 and central neck, level 6 should be carefully evaluated.
  - Nodes >1 cm should be prompt suspicion for metastatic disease.

## Squamous Cell Carcinoma of the Larynx

- Larynx cancer represents one third of all head and neck cancers, with 90% being SCC. It is most commonly seen in patients with significant smoking history but increasing evidence shows up to 19% hr-HPV association. Males are more affected during the fifth to seventh decades of life.
  - It can originate at different subsites of the larynx, with different implications in clinical presentation, patterns of spread, and disease management. Larynx-preserving curative success is high in early-stage disease with either surgical or radiation monotherapy, whereas late-stage disease has a worse outcome and warrants multimodal therapy with poor functional outcomes. In locally limited larynx cancer, 5-year survival rate is 78%. Nodal and locoregional spread drops the 5-year survival rate to 46% and distant organ metastasis to 34%.
  - Subsite specific survival data of the larynx shows the following:
    - Supraglottis: The second most common subsite, harboring 35% of laryngeal cancer. It has a rich lymphatic network and commonly presents with nodal disease even in early stages. Therefore the survival rates are lower than glottis, with 80% for the earliest stage and 34% for the most advanced stage.
    - Glottis: The most common subsite, harboring 60% of laryngeal cancer. Almost 80% of cases are found in early stages because it induces symptoms with voice changes. Early disease has a survival rate of 90%, which drops to 44% with distant metastasis.
    - Subglottis: The least common larynx subsite, harboring 5% of laryngeal cancers. Survival rates range from 65% at the earliest stage to 32% at the most advanced stage.
- CT is the mainstay of imaging because many of the larynx cancer patients have swallowing and breathing problems that cause motion-related artifacts,

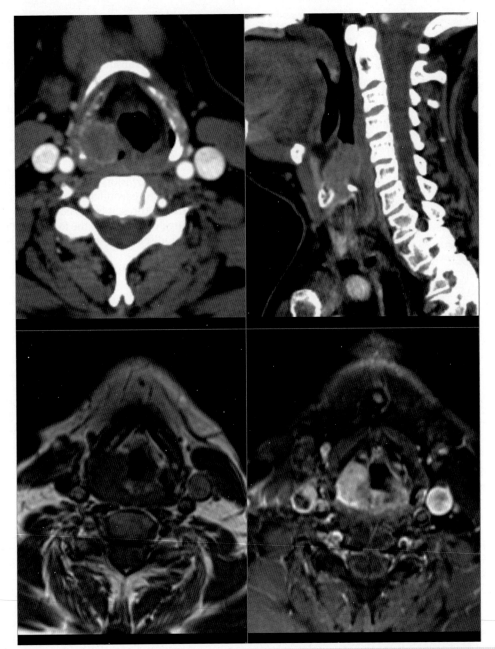

**Fig. 13.26 Hypopharyngeal cancer.** (A) Axial contrast-enhanced computed tomography (CT) demonstrates right pyriform sinus enhancing mass infiltrating the right false vocal fold and paraglottic space. (B) Coronal CT shows the mass abutting but not definitively invading the right thyroid cartilage. The pre- (C) and postcontrast (D) axial T1-weighted imaging (T1WI) also show the paraglottic space infiltration.

making MRI a challenge. The irregular ossification-calcification of the thyroid cartilage is particularly troublesome, but the absolute convincing finding of invasion is through-and-through erosion with extension of the mass into the strap muscles.

- Sclerosis of the cartilage may be a harbinger of cartilaginous invasion; however, arytenoid sclerosis can occur in 16% of normal subjects, especially in the body of the arytenoid and more commonly in females. Other CT findings include lysis or destruction of cartilage or obliteration of the marrow space of ossified cartilage. Unfortunately, CT tends to be relatively insensitive to early cartilage invasion (Fig. 13.27).

- Although MRI is advocated to provide better cartilage detail for invasion using dedicated larynx protocols, the quality is very much dependent on the patient motion. In an ideal postcontrast T1 with fat saturation, you can see the abnormal enhancement of the cartilage. Using these criteria, MR is very sensitive (85%) to cartilage invasion but with poor specificity.

- The suspected locally advanced disease should prompt contrast-enhanced CT of the chest and FDG-PET/CT to rule out distant metastases.

- Suspected invasion into the hypopharynx may prompt esophagogastroduodenoscopy (EGD) and/or barium swallow.

**Table 13.10** Hypopharynx (p16 -) Carcinoma T Staging (AJCC 8th ed.)

| ✓ T Category | T Criteria |
|---|---|
| TX | Primary tumor cannot be assessed |
| Tis | Carcinoma in situ |
| T1 | Tumor limited to one subsite of hypopharynx and/or 2 cm or smaller in greatest dimension |
| T2 | Tumor invades more than one subsite of hypopharynx or an adjacent site, or measures larger than 2 cm but not larger than 4 cm in greatest dimension without fixation of hemilarynx |
| T3 | Tumor larger than 4 cm in greatest dimension or with fixation of hemilarynx or extension to esophageal mucosa |
| T4a | Moderately advanced local disease |
| | Tumor invades thyroid/cricoid cartilage, hyoid bone, thyroid gland, esophageal muscle or central compartment soft tissue* |
| T4b | Very advanced local disease |
| | Tumor invades prevertebral fascia, encases carotid artery, or involves mediastinal structures |

*AJCC*, American Joint Commission on Cancer.

(From Amin MB, Greene FL, Edge SB, et al., eds. AJCC Cancer Staging Manual. Springer International Publishing: American Joint Commission on Cancer; 8th ed. New York; 2017.)

*Note: Central compartment soft tissue includes prelaryngeal strap muscles and subcutaneous fat.

**Table 13.11** Hypopharynx (p16 -) Carcinoma N Staging (AJCC 8th ed.)

| ✓ N Category | N Criteria |
|---|---|
| NX | Regional lymph nodes cannot be assessed |
| N0 | No regional lymph node metastasis |
| N1 | Metastasis in a single ipsilateral lymph node, 3 cm or smaller in greatest dimension and ENE(-) |
| N2a | Metastasis in a single ipsilateral node larger than 3 cm but not larger than 6 cm in greatest dimension and ENE(-) |
| N2b | Metastases in multiple ipsilateral nodes, none larger than 6 cm in greatest dimension and ENE(-) |
| N2c | Metastases in bilateral or contralateral lymph nodes, none larger than 6 cm in greatest dimension and ENE(-) |
| N3a | Metastasis in a lymph node larger than 6 cm in greatest dimension and ENE(-) |
| N3b | Metastasis in any node(s) and clinically overt ENE(-) |

Note: A designation of "U" or "L" may be used for any N category to indicate metastasis above the lower border of the cricoid (U) or below the lower border of the cricoid (L). Similarly, clinical and pathologic ENE should be recorded as ENE(-) or ENE(+).

*AJCC*, American Joint Commission on Cancer.

(From Amin MB, Greene FL, Edge SB, et al., eds. AJCC Cancer Staging Manual. Springer International Publishing: American Joint Commission on Cancer; 8th ed. New York; 2017.)

## Supraglottic Squamous Cell Carcinoma.

- The supraglottis is subdivided into suprahyoid epiglottis, infrahyoid epiglottis, false vocal cords, aryepiglottic folds, and the arytenoids.

- Suprahyoid epiglottic tumors may grow exophytically and superiorly into vallecula and the base of the tongue, reaching a locally advanced large volume before becoming symptomatic (Fig. 13.28).
- Infrahyoid epiglottic tumors tend to grow circumferentially, involving the aryepiglottic folds, false vocal folds, pre-epiglottic fat, and pyriform sinus.
- Lymphatic involvement is a pathologic hallmark of supraglottic cancers, with decreasing order of risk of spread to levels II, III, and IV lymph nodes.
- Organ-preserving therapies are becoming the main elements maintaining the quality of life. In contemplating supraglottic laryngectomy, presence of tumor at the upper margin of the true vocal cord becomes a critical question in the surgical decision-making tree.
- If there is cartilaginous, postcricoid, or anterior commissure invasion, a supraglottic laryngectomy is not possible.
- The incidence of thyroid cartilage invasion is much higher than that of hyoid bone, arytenoid cartilage, or cricoid cartilage invasion, but thyroid cartilage extension usually occurs when the tumor is transglottic.
- Other contraindications to supraglottic laryngectomy include involvement of both arytenoid cartilages, arytenoid fixation (which implies cricoid cartilage invasion), or extensive bilateral involvement of the base of tongue and/or pre-epiglottic fat.
- The distinction between supraglottic and hypopharyngeal lesions gets blurred when the tumor extends from the aryepiglottic fold to the pyriform sinus and/or the posterior pharyngeal wall. Often it is difficult to determine the site of origin of a cancer that has spread in this fashion, but in either case, an extended resection (partial laryngectomy), taking the pyriform sinus, may be required.

## Glottic Squamous Cell Carcinoma.

- The apex of the ventricle represents the transition from supraglottic to the glottic larynx. The vocal folds are 3 to 5 mm thick and terminate at the posterior commissure with the vocal processes of arytenoid cartilages (Fig. 13.29).
- The paraglottic space soft tissue at the true cord level is the thyroarytenoid muscle and is readily separable from the fat above. The true cord is below the laryngeal ventricle. These structures need to be clarified on axial and coronal imaging planes.
- Glottic cancers typically present confined to the anterior portion of the upper free margin of one vocal cord. The vocal cord can be fixed by size of the mass, intrinsic muscles and ligament infiltration, or involvement of the recurrent laryngeal nerve. Tumor can spread to the contralateral vocal cord along the anterior commissure (Broyles' ligament).
- The glottis has a sparse lymphatic supply. If there is nodal metastasis with a glottis cancer, check CT and MRI to evaluate the supraglottic or glottic extension.
- A potential surgical treatment for primary glottic carcinoma is the vertical hemilaryngectomy (unilateral removal of the cord and supraglottic structures, sparing the contralateral side). This surgery leaves the patient with a working voice and is the preferred modality of treatment in the appropriate patient population.

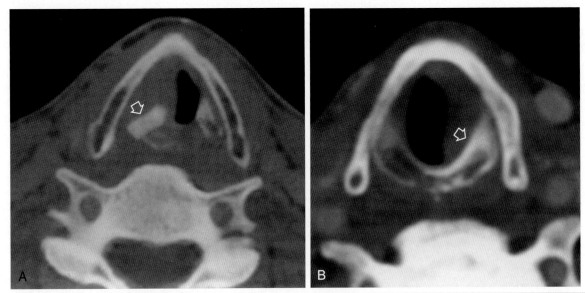

**Fig. 13.27 Cartilage sclerosis.** (A) This glottic carcinoma has led to arytenoid sclerosis *(arrow)* on the *right* side. Although that is pretty obvious, the density change in the anterior half of the thyroid cartilage may be entirely normal. (B) Do you buy the left cricoid sclerosis *(arrow)* in this patient with left vocal cord carcinoma?

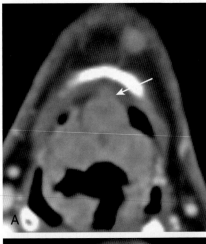

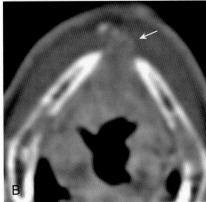

**Fig. 13.28 Supraglottic carcinoma considerations.** (A) Note the pre-epiglottic fat infiltration *(arrow)* from this epiglottic carcinoma. (B) Invasion through the anterior commissure into adjacent soft tissues *(arrow)* from this epiglottis tumor in a different patient also renders it unacceptable for supraglottic laryngectomy.

- Consideration of this therapy is contingent on the tumor not extending contralaterally beyond the anterior third of the opposite true vocal fold.
  - Posterior extension into the arytenoid cartilages or the cricoid cartilage is also a contraindication to the vertical hemilaryngectomy.
- Glottic carcinomas may spread from the anterior commissure, via the neurovascular perforations through the thyrohyoid membrane to the soft tissues of the neck, to the paraglottic space, or to the subglottic compartment. This is difficult to visualize at endoscopy and sometimes the presence of subglottic disease is initially borne out by imaging studies showing thickening in this location.
- Supracricoid laryngectomies remove the supraglottic structures and the entire thyroid cartilage. This surgery requires at least one freely mobile arytenoid with no interarytenoid tumor and a clean cricoid cartilage for providing this option to the patient.
- Pharyngeal involvement and subglottic spread also are surgical contraindications in most settings.
- T1 and T2 glottic carcinomas can be successfully treated with radiation therapy alone in some instances. The cure rates for T1 glottic carcinoma with either surgery or radiation are approximately 90%. However, the quality of the voice is generally better after focal localized radiation therapy. The radiation therapy usually does not include the lymph node chains because of the sparse lymphatics involved.

**Subglottic Squamous Cell Carcinoma.**
- The subglottis spans 10 mm below the apex of the ventricle extending 5 mm below the free margin of the vocal cord to the inferior border of the cricoid cartilage. Below the inferior surface of the cricoid cartilage, the tumors are referred to as tracheal lesions rather than subglottic laryngeal lesions. Like the glottis, it has a sparse lymphatic supply, draining into levels IV and VI lymph nodes.

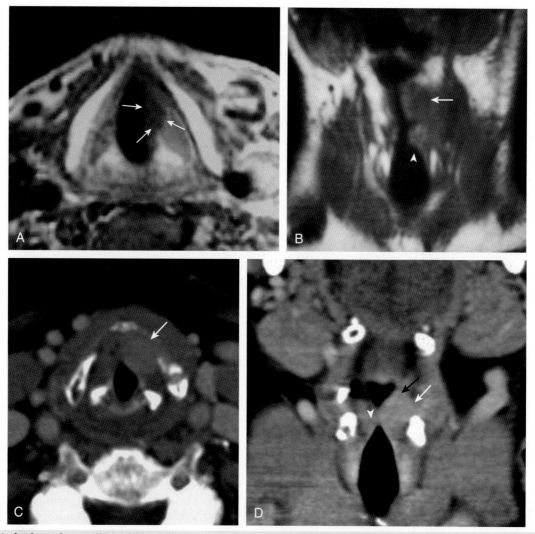

**Fig. 13.29 T1 glottic carcinoma.** (A) Axial T1-weighted imaging delineates a small focal mass *(arrows)* in the left true vocal cord. The mass did not impair cord mobility and was localized to the *left* side, thereby classifying it as a T1a lesion. (B) This case endoscopically appeared to be a small true vocal cord lesion *(arrowhead)*. However, deep to the endoscopist's view, there was extensive paraglottic spread upward *(arrow)*, rendering a T3 designation. (C) Axial computed tomographic image shows a left glottic cancer that has invaded the paraglottic soft tissues *(arrow)*. (D) Coronal reconstruction shows that in the paraglottic tissues, the left vocal cord cancer *(white arrow)* has ascended above the laryngeal ventricle level *(arrowhead)* and therefore this part of the cancer *(black arrow)* is considered "transglottic."

■ The mucosa of the subglottis is pencil thin. Any nodularity or thickening must be suspected of being cancerous on any imaging modality (Fig. 13.30).

■ The major diagnostic issue when examining a patient for subglottic carcinoma is whether there is paraglottic, glottic, and/or supraglottic extension at the time of diagnosis. These lesions are very difficult to identify at endoscopy because visualization of the undersurface of the vocal cord or the proximal trachea may be obscured by the shadow of apposed true vocal cords.

■ Because surgical resection of subglottic carcinomas nearly always requires cricoid cartilage resection, total laryngectomy is usually performed.

■ As with other sites of larynx, early T1 to T2 cancers are successfully managed by radiotherapy alone.

■ T staging pearls include the following (Tables 13.12 to 13.14):

  ■ In which subsite is the mass located? (supraglottis, glottis, subglottis?)

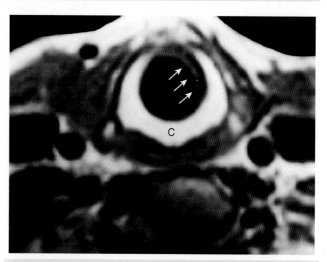

**Fig. 13.30 Subglottic carcinoma.** Axial T1-weighted imaging demonstrates thickening of the mucosa *(arrows)* along the left subglottic region. At this level, one should not see any thickness to the mucosa of the subglottic larynx. Note the normal high signal of the cricoid cartilage *(C)*.

**Table 13.12** Supraglottic Larynx Carcinoma T Staging (AJCC 8th ed.)

| ✓ | T Category | T Criteria |
|---|---|---|
| | Tx | Primary tumor cannot be assessed |
| | Tis | Carcinoma in *situ* |
| | T1 | Tumor limited to one subsite of supraglottis with normal vocal cord mobility |
| | T2 | Tumor invades mucosa of more than one adjacent subsite of supraglottis or glottis or region outside the supraglottis (e.g., mucosa of base of tongue, vallecula, medial wall of pyriform sinus) without fixation of the larynx |
| | T3 | Tumor limited to larynx with vocal cord fixation and or invades any of the following: postcricoid area, pre-epiglottic space, paraglottic space, and/or inner cortex of thyroid cartilage |
| | T4a | Moderately advanced local disease Tumor invades through the outer cortex of the thyroid cartilage and/or invades tissues beyond the larynx (e.g., trachea, soft tissues of neck including deep extrinsic muscle of the tongue, strap muscles, thyroid gland, or esophagus) |
| | T4b | Very advanced local disease Tumor invades prevertebral space, encases carotid artery, or invades mediastinal structures. |

*AJCC*, American Joint Commission on Cancer.

(From Amin MB, Greene FL, Edge SB, et al., eds. AJCC Cancer Staging Manual. Springer International Publishing: American Joint Commission on Cancer; 8th ed. New York; 2017.)

**Table 13.13** Glottic Larynx Carcinoma T Staging (AJCC 8th ed.)

| ✓ | T Category | T Criteria |
|---|---|---|
| | TX | Primary tumor cannot be assessed |
| | Tis | Carcinoma in *situ* |
| | T1a | Tumor limited to one vocal cord (may involve anterior or posterior commissure) with normal mobility |
| | T1b | Tumor involves both vocal cords (may involve anterior or posterior commissure) with normal mobility |
| | T2 | Tumor extends to supraglottis and/or subglottis, and/or with impaired vocal cord mobility |
| | T3 | Tumor limited to the larynx with vocal cord fixation and/or invasion of paraglottic space and/or inner cortex of the thyroid cartilage |
| | T4a | Moderately advanced local disease Tumor invades through the outer cortex of the thyroid cartilage and/or invades tissues beyond the larynx (e.g., trachea, cricoid cartilage, soft tissues of neck including deep extrinsic muscle of the tongue, strap muscles, thyroid, or esophagus) |
| | T4b | Very advanced local disease Tumor invades prevertebral space, encases carotid artery, or invades mediastinal structures |

*AJCC*, American Joint Commission on Cancer.

(From Amin MB, Greene FL, Edge SB, et al., eds. AJCC Cancer Staging Manual. Springer International Publishing: American Joint Commission on Cancer; 8th ed. New York; 2017.)

**Table 13.14** Subglottic Larynx Carcinoma T Staging (AJCC 8th ed.)

| ✓ | T Category | T Criteria |
|---|---|---|
| | TX | Primary tumor cannot be assessed |
| | Tis | Carcinoma in *situ* |
| | T1 | Tumor limited to the subglottis |
| | T2 | Tumor extends to vocal cord(s) with normal or impaired mobility. |
| | T3 | Tumor limited to larynx with vocal cord fixation and/or invasion of paraglottic space and/or inner cortex of the thyroid cartilage |
| | T4a | Moderately advanced local disease Tumor invades cricoid or thyroid cartilage and/or invades tissues beyond the larynx (e.g., trachea, soft tissues of neck including deep extrinsic muscles of the tongue, strap muscles, thyroid, or esophagus) |
| | T4b | Very advanced local disease Tumor invades prevertebral space, encases carotid artery, or invades mediastinal structures |

*AJCC*, American Joint Commission on Cancer.

(From Amin MB, Greene FL, Edge SB, et al., eds. AJCC Cancer Staging Manual. Springer International Publishing: American Joint Commission on Cancer; 8th ed. New York; 2017.)

- Does the mass cross between the subsites of the larynx? *Transglottic is reserved for masses involving at least two subsites (commonly glottis and supraglottis).*
- Are the cartilages infiltrated?
- Are the thyroid gland, esophagus, and/or trachea infiltrated?
- Is the base of tongue or extrinsic oral tongue muscle infiltrated?
- Are paraglottic and pre-epiglottic space fat clear on axial and coronal imaging plane?
- Is the carotid artery or sheath encased?
- Are the laryngeal muscles involved?

- N staging pearls include the following (Table 13.15):
  - If a metastatic lymph node is found with glottic or subglottic tumor, suspicion should be raised for supraglottic and therefore transglottic extent.
  - Be mindful of RP lymph nodes.

### Other Rare Considerations.

CHONDRORADIONECROSIS.

- Chondroradionecrosis can occur after standard doses of radiotherapy. CT findings are varied, including soft tissue swelling, loss of cartilage density because of sloughing with subluxation, fragmentation, sclerosis, and collapse of the involved cartilage (Fig. 13.31). Presence of gas bubbles around the cartilage may indicate infection.

CARCINOSARCOMA.

- A neoplasm that has characteristics of both SCC and sarcoma is known as the spindle cell sarcoma or carcinosarcoma. This lesion is rarely seen elsewhere in the aerodigestive tract besides the larynx.

### Other Mucosal-Based Malignancies

### Lymphoma.

- The most common noninflammatory cause for a unilateral neck mass in a patient between 20 and 40 years old

**Table 13.15** Larynx Carcinoma N Staging (AJCC 8th ed).

| ✓ | N Category | N Criteria |
|---|---|---|
| | NX | Regional lymph nodes cannot be assessed |
| | N0 | No regional lymph node metastasis |
| | N1 | Metastasis in a single ipsilateral lymph node, 3 cm or smaller in greatest dimension and ENE(-) |
| | N2a | Metastasis in a single ipsilateral node, larger than 3 cm but not larger than 6 cm in greatest dimension and ENE(-) |
| | N2b | Metastases in multiple ipsilateral nodes, none larger than 6 cm in greatest dimension and ENE(-) |
| | N2c | Metastases in bilateral or contralateral lymph nodes, none larger than 6 cm in greatest dimension and ENE(-) |
| | N3a | Metastasis in a lymph node, larger than 6 cm in greatest dimension and ENE(-) |
| | N3b | Metastasis in any lymph node(s) with clinically overt ENE(+) |

Note: A designation of "U" or "L" may be used for any N category to indicate metastasis above the lower border of the cricoid (U) or below the lower border of the cricoid (L). Similarly, clinical and pathologic ENE should be recorded as ENE(-) or ENE(+).

*AJCC,* American Joint Commission on Cancer.

(From Amin MB, Greene FL, Edge SB, et al., eds. AJCC Cancer Staging Manual. Springer International Publishing: American Joint Commission on Cancer; 8th ed. New York; 2017.)

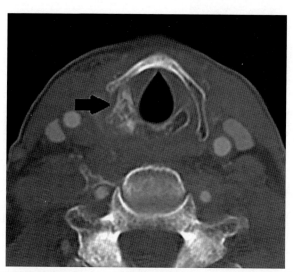

**Fig. 13.31 Chondronecrosis of the laryngeal cartilage.** Axial computed tomography (CT) image from surveillance CT after surgery, chemotherapy, and radiation for pyriform sinus squamous cell carcinoma shows mottled sclerosis of the right aspect of the cricoid cartilage *(arrow).* This could reflect tumor recurrence, but absence of associated soft-tissue mass made chondronecrosis a more likely diagnostic consideration. Absence of metabolic activity on subsequent positron emission tomography (PET)-CT helped make the diagnosis in this case.

is lymphoma. Non-Hodgkin lymphoma (NHL; 75% of lymphomas) is more common in the head and neck than Hodgkin lymphoma (25%), and usually Waldeyer ring is also involved with NHL. Fifty percent of patients with Waldeyer ring NHL have nodes at presentation. When one has isolated nodal disease in the neck or mediastinal involvement, the odds shift more in favor of Hodgkin disease (HD).

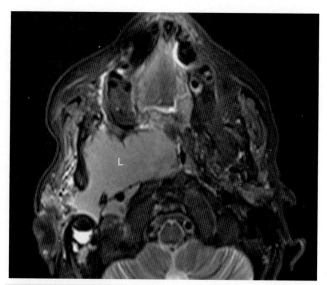

**Fig. 13.32 Oropharyngeal lymphoma.** The oropharyngeal lymphoma *(L)* centered at the palatine tonsil is spilling into the parapharyngeal, masticator, carotid, and retropharyngeal spaces.

- Lymphoma can develop in the abundant lymphoid tissue in the Waldeyer ring in both nodal and extranodal forms. It is usually in the form of NHL and affects young adults. Its appearance is identical to that of carcinoma, except that necrosis is uncommon in lymphoma (Fig. 13.32).
- Lymphoma in the nasopharynx can spread to the skull base and cranial nerve foramina.

### Minor Salivary Gland Malignancies.
- Nearly half of minor salivary gland tumors of the pharynx are pleomorphic adenomas, with the other half being malignant. Minor salivary gland malignancies most commonly occur at soft palate, with adenoid cystic carcinoma being the most common and more difficult to treat because of propensity for perineural spread (60%). Distinction between carcinoma, lymphoma, or minor salivary gland neoplasm is almost impossible with imaging.
- The extensive minor salivary gland tissue accounts for neoplasms such as adenoid cystic carcinoma (the most common minor salivary gland malignancy), mucoepidermoid carcinoma, acinic cell carcinoma, adenocarcinoma, pleomorphic low-grade adenocarcinoma, and undifferentiated carcinoma.
- Perineural progression portends a poor prognosis. It is commonly seen with nasopharyngeal and minor salivary gland cancers and ultimately leads to intracranial tumor extension.

### Plasmacytomas.
- Plasmacytomas can occur in the nasopharynx, palatine tonsils, and base of tongue. They are usually oval in shape and have similar intensity to muscle on T1WI and are only slightly hyperintense on T2WI. They enhance notably, often with a heterogeneous center.

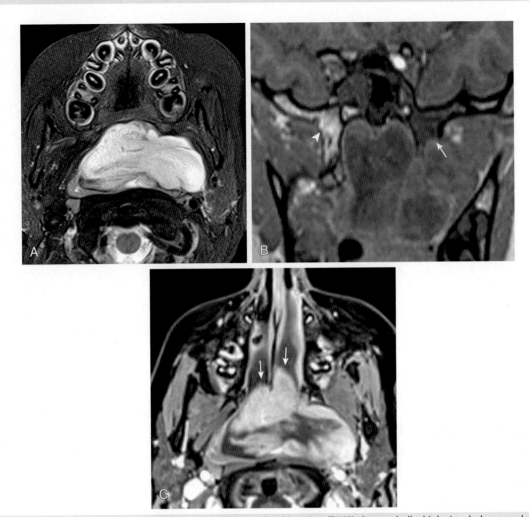

**Fig. 13.33 Rhabdomyosarcoma of the nasopharynx.** (A) Axial T2-weighted imaging (T2WI) shows a bulky high signal pharyngeal mass obliterating the airway. (B) Coronal T1-weighted imaging (T1WI) shows loss of the normal fatty signal and loss of cortical definition indicating invasion of the pterygoid plates *(arrow)*. Compare to normal right side *(arrowhead)*. (C) The tumor enhances heterogeneously on postcontrast T1WI. Extension into the posterior nasal cavity bilaterally is seen *(arrows)*.

**Sarcomas.**

- In children, the predominant tumor of the upper aerodigestive tract and particularly nasopharynx and oral tongue is rhabdomyosarcoma, typically treated with chemotherapy (Fig. 13.33). Intracranial extension is common with rhabdomyosarcomas, and rhinorrhea may be a presenting symptom. The survival rate with combined chemotherapy and radiation is more than 50% at 5 years.
- Other rare mesenchymal tumors, including hemangiopericytoma-solitary fibrous tumor and synovial sarcomas, may occur in the pharynx and larynx.
- The cricoid cartilage is associated with chondromas and chondrosarcomas. These lesions are identified on CT by their "popcorn-like" whorls of calcification caused by the chondroid matrix of the tumor (Fig. 13.34). Distinguishing a benign from a malignant chondroid tumor is sometimes difficult, but most are low grade. Chondrosarcomas account for less than 1% of laryngeal malignancies, are seen in the 40 to 60 year age range, and occurs more commonly in males by 5–10:1 ratio. Over 70% arise in the cricoid cartilage.

## MALIGNANT LYMPHADENOPATHY

- Metastasis to the regional lymph nodes is the most powerful predictor of outcome in head and neck cancers, decreasing 5-year survival by 50% when present. The 5-year prognosis is 50% decreased by having bilateral nodes and furthermore by extranodal spread of tumor or fixation to vital structures (carotids, vertebral arteries, paraspinal muscles, transverse processes, brachial plexi).

**TEACHING POINTS**

Features of Nodes that Have Prognostic Significance

- Unilateral adenopathy
- Bilateral adenopathy
- Extracapsular spread of tumor
- Fixation to vital structures (e.g., carotid artery, prevertebral musculature)

- Previous editions of the AJCC Cancer Staging manual always incorporated number, size, and laterality of the

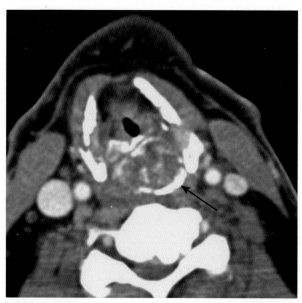

**Fig. 13.34 Chondrosarcoma of the larynx.** Note the cricoid origin *(arrow)*, popcorn-like appearance with ring and arcs calcifying matrix that characterize this tumor.

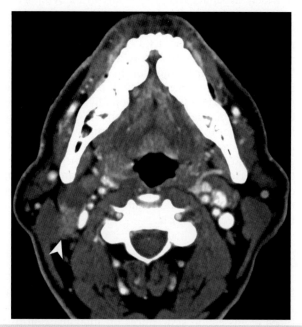

**Fig. 13.35 Metastatic extranodal extension.** Axial computed tomography (CT) image from patient with oropharyngeal cancer shows level 2 mixed cystic and solid metastatic lymph node on the right *(arrowhead)*. Notice the blurred margin of the metastatic lymph node with the adjacent fat and the adjacent sternocleidomastoid muscle, suggesting extracapsular extension, which was later confirmed histopathologically. We are not great at diagnosing extracapsular extension, so we should only call when certain, and if not, err on the side of caution, leaving the final decision to our colleagues in pathology.

lymph nodes involved. However, extranodal extent (ENE), which has long been known to be an important feature of nodal metastases in non-HPV mediated tumors, was recently incorporated in the latest eighth edition for both clinical and pathologic staging. Impact of ENE on HPV-positive OPC staging is still unclear and therefore not incorporated in the eighth edition.

- Early or microscopic ENE can be identified only on pathologic examination and cannot be detected reliably on clinical exam.
- The AJCC committee has therefore defined the clinical ENE to reflect unambiguous radiologic signs with dysfunction of a cranial nerve, the brachial plexus, the sympathetic trunk, phrenic nerve, and unequivocal clinical signs of gross ENE, such as skin involvement or muscle invasion causing tethering of nodal mass.
- The pathologic ENE is subcategorized as macroscopic ENE greater than 2 mm beyond the nodal capsule under the microscope or complete loss of the nodal architecture.
- The pathologic microscopic ENE is defined as up to 2 mm infiltration from the nodal capsule.
- Critical numbers to remember for most mucosal based SCC are less than or equal to 3 cm for N1, 3 to 6 cm for N2, and greater than 6 cm for the N3 classification. The exceptions are for hr-HPV-related OPC and for NPC, where nodes less than or greater than 6 cm distinguish N1 from N3 disease and laterality affecting N2 designation (see Table 13.3 and 13.6).
- The incidence of extracapsular spread of tumor correlates with the nodal size. Histopathologically, 23% of nodes less than 1 cm, 53% of nodes 2 to 3 cm, and 74% of nodes greater than 3 cm in transverse diameter have ENE (Fig. 13.35). We are not great at calling extracapsular extension on imaging, and making the finding has critical treatment strategy implications. For this reason, we should only call ENE if there is no doubt on imaging; if there is doubt, then err on the side of caution, and leave the final call to our colleagues in pathology.
- Some lymph nodes that are located deep in the head and neck are not clinically palpable. Retropharyngeal lymph nodes, which commonly accompany nasopharyngeal carcinoma, are impossible to detect clinically (Fig. 13.36). For this reason, it is generally accepted that 15% to 30% of all malignant lymph nodes escape clinical detection.
- Most head and neck radiologists agree that CT is the most efficient method for identifying metastatic lymph nodes in the neck, provided that a large bolus of contrast has been delivered to the blood vessels to distinguish them from lymph nodes. Sensitivity and specificity for nodal metastases is highly variable on MRI and CT, and unfortunately neither is 100%. However, there are certain imaging features that can raise concern for metastatic involvement.
  - Consensus is that if greater than 15 mm (longest measurement in the axial plane), the node should be considered suspicious until proven otherwise.
  - Retropharyngeal nodes should generally not exceed 8 mm in diameter.
  - The shape of the lymph node is also helpful in detecting involvement by tumor. More rounded lymph nodes have a greater chance of being neoplastic than those that have a kidney bean shape.
  - A lymph node that has central necrosis no matter its size should be considered malignant until proven otherwise.
  - Heterogeneous contrast enhancement, calcifications, asymmetric clustering, and perinodal stranding should help improve your odds in detecting malignant adenopathy.

Expected Nodal Drainage Patterns

| Nodal Level | Primary Malignancy Site |
|---|---|
| I | Anterior oral, lip, sinonasal |
| II | Nasopharynx, oropharynx, posterior oral cavity, supraglottic larynx, parotid gland |
| III | Nasopharynx, larynx, hypopharynx |
| IV | Nasopharynx, larynx, thyroid, cervical esophagus |
| V | Nasopharynx, skin |
| VI | Nasopharynx, subglottic, thyroid, cervical esophagus |
| VII | Subglottic, thyroid, cervical esophagus |
| Retropharyngeal | Nasopharynx, oral cavity, sinonasal, thyroid, posterior pharyngeal/laryngeal |
| Intraparotid | Scalp, orbit, nasopharynx |

Adapted from Hoang JK, Vanka J, Ludswig BJ, Glastonbury CM. Evaluation of cervical lymph nodes in head and neck cancer with CT and MRI: tips, traps, and a systematic approach. *AJR Am J Roentgenol.* 2013;200(1):W17-25.

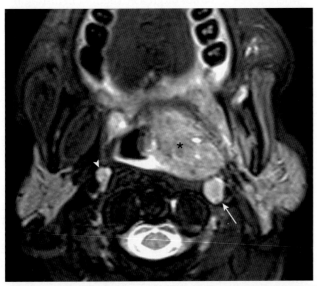

**Fig. 13.36 Retropharyngeal lymph node.** Axial T2-weighted image shows a bulky oropharyngeal mass (you guessed it, squamous cell carcinoma), clearly visible on endoscopy. What the clinician can't see is the asymmetrically enlarged left retropharyngeal lymph node *(arrow)* indicating nodal metastasis. Compare to more normal size on the right *(arrowhead).*

### Malignant Adenopathy: Other Considerations

- Another important issue to consider when you are dealing with internal jugular chain lymph nodes is the presence or absence of carotid invasion by lymphadenopathy. Although it has not been incorporated into the eighth edition of the AJCC, it has critical impact on surgical success. Presently, no ideal radiographic study can predict whether the carotid artery is invaded by tumor when there is contiguous lymphadenopathy. It has generally been accepted that if less than 270 degrees of the circumference of the carotid artery is encircled by SCC, the likelihood of carotid wall invasion is less than if greater than 270 encasement is present.
- Extension of lymph nodes into the posterior musculature of the neck, paraspinal soft tissue, and/or the base of the skull also makes surgical resection much more difficult

if not impossible. The presence of these findings suggests that the tumor may be extensive beyond visible dimensions and may require heroic surgery for a small chance of cure.

- A widely accepted fact is that any cystic lymph node, or cystic neck mass for that matter, in an adult patient should be managed as metastatic lymphadenopathy until proven otherwise (Fig. 13.37). This has become even more apparent with HPV-16-related primary tumors.
- "Unknown primary tumor" of the head and neck occurs in the scenario in which a patient presents with a neck mass proven to be a lymphadenopathy on imaging. PET/CT and, if available, PET/MRI with 18F-FDG is indicated in those cases to search for the primary, which is commonly not apparent on routine CT or MRI. The AJCC endorses to check for p16 and EBV, which would help treat those cases per viral status. Clinical and endoscopic examination and imaging will identify the primary tumor in 25% of cases. In many instances, the primary tumor is never discovered.

## Posttreatment Imaging

- Neck dissections are performed to remove suspected adenopathy; it's important to be familiar with the different types of dissection procedures on imaging. Soft-tissue matting, subcutaneous stranding, and tissue distortions are commonly seen after neck dissection and can be confused with tumor recurrence (Fig. 13.38).

Types of Neck Dissection

- **Radical neck dissection:** The sternocleidomastoid muscle, the spinal accessory nerve (XI), the jugular vein, and the submandibular gland are removed with level I to V nodal chains.
- **Modified neck dissection:** Either the spinal accessory nerve (allowing a functional trapezius muscle), the sternocleidomastoid muscle, and/or the internal jugular vein are spared. Level I to V nodal chains can be removed.

Continued

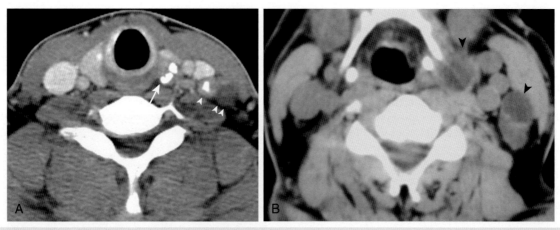

**Fig. 13.37 Metastatic papillary thyroid cancer to lymph nodes.** (A) Axial contrast-enhanced computed tomography (CT) image shows a calcified nodule in the left thyroid gland *(arrow)* with calcified *(single arrowhead)* and cystic *(double arrowheads)* metastatic lymph nodes. (B) A different patient with cystic nodal metastases.

- **Supraomohyoid neck dissection:** Level I to III nodes above the cricoid cartilage are removed. It usually spares the sternocleidomastoid muscle, internal jugular vein and spinal accessory nerve. This dissection is commonly performed for N0 primary tumors high in the aerodigestive system, with a low to intermediate rate of occult metastases.
- **Anterior neck dissection** may be performed for thyroid cancer to remove anterior visceral chain nodes (level VI).

---

- Keep in mind that once the normal pathway of lymphatic drainage from a primary site has been removed surgically, nodal metastases may subsequently occur in unusual locations for that particularly primary tumor.
- After both nodal chains have been removed, watch out for dermal lymphatic drainage of tumor cells because the nodes are no longer available to sequester the neoplasm. This is identifiable as subcutaneous stranding and thickening on CT or MRI. Unfortunately, this may be indistinguishable from the edema associated with radiation treatment.
- Surgical reconstruction of defects in the head and neck after operation requires the interposition of flaps and grafts. Flaps are usually separated into several categories.
  - Site: Local, regional, or distant
  - Tissue: Cutaneous, fasciocutaneous, musculocutaneous, or osteomusculocutaneous
  - Blood supply: Random, axial, pedicled, or free
  - Modern techniques of inserting osteointegrated implants into bone grafts (often distant osteomusculocutaneous free flaps of the fibula) afford the patient an opportunity to have a dental surface capable of chewing.
  - All flaps, regardless of how simple or complex they are, undergo denervation and atrophy involving fat, soft tissue (muscle), and fat components.
  - The site from which the flap is taken precedes the description of what is taken. A fibular free flap may be used to reconstruct the mandible, or a radial forearm

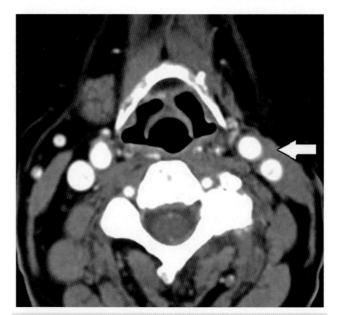

**Fig. 13.38 Surgical change.** Axial contrast-enhanced computed tomography (CT) neck after left neck dissection shows confluent soft-tissue matting surrounding the left carotid artery and jugular vein *(arrow)*, an expected postsurgical finding not to be confused with tumor recurrence. Note surgical absence of the left sublingual gland.

free (cutaneous) flap frequently fixes defects in the floor of the mouth.
  - Free flaps require anastomoses of blood vessels (and sometimes nerves) from the donor site to the surgical bed with microvascularization techniques.
  - A local or regional flap requires rotation or "pedicling" a piece of adjacent tissue into a surgical gap without disrupting the original blood supply of the flap. Thus, a local muscular (myocutaneous) temporalis flap may be rotated down to fill the gap of an infratemporal fossa resection, or a pedicled pectoralis major flap may reconstruct a large base of tongue or floor-of-mouth defect.
  - Often on imaging the most striking feature of these flaps is the dominance of the fat in the graft. Granted,

some of the appearance varies with patient habitus, but the muscle of the graft often atrophies to a greater extent than the fat.

- A graft that has been irradiated often has a denser appearance on CT and MRI than one that has not been irradiated and may appear as a sheet of fibrous-like tissue without clearly defined tissue planes.
- Recurrences of malignancies most often occur at the cut planes of flaps and grafts or at the margins with native intrinsic tissues.

- Radiation changes can occur early (< 6 months) or late (>6 months) after treatment. Early changes of mucositis are not unexpected and do not typically require imaging. Reliable radiation changes on imaging include subcutaneous fat stranding, atrophy or hyperenhancement of salivary glands, and generalized mucosal thickening of the aerodigestive tract (Fig. 13.39).
  - After radiation therapy and/or in individuals who have carious teeth, marrow changes may occur that might simulate tumoral infiltration but may actually represent radiation fibrosis, osteoradionecrosis (Fig. 13.40), osteomyelitis, or periodontal disease.
- Ninety percent of head and neck cancer recurrences take place within the first 12 months and 96% within 2 years. Recurrences are usually split evenly between primary site, nodes, and combined primary site and nodes. For this reason, patients are not considered cured of their tumor until 5 years have passed and no evidence of tumor is identified.
- The survey for residual or recurrent disease should be performed frequently within the first 2 years, usually at 6-month intervals, and must cover the primary site and the cervical lymph nodes. The best time to image the posttreatment neck is typically considered 8 weeks after surgery and 12 weeks after radiotherapy.

- A general adage among head and neck clinicians is that tumors recur at surgical margins (Fig. 13.41), whereas they recur centrally within the tumor bed when radiation therapy is the primary modality of treatment. Recurrent SCC may be very difficult to identify when

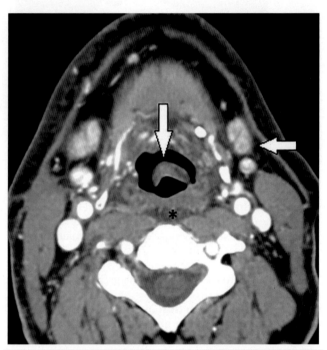

**Fig. 13.39 Radiation change.** Axial postcontrast computed tomography (CT) image shows expected findings after radiation treatment, including hyperenhancement of the salivary glands (*horizonal arrow*), thickening of the epiglottis (*vertical arrow*) and pharyngeal mucosa, and retropharyngeal edema (*asterisk*). Generalized thickening of the platysma musculature and stranding of the subcutaneous tissues are also expected features of the postradiation picture.

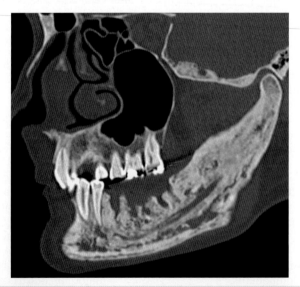

**Fig. 13.40 Osteoradionecrosis of the mandible.** Sagittal oblique reconstructed computed tomography (CT) image shows mixed lucent and sclerotic change in the mandible with loss of cortical definition. Absence of soft-tissue mass in conjunction with history of oral cancer and radiation treatment help make the diagnosis of osteoradionecrosis. Pathologic fracture can coexist. This is an infrequent treatment-related effect thanks to improved radiotherapy technology. (*Courtesy Nafi Aygun, MD*).

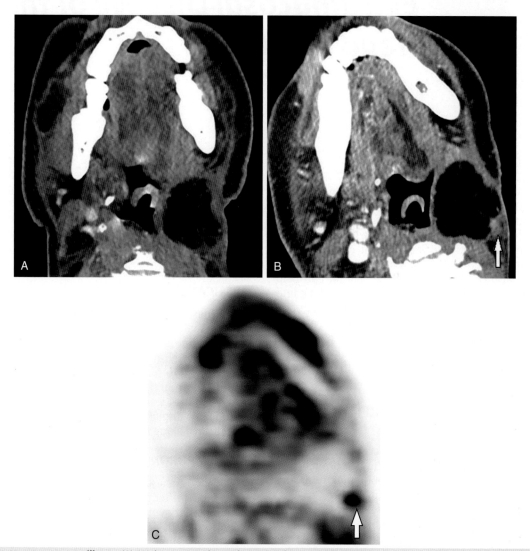

**Fig. 13.41 Posttreatment surveillance.** (A) Axial contrast-enhanced computed tomography (CT) image from surveillance CT in patient after left pectoralis pedicle flap reconstruction of the left neck shows fatty attenuation of the graft. (B) One year later, axial CT images shows new nodular soft tissue *(arrow)* along the periphery of the fat graft, which is concerning for tumor recurrence. (C) Nodular soft tissue shows marked metabolic activity on subsequent positron emission tomography (PET) exam *(arrow)*, confirming tumor recurrence.

small, and this has been another area where FDG PET has shown value.

■ MR intensity, CT density, and enhancement features are difficult to rely on for recurrence, particularly after radiotherapy. Growth with time is the only surefire sign to hang your hat on for recurrence!

## Future Cancer Risk

■ For the rest of their lives, patients with head and neck cancers generally are surveyed for the possibility of a secondary malignancy. Incidence of synchronous or metachronous oral cavity cancers in a patient who has had a previous cancer is approximately 40%. In patients who have head and neck cancers outside the oral cavity, the metachronous rate is still 15%. This includes the lungs and esophagus, so be sure to carefully survey the lower most images of the neck CT scan.

■ The primary sites of the head and neck cancers that have second lesions are fairly evenly distributed between larynx, pharynx, and oral cavity and most have associated lymphadenopathy.

■ Most series of patients with head and neck cancers report a second lung primary incidence of 0.8% to 6% and lung metastases incidence of 5% to 7%. So be sure to check for that second primary even as you scrutinize images for recurrence of the first!

# Extramucosal Disease of the Head and Neck

KAREN BUCH

## Relevant Anatomy

The extramucosal neck can be divided into several anatomic compartments that are subject to varied pathology. In addition to intrinsic imaging features of disease processes, the effect of these processes on structures within individual anatomic compartments and on adjacent compartments can help narrow the differential diagnosis, For example, the displaced appearance of the parapharyngeal fat can help identify the space a lesion is centered in (Table 14.1), and from there we can figure out the best differential diagnosis based on expected pathology in that location. This chapter begins with an anatomic description of these different spaces, then reviews several pathologic entities that are common to these compartments, and ends with pathologies that are unique to individual compartments.

### PAROTID, SUBMANDIBULAR, AND SUBLINGUAL SPACES

- The parotid space is enclosed in deep cervical fascia and houses the parotid gland, facial nerve, branches of the external carotid artery, retromandibular vein, and branches of the auriculotemporal rami of V3.
  - The parotid gland (Fig. 14.1) is the largest of the paired salivary glands, is divided into two lobes that are separated by the facial nerve, and secretes serous saliva. Unlike other salivary glands, the parotid encapsulates later and contains lymphoid tissue.
  - The parotid duct (Stensen duct) passes over the masseter muscle before curving medially and inserting in the cheek at the second maxillary molar.
- The submandibular space includes tissue below the mucosa of the floor of mouth and above the fascia connecting the mandible to the hyoid bone. The adjacent sublingual space contains the mylohyoid muscle, sublingual gland, portions of the submandibular gland, the associated ducts, and the corresponding neurovascular structures (lingual artery and lingual, hypoglossal, and glossopharyngeal nerves). The sublingual space communicates with the submandibular space along the posterior margin of the mylohyoid muscle.
  - The submandibular gland is located in the floor of the mouth, deep to the angle of the mandible (Fig. 14.2) and secretes seromucinous saliva.
  - The submandibular duct (Wharton duct) courses anteriorly and superiorly before reaching its orifice at the floor of mouth.
  - The sublingual gland is the smallest of the major salivary glands and secretes seromucinous saliva. It is located in the sublingual space at the floor of mouth, medial to the mylohyoid muscle, and has many draining ducts opening below the tongue.

- Minor salivary glands are scattered throughout the aerodigestive mucosal space, mainly in the oral cavity (especially the hard and soft palate), but may also be found in the oropharynx, the nasopharynx, the sinonasal cavity, the parapharyngeal space, the larynx, the trachea, the lungs, and even into the middle ear and eustachian tube.

### MASTICATOR SPACE

- The masticator space is defined by layers of deep cervical fascia and encompasses muscles of mastication (medial and lateral pterygoid, masseter, and temporalis), mandibular body and ramus, branches of external carotid artery and third division of cranial nerve V, and venous branches from the jugular system (Fig. 14.3).
- When a masticator space lesion is present, parapharyngeal fat is displaced posteromedially, and this fat may be infiltrated along its anterolateral aspect (see Table 14.1).

### JAW/TEMPOROMANDIBULAR JOINT

- The jaw consists of the mandible, its dentition, and the bilateral temporomandibular joint (TMJ) space. The mandibular symphysis is at the midline and houses the incisor teeth. The mandibular bodies extend laterally from the symphysis to the mandibular angle and house the remainder of the dentition. From the angles, the wider mandibular rami extend vertically and split into the coronoid process anteriorly (upon which the temporalis and masseter muscles insert) and the mandibular condyle posteriorly. The condyle is centered within the

---

**TEACHING POINTS**

Anatomy of the Temporomandibular Joint (see Fig. 14.4)

- The condyle sits centered in the glenoid fossa on closed mouth positioning but "translates" anteriorly to its resting place just below the articular eminence on mouth opening.
- The articular disc should always be interposed between the condyle and the temporal bone regardless of open versus closed mouth positioning.
- The articular disk has an anterior band and a larger posterior band, which are joined in the middle by an intermediate zone.
- The posterior band is attached to the posterior joint by the retrodiskal tissue or bilaminar zone.
- The joint capsule has an anterosuperior compartment and an inferior compartment separated by the disk.
- The lateral pterygoid muscle opens the jaw and inserts on the anterior portion of the disk. Medial pterygoid, temporalis, and masseter muscles close the jaw.

**Table 14.1** How to Place a Lesion

| Lesion Location (Space) | Displacement of Parapharyngeal Fat | Displacement of Styloid Musculature | Displacement of Longus Musculature |
|---|---|---|---|
| Parotid deep portion | Anteromedial | Posterior | Posterior |
| Masticator | Posteromedial | Posterior | Posterior |
| Carotid | Anterior | Anterior | Posterior |
| Mucosal | Posterolateral | Posterior | Posterior |
| Retropharyngeal | Anterolateral | Anterior | Posterior |
| Perivertebral | Rarely displaced | Anterior | Anterior |
| Parapharyngeal | N/A | Posterior | Posterior |

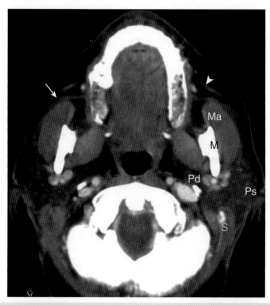

**Fig. 14.1 Normal parotid anatomy.** Computed tomography (CT): The plane between the styloid process (S) and the mandible (M) defines the superficial portion of the parotid gland (Ps) from its deep portion (Pd) on CT. The parotid duct (white arrow) on the right is distinguished from the zygomaticus muscle (white arrowhead) on the left. Note parotid tissue superficial to the masseter muscle (Ma).

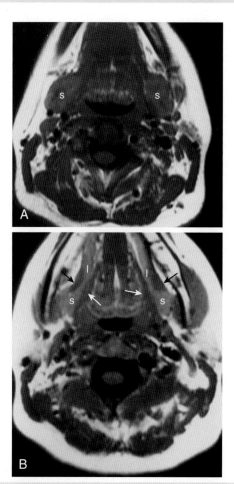

**Fig. 14.2 Normal submandibular-sublingual anatomy.** (A) Submandibular glands (s) can be seen on this T1-weighted image. Note that normally there is some heterogeneity to the gland because of its hilum and ductal system. (B) Superior portion of the submandibular gland (s) can be seen on this section, which also nicely demonstrates the sublingual gland tissue (l). Note that the sublingual space is bounded by the mylohyoid musculature (black arrows) laterally and the styloglossus-hyoglossus complex (white arrows) medially.

temporomandibular fossa (or glenoid fossa) on mouth closing and translates anteriorly on mouth opening with help from an elaborate pulley system involving an articular disk, ligaments, and muscle tendons (Fig. 14.4).

## DENTITION

■ Dental-related pathologies are centered about the tooth and can affect the tooth itself, the periapical regions (the tissues surrounding the root of the tooth), the crown (the part of the tooth that does the chomping), and/or the adjacent marrow space.

## PARAPHARYNGEAL SPACE: PRESTYLOID AND POSTSTYLOID

■ Parapharyngeal fat is readily mobile and readily displaced and infiltrated by adjacent disease. By observing the direction of displacement of this fat, you can

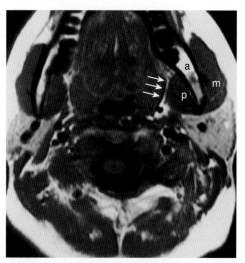

**Fig. 14.3 Normal masticator space.** Masseter muscle (m), pterygoid muscle (p), and angle of the mandible (a) are well visualized on this T1-weighted imaging scan. Note that a masticator space lesion would displace parapharyngeal fat (arrows) medially and/or posteriorly.

Differential Diagnosis of Prestyloid Parapharyngeal Space Lesions

Direct spread of tumors in adjacent spaces
Lymph nodes (normal and abnormal)
Branchial cleft cysts
Neurogenic tumors
Paragangliomas
Parapharyngeal space abscesses
Salivary gland neoplasms (e.g., pleomorphic adenomas)

identify a lesion as arising from one of the deep spaces of the head and neck (see Table 14.1).

- The parapharyngeal space is separated into two compartments: the prestyloid compartment and a poststyloid compartment (Fig. 14.5).
- The fascia of the stylopharyngeus, styloglossus, and tensor veli palatini muscle separate the prestyloid and poststyloid spaces. The styloid process can also be used to delineate this boundary on computed tomography (CT).
- The compartment contains fat and lymphatics. Very small branches of the internal maxillary artery, ascending pharyngeal artery, and mandibular (V3) nerve lie within the parapharyngeal space. Occasionally, you may find ectopic minor salivary gland tissue. Based on

contents and neighbors, the differential diagnosis of parapharyngeal space lesions is predictable.

- The *poststyloid* compartment is also referred to as the carotid space and contains the carotid sheath.
- Parapharyngeal fat is readily mobile and readily displaced and infiltrated by adjacent disease. By observing the direction of displacement of this fat, you can identify a lesion as arising from one of the deep spaces of the head and neck (see Table 14.1).

## CAROTID SPACE/POSTSTYLOID PARAPHARYNGEAL SPACE

- The carotid space courses down the entire length of the neck, beginning at the level of the skull base. This space is partially encapsulated by deep cervical fascia and may be incomplete in parts or even absent in some people. This fascia is uniformly intact only below the level of the carotid bifurcation.
- Above the hyoid bone, the carotid space is part of the poststyloid parapharyngeal space and is separated from the prestyloid parapharyngeal space by the styloid musculature (styloglossus and stylopharyngeus) just anterior to the carotid sheath but posterior to the parapharyngeal fat (see Fig. 14.5).
- The contents of the carotid space include the carotid artery, internal jugular vein, cranial nerves IX-XII,

**Normal TMJ**

1. Condyle
2. Temporal bone, articular eminence
3. Temporal bone, mandibular fossa
4. Disk, anterior band
5. Disk, intermediate zone
6. Disk, posterior band
7. Superior retrodiscal layer
8. Inferior retrodiscal layer
9. Capsular superior attachment
10. Capsular inferior attachment
11. Superior joint space
12. Inferior joint space
13. Superior head of the lateral pterygoid muscle (LPM)
14. Inferior head of the LPM

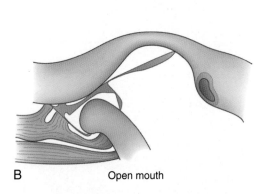

A    Closed mouth

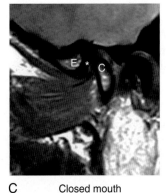

B    Open mouth

C    Closed mouth

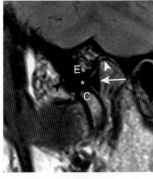

D    Open mouth

**Fig. 14.4  Normal temporomandibular joint (TMJ) anatomy.** Schematic of the TMJ in sagittal oblique plane demonstrates normal anatomic relationships in the (A) closed- and (B) open-mouth positions. Note how the mandibular condyle translates forward anteriorly on mouth opening to allow for disk recapture. (C) Sagittal oblique proton density (PD) image in closed-mouth position shows the mandibular condyle *(C)*, articular eminence *(E)*, and normal disk position *(asterisk)* relative to these structures. (D) Sagittal oblique PD image in the open-mouth position shows the normal position of the articular disk *(asterisk)* juxtaposed between the articular eminence *(E)* and condyle *(C)*, indicating appropriate recapture of the disk. The posterior band *(white arrow)*, superior retrodiskal later *(white arrowhead)*, and superior *(black arrowhead)* and inferior capsular *(black arrow)* attachments, are shown. From Mukherji SK, Fatterpekar G, Castillo M, et al. Imaging of congenital anomalies of the branchial apparatus. *Neuroimaging Clin North Am.* 2000;10:76–77.)

sympathetic nervous plexus, branches of the ansa cervi-calis (C1–C3 roots), and cranial and lymph nodes within and around the carotid sheath.

## RETROPHARYNGEAL SPACE

■ The retropharyngeal space is defined by the deep cervical fascia and is located deep to the pharyngeal mucosa and anterior to the longus colli and capitis muscles. The normal contents of the retropharyngeal space include fat and lymph nodes above the hyoid bone and fat alone below the hyoid bone, with the occasional carotid artery making an appearance (Fig. 14.6). The retropharyngeal space extends from the base of the skull to the upper thoracic spinal level. This is a site for potential spread of disease from pharyngeal or esophageal lesions.

■ The "danger space" refers to a potential space associated with the retropharyngeal space. It arises from splitting of layers of the deep cervical fascia's deep layer into the

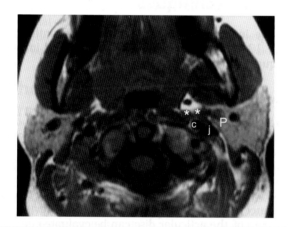

**Fig. 14.5 Normal parapharyngeal space.** Axial T1-weighted imaging shows the high signal intensity of the prestyloid parapharyngeal space fat *(arrowhead)*, anteromedial to the deep lobe of the parotid gland *(P)*. Separating the prestyloid and poststyloid parapharyngeal space is the styloid musculature *(asterisks)*. Directly behind the styloid musculature, one can identify the carotid artery *(c)* and jugular vein *(j)* within the carotid space. On computed tomography, the styloid process may be the best anatomic landmark to separate the two spaces.

alar fascia, ventral to the perivertebral space. Whereas the middle layer of the deep cervical fascia fuses with the deep layer at T6, the split in the deep layer may track to the level of the diaphragm.

■ Distinguishing this anatomic location from its neighbor the prevertebral space can be tricky. Lesions in retropharyngeal space displace fat anterolaterally and remain anterior to longus musculature, whereas a prevertebral space mass displaces the muscle anteriorly or is intrinsic to them.

## PERIVERTEBRAL SPACE

■ The perivertebral space refers to space in front of (prevertebral) and within, behind, and on the side of the cervical spine (posterolateral neck). The deep cervical fascia of the perivertebral space encircles the paraspinal and prevertebral muscles, the vertebral bodies, the nerves, and vessels.

■ Contents include the longus colli-capitis muscle complex, the paraspinal musculature, the vertebral body, the posterior triangles of the neck, the neurovascular structures within the spinal canal, and the brachial plexus.

■ Perivertebral space lesions displace the longus colli musculature anteriorly and, when large enough, displace the parapharyngeal fat anterolaterally.

## BRACHIAL PLEXUS

■ The *brachial plexus* is considered a part of the perivertebral space. The brachial plexus is derived from the C5-T1 cervical nerve roots and runs between the anterior and middle scalene muscles and then with the subclavian artery to the level of the clavicles to supply the upper extremity (Fig. 14.7). At that point, the plexus runs with the axillary artery, posterior to the larger axillary vein.

■ Try this mnemonic for remembering brachial plexus anatomy: "Rad Techs Drink Cold Beer." Roots merge into Trunks (upper, middle, and lower) at the scalene muscular triangle. Trunks divide into Divisions (anterior and posterior) and form Cords (lateral, posterior, and middle) at the clavicle. Cords form Branches in a painfully complicated manner.

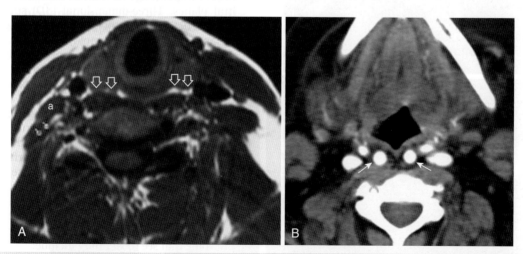

**Fig. 14.6 Retropharyngeal space.** (A) The normal fat of the retropharyngeal space is indicated with *open arrows*. The prevertebral musculature is located posterior to the retropharyngeal space. As a prequel to the brachial plexus section in this chapter, also noted on this image are the anterior scalene muscle *(a)* and the brachial plexus coursing posteriorly to this muscle *(open small arrows)*. (B) Note the medial location of both internal carotid arteries *(arrows)* in the retropharyngeal space. Careful, spine surgeons, take note before you start your anterior approach spinal fusion!

- **A first branchial cleft anomaly** classically occurs in the parotid gland or around the external auditory canal (EAC). Patients present in adulthood with recurrent facial swelling that can become painful if infected.
  - On CT and MRI, these typically show fluid density and intensity characteristics, but if infected or traumatized, their appearance may be a bit more complex with thick rim enhancement (Fig. 14.9).
- **A second branchial cleft anomaly** is the most common of the four branchial cleft anomalies and may occur anywhere from the palatine tonsil to the supraclavicular region, but most are found near the angle of the mandible lateral to the carotid sheath (Fig. 14.10). The Bailey classification (type I–IV) can help characterize location of 2nd branchial cleft, including cysts superficial to sternocleidomastoid muscle (type I), tucked in the space bounded by sternocleidomastoid muscle, submandibular gland and carotid sheath (type II, most common), between internal and external carotid arteries (type III) and medial to carotid sheath within the parapharyngeal or pharyngeal mucosal space (type IV).
  - On CT and MRI, look for a fluid attenuation/signal well-circumscribed rounded lesion tucked behind the submandibular gland, deep to the sternocleidomastoid muscle, with the carotid sheath along its anteromedial aspect. Rim enhancement can indicate

superinfection, a common scenario that can bring these cysts to clinical attention.
- **Third and fourth branchial cleft anomalies** are very rare, more common on the left side near the thyroid gland, and not easily distinguishable from each other on imaging (Fig. 14.11). Suppurative thyroiditis may occur from bacterial infection or complication of the third and fourth branchial cleft fistulae from the piriform sinus that inflame the adjacent thyroid gland. These can be associated with a small cutaneous opening at the level of the clavicle.
  - An inflamed thyroid gland can be diffusely enlarged with surrounding stranding. Look for adjacent organized rim-enhancing fluid collection. The abscess can be clinically managed, and once the infection is under control, the culprit branchial cleft anomaly can be identified on a swallow study as a fistulous or sinus tract originating from the piriform sinus.

## BENIGN NEOPLASMS

- **Neurogenic tumors** (*schwannomas and neurofibromas*) are benign neoplasms that can be seen in multiple head and neck spaces, including masticator, carotid, and perivertebral spaces.
  - Isolated schwannomas are the most common neurogenic tumor of the masticator space.

**Table 14.2**    Branchial Cleft Cysts

| Features | BCC type 1 | BCC type 2 | BCC type 3 | BCC type 4 |
|---|---|---|---|---|
| % of all BCCs | 7 | 90 | 2 | 1 |
| Location | Inferoposteromedial to pinna | Anterior to mid SCM, deep to ICA | Anterior to lower SCM, superficial | Low, anterior to SCM |
| | Angle of mandible to EAC | Angle of mandible | | Left side in 90% |
| | Periparotid | At CCA bifurcation | | Follows recurrent laryngeal nerve |
| | | Parapharyngeal | | |
| Sinus drainage | Ear, skin | Tonsillar fossa, skin | Pyriform sinus | Pyriform apex |
| Etiology | Persistent cleft | Failure of arch to proliferate, persistent cervical sinus | Persistent cervical sinus | Persistent cervical sinus |

*BCC*, Branchial cleft cyst; *CCA*, common carotid artery; *EAC*, external auditory canal; *ICA*, internal carotid artery; *SCM*, sternocleidomastoid muscle.

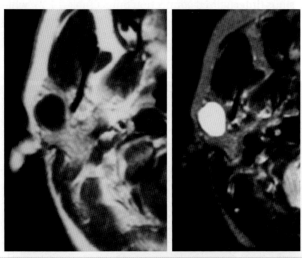

**Fig. 14.9  First branchial cleft cyst (BCC).** This intraparotid cyst with a sharply defined wall is dark on T1-weighted imaging (T1WI) (to the *left*) and very bright on T2WI (image on the *right*). There is no way of knowing whether this is an inflammatory cyst, a posttraumatic sialocele, or a BCC based on imaging alone.

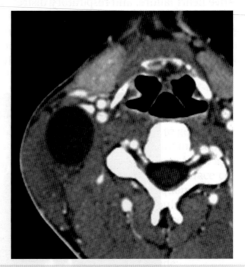

**Fig. 14.10  Second branchial cleft cyst (BCC).** On this axial contrast-enhanced computed tomography (CT) image, this cyst lies deep to the sternocleidomastoid muscle, posterior to the submandibular gland, and posterolateral to the carotid space, a typical location for 2nd BCC, Bailey type II.

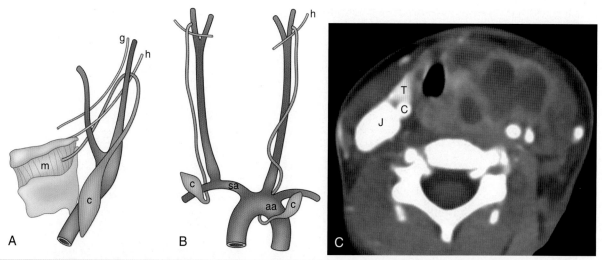

**Fig. 14.11 Third and fourth branchial cleft cysts.** (A) Third branchial cleft cyst anomaly. The cyst tract typically ascends posterior to the internal carotid artery. It then courses medially to pass over the hypoglossal nerve *(h)* and below the glossopharyngeal nerve *(g)*. It then pierces the posterolateral thyrohyoid membrane *(m)* to communicate with the pyriform sinus. (B) Fourth branchial cleft cyst anomaly. The nonkeratinized stratified squamous epithelium-lined cysts are located anterior to the aortic arch on the *left* and the subclavian artery on the *right,* respectively. The sinus tract is seen to hook inferiorly around the adjacent vascular structures (like the recurrent laryngeal nerve) and ascends to the level of the hypoglossal nerve posterior to the common and internal carotid arteries. It then loops over the hypoglossal nerve to pass deep to the internal carotid artery. (C) This patient had a fourth branchial cleft cyst that got recurrently infected. There is a rim-enhancing fluid collection in the left perithyroidal soft tissues, displacing the trachea to the right. The normal thyroid gland *(T)*, carotid artery *(C)*, and jugular vein *(J)* are indicated on the *right. aa,* Aortic arch; *c,* cyst; *h,* hypoglossal nerve; *sa,* subclavian artery. (A and B from Mukherji SK, Fatterpekar G, Castillo M, et al. Imaging of congenital anomalies of the branchial apparatus. *Neuroimaging Clin North Am.* 2000;10:89, 92.)

- Schwannomas can be seen in the carotid space, arising from cranial nerves IX to XII, the sympathetic plexus, or cervical spine nerve roots. These are often situated posterior to the carotid artery. Vagus nerve schwannomas tend to displace the carotid artery and parapharyngeal fat in an anteromedial direction (Fig. 14.12). Clues that the lesion may arise from a specific nerve other than the vagus include tongue atrophy (XII), sternocleidomastoid or trapezius atrophy (XI), neural foraminal enlargement (cervical root origin), or Horner syndrome (sympathetic plexus origin). Uvular deviation suggests the vagus, and IX may affect smaller pharyngeal muscles.
- Neurofibromas can be isolated or multiple or plexiform (permeative, involving multiple head and neck spaces). Plexiform neurofibromas occur in patients with neurofibromatosis type 1 (NF1) and can be very extensive (Fig. 14.13). Neurofibromas of the brachial plexus outnumber schwannomas.
  - On MRI, both schwannomas and neurofibromas can appear as T1 dark, centrally T2 dark, and peripherally T2 bright (target sign). Both tumor types enhance, and enhancement of neurofibromas tend to be more limited compared with schwannomas in general, although this is not always the case.
  - On CT, these tumors can be isodense to muscle, and there can be remodeling changes of the adjacent bony structures (not erosion, which would imply a more aggressive process).
  - Occasionally, schwannomas may be cystic and demonstrate characteristic density and intensity features for cyst fluid. Schwannomas also may show internal hemorrhage.

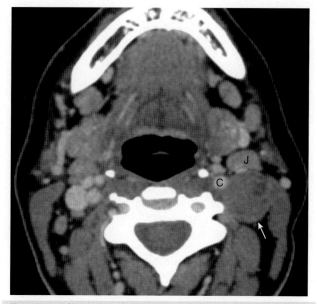

**Fig. 14.12 Schwannoma in carotid space.** Axial computed tomography shows a low-density schwannoma *(arrow)*. The carotid artery *(C)* is displaced anteromedially and the jugular vein *(J)* anteriorly by the mass. The mass is relatively isoattenuating to muscle.

- **Lipomas** are fatty tumors that can occur anywhere in the head and neck (Fig. 14.14) but have a predilection for the lateral subcutaneous tissues, the supraclavicular fossa, and the posterior perivertebral space.
  - Lipomas on imaging appear as localized, homogeneously fat density/intensity masses with or without a capsule. Fat suppression techniques on MRI can make

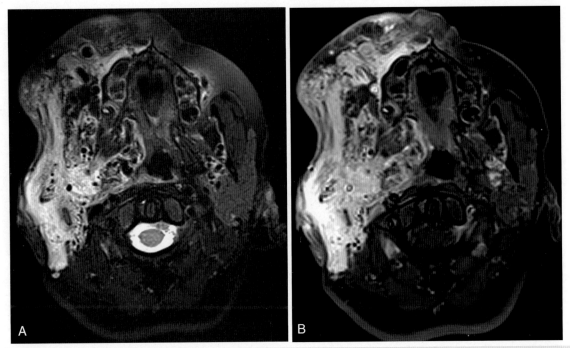

**Fig. 14.13 Plexiform neurofibroma in patient with neurofibromatosis type 1 (NF1).** (A) Axial fat-suppressed T2-weighted imaging (T2WI) and (B) axial fat-suppressed T1-weighted imaging (T1WI) shows extensively infiltrative T2 bright, avidly enhancing mass involving the parotid, masticator, carotid, parapharyngeal and perivertebral spaces, consistent with plexiform neurofibroma.

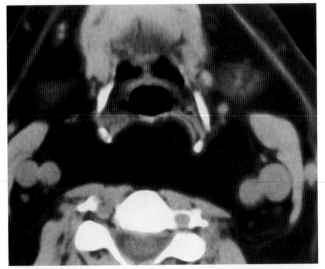

**Fig. 14.14 Lipoma of the retropharyngeal space.** The computed tomography shows a mass anterior to the longus muscles, which has fat density. It is posterior to the pharyngeal musculature and resides in the retropharyngeal space.

this a slam dunk diagnosis. There should be no enhancement. If nodular areas of soft tissue or enhancement are seen, then liposarcoma should be suspected.

■ Madelung disease is a massive lipomatosis predominantly affecting the posterior part of the neck, seen most typically in the context of chronic alcohol use. Fatty deposition is focused in the neck and trunk, giving an overall "athletic" appearance, but it's not muscle! Patients present with respiratory symptoms secondary to tracheal compression, neuropathies, weakness, macrocytic anemia, and venous stasis.

## LYMPHADENOPATHY

■ Lymph nodes are present throughout the neck and, as such, nodal disease can be seen in just about every anatomy space in the neck. Adenopathy may be associated with either infectious, inflammatory, or neoplastic disease.

■ Sources of malignant adenopathy can be from nasopharyngeal (most common) and oropharyngeal cancers , lymphoma and leukemia. Other sources of lymphadenopathy include papillary carcinoma of the thyroid gland and malignant melanoma. Invasion or encasement of the carotid artery or jugular vein by malignant lymphadenopathy can be seen (Fig. 14.15).

■ Because the parotid gland contains lymph nodes that drain the scalp and external auditory canal, it is not usual for dermal-based neoplasms (e.g., melanoma, squamous cell carcinoma [SCC]) to metastasize to the parotid lymph nodes. Look for enlarged enhancing masses within the parotid gland and then check the adjacent skin for the primary lesion.

■ Clinical and imaging features of nodal disease are discussed in detail in Chapter 13, but generally heterogeneously enhancing, necroticlymph nodes with loss of fatty hilum should raise suspicion for nodal disease. Lymphoma can appear as enlarged lymph nodes with low T2 signal and low apparent diffusion coefficient (ADC) values. Although it is often difficult to identify subtle extranodal tumor extension on imaging, if we see breach of the nodal capsule and/or tumor extension into the perinodal soft tissues, we should raise concern for radiographic extranodal tumor extension, which can have implications for treatment and prognosis.

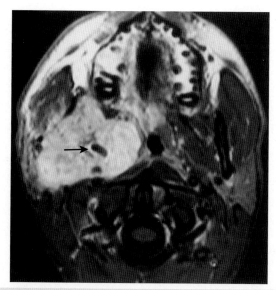

**Fig. 14.15 Carotid space adenopathy encasing the carotid artery.** When the carotid artery is encircled by tumor *(arrow)*, you can bet that the surgeons will call the mass unresectable. If the tumor envelops less than 270 degrees of the vessel's circumference, it may be saved.

## Pathology Isolated to Specific Extramucosal Spaces

### PAROTID, SUBMANDIBULAR, AND SUBLINGUAL SPACES

#### Inflammatory Disorders

- **Calculous disease** is the most common benign condition to affect the salivary glands, and calculi are most common in the Wharton duct because of the alkaline nature of the secretions and because of the anatomic course of the duct, with the dependent portion prone to accumulation of stone precursors. Sublingual gland

calculi and minor salivary gland calculi are extremely uncommon. Parenchymal calculi can also occur and can be associated with human immunodeficiency virus (HIV) infection, chronic kidney disease, alcoholism, and autoimmune disease, including sarcoidosis and systemic lupus erythematosus.

- Patients with intraductal calculi can present with painful facial swelling, exacerbated by chewing foods that precipitate salivation.
- CT is often performed for the detection of calcification and associated inflammation within and around the affected salivary gland (sialadenitis). Some advocate for noncontrast CT to identify the stone and contrast-enhanced CT to identify the associated inflammation, but in most cases, the stone can be detected on post-contrast images, obviating the need for a noncontrast CT (Fig. 14.16). The inflamed gland is enlarged and hyperenhancing, and microabscesses may be present.
- Thin section imaging by MRI can show ductal filling defects or stenosis that can cause salivary gland inflammation (Fig. 14.17). This is a bit more palatable than the sialogram option, in which contrast is injected into the parotid gland ductal system under fluoroscopy.
- Treatment consistent of sour solutions to stimulate saliva product, and sialodochoplasty can be performed for isolated distal duct (close to ampulla) sialoliths.
- Chronic sialadenitis from sialolithiasis of the submandibular gland can result in a sclerosing sialadenitis appearing as a firm benign inflammatory pseudomass associated with calcifications (Kuttner tumor).
- Rarely, mucus plugging can cause a painful swollen gland (Kussmaul disease).
- **Sialosis** is painless enlargement of the parotid glands, usually bilateral and symmetric, with numerous causes, including diabetes, alcoholism, hypothyroidism, medications like phenothiazines and some diuretics, obesity, starvation, radiation, and idiopathic causes.

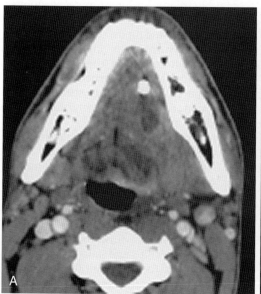
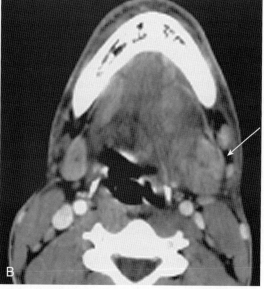

**Fig. 14.16 Submandibular sialadenitis.** (A) A large stone with a dilated Wharton duct is seen in the left sublingual space. (B) Note the swollen submandibular gland *(arrow)* with the effaced sublingual space fat planes.

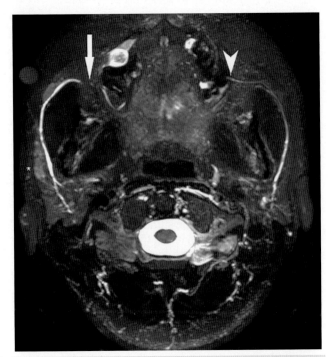

**Fig. 14.17 Parotid ductal obstruction.** Axial T2-weighted imaging (T2WI) shows a normal thin gracile left parotid duct terminating at its expected location at the maxillary molar tooth level *(arrowhead)*. On the other side, however, the duct is enlarged, and terminates abruptly at a point of stenosis *(arrow)*. The anterior aspect of the right parotid gland *(*)* is hyperintense, from chronic inflammation. On interrogation of the duct by an ear, nose, and throat specialist, debris was found to the cause of obstruction, and the patient got much need relief after debris was removed.

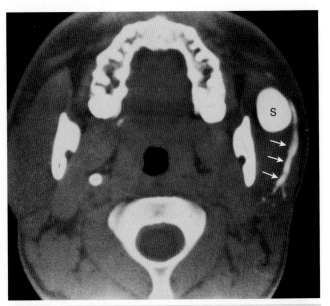

**Fig. 14.18 Posttraumatic sialocele.** Axial computed tomography after left parotid sialography demonstrates opacification of a sialocele *(s)*. One can see the normal parotid duct *(arrows)* coursing to and communicating with the sialocele on the left side. This patient had been punched in the left side of the face.

- On imaging, patients generally have a CT density and signal intensity on T2WI slightly greater than that of normal parotid glands. Glands in sialosis usually are not as bright on T2WI as glands that are infected.
- **Sialadenitis** is a common reason for imaging the salivary glands, usually by CT. Pathogens include mumps, HIV, Coxsackie, and influenza viruses resulting in bilateral inflammation. Bacterial infection can be unilateral or bilateral, most often by *Streptococcus*, *Haemophilus*, and *Staphylococcus*.
  - An infected gland will be enlarged and hyperenhancing with surrounding fat stranding. Look for associated rim-enhancing fluid collections because abscesses will likely require surgical drainage.
- **Sialoceles** are collections of salivary secretions that communicate with the parent duct, similar to that of a pharyngocele or a laryngocele filled with fluid (Fig. 14.18). The most common cause is penetrating trauma (punch or stab wounds), and these most commonly occur in the parotid gland. These are distinguished from pseudocysts because they communicate with the parent duct and are not lined by fibrous tissue.
  - A fluid density/intensity cyst in and around the salivary gland in the proper clinical setting can indicate the presence of sialocele.
- **Ranula**, on the other hand, is a postinflammatory pseudocystic lesion caused by obstruction and focal rupture of either the sublingual or submandibular duct producing a cystic mass.

- Ranulas are fluid density/intensity well circumscribed collections confined by the mylohyoid muscle (simple ranula) or extending to the submandibular region (plunging ranula) by passing through the mylohyoid dehiscence known as the "boutonniere" (see Fig. 13.9).
- Treatment for simple ranula involves transoral resection or marsupialization, while for a plunging ranula, it requires transcervical submandibular incision with a neck dissection.
- **Sarcoidosis** in one of several inflammatory processes that can affect the salivary glands. Sarcoidosis may manifest as bilaterally enlarged glands with multifocal nodules, and gallium uptake on nuclear medicine scans may be striking. Multiple tiny calcifications in the parotid glands may be seen in sarcoidosis, Sjögren syndrome, tuberculosis, and lupus.
- **Sjögren syndrome** is another systemic autoimmune disease that can affect the salivary glands. Punctate, globular, cavitary, or destructive appearance of the ducts of the parotid glands can be seen. Parotid gland appearance may range from normal to a dried-up, scarred-down, atrophic gland.
  - In Sjögren syndrome, imaging can show a gland with lots of benign, large, and/or tiny cysts and nodules (lymphoepithelial lesions), a finding that can also be seen with HIV (Fig. 14.19).
  - Occasionally, a dominant mass may be seen in the background of chronic inflammation, which can represent aggressive lymphoma.
- **Mikulicz disease** is an autoimmune disease that causes chronic sialadenitis and sialodochitis and leads to fibrous salivary gland tissue (primarily of the minor glands) with resultant dry mouth. It most often occurs among middle-aged females and may be seen in the setting of collagen-vascular disease (rheumatoid arthritis, systemic lupus

erythematosus). Involvement of the lacrimal glands can coexist. These patients have a tenfold increased risk of developing lymphoma (non-Hodgkin variety).

## Benign Neoplasms

- **Pleomorphic adenoma**, also known as benign mixed tumor, is the most common salivary gland neoplasm and most commonly occurs in middle-aged females. Pleomorphic adenomas are often unicentric but may be multicentric in approximately 0.5% of cases.
  - On MRI, the large majority (80%) of pleomorphic adenomas are typically very bright on T2WI, reflecting its myxoid component (Fig. 14.20). A complete surrounding capsule is associated with these lesions, with the capsule often appearing as a rim of low signal

intensity on T2WI. They usually enhance homogeneously. On an ADC map, these lesions typically have higher ADC values compared with other benign and malignant salivary gland masses.
  - On CT, these lesions are isodense to muscle and demonstrate mild to moderate enhancement.
  - These lesions are challenging to excise and there can be recurrence at the surgical site following resection. Additionally, pleomorphic adenomas may degenerate into or coexist with a carcinoma ex pleomorphic adenoma in approximately 10% to 25% of cases within 25 years, and for this reason, despite overall likelihood of benignity, these tumors need to be completely excised. It is currently not known whether carcinoma is present within the pleomorphic adenoma from its outset (malignant mixed tumor) or whether this is a manifestation of malignant transformation (carcinoma ex pleomorphic adenoma) (Fig. 14.21).
- **Warthin tumor** (also known as cystadenoma lymphomatosum) is a benign tumor that can be cystic or lymphoma-like in appearance. It is most commonly seen in elderly men and smokers and almost exclusively occurs in the parotid gland, with preference for the parotid tail. Warthin tumors most commonly occur as multicentric and bilateral tumors in the parotid glands. These are entirely benign and show no evidence of malignant transformation.

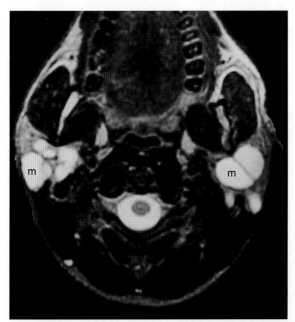

**Fig. 14.19 Lymphoepithelial lesions associated with human immunodeficiency virus (HIV).** Both parotid glands have multiple high intensity masses *(m)* on this fat-suppressed fast spin-echo T2-weighted imaging, typical of lymphoepithelial .

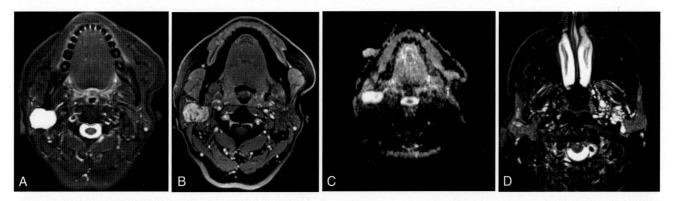

**Fig. 14.20 Pleomorphic adenoma.** (A) T2-weighted image (T2WI) shows T2 hyperintense mass in the right parotid gland which could be mistaken for cyst if not for postcontrast T1-weighted image (T1WI), (B) which shows the mass to be solid and heterogeneously enhancing. (C) ADC values in the lesion are noted to be very high. This was a pathologically proven pleomorphic adenoma. (D) T2WI in a different patient status postresection of pleomorphic adenoma years ago who now presents with neck swelling. This image demonstrates recurrent pleomorphic adenoma at the operative site, shows as T2 bright nodules in the left parapharyngeal space.

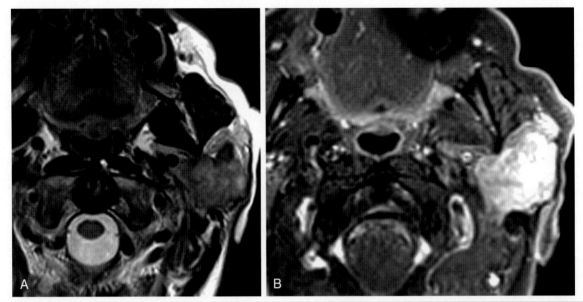

**Fig. 14.21 Meet the ex: carcinoma ex pleomorphic adenoma, that is.** (A) Axial T2-weighted image (T2WI) shows a heterogeneous signal mass replacing most of the left parotid gland. (B) The mass enhances on postcontrast fat-suppressed T1-weighted image (T1WI). On resection, carcinoma was seen arising from a pleomorphic adenoma histopathologically.

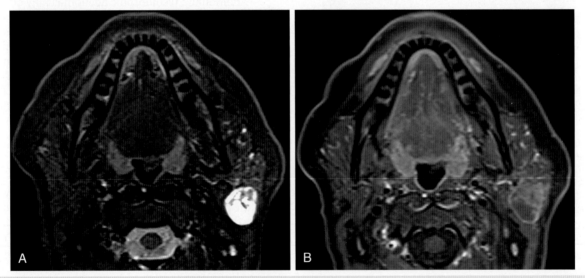

**Fig. 14.22 Warthin tumor.** (A) Axial T2-weighted imaging (T2WI) shows heterogenous but predominantly bright mass in the left parotid gland. (B) Postcontrast T1-weighted imaging (T1WI) demonstrates heterogeneous enhancement. Histopathology revealed Warthin tumor.

**TEACHING POINTS**

Differential Diagnosis for Multiple Masses in the Parotid Gland

Oncocytomas
Lymph nodes (normal or abnormal)
Lymphoepithelial lesions
Lymphoma
Pleomorphic adenomas
Metastases
Warthin tumors
Sarcoidosis
Sjogren syndrome
Acinic cell carcinomas

- On MRI, these lesions appear as hyperintense masses on T1WI, with heterogeneous signal intensity on T2WI. The bright signal on T2WI overlaps with the appearance of the bright signal of pleomorphic adenomas (Fig. 14.22). Warthin tumors can also have low T2 signal intensity sharing overlap with the darker intensity of malignancies of the parotid gland (see the next section).

- Warthin tumors have increased uptake on technetium 99 m pertechnetate nuclear medicine scans. Therefore, if a fine-needle aspiration (FNA) is equivocal or nondiagnostic, you could recommend a nuclear medicine technetium scan to make the diagnosis of Warthin tumor.

- **Oncocytomas** are a relatively rare benign tumor, almost exclusively seen in the parotid gland and can be single or multiple, unilateral or bilateral. These are called the "vanishing parotid mass" because they are often hypointense on T1WI to parotid gland tissue but are isointense to parotid tissue (and therefore imperceptible) on fat saturated T2 and postcontrast T1 imaging. These tumors may also take up technetium on nuclear medicine scans.

## Malignant Neoplasms

- In the adult population, sublingual gland lesions have a higher rate of malignancy than submandibular gland lesions, with parotid gland lesions having the lowest rate of malignancy. In the pediatric population, parotid gland lesions have higher rates of malignancy than submandibular and sublingual gland lesions.

- Malignant parotid gland lesions often present as palpable, discrete, and painless masses (98% of the time); however, patients may present with facial nerve dysfunction (24%) and cervical lymphadenopathy (6%). Facial nerve paralysis is a worrisome finding concerning for perineural tumor spread, a feature most commonly associated with adenoid cystic carcinoma and undifferentiated carcinoma.

- When evaluating a potentially malignant lesion in the parotid gland, it is important to delineate superficial versus deep parotid malignancies. This delineation helps to determine the extent of dissection needed to separate the nerve from the tumor and the surgical approach. It is important for the radiologist to evaluate for perineural extension of tumor at the stylomastoid foramen (or above), which will prod the surgeon to plan for transmastoid (temporal bone) surgery. Additionally, if the skull base is invaded, the cartilaginous external auditory canal may have to be resected.

- Keep in mind that although T2 hyperintensity and high ADC values can strongly favor pleomorphic adenoma, there are no reliable imaging features to determine the histopathology of salivary gland neoplasms. In particular, assessment of lesion margins is not reliable because both benign and malignant processes in the salivary glands can present as either circumscribed or infiltrative lesions. Similarly, T2 signal is variable among these malignant processes, although mucoepidermoid cancer may have higher T2 signal compared with other malignancies. Malignant tumors often enhance, have lower ADC values, and have lower blood flow and blood volume on perfusion imaging (compared with benign parotid tumors and in contradistinction to brain tumors).

- Rather than making histopathologic diagnoses, the role of the radiologist in these cases is to identify the location of the lesion (e.g., superficial versus deep parotid gland) and to assess for extraglandular spread, perineural tumor spread, intracranial involvement, and lymphadenopathy, as can be seen in the setting of malignant disease.

- Metastatic adenopathy is uncommon with primary salivary neoplasms, but mucoepidermoid carcinoma and SCC can metastasize to nodes in 37% to 44% of cases.

- **Mucoepidermoid carcinoma** represents 30% of all salivary gland malignancies and is the most common malignant lesion of the parotid gland (60% occur in the parotid gland; Fig. 14.23). Like SCC, mucoepidermoid carcinoma can be graded from low to high grade, with prognosis varying with tumor grade. This is also the most common pediatric salivary gland malignancy.

- **Adenoid cystic carcinoma** (ACC) is the second most common primary malignancy of the parotid and the most common tumor of the submandibular, sublingual,

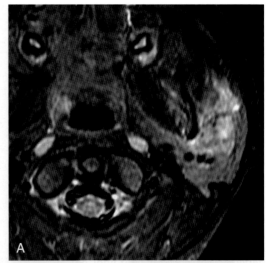

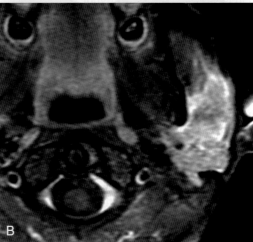

**Fig. 14.23 Mucoepidermoid carcinoma.** (A) Axial T2-weighted imaging (T2WI) scan shows a poorly defined heterogeneous signal lesion in the parotid gland focally invading the adjacent masseter and pterygoid musculature. (B) Axial fat-suppressed contrast-enhanced T1-weighted imaging (T1WI) shows heterogeneous enhancement in the mass and the invasive component in the masseter muscle. Invasive mass in the parotid in a kid? Best guess is mucoepidermoid carcinoma, which this turned out to be.

and minor salivary glands. Persistent disease is often noted with ACC despite "complete surgical resection" often being described at the time of surgery. This is a relentless, slow-growing tumor. Prognosis is generally measured in decades because of its prolonged course.

- ACC is notorious for perineural tumor spread (seen in 50%–60% of cases). It may spread via the facial nerve in retrograde fashion into the temporal bone. It may also spread via the auriculotemporal branches of cranial nerve V to the Meckel cave region through the foramen ovale (Fig. 14.24). Tumor can also spread from from the facial nerve intracranially along the greater superficial petrosal nerve to gain access to the vidian canal and pterygopalatine fossa. When ACC occurs in the other salivary glands, it may extend along branches of the second and third divisions of cranial nerve V and head intracranially.

- **SCC** can be seen in the parotid gland. It can be difficult to tell if SCC is present secondarily because of invasion of

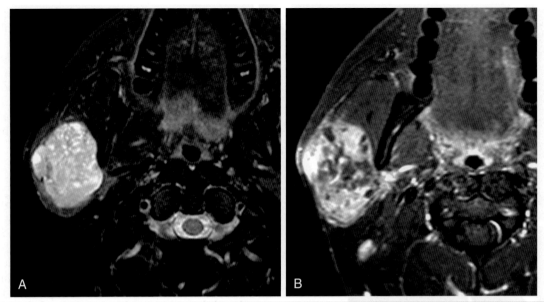

**Fig. 14.26 Acinic cell carcinoma.** (A) Axial T2-weighted image (T2WI) shows a well-circumscribed mass in the right parotid gland. So you're thinking pleo, right? (B) The mass enhances heterogeneously on T1-weighted image (T1WI). This turned out to be acinic cell carcinoma. Thank goodness for fine-needle aspirations!

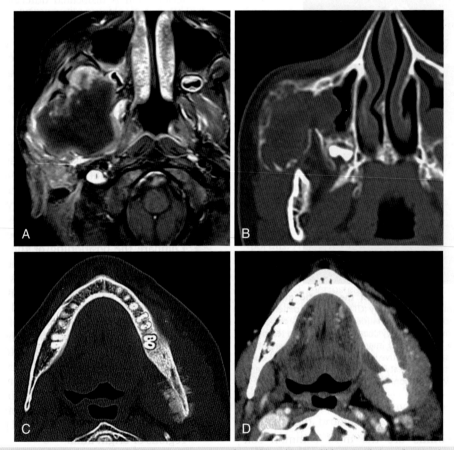

**Fig. 14.27 Sarcomas at the masticator space.** (A) Ewing sarcoma arising from the right mandible extends into the masticator space on this post-contrast axial T1-weighted image (T1WI). (B) Axial computed tomography (CT) in a different patient with Ewing sarcoma shows expansile destructive mass arising from the right zygoma projecting posteriorly towards the masticator space. (C) Axial CT in bone window in another patient shows marked sclerosis of the left mandible with striking periosteal reaction. This was an osteosarcoma that developed in a patient who underwent radiation therapy for oral squamous cell carcinoma (double bummer). (D) CT in soft-tissue window in this same patient shows soft-tissue tumor involvement of the masseter and pterygoid muscles (compare to size on the normal right side) and fluid component along the buccal and lingual surfaces of the mandible.

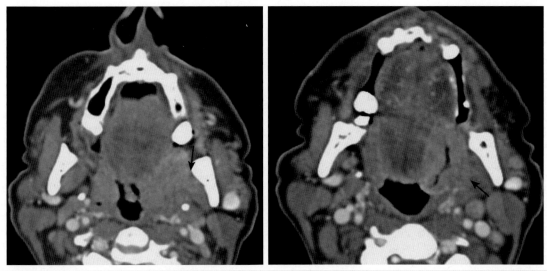

**Fig. 14.28 Squamous cell carcinoma extending into the masticator space.** This left tonsil/lateral base of tongue squamous cell carcinoma grew into the pterygoid musculature *(arrows)*, thereby invading the masticator space.

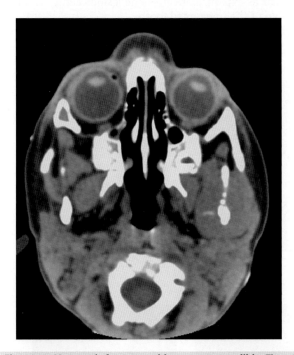

**Fig. 14.29 Metastasis from neuroblastoma to mandible.** There is a soft-tissue mass centered about the left mandible on this scan. Note that this is a child. Diagnosis: neuroblastoma metastasis.

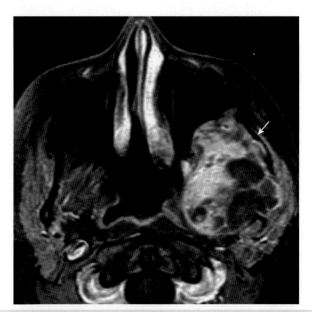

**Fig. 14.30 Rhabdomyosarcoma of masticator space.** Postcontrast T1-weighted imaging scan shows diffuse infiltration of the left masticator space by rhabdomyosarcoma. Note the remodeling of the left mandible *(arrow)* and posterolateral wall of the maxillary sinus.

- **Rheumatoid arthritis** in an inflammatory arthritis that can affect the TMJ and may appear as erosions of the mandibular condyle with an associated soft-tissue component (see Fig. 14.32B). Effusions, retrodiskal edema and meniscal perforations also complicate the rheumatoid joint. Postcontrast images can show the enhancing synovial proliferation.

- Additional disorders of the TMJ include synovial chondromatosis, characterized by calcified and ossified fragments within the joint space; calcium pyrophosphate dihydrate (CPPD) deposition disease, characterized by heterogeneous calcification within an expanded joint space (Fig. 14.33); and pigmented villonodular synovitis,

characterized by hemosiderin or other blood products seen as dark signal on T2* MR.

- **Bruxism** may manifest as bilateral enlargement of the muscles of mastication. It is most commonly idiopathic but may develop as a result of malocclusion, excessive chewing, or clenching the teeth. Rarely, this may be a unilateral phenomenon. Conditions that can result in an enlarged appearance of the muscles of mastication are listed.

- **Atrophy** of the muscles of mastication can occur in the setting of cranial nerve V abnormality (Fig. 14.34). This may occur as a result of neurogenic tumors or perineural spread of disease occurring along the peripheral branches of the third division of cranial nerve V, operative injury, and trauma.

- **Fibrous dysplasia** can affect any bone in the skeleton and has a similar appearance at the jaw with expansion of the marrow space by ground glass attenuation and cortical thinning. There is usually no erosion through the bone. McCune-Albright syndrome includes precocious puberty, café-au-lait spots, and polyostotic fibrous dysplasia. This often may affect the mandible.

## Dentition/Jaw

- The **periapical or radicular cyst** is the most common dental-related cyst (Table 14.3). This is a lucent lesion of either the mandible or the maxilla and is associated

with an infected tooth (Fig. 14.35). Sequelae include osteomyelitis of the mandible or maxilla, subperiosteal abscesses, and facial cellulitis. If not addressed, the infection can become extensive, involving other soft tissues of the face and neck, causing airway compromise (Ludwig angina), thrombophlebitis, and vision loss (from orbital extension).

- On CT, look at the teeth for lucencies surrounding the suspected tooth root. There may also be dehiscence of the adjacent maxillary or mandibular cortex, and there might be an accompanying subperiosteal abscess. These can be tricky to spot but should appear as a lenticular-shaped fluid collection hugging the bony margin of the jaw with rim enhancement. Look for associated bony dehiscence and extension of inflammation into the adjacent soft tissues.

- Among the more common dental cysts (Fig. 14.36), the **dentigerous cyst** is a benign unilocular cyst associated with an unerupted tooth and is usually seen in the mandible, particularly around the molar region. On CT, these appear as expansile lucent bone lesions centered on the crown of the unerupted tooth.

- **Odontogenic keratocysts** (previously *keratocystic odontogenic tumor*) are benign but aggressive cystic

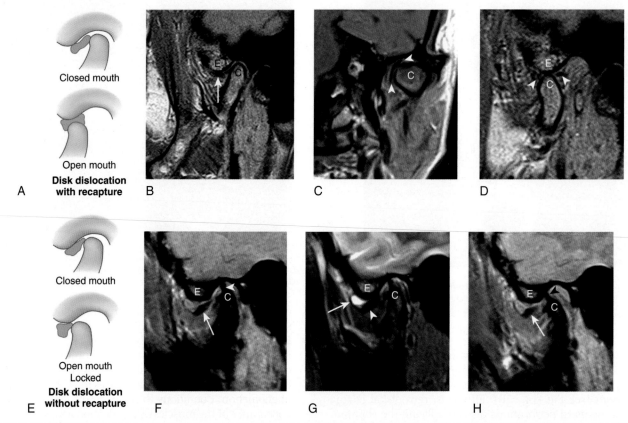

**Fig. 14.31** (A) Schematic representation of anterior disk dislocation on closed mouth view with appropriate recapture despite the dislocation on mouth opening. (B) PD image in closed-mouth position shows a thinned irregular anteriorly displaced disk *(arrow)* relative to the condyle *(C)*. Note relationship of the disk to the articular eminence *(E)*. (C) A coronal T1-weighted image shows that the disk *(between arrowheads)* is also medially dislocated relative to the condylar head *(C)*. (D) On mouth opening, despite its degenerative appearance, this disk *(between arrowheads)* does recapture appropriately between the condyle *(C)* and eminence *(E)*. (E) Schematic representation of anterior disk dislocation on closed-mouth view without appropriate recapture on mouth opening. Note how the condyle shows very limited anterior translation, giving the "locked" appearance. (F) PD image shows anteriorly displaced irregular disk on closed-mouth position *(arrow)*. The eminence *(E)* and condyle *(C)* position are noted. Note the osteophyte at the joint space *(arrowhead)* that's got to be very annoying. (G) Sagittal oblique T2 image shows the same anteriorly displaced disk *(arrowhead)*, condyle *(C)*, and eminence *(E)* on closed-mouth view. There is joint fluid present *(arrow)*, which can correlate with patient pain. (H) On mouth opening, the pesky osteophyte *(arrowhead)* limits anterior translation of the condyle *(C)*, and the displaced disk *(arrow)* does not recapture. Eminence indicated by E.

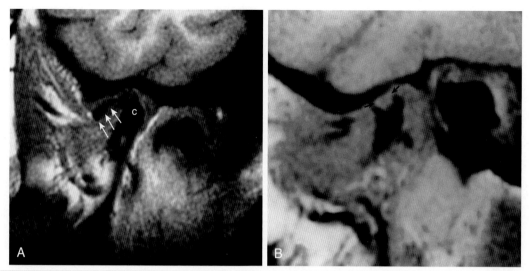

**Fig. 14.32 Avascular necrosis of the temporomandibular joint (TMJ).** (A) Sagittal T1-weighted imaging (T1WI) shows decreased intensity in the mandibular condyle marrow *(c)* in this patient with chronic TMJ syndrome. Note that the disk *(arrows)* is anteriorly dislocated in this closed mouth view. This patient had avascular necrosis of the condyle, confirmed by wedge resection. (B) Erosive synovitis of the TMJ. Note the erosion *(arrows)* of the condylar head on the sagittal T1WI in this patient with rheumatoid arthritis.

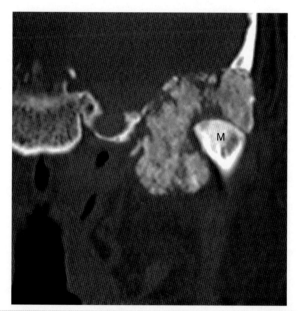

**Fig. 14.33 Calcium pyrophosphate dihydrate deposition disease (CPPD) of the TMJ.** Temporomandibular joint lesion shows a calcified matrix and destruction of the temporal bone making up the glenoid fossa. The differential diagnosis would include CPPD, synovial chondromatosis, chondrosarcoma, chondroblastoma, tumoral calcinosis, and Brown tumor. Final diagnosis: CPPD.

lesions most commonly affecting the mandible. They are associated with the basal cell nevus (Gorlin) syndrome, in which patients have proliferative falcine calcification, multiple basal cell carcinomas of the skin, scoliosis, ribbon-shaped ribs, central nervous system tumors, and keratocysts of the mandible Fig 14.36C. On CT, they appear as expansile, well-defined, lucent lesion of the jaws and, if large enough, can resorb roots of adjacent teeth. They are more commonly unilocular but can be multilocular too.

- **Ameloblastoma** is a benign neoplasm of the jaw that is hard to remove completely and has a high rate of recurrence (Fig. 14.37). Ameloblastoma is the second most common odontogenic tumor and arises in the mandible in 81% of cases. The molar region is affected in 70% of cases. The lesion is painless unless superinfected and has scalloped margins, multiloculation, and expanded cortical surfaces. Solid and cystic components are seen on MR with frequent mural nodules. Enhancement is marked in the periphery, not in the cysts. High intensity on T1WI sometimes occurs and may be because of hemorrhage or cholesterol crystal accumulation.
- **Sclerotic dental lesions** also span the spectrum of inflammatory, benign neoplastic, and malignant lesions (Table 14.4; Fig. 14.38). These are often challenging to come down hard on making a precise diagnosis (a task best left for pathologists), but it can be helpful to favor aggressive or nonaggressive processes by assessing margins (well defined favors nonaggressive lesions) and presence of extraosseous soft tissue (which implies a more aggressive nature).

# Prestyloid Parapharyngeal Space

- In the prestyloid parapharyngeal space, primary lesions are extremely uncommon, given the limited tissue types in this location (fat, ectopic minor salivary gland tissue, and lymph nodes). The most common intrinsic lesion involves enlarged lymph nodes, either inflammatory or neoplastic, followed by minor salivary gland tumors (with pleomorphic adenomas being the most common), and lipomas.

## INFECTIONS

- Infections may spread secondarily from (1) mucosal infections, such as tonsillitis or pharyngitis (Fig. 14.39); (2) masticator space lesions, such as odontogenic

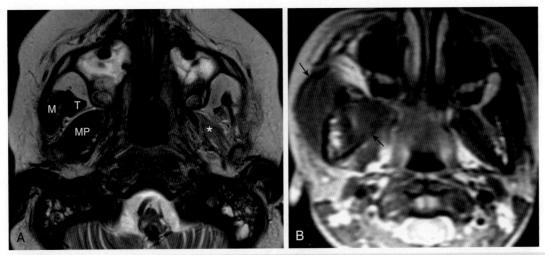

**Fig. 14.34 Unhappy muscles.** (A) Axial T2-weighted image in a young child with metastatic medulloblastoma involving the trigeminal nerve intracranially. There is marked atrophy of the left muscles of mastication *(asterisk)* because of V3 disease. Compare to the normal bulk of the medial pterygoid *(MP)*, and the insertions of the temporalis *(T)* and masseter *(M)* muscles on the right. (B) The muscles *(arrows)* on the right in a different patient are larger than the left (the normal side). This could be from malocclusion or a glycogen storage disease infiltration.

**Table 14.3**    Benign Lytic Dental Lesions

| Lesion | Imaging Appearance | Typical Clinical Findings |
|---|---|---|
| Ameloblastoma | Multiloculated (60% of cases) lytic lesion often associated with dentigerous cysts; hyperostotic margins; cortex eroded or penetrated | 85% in mandibular molar area with expanded jaw; painless, male predominance |
| Brown tumor | Lytic lesion with erosion of lamina dura; ill-defined borders | Hyperparathyroidism |
| Central odontogenic fibroma | Multilocular lesion with sclerotic borders | Expanded mandible |
| Cherubism | Bilateral, symmetric multilocular lucencies (soap bubble) in posterior mandible; expanded cortex without perforation; simulates fibrous dysplasia | Painless; bilateral enlargement of lower part of face; angelic appearance; autosomal dominant inheritance; regression after adolescence |
| Dentigerous (follicular) cyst | Lytic, lucent, expansile lesion adjacent to unerupted tooth; spares cortex; sclerotic margins | Unerupted asymptomatic third molar or canine tooth |
| Giant cell granuloma | Well-defined multilocular lucency with sclerotic margins involving mandible | Asymptomatic in children and young adults |
| Globulomaxillary cyst | Lucent lesion between lateral incisor and canine in maxilla | Asymptomatic |
| Incisive canal cyst (nasopalatine duct cyst) | Lucent lesion in midline hard palate with hyperostotic borders at canal | Usually asymptomatic |
| Keratocyst (primordial cyst) | Unilocular or multilocular expansile lucent lesion; erodes cortex but does not perforate it | Recurrent posterior mandibular lesion with thin walls; associated with basal cell nevus syndrome |
| Radicular (periapical) cyst | Lytic; lucent at apex of erupted tooth; loss of lamina dura; hyperostotic borders | Carious, tender nonvital tooth |

abscesses; or (3) parotid infections. Additionally, adenitis related to any of these primary infections may coexist.

## MALIGNANT NEOPLASMS

- Typically, malignant disease of the parapharyngeal space occurs secondary to spread from a mucosal space carcinoma. The nasopharynx and tonsils are the most frequent sources of secondary invasion of the parapharyngeal space.
- **Nasopharyngeal carcinoma** can invade the parapharyngeal space in 65% of cases at the time of diagnosis. This propensity for submucosal growth extending from the nasopharyngeal space means that the infiltration of the parapharyngeal fat may be the only indicator of a nasopharyngeal primary cancer.
- **Tonsillar carcinoma** can grow laterally with extension into the parapharyngeal fat. A tumor deep within the tonsillar crypts may escape the endoscopist's attention, and the radiologist may be the only one who can identify the primary tumor, on the basis of its infiltration of the parapharyngeal fat.
- **Synovial sarcomas** can occur in this locale. These lesions are not derived from the synovium and are unrelated to joints. These tumors may be well defined, with a propensity for fluid-fluid levels, intratumoral hemorrhage, calcifications, and cysts.

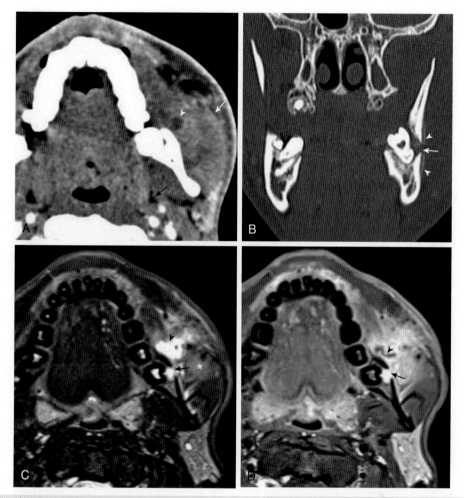

**Fig. 14.35  A plea to brush regularly.** (A) Axial contrast-enhanced computed tomography *(CT)* shows marked fullness of the left masseter muscle *(white arrow)* with low density, possibly necrotic component *(arrowhead)*. There is also fullness of the pterygoid musculature resulting in displacement of the parapharyngeal fat *(black arrow)*. Could this be a tumor? (B) Coronal CT shows periapical lucency surrounding the left mandibular molar tooth, with dehiscence of the buccal cortex *(arrow)* and periosteal reaction along the mandibular ramus *(arrowheads)*. Hmmm, this looks like a case of dental infection gone really bad, with extraosseous extension into the masticator soft tissues, abscess in the masseter, and osteomyelitis of the mandible. (C) Axial T2-weighted and (D) postcontrast T1-weighted images show the sinus tract from mandible to overlying soft tissues *(arrows)*, as well as the abscess *(arrowhead)*, and edema *(asterisk in C)* in the masseter muscle.

# Carotid Space/Poststyloid Parapharyngeal Space

### INFLAMMATORY LESIONS

- **Lemierre syndrome** refers to internal jugular vein thrombophlebitis and can be complicated by septic pulmonary emboli. This may occur because of pharyngitis or iatrogenic causes (e.g., secondary to venous line placement or surgery) (Fig. 14.40).
  - On CT and MRI, there will be absent opacification/flow-related signal within the jugular vein and branches. There can be a halo of edema around the thrombosed vein and enhancement of the vessel wall and the adjacent soft tissues.
- **Pseudoaneurysms** of the carotid artery may present as a neck mass and may be caused by parapharyngeal space abscesses, fibromuscular dysplasia, Ehlers-Danlos syndrome, trauma, surgery, neoplastic "blow-out" after radiation treatment in the setting of head and neck cancer (Fig. 14.41), or idiopathic etiologies.

- These can appear as soft-tissue masses abutting the carotid artery and can show variable enhancement if partially thrombosed. Mixed signal on MRI is common on the basis of partial thrombosis and flow-related signal. Look for pulsation artifacts on MRI that can indicate the vascular nature of this lesion.
- **Carotidynia** is a syndrome with symptoms including tenderness, swelling, or increased pulsations over the affected carotid artery. This is often a self-limited syndrome, lasting less than 2 weeks in duration and treated conservatively with nonsteroidal antiinflammatory medication. There is some controversy as to the precise terminology of this condition with some advocating the term be used to describe the clinical features and transient perivascular inflammation of the carotid artery (TIPIC) syndrome be used when imaging features are present.
  - On CT and MRI, this appears as an enhancing soft tissue around the distal common carotid artery and bifurcation region. Minimal vessel narrowing may be seen.
- **Glomus tumors**, also known as *paragangliomas*, are highly vascular tumors that demonstrate dramatic

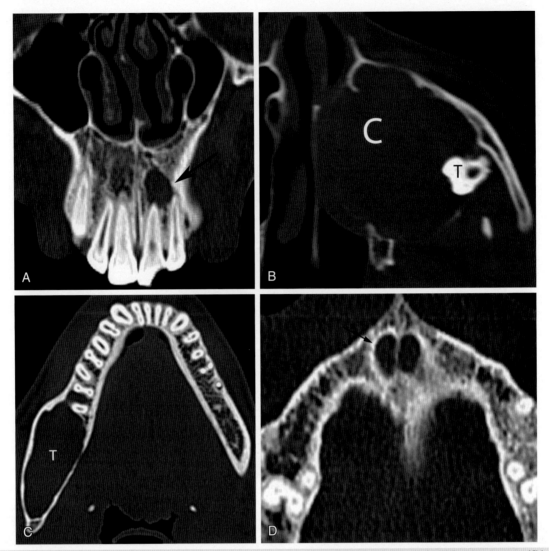

**Fig. 14.36 Common dental cysts.** (A) Radicular cyst *(arrow)* is at the root of a carious left central incisor tooth. (B) Dentigerous cyst *(C)* is associated with the crown of unerupted tooth *(T)*. (C) An odontogenic keratocyst may be oriented horizontally along the long plane of the mandible *(T)*. Note that the lesion splays the dentition rather than arising from the teeth and causes expansion of the medullary compartment with cortical remodeling. (D) Nasopalatine cyst *(arrow)* is a congenital cyst of the incisive canal and will therefore be midline in the maxilla.

enhancement and can present in the carotid space as glomus jugulare, glomus vagale, or carotid body tumors. A small percentage of patients have a familial incidence of glomus tumors. Rare reports of head and neck paragangliomas have been linked to multiple endocrine neoplasia (MEN) type 2 and von Hippel–Lindau disease. The multiplicity rate, including bilateral involvement, may be as high as 30%.

- Carotid body tumors (Fig. 14.42) arise at the carotid bulb and splay the internal and external carotid arteries away from each other. The external carotid artery is typically pushed posterolaterally, away from the internal carotid artery.
- Glomus jugulare tumors may grow through the skull base to involve the carotid space and may infiltrate the lumen of the jugular vein. Often, erosion of the jugular spine is the sine qua non at the skull base.
- Glomus vagale tumors may also present in the poststyloid parapharyngeal space (Fig. 14.43). These displace the carotid artery and external carotid artery anteriorly (as opposed to splaying it at the bifurcation like the carotid

body tumor). The internal jugular vein is displaced posteriorly. These tumors are from the nodose ganglion (one of the vagal ganglia in the upper neck) and lie in the carotid sheath. The most common level of involvement is near angle of the mandible and above the hyoid bone.

- Cranial nerves IX to XII may be affected, or the patient may present with a Horner syndrome. Treatment of these lesions almost always results in sacrifice of the vagus nerve and subsequent vocal cord paralysis. You may see a medialized ipsilateral true vocal cord after such surgery, as well as implants, silastic or otherwise, in the vocal cord.
- On CT, avid enhancement of glomus tumors is expected. On MR, numerous flow voids within the lesion are the norm along with marked enhancement. These features help distinguish these masses from schwannomas, which can also present in this anatomic region. Remember that schwannomas can occur in the carotid space too, and there are some imaging features that help distinguish these from glomus tumors (Table 14.5).
- Nuclear medicine: Indium 111 octreotide scintigraphy enables the distinction of glomus tumors from

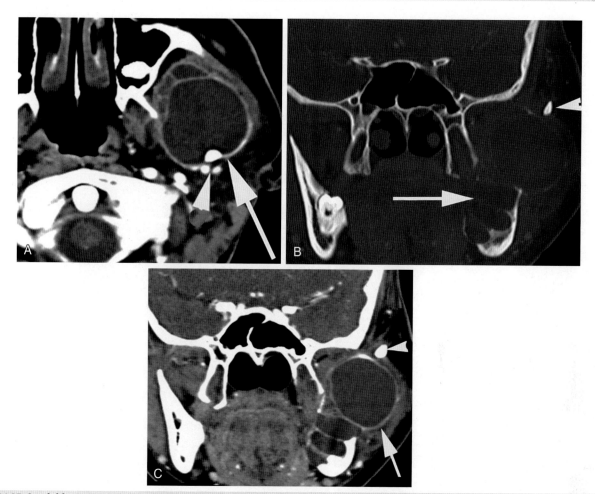

**Fig. 14.37 Ameloblastoma.** (A–C) This mass arose in the mandible and has multiple cystic loculations *(arrows)*; residual tooth remnants and bone erosions *(arrowheads)*.

**Table 14.4**    Sclerotic Dental Lesions

| Lesion | Imaging Appearance | Typical Clinical Findings |
|---|---|---|
| Adenomatoid odontogenic tumor | Calcified well-defined lesions with thick capsule; associated with impacted tooth; involves crown of tooth | Teenagers with impacted maxillary front teeth; painless; female predominance |
| Cementoblastoma | Circular radiodensity attached to a mandibular tooth with pencil-thin border; surrounded by lucency; radial spicules | Expanded mandible with vital tooth; occurs first to third decades of life |
| Chondrosarcoma | "Moth-eaten" appearance with chondroid whorls; may be lucent or dense | Maxillary swelling; painful in adults |
| Ewing sarcoma | Onion-skinning; destructive lesion; poorly defined | 5–25 years of age with painful mandibular mass, fever, rapid growth, loose teeth |
| Fibrous dysplasia | Ground-glass appearance, homogeneous in later stages | Focal painless mass; slow growth; posterior maxilla |
| Garré sclerosing osteomyelitis | Predominantly sclerotic bony lesion; hot on scintigrams; often with periosteal reaction and apical lucency | Bony-hard cortical swelling of mandible; carious molars; nonvital teeth |
| Lymphoma | "Moth-eaten," sclerotic bone | Often systemic symptoms |
| Metastases | Dense or lytic permeative lesions | Lung, breast, prostate, colon, kidney, thyroid primary tumors; loose teeth; often painful |
| Odontoma | Compound: Miniature teeth (enamel) in mandibular with peripheral lucent zone<br><br>Complex: Irregular opaque mass in mandibular molar region | Young patient with mass between canines or in mandible; painless; young adults or children |
| Osteoma | Dense benign excrescence; well-defined | Associated with Gardner syndrome with colonic polyps, supernumerary teeth, cysts; seen as a torus on palate; painless, slow-growing |
| Osteosarcoma | Sclerotic or lytic; poorly defined with opaque spicules with sunray appearance; resorbs roots | Maxillary or mandibular mass; rapid growth; painful; loose teeth |
| Paget disease | Dense thickened bone with risk of osteosarcoma; cotton-wool appearance in maxilla; loss of lamina dura | Elderly patient with dentures no longer fitting commonly in maxilla |
| Pindborg tumor (i.e., calcifying epithelial odontogenic tumor) | Multiple small calcifications within lytic lesion associated with impacted teeth | Mass in posterior mandible |

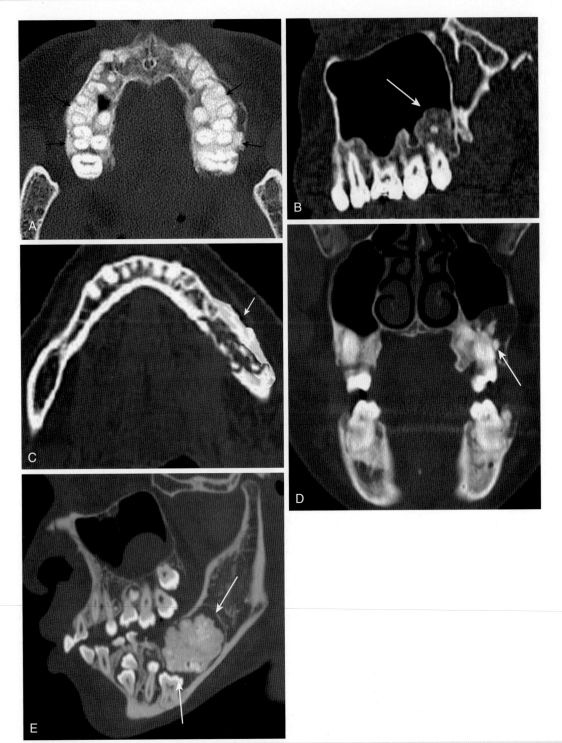

**Fig. 14.38 Common sclerotic dental lesions.** (A) Axial computed tomography (CT) image shows periapical cemetal dysplasia, which occurs near the roots of teeth with dense sclerotic appearance without bony destruction *(arrows)*. (B) Fibrous dysplasia is more common in the maxilla than the mandible. Note expansile nature of this lesion with ground glass matrix. (C) There is sclerosing osteomyelitis with thickened outer bone *(arrow)* and lytic lingual surface of the mandible from chronic infection. Odontomas can be complex, presenting as calcified lesions without discrete tooth components (D) or compound, presenting with tooth elements (E). Note crown like material at the base of the lesion in (E). Radiolucent rim can be seen in more mature odontomas *(top arrow in E)*.

schwannomas and other masses of the carotid space because uptake occurs in the former but not the latter. Beware that false-positive cases can be seen in other neuroendocrine-like lesions such as medullary thyroid carcinomas, thyroid adenomas, Merkel cell tumors, and carcinoid lesions.

# Retropharyngeal Space

## CONGENITAL

- **Retropharyngeal carotid artery** is a potentially dangerous normal variant (see Fig. 14.6B). It may simulate

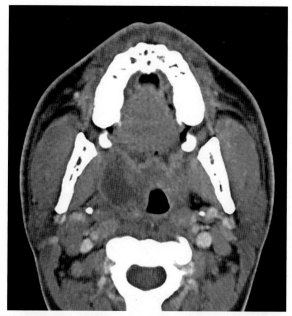

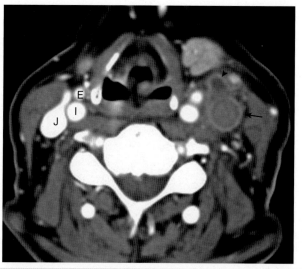

Fig. 14.40 **Thrombophlebitis.** This axial contrast-enhanced computed tomographic image shows an occluded left internal jugular vein *(arrow)* and external jugular vein *(arrowhead).* There is enhancement of the vessel margins and stranding of the soft tissues surrounding these vessels. The normally enhancing jugular vein *(J)*, internal *(I)*, and external *(E)* carotid arteries are indicated on the patient's right side.

Fig. 14.39 **Peritonsillar abscess affecting the parapharyngeal space.** Axial contrast-enhanced computed tomography (CT) image shows an organized abscess in the right pertonsillar tissues with adjacent fat stranding effacing the right parapharyngeal space. Note the clean appearance of the fat in the left parapharyngeal space for comparison.

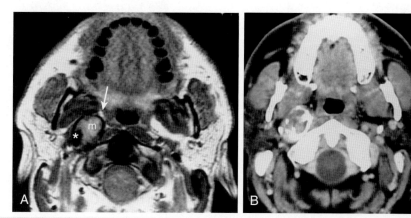

Fig. 14.41 **Pseudoaneurysm of the right internal carotid artery.** (A) Axial proton density (PD) image shows a right carotid space mass *(m)* that has variable signal intensity. Note the peripheral rim of signal void and the posterolateral area of dark signal *(asterisk).* Is that because of flow void, calcification, or hematoma? Only the surgeon will know for sure if you are unfortunate enough to recommend biopsy. Note also that the parapharyngeal fat *(arrow)* is displaced anteromedially by this carotid space lesion. (B) Axial computed tomography (CT) shows that its rim. There is partial enhancement centrally, indicating that this pseudoaneurysm is only partially thrombosed.

a deep submucosal mass to the endoscopist looking from within. Biopsy may lead to a catastrophic complication; the vessel can also be injured in anterior cervical spinal fusion. These vessels are not fixed in location; rarely, the carotid can be mobile, sitting in the retropharyngeal space on one scan, and back to the carotid space on the next!

## INFECTIOUS PROCESSES

- Retropharyngeal abscesses, suppurative (necrotizing) adenitis, and cellulitis are usually sequelae of pharyngitis (adenoidal or tonsillar infections), sinusitis, or intrinsic lymphadenitis (in children). Initially the infection

spreads to a retropharyngeal lymph node (Fig. 14.44) then may spread into the retropharyngeal space as the capsule of the node is violated.
- Retropharyngeal fat may become quite edematous with adjacent inflammatory masses. Be careful not to jump to the conclusion that low density in this space represents an abscess, unless there is a ring-enhancement picture. An infected, ill-defined fluid density may be a phlegmon, which is not readily drainable.
- Internal carotid artery thickening, spasm, and even thrombosis may accompany retropharyngitis and/or lymphadenitis in children. Vasospasm is considered benign and self-limiting in this setting. Neurologic findings may be absent or subtle despite the carotid changes.

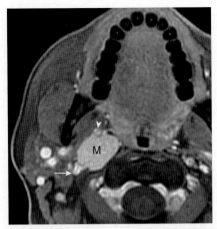

**Fig. 14.42 Carotid body tumor.** Axial postcontrast T1-weighted image (T1WI) shows an avidly enhancing mass *(M)* at a high right carotid bifurcation, splaying the internal carotid artery (ICA) *(arrowhead)* and external carotid artery *(arrow)*.

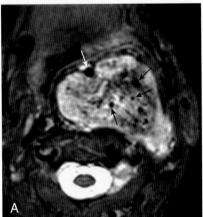

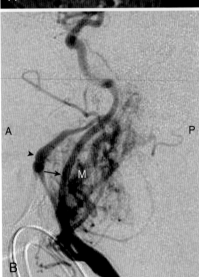

**Fig. 14.43 Glomus tumor.** (A) Axial T2-weighted image (T2WI) shows an enormous mass in the deep left neck—it's so big it's really hard to tell where it's originating from. The displaced internal carotid artery flow void *(white arrow)*, numerous serpentine flow voids in the lesion proper *(black arrows)*, and "salt-n-pepper" appearance helps us a lot in the diagnosis of glomus tumor. Yikes, where's the airway? (B) Conventional catheter angiogram of the left common carotid in lateral projection (A, anterior; P, posterior) shows the avidly enhancing mass *(M)* displacing the internal *(arrow)* and external *(arrowhead)* arteries anteriorly, typical of glomus vagale.

**Table 14.5**  Differentiation of Carotid Space Glomus Tumors from Schwannomas

| Feature | Schwannoma | Glomus Tumor |
|---|---|---|
| Carotid displacement | Pushes anteriorly | Splays internal and external carotid arteries apart and displaces them anteriorly |
| Contrast uptake | Slow uptake | Rapid uptake dynamically, early dip |
| Flow voids on magnetic resonance imaging | No | Yes |
| Vascularity on angiography | Variable | Hypervascular |
| Density on unenhanced computed tomography | Usually hypodense to muscle | Usually isodense to muscle |
| Morphology | May have cysts | Speckled |

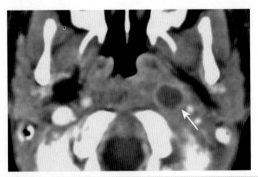

**Fig. 14.44 Retropharyngeal adenitis.** Positioned as it is anterior to the longus colli muscles and lateral to the pharynx, this represents a necrotic suppurative left retropharyngeal node *(arrow)*. Note the associated pharyngitis and loss of fat planes. Is the left carotid artery smaller than the right at the level of the head of the arrow? Vasospasm!

## Perivertebral Space

### CONGENITAL DISORDERS

- **Cystic hygroma** is a classic congenital mass in perivertebral space, often located in the posterior triangle of the neck and associated with Turner syndrome, Noonan syndrome, Down syndrome, and fetal alcohol syndrome. Most lesions are apparent at birth (50%–60%) and are most common in the neck (75%) and axilla (20%) (see Fig. 14.45). These are thought to result from obstruction of primitive lymphatic channels that are derived from the venous system early in gestation. These may be diagnosed in utero in the setting of polyhydramnios or may present acutely as a result of spontaneous or posttraumatic intralesional hemorrhage with fluid-fluid levels or infection. These are benign but can be infiltrative.
  - On ultrasound (US), these cysts can transilluminate and be centrally anechoic to hypoechoic. On CT, they are usually hypodense, multiloculated, and nonenhancing. On MR, these can show variable intensity on T1WI and T2WI, related to proteinaceous-chylous-hemorrhagic content. No solid enhancement should be seen.

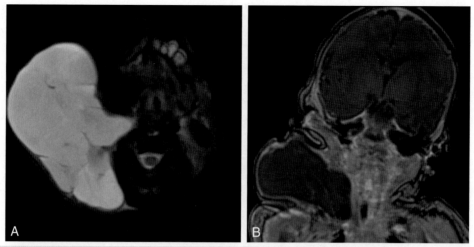

**Fig. 14.45  Cystic hygroma.** (A) Axial T2-weighted image shows a large right fluid intensity neck mass with multiple septations in this newborn corresponding to cystic lesion seen on prenatal ultrasound, fluctuant to touch on exam after delivery. (B) On coronal post-contrast T1-weighted image, there is no enhancement, confirming fluid nature.

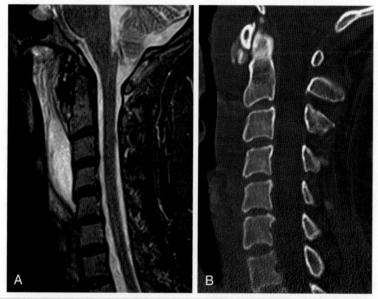

**Fig. 14.46  Acute calcific tendinitis.** (A) Sagittal short tau inversion recovery (STIR) image shows what looks like a nasty brewing prevertebral infection, but interestingly, no evidence of discitis or osteomyelitis. (B) Sagittal computed tomography (CT) of the spine shows again the prevertebral swelling but also elegantly demonstrates the hydroxyapatite deposition in the longus coli muscle insertions, just inferior to the anterior arch of C1. Just like that, case just went from concern for rip-roaring infection to go home, take an aspirin, and call me in the morning!

## INFLAMMATORY LESIONS

■ **Acute calcific tendinitis** (Fig. 14.46) occurs as a result of hydroxyapatite deposition within the tendons of the longus coli muscles. There can be swelling of the longus coli musculature, and there may be associated retropharyngeal effusion. The key here is not to overcall retropharyngeal abscess, which requires urgent surgical debridement; calcific tendinitis is a self-limited process that can be conservatively managed.

■ Infections of the perivertebral space center on **diskitis** and **osteomyelitis**. This may occur in patients after cervical spine surgery, with compromised immune system, bacteremic patients, or in intravenous (IV) drug abusers. The radiographic findings of diskitis and osteomyelitis are discussed fully in Chapter 16.

■ Rotatory subluxation of the atlantoaxial joint may coexist with retropharyngitis in the entity known as Grisel syndrome.

■ Esophageal perforation may lead to mediastinitis and infection of the perivertebral space. Symptoms include neck pain, fever, and swollen prevertebral muscles.

## NEOPLASMS

■ **Chordomas** are notochordal remnant tumors that are considered benign bony neoplasms but are very aggressive. When they involve the craniocervical junction, the perivertebral space can be affected.

　■ These tumors are destructive and lytic and are often associated with calcifications best depicted on CT. On MRI, they are classically bright on T2WI (Fig. 14.47) with variable degrees of enhancement.

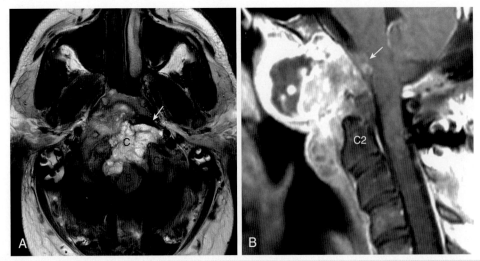

**Fig. 14.47 Chordoma of the perivertebral space.** (A) This T2-weighted image (T2WI) demonstrates a high-intensity chordoma *(C)*, arising at the level of the atlas *(C1)*, anteriorly displacing and stretching the longus coli muscle on the left *(arrow)* and infiltrating the muscle on the right with elevation of the nasopharyngeal soft tissues. Posterior extension at the craniocervical junction results in displacement and distortion of the brain stem *(B)*. (B), on post-contrast T1-weighted image, the mass is heterogeneously enhancing with destruction of C3 dens and bulky nasopharyngeal, prevertebral and retroclival (arrow) components.

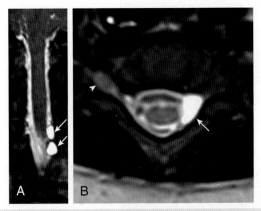

**Fig. 14.48** (A) Coronal and (B) axial T2-weighted images show left-sided pseudomeningoceles *(arrows)* because of avulsion of the left C7 and C8 nerve roots from birth trauma. The expected signal of the C7 nerve root within the neural foramen is present on the right *(arrowhead)* but absent on the left.

- **Osseous metastases** become a perivertebral problem when there is extraosseous extension of disease from the affected vertebral body level into the surrounding soft tissues, often from breast, lung, or kidney primary tumors. Primary vertebral body malignancies include osteosarcomas and Ewing sarcomas in addition to plasmacytomas. Multiple myeloma may affect the cervical spine as well.
- **Soft-tissue malignant masses** in the perivertebral musculature include lymphoma, rhabdomyosarcoma, malignant fibrous histiocytoma, neurofibrosarcoma, and malignant peripheral nerve sheath tumor.
- **Local invasion** by Pancoast tumors extending from the lung apex may also present as a perivertebral or supraclavicular mass and may cause a brachial plexopathy.

## Brachial Plexus

- **Traumatic injury** to the brachial plexus can occur in both the adult and pediatric (perinatal) populations.

Perinatal injuries include two main types of injury caused by shoulder dystocia at the time of delivery.
- Erb palsy results from an avulsion of C5 and C6 nerve roots with weakness at the level of the shoulder. This does not affect intrinsic muscles of the hand.
- Klumpke palsy results from an avulsion of the C8 and T1 nerve roots (Fig. 14.48). There is weakness of the intrinsic muscles of hand, and patients may have coincident Horner syndrome from involvement of sympathetic structures and/or stellate ganglion at the C7-T1 level.
- Traumatic adult injuries result from avulsion of the brachial plexus nerve roots, usually in the setting of motor vehicle accidents.
- On MRI, look for absent nerve roots that ought to be arising from the cord, dilated cerebrospinal fluid (CSF) spaces at the level of injury (pseudomeningoceles), displacement of the cord contralateral to the side the avulsed nerve roots, and, in some cases, concurrent injury to the spinal cord.
- **Plexopathy** may also occur because of injury from cervical ribs (Fig. 14.49) which often have a band leading to the clavicle, unilateral in majority of cases, trapping the brachial plexus. This results in a thoracic outlet syndrome and more commonly affects females than males.

## INFLAMMATORY LESIONS

- **Brachial plexitis** is most commonly viral in origin (Fig. 14.50) but may also occur as a complication of radiotherapy (especially after treatment of supraclavicular adenopathy and/or breast cancer axillary nodes).
  - On MR, findings of brachial plexitis include thickening of nerve roots, asymmetric high signal on fat-suppressed T2WI, and variable enhancement. Imaging findings of perineural tumor extension are similar, and often making the distinction requires clinical and imaging follow-up.

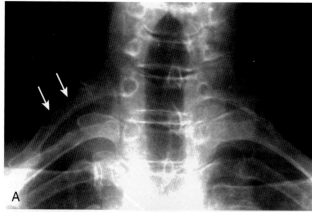

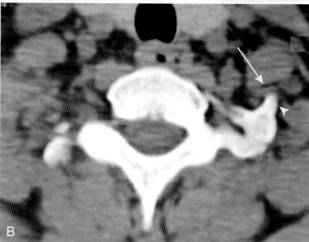

**Fig. 14.49 Cervical rib.** (A) There is a complete cervical rib on the right *(arrows)* and an incomplete one on the left. The patient had a left brachial plexopathy. At surgery, a fibrous band across the left brachial plexus from the cervical rib stump to the manubrium was present. (B) Left cervical rib attaching to C7 transverse process with an exostosis-like process *(arrowhead)* compressing the brachial plexus *(long arrow)*.

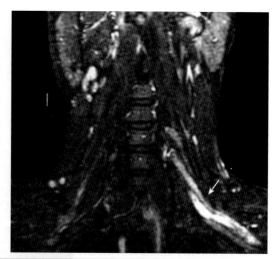

**Fig. 14.50 Brachial plexitis.** Fat-suppressed T2-weighted imaging shows left-sided brachial plexus *(arrow)* inflammation that was viral in etiology. Brachial plexitis may or may not show enhancement.

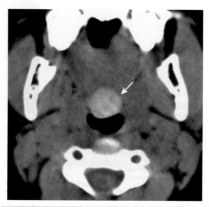

**Fig. 14.51 Lingual thyroid.** This axial computed tomography (CT) image shows a mass in the base of the tongue that is hyperdense on a noncontrast scan.

## MALIGNANT NEOPLASMS

- **Primary malignancies** include malignant fibrous histiocytoma, fibrosarcoma, liposarcomas, and, in children, rhabdomyosarcomas and neurofibrosarcomas (in the NF-1 population).
- **Secondary invasion** may be caused by contiguous involvement or lymphadenopathy. Direct invasion may occur via may Pancoast tumors or chest wall sarcomas leading to a brachial plexopathy. Often there is an associated Horner syndrome. The most common sources of lymphadenopathy leading to a brachial plexopathy are lymphoma, breast, lung, esophagus, and head and neck cancers.

## Thyroid Gland

### CONGENITAL DISORDERS

- **Ectopic thyroid gland** is more common than total agenesis of the thyroid gland. Approximately 50% are located at the base of the tongue (lingual thyroid,

Fig. 14.51), whereas the remaining 50% resides between the tongue and the normal location of the gland, along the expected developmental migration of this tissue from base of tongue to thyroid bed.

- In 80% of cases, the lingual thyroid gland is the only source of thyroid hormone in the individual, so ideally it should be left alone. However, just as with the thyroid gland positioned where it ought to be, the incidence of papillary carcinoma runs as high as 3% to 5%.
- On CT, ectopic tissue appears as hyperattenuating material in an unexpected place, with absence of thyroid tissue in an expected place.
- On nuclear medicine scintigraphy, work-up of lingual thyroid gland requires an iodine-based nuclear medicine study to search for other thyroid tissue.
- **Thyroglossal duct cysts** (TGDCs) are the most common nonodontogenic cysts in the head and neck, behind Tornwaldt cysts. These make up approximately 70% of congenital neck masses. TGDCs are caused by a remnant of the duct along the pathway of embryologic descent of the thyroid gland and may occur anywhere from the

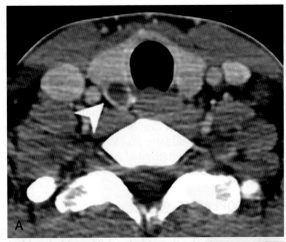

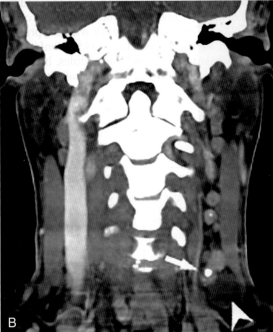

**Fig. 14.54 Metastatic papillary thyroid cancer.** (A) Axial computed tomography (CT) image shows an innocent looking nodule in the right thyroid gland *(arrowhead)*. (B) In the left neck, there are numerous suspicious looking lymph nodes including a large cystic node *(arrowhead)* and several nodes with internal calcification *(arrow points* at one of these). The constellation of findings is very suspicious for metastatic papillary thyroid cancer, even though the nodes are on the contralateral side. Even if no thyroid nodule was evident, the conclusion should be the same.

cause. Cold nodules are more worrisome for malignancy. Malignancy occurs in less than 14% of cases.

- Thyroid **adenoma** is the most common benign tumor of the thyroid gland. More than 70% of solitary neoplasms in the thyroid glands are benign adenomas (follicular or papillary). Colloid cysts are another common benign lesion in the thyroid gland and may be multifocal.
  - On nuclear medicine, more highly differentiated adenomas may concentrate radiotracers and appear as hot or warm nodules, whereas colloid cysts can appear cold.
  - Don't bet the farm on CT and MRI features of thyroid adenoma or colloid cyst as they are nonspecific, but

they are commonly seen incidentally as focal nodules within the gland.
  - That said, the incidental thyroid nodule is painfully common on CT and MRI, and because of the small possibility the nodule could be malignant, management of these pesky lesions has become a hot topic. The American Thyroid Association recommends that a nodule larger than 1 cm in size be correlated with thyroid-stimulating hormone (TSH) level, and if low, radionuclide thyroid scan should follow, and biopsy can be considered based on those results. The American College of Radiology (ACR) recommends further evaluation by US for any incidental nodule that shows invasive appearance, suspicious adenopathy, size of at least 1 cm axially in patients younger than 35 years of age and at least 1.5 cm in patients older than 35 years; suspicious US features that should prompt biopsy are described in the TI-RADS system proposed by the ACR in 2017 (Fig. 14.53).

## MALIGNANT NEOPLASMS

- Thyroid nodules are exceedingly common, and the vast majority of thyroid nodules are benign, with only 4 % of nodules malignant in nature. A history of radiation exposure, male sex, and younger age can increase likelihood of a nodule being cancerous. Papillary, follicular, and mixed papillary-follicular carcinomas account for 80% of thyroid malignancies.
- **Papillary carcinoma** is by far the most common malignancy of the thyroid gland, making up approximately 50% of all thyroid cancers. Medullary carcinoma (10% of thyroid malignancies), undifferentiated or anaplastic carcinoma (3%), and Hürthle cell (2%) are less common cancers of the thyroid gland.
- The prognosis of papillary carcinoma is the best of the thyroid malignancies. Age is the most important prognostic factor, even with distant metastases. Patients under 45 years of age can have an excellent prognosis.
  - When metastatic to lymph nodes, papillary carcinoma has a propensity for cystic-appearing and/or calcified lymph nodes (best appreciated on CT) (Fig. 14.54). On MRI, metastatic nodes may be bright on T1WI because of thyroglobulin content.
- **Follicular carcinoma** tends to spread hematogenously. Prognosis is almost as good as papillary carcinoma. Age is a critical factor in prognosis, and younger patients have better long-term prognosis than older patients.
- **Medullary carcinoma** is derived from parafollicular cells that secrete calcitonin, and approximately 10% of cases are associated with MEN II syndrome (Table 14.6). Some cases are familial without other endocrine lesions.
- **Anaplastic carcinoma** is a highly aggressive carcinoma that typically affects older patient populations and carries a grim prognosis (Fig. 14.55). Lesions are typically large and bulky in appearance. At the time of diagnosis, there is usually infiltration of adjacent trachea, esophagus, or extrathyroidal tissues. The larger the tumor, the higher the rate of invasion. Greater than 80% of cases with anaplastic carcinoma have tracheal invasion at the time of diagnosis.

**Table 14.6**   Multiple Endocrine Neoplasia Syndromes

| Feature | MEN I | MEN II or IIa | MEN III or IIb |
|---|---|---|---|
| Eponym | Wermer syndrome | Sipple syndrome | Mucosal neuroma syndrome, Froboese syndrome |
| Parathyroid abnormality | Hyperparathyroidism (90% of cases) more commonly caused by hyperplasia than by adenoma | Parathyroid hyperplasia in 20%–50% | Very rare |
| Thyroid lesion | Goiter, adenomas, thyroiditis are rare | Medullary thyroid carcinoma (100%) | Medullary thyroid carcinoma (100%) |
| Pituitary lesions | Adenomas (20%–65%) | No | No |
| Pheochromocytoma | No | Yes (50%, bilateral) | Yes (50%) |
| Other manifestations | 1. Pancreatic islet cell adenomas (insulinoma or gastrinoma) in 30%–80%<br>2. Adrenal cortex adenomas or carcinomas (30%–40%)<br>3. Rarely glucagonomas, VIP-omas, carcinoid tumors<br>4. Zollinger-Ellison syndrome | 1. Pheochromocytoma<br>2. Scoliosis | 1. Mucocutaneous neuromas (100%)<br>2. Marfanoid facies<br>3. Café-au-lait spots<br>4. Intestinal ganglioneuromatosis (100%) |
| Chromosomal linkage | Autosomal dominant, chromosome 11 | Autosomal dominant, chromosome 10 | Autosomal dominant, chromosome 10 |

*MEN,* Multiple endocrine neoplasia; *VIP,* vasoactive intestinal polypeptide.

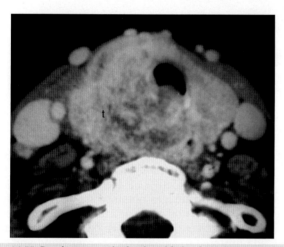

**Fig. 14.55  Dominant mass in the thyroid gland.** The large size of this right thyroid mass *(t)*, the degree of tracheal displacement, the effacement of the wall of the esophagus, and the heterogeneous density in an elderly male patient makes one write a run-on sentence and suspicious of the correct diagnosis of anaplastic carcinoma.

- **Non-Hodgkin lymphoma** may be primary to the thyroid gland or may result from systemic dissemination. Hashimoto thyroiditis may be a predisposing risk factor and approximately 20% to 50% of patients are hypothyroid. The disease can present as solitary nodules (most common), multiple nodules, or diffuse enlargement (least common). Tumor often invades outside the thyroid gland into the carotid sheath.
- These malignancies do not have unique image features that can render an accurate histopathologic diagnosis; however, in a patient younger than 40 years old, papillary carcinomas outnumber all other cancers of the thyroid by a 5-to-1 margin, with females more commonly affected than males.
  - Lesions may have well-circumscribed or poorly circumscribed margins and do not have a characteristic CT or MR appearance to distinguish them from adenomas.

- The presence of adenopathy in the neck, especially when cystic or calcified, should raise concern for possible thyroid primary malignancy (though metastatic HPV-related oropharyngeal cancer can share these imaging findings).
- Larger tumors, esophageal invasion, tracheal invasion, lymphadenopathy, and carotid encasement are findings that can be seen in malignant thyroid disease.
- **Metastatic disease** from lung, breast, and renal cell carcinoma can occur within the thyroid gland.

## Parathyroid Gland

### BENIGN NEOPLASMS

- Parathyroid **adenomas** are a benign tumor of the parathyroid gland that induces elevated parathyroid hormone production. Patients often present with signs and symptoms of hypercalcemia. These can occur spontaneously but can also be seen in MEN syndromes (see Table 14.6). Treatment is with surgical resection.
  - Although surgical success rate for adenoma resection approaches 95% without imaging, preoperative imaging is playing an increasing role these days to keep the surgical exploration as minimally invasive as possible. In a patient with persistent hypercalcemia after initial surgery for resection of the parathyroid glands, imaging may be helpful because the reoperation success rate drops to as low as 62% without imaging.
  - 4-D CT has been advocated for showing early arterial type enhancement of parathyroid hormone adenomas that can be differentiated from veins, nodes, and thyroid lesions (Fig. 14.56). The classic adenoma will show washout or decreased enhancement on later phase images. Hunt for these lesions in and around the thyroid gland, in the tracheoesophageal groove, retropharynx, and the anterior mediastinum, and keep in mind there may be more than one. Remember to check the attenuation of the enhancing candidate

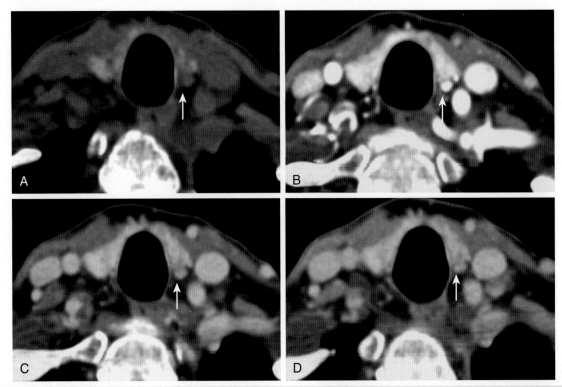

**Fig. 14.56  Parathyroid adenoma on four-dimensional computed tomography.** The left-sided adenoma *(arrows)* is seen as less dense than thyroid gland on unenhanced scan (A), more dense than thyroid, simulating vessel enhancement on arterial phase (B), and denser than lymph nodes on venous (C) and delayed (D) phases *(arrow)*.

lesion with the noncontrast imaging; thyroidal tissue will be hyperattenuating on noncontrast CT and adenomas should be hypoattenuating. Classic adenomas have associated polar vessel sign, which is a prominent artery or vein closely apposed to either pole of the adenoma, which can be a helpful clue when present. Similar enhancement features can be seen on time-resolved contrast enhanced MRA as well.

■ On MR, parathyroid adenomas are typically very bright on T2WI and can usually be readily distinguished from normal glands. In 30% of cases, the MR findings may be atypical with high intensity on T1WI or intermediate on T2WI. These atypical cases have been correlated histopathologically with cellular degeneration, intratumoral hemorrhage, fibrosis, and hemosiderin deposition. Parathyroid adenomas enhance avidly on MRI.

■ On US, adenomas larger than 1 cm in size can be visualized and are generally homogeneous in echotexture, usually less echogenic that the thyroid gland. Doppler US can show the polar vessel sign too, with associated rim of hypervascularity.

■ On nuclear medicine, technetium sestamibi (99 m technetium 2-methoxy-isobutyl-isonitrile [MIBI]) scans, 10 to 25 mCi of technetium-labeled MIBI is given with images obtained in the first minutes after injection and again at 2 hours after injection of the radiotracer. If needed, Tc pertechnetate can be administered to localize the thyroid gland and even subtract the pertechnetate activity in the thyroid from the MIBI activity in the parathyroids and thyroid. With this technique, accuracy approaches 80% to 90% for adenomas, with equally high specificity when applying single-photon emission CT (SPECT) technology. For parathyroid hyperplasia, the sensitivity is only 60%.

■ **Parathyroid carcinomas** are super rare, occurring in 1% of cases of hyperparathyroidism. There are no specific imaging features to separate this lesion from a large adenoma unless invasive features are present. These tumors show rapid growth with nodal metastases.

# PART III

# SPINE

# 15 *Degenerative Disease of the Spine*

ROHINI NADGIR

## Relevant Anatomy

### BONY SPINE

- The bony spine is divided into the cervical spine containing seven vertebrae (the first two of which are rather unique and are discussed further); the thoracic spine, consisting of 12 vertebral bodies; and the lumbar spine, with 5 vertebral bodies. The lower spine consists of the sacrum and coccyx.
- The spine encases the spinal cord, which normally terminates at a variable level from approximately T12 to L2 in adults.
- The generic vertebra is composed of the cylindric vertebral body, which contains cancellous bone with marrow and fat, covered by a thin layer of compact bone, and the vertebral arch or posterior elements, covered by a thick layer of compact bone (cortex), including the pedicles, laminae, superior and inferior facets, transverse processes, and spinous process (Fig. 15.1). The vertebral configuration is modified in the different regions of the spine.
  - The C1 and C2 bodies are unique in their configuration (Fig. 15.2).

---

#### TEACHING POINTS

Getting to Know C1

- The first cervical vertebra (*atlas*) has no body, just an anterior arch connected to two lateral masses and a posterior arch.
- On the upper surface of the posterior arch is a groove over which the vertebral artery courses after it leaves the foramen transversarium of C1.
- The vertebral arteries pass through the posterior atlantooccipital membrane and course anteriorly superiorly upward through the foramen magnum.
- As it pierces the dura, the vertebral artery may be slightly narrowed, and this caliber change can serve as a marker for the beginning of the intradural segment of the vertebral artery. The first spinal nerve exits here as well.

---

#### TEACHING POINTS

Getting to Know C2

- The second cervical vertebra, the *axis*, is unique, with a superior extension from its body termed the *dens* (odontoid process).
- The articulation between the atlas and axis is composed of multiple synovial joints: one medial between the dens

and the anterior arch, one on each side between the inferior articular facet of the lateral mass of the atlas and the superior facet of the axis.
- The cruciate, alar and apical ligaments and the tectorial membrane help secure the axis to the occipital bone while transverse ligament helps secure the C1-C2 relationship at the dens level (see Fig 16.45).

---

- The cervical vertebrae have their neural foramina between the transverse processes. The superior and inferior articular facets have joints between them (zygapophyseal) and form the articular pillar. The uncovertebral (Luschka) joints originate from the lateral posterior portion of the vertebral body, articulate with the contiguous vertebral body, and insinuate themselves between the disk and the nerve root canal. These joints have no synovium and no hyaline cartilage, but clefts can develop in the fibrocartilage with age and degeneration. The vertebral artery enters the foramen transversarium (in the cervical transverse process, naturally) at approximately C6 and travels superiorly.
- The thoracic vertebrae have an articulation on the transverse process for the rib and no foramen transversarium, whereas the lumbar vertebrae have neither a foramen transversarium nor a facet for the rib articulation.
- The lumbar vertebral articulations are composed of the lumbar disk and two facet joints posteriorly. The lateral recess of the lumbar spine is in the anterolateral portion of the spinal canal, with boundaries consisting of the posterior margin of the vertebral body and disk anteriorly, the medial margin of the pedicle laterally, and the superior articular facet, the medial insertion of the ligamentum flavum, the lamina, and the pars interarticularis posteriorly (Fig. 15.3).

### SPINAL CONTENTS

- The spinal cord contains 8 cervical, 12 thoracic, 5 lumbar, 5 sacral, and 1 coccygeal paired spinal nerves. It is important to appreciate that C1 exits above the C1 and C2 interspace so that the C2 nerve exits between C1 and C2, the C3 nerve exits between C2 and C3, and so on. The C8 nerve root exits between C7 and T1. In the thoracic region, the T1 root exits between T1 and T2, and T12 root exits between T12 and L1. In the lumbar spine the L1 root exits between L1 and L2, and so forth, so that the L5 root exits between L5 and S1. (Fig. 15.4).
  - Each spinal nerve is divided into a dorsal or sensory root and a ventral or motor root. The dorsal root ganglion is a distal dilatation of the dorsal root just

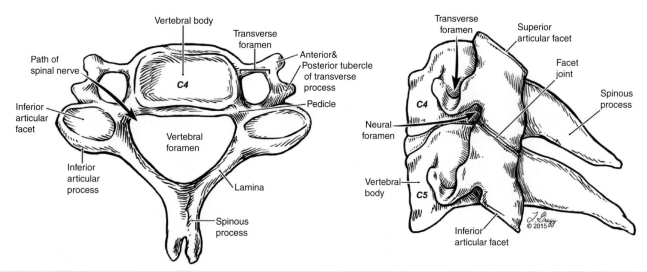

Fig. 15.1 Cervical vertebra illustration shows vertebral parts and relationships (Courtesy Lydia Gregg.)

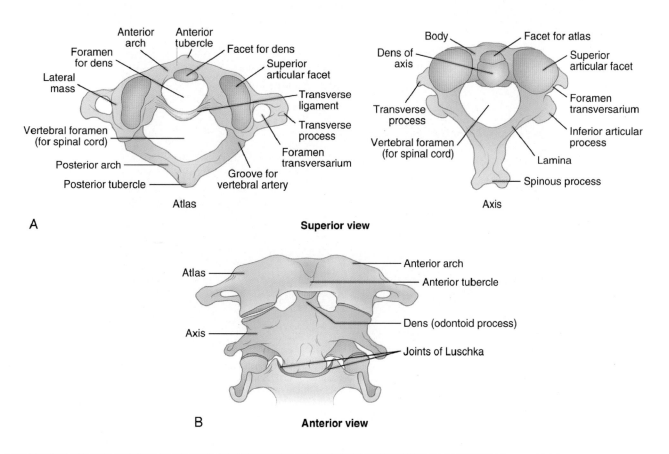

Fig. 15.2 Schematic representation of the atlas and axis from a (A) superior view and (B) anterior view.

proximal to its joining with the ventral root to form the spinal nerve (Fig. 15.5).

■ An anatomic variation is the conjoined nerve root, which occurs in less than 5% of patients, with L5-S1 being the most commonly affected level. This normal variation consists usually of two nerve roots traveling in the same dural pouch and exiting through the same or through different foramina.

## INTERVERTEBRAL DISKS

■ The diskovertebral complex is composed of three components: the cartilaginous endplate, annulus fibrosus, and nucleus pulposus. The endplate consists of a flat bony disk with an elevated rim (attached ring apophysis), which produces a central depression in the endplate occupied by hyaline cartilage.

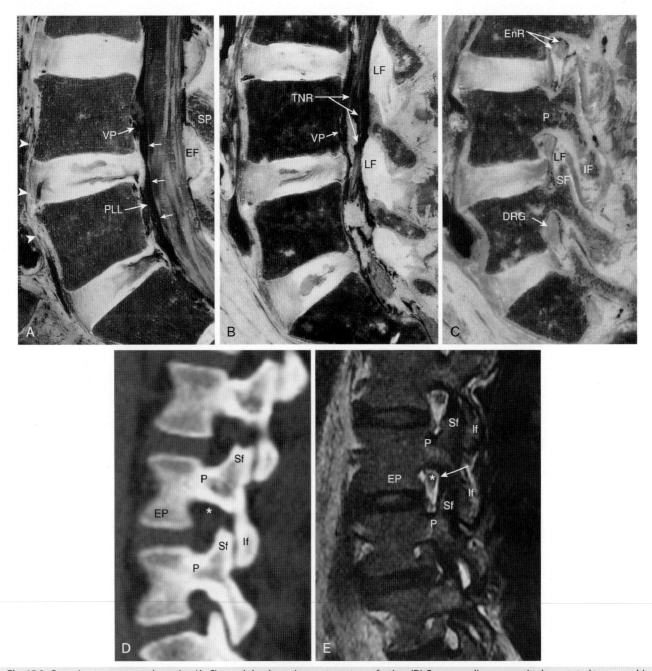

**Fig. 15.3** Cryomicrotome anatomic section (A–C) reveals lumbar spine anatomy to perfection. (D) Corresponding parasagittal computed tomographic scans shows dorsal root ganglion *(asterisk)* surrounded by bony margins of the pedicle *(P),* superior *(Sf)* and inferior *(If)* facets and the endplace *(EP)* of the vertebral body. Similar anatomy on T2-weighted magnetic resonance (E) with the dorsal root ganglion in the neural foramen *(arrow)* surrounded by fat. Anterior longitudinal ligament *(long arrows);* dura mater *(short arrows). DRG,* Dorsal root ganglion; *EF,* epidural fat; *EnR,* exiting nerve root; *IF,* inferior facet; *LF,* ligamentum flavum; *P,* pedicle; *PLL,* posterior longitudinal ligament; *SF,* superior facet; *SP,* spinous process; *TNR,* traversing nerve root; *VP,* venous plexus.

■ The annulus fibrosus surrounds the nucleus pulposus (the remnant of the notochord). The nucleus is eccentrically located near the posterior surface of the disk. The lamellae of the annulus are fewer in number, thinner, and more closely packed posteriorly than anteriorly. This anatomic arrangement may account for the propensity for posterior herniation. The external fibers of the annulus are connected to the bone of the vertebral bodies by Sharpey fibers, which usually cannot be distinguished by imaging. Annular fibers also merge with both anterior and posterior longitudinal ligaments.

## SPINAL LIGAMENTS

■ Important ligaments of the vertebral column are: (1) the anterior longitudinal ligament, running along the anterior aspect of the vertebral bodies; (2) the posterior longitudinal ligament, running along the posterior aspect of the vertebral bodies anterior to the thecal sac; (3) the

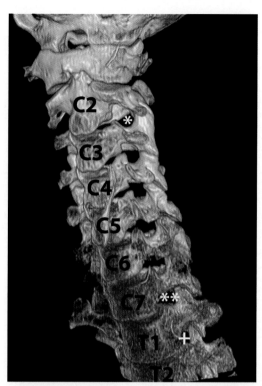

**Fig. 15.4 The root of it all.** Three-dimensional (3D) reconstruction from cervical spine computed tomography (CT) shows individual vertebral body levels (as labeled) and associated neural foramina. The sites of exiting C3, C8, and T1 nerve roots are indicated (*asterisk, double asterisk, plus sign,* respectively).

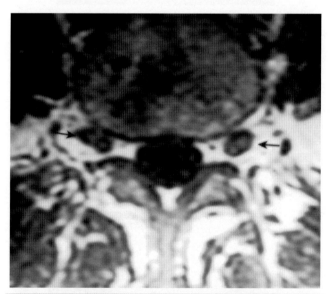

**Fig. 15.5 These ganglia of dorsal root supply sensation to the foot.** Axial T1-weighted imaging demonstrates normal appearance of the dorsal root ganglia *(arrows)*. Do not mistake this for a foraminal disk herniation. Note normal appearance of surrounding hyperintense fat within the foramen.

ligamentum flavum, connecting the laminae and extending from the midline laterally to the facets; and (4) the interspinous ligament, joining the superior portion of the spinous process below to the inferior portion of the spinous process above and meeting the ligamentum flavum in the midline (see Fig. 15.3). Stabilizing ligaments at the craniocervical junction are discussed in Chapter 16.

# Imaging Techniques/Protocols

- There are numerous imaging techniques for spinal imaging, and from the clinician's perspective, the decision about which, if any, to use can be challenging. In general, most cases of run-of-the-mill neck and back pain can be managed conservatively, without imaging. If there are red flags present, such as recent trauma, corticosteroid use, cancer history, and concern for cord compression or myelopathy, imaging should play a role in the workup. Current protocols require 6 weeks of maximal medical management (bed rest, nonsteroidal anti-inflammatory medications, physical therapy) before cross-sectional spine imaging for pain complaints alone.

## RADIOGRAPHS

- Radiographs are useful, particularly when looking for fractures in cases of trauma and to check alignment of the vertebral bodies, (ab)normal motion on flexion and extension for assessment of instability or fusion status, and the position of bone grafts, pedicle screws, cages, and plates. Subsidence (settling/sinking of the interbody spacer device into the endplate), pseudarthrosis (incomplete or absent fusion leading to a mobile and often painful segment), and spinal stability can be evaluated with flexion/extension plain radiographs.
- The lateral spine radiograph provides an excellent overview of spinal alignment and disk heights. Anterior and posterior aspects of vertebral bodies as well as spinous process tips should be in reasonable alignment and facet relationships should be preserved on this view (Fig. 15.6).
  - In the cervical spine, it is important to address the relationship between the odontoid process and the anterior arch of C1. The distance between the anterior aspect of the odontoid and the posterior surface of the anterior arch of C1 should not be greater than 3 mm in an adult and 5 mm in a child.
  - A "swimmer's" view is used to study C7-T1 if it cannot be visualized on the lateral and consists of a lateral view with the tube-side arm depressed and the film-side arm elevated.
- The anteroposterior (AP) view aids in addressing alignment of lateral masses at the level of spinal interest, and the odontoid view shows the relationship of the C1 and C2 vertebrae (Fig. 15.7).
- Oblique radiographs are obtained to view the neural foramina and the facets (Fig. 15.8).
  - In the cervical spine, these views additionally provide a more detailed evaluation of the uncovertebral joint and potential impact of degenerative change here on foraminal patency. The foramina are directed anteriorly and laterally; therefore, in the right posterior oblique projection with the film behind the neck, the left foramina are being visualized. Of course, the opposite is true for the left posterior oblique film.
  - In the lumbar spine, oblique radiographs produce the well-known "Scottie dog," which provides an excellent view of the pars interarticularis. Fractures of the "neck" of the dog indicate spondylolysis (Fig. 15.9). There may be associated anterolisthesis of the "spondylolysed" vertebral body above with respect to the vertebra below.

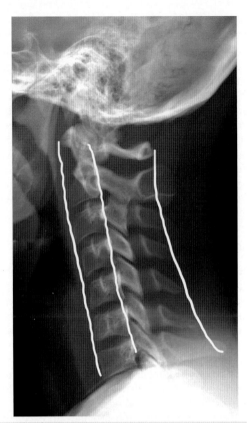

**Fig. 15.6** Lateral view of cervical spine shows reasonable straight alignment of the anterior and posterior aspects of the cervical vertebral body, and the spinous processes show expected mild curvilinear alignment, noting increased bulk of C2 spinous process relative to the others (indicated by white drawn lines *drawn lines*).

## MAGNETIC RESONANCE IMAGING

- The beauty of magnetic resonance (MR) is its ability to provide multiplanar images of both the bone and soft tissues of the spine. Loss or change of expected signal in marrow, disk, ligamentous, cord, and peripheral neural tissue indicates the presence of pathology. Multiplanar imaging aids in localizing pathology and its neural impact with greater accuracy.

### TEACHING POINTS

Magnetic Resonance Imaging and Marrow

- T1-weighted imaging (T1WI) is your best sequence for detecting marrow signal abnormality; in general, abnormal marrow (focal or diffuse) is as dark or darker than the adjacent disk on T1.
- In children, the marrow is lower in intensity on T1 than in adults because of the low-fat content of hematopoietic marrow.
- A small region of high intensity on T1WI is observed at the entry of the basivertebral veins.
- In the adult, the normal vertebral marrow generally has intermediate-to-high signal intensity on T1WI.
- On T2-weighted imaging (T2WI) fast spin echo (FSE) images, the normal vertebral marrow is high intensity, making lesion detection in the vertebral body more challenging.
- Fat saturation in the form of short tau inversion recovery (STIR) imaging is important when vertebral body lesions are suspected and FSE techniques are being employed.

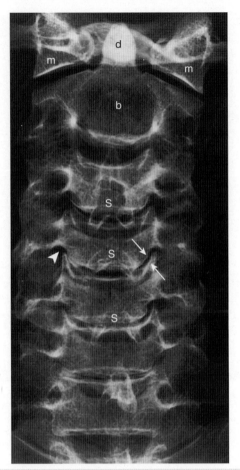

**Fig. 15.7** Anteroposterior view of cervical spine confirms the bodies are in line. Lateral masses of C-1 *(m)*, dens *(d)*, body of C-2 *(b)*, bifid spinous processes *(S)*, C4-C5 left uncovertebral joint *(arrows)*, and a neural foramen *(arrowhead)* are identified.

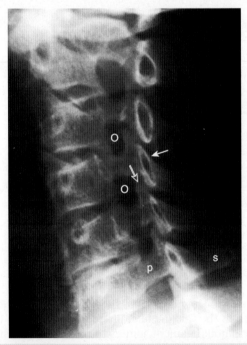

**Fig. 15.8 Oblique radiograph of the cervical spine.** Right posterior oblique demonstrates the left neural foramina *(O)*, the pedicle *(p)*, the superior articular facet *(open arrow)*, the lamina *(arrow)*, and the spinous process *(s)*.

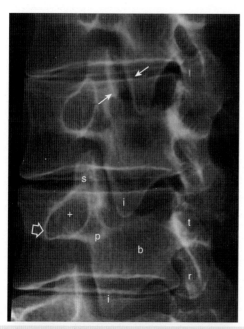

**Fig. 15.9** Anatomy on oblique scan explains the "Scottie dog" diagram. Facet joint is seen *(arrows)*. At the disk space below, components of the Scottie dog are identified: *face*, pedicle (+); *neck*, pars interarticularis *(p)*; *ear*, superior articular facet *(s)*; *front leg*, inferior articular facet *(i)*; *body*, lamina *(b)*; *nose*, transverse process *(open arrow)*; *tail*, contralateral superior articular facet *(t)*; *rear leg*, contralateral inferior articular facet *(r)*. A broken "neck" at the pars would indicate a pars interarticularis defect.

- Complete MR examination requires an excellent sagittal image. Use sagittal sequences, including T1-weighted imaging (T1WI), T2-weighted imaging (T2WI), and short tau inversion recovery (STIR) scans with thin sections, with the minimum inter-slice gap that your particular instrument permits, Use sagittal sequences, including to assess for disk/endplate/body/ligamentous signal abnormalities.

- Assess the foramina for bony constriction and the normal fat and nerves both in the axial and sagittal plane. The axial plane, because of the oblique orientation of the neck foramina, is better for such an evaluation in the cervical region. In the thoracic and lumbar regions, the foramina have a vertical orientation and are filled in part with fat, so they are well visualized in the sagittal plane on T1WI. The nerve root is in the superior portion of the foramen under the pedicle in the lumbar zone.

- In the cervical region, thin-section axial T2WI are necessary, but axial T1WI not essential in the setting of degenerative pathology.

  - Look for osteophytic and disk compression of the roots or spinal canal. Being able to distinguish osteophyte from disk is critical; otherwise, you default to the lazy "disk-osteophyte complex" phrase that plagues our specialty (Fig. 15.10).

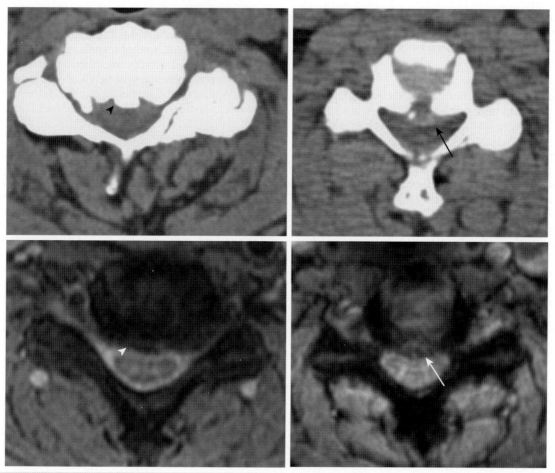

**Fig. 15.10** Gradient echo magnetic resonance separates disk from osteophyte. Axial computed tomographic images are above and gradient echo images below. Note the difference of CT density and MR intensity in the disk herniation *(arrows)* versus osteophyte *(arrowheads)*.

The gradient echo sequence is a low flip angle volumetric acquisition through the cervical spine which enables sections of 1.5 mm or less with enough tissue contrast such that the cerebrospinal fluid (CSF) is high signal, disk material is intermediate signal, and osteophytes are low signal intensity (see Fig. 15.10). It can really help distinguish dark osteophyte from less dark disk herniation.

- Axial gradient echo images are often employed in the cervical spine. Note that these may tend to exaggerate foraminal or bony canal stenosis of the spine, and what appears as high-grade or complete blocks on MR imaging (MRI) may not be as severe on myelography, computed tomography (CT) myelography, or T1WI.
- Fast spin echo (FSE) T2WI is the routine technique used for imaging the cerebrospinal fluid (CSF), spinal cord, and nerve roots.

One advantage of fast spin echo (FSE) imaging derives from its relative insensitivity to susceptibility effects compared with gradient and conventional spin echo techniques. Thus, spinal osteophytes are not as exaggerated on sagittal images as with the other techniques, and there is better visualization of the extent of thecal sac compression, cord compression, and intrinsic cord pathology.

- STIR images are excellent for detection of ligamentous injury and bone edema that otherwise is lost on FSE T2WI where fat and edema are both bright in the bone.
- Intravenous (IV) contrast on MRI becomes necessary in the postoperative back to distinguish between scar and disk, in infectious and inflammatory conditions of the spine, and in the evaluation of the spine to in tumor workup.
  - Although enhancement with fat suppression is in many cases useful in detecting metastatic disease to the vertebral bodies, it is not always necessary, especially with good-quality T1-weighted and STIR images, and many times, replacement of the fatty marrow by tumor is obvious on unenhanced images.
  - Furthermore, because both benign and malignant marrow processes enhance, in many cases contrast enhancement of a marrow lesion will not help you make a distinction between the two.

## COMPUTED TOMOGRAPHY

- CT provides excellent bony anatomic definition far greater than radiographs as well as the ability to reconstruct imaging data sets in multiple planes.
- CT without intrathecal contrast can be adequate for the lumbar region, where natural contrast exists between epidural fat, disk, and bone (Fig. 15.11).

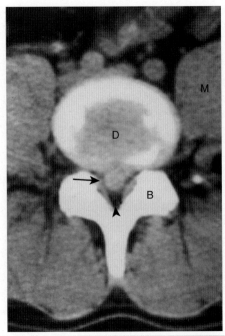

Fig. 15.11 Don't discount the value of computed tomography (CT) in diagnosing disk disease in the lumbar spine. Huge central herniated disk *(arrow)* is squashing the thecal sac. Herniated disk and the parent disk (D) have the same density. Note the array of densities from disk (D), bone (B), muscle (M), and posterior epidural fat *(arrowhead)*.

- There is usually little soft tissue contrast between the spinal cord and the subarachnoid space in the cervical and thoracic regions, so that intradural processes are suboptimally imaged without intrathecal contrast.
- In the postoperative setting, CT is favored over MRI for evaluating metallic hardware for spine stabilization, such as pedicle screws and anterior metallic plates.

## MYELOGRAPHY

- Myelography is a good option to consider when canal or foraminal stenosis is suspected, but routine noncontrast CT and MRI do not provide adequate detail or if MRI is contraindicated. Although not performed as often as it once was, myelography, almost always combined with CT (myelo-CT), is still a sensitive and useful technique for disk herniation and, more importantly, osteophytic impingement on nerve roots. The search for CSF leakage sites in patients with intracranial hypotension is another indication for postmyelogram CT of the brain and spine.
- The procedure involves injection of intrathecal contrast into the spinal canal under fluoroscopic guidance, via lumbar or cervical puncture, followed by fluoroscopic and/or CT imaging after contrast has made its way within the thecal sac in the region of interest. The advantage of the myelo-CT is the exquisite bone detail superimposed upon the subarachnoid contrast (Fig. 15.12).
- In patients who are candidates for MRI, thin section (1–2 mm) T2 images of the entire spine obtained in multiple planes can provide very high-resolution images and are useful for detecting sources of CSF leak noninvasively.

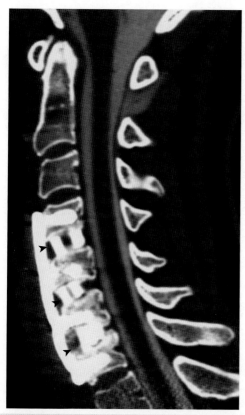

**Fig. 15.12 Postoperative myelogram.** Computed tomography sagittal reconstruction from thin section axial data nicely shows good alignment, fusion from C4 to C7, and use of autologous bone interbody spacers *(arrowheads)*. There is no impingement on the cord.

## DISKOGRAPHY

- This procedure is performed (rarely) in the hopes of finding a culprit disk causing pain when no definitive imaging findings have been identified. Potentially, you can find the disk level that is producing the symptoms or in cases with multiple disk herniations and no definitive notion of which level is the symptomatic one.
- The procedure involves injection of contrast material within the disk nucleus itself and assessing reproducibility of pain by the patient's response. After injection, plain radiographs are made and additional CT images can be performed to assess whether the contrast is appropriately confined by the annulus, or if an annular tear is present, evidenced by streaks into the annulus or leaks into the epidural space.

# Pathology

## SPONDYLOSIS

- Unlike great wines, the spinal column does not improve with age—it degenerates. Low back pain is very common and occurs in more than 60% of all adults. Although practice patterns vary, most agree that imaging should not be performed within 6 weeks of pain onset because radicular symptoms tend to improve over time with conservative management. However, if you actually have

weakness and muscle loss, or other red flags such as new pain after trauma, corticosteroid use, or cancer history, best to image sooner rather than later.
- *Spondylosis deformans* refers to the typical aging process in which the annulus fibrosis and adjacent apophyses form bone spurs/osteophytes from the endplates or adjacent joints, and the nucleus pulposus degenerates.
- It is important to separate the process of disk degeneration from disk herniation. The pathophysiology of the degenerative process consists of dehydration of the nucleus pulposus and decreased tissue resiliency with decrease in the height of the disk space and endplate changes.
  - Initially, the nucleus pulposus is soft and gelatinous; however, with aging, it is replaced by fibrocartilage, and the distinction between the nucleus and annulus fibrosus becomes less well defined. The cartilaginous endplate becomes fissured and more hyalinized. The annulus, which is initially attached to the anterior and posterior longitudinal ligaments, loses its lamellar configuration and develops fissures. The cracks have negative pressure so that gas, primarily nitrogen, comes out of solution and deposits in the intervertebral disk, close to the subchondral bone plate or in other locations. This is termed the "vacuum" (cleft) phenomenon (Fig. 15.13).
  - Early MR abnormalities representing disk degeneration include an infolding of the anterior annulus and a hypointense central dot within the disk on T2WI. With time, the disk degeneration is manifested on MR by decreased signal intensity on T2WI. Disk calcification commonly occurs in the elderly and is part of the normal aging process. It is also associated with other, often systemic conditions.
  - Increased intensity on T1WI of the disk can be seen uncommonly with mild calcification associated with degeneration. As calcification increases, the intensity on T1WI decreases. Ultimately, the degenerative

---

**TEACHING POINTS**

Calcify This! Diseases Associated with Disk Calcification

- Acromegaly
- Amyloidosis
- Ankylosing spondylitis
- Calcium pyrophosphate deposition disease (CPDD)
- Chondrocalcinosis
- Diabetes mellitus
- Degenerative disk disease
- Diffuse idiopathic skeletal hyperostosis (DISH)
- Gout
- Hemochromatosis
- Homocystinuria
- Hyperparathyroidism
- Hypothyroidism
- Ochronosis
- Osteoarthritis
- Poliomyelitis
- Sequelae of disk infection

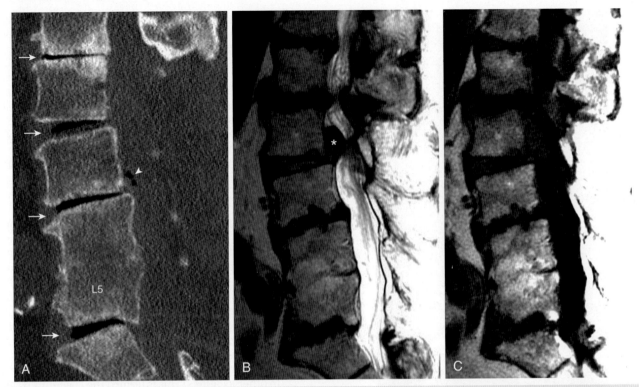

**Fig. 15.13 Vacuum clefts.** (A) Sagittal reconstruction of a computed tomography (CT) lumbar spine in a patient after lumbar laminectomy from L2 through L5 shows multilevel vacuum disks at L1-L2 through L5-S1 *(arrows)* with the exception of L4-L5 where bony fusion has developed across the disk level. Note disk herniation at L3-L4 into the spinal canal is evident by virtue of the associated vacuum phenomenon *(arrowhead)*. (B) Sagittal T2 and (C) T1 images from the same patient demonstrate how challenging it is to appreciate the vacuum phenomenon *(dark intensity* on both sequences) by magnetic resonance imaging. The giant disk herniation at L1-L2 on the other hand is obvious on T2-weighted image *(asterisk)* but not appreciable on the CT bone window.

changes permit disk material to bulge and subsequently to herniate, but disk herniation may occur in the absence of significant disk degeneration, especially with acute trauma.

## DISK HERNIATION

- Degenerative processes may be accompanied by disk herniation, wherein nuclear material squeezes itself through the annular fissures, and can occur at any spinal level, although it most frequently occurs at the lumbar and cervical spine.
- Disk herniations can occur acutely (from moving that heavy sofa across the room) or over a prolonged time course in a degenerating spine. Unfortunately, there are no specific imaging criteria for determining whether a herniation is acute or not. We have to rely on our clinical colleagues' evaluations to make that determination.
- Disks can improve over time and spontaneous reduction of herniations, particularly those larger than 6 mm, are reported 6 to 12 months after the initial event. This is associated with clinical improvement (if you have a high pain threshold and no significant neurologic deficit to tolerate the wait).
  - Exactly how this occurs is unknown, but investigators have hypothesized about dehydration with disk shrinkage, fragmentation, and phagocytosis as possible factors in the reduction of disk herniation. With the onset of herniation, there is an associated inflammatory response. Neovascularity occurs at the periphery of the herniated disk, and the combination of inflammation and neovascularity may contribute to resorption of the disk material and better clinical outcomes. The inflammatory component has also been suggested for the reason why epidural steroids have been used successfully for the nonsurgical treatment of herniated disks.
- The radiologic descriptions that are associated with various imaging findings of disk herniation were imprecise and confusing until a consortium of radiologists and orthopods and neurosurgeons agreed on a common lumbar disk nomenclature, accepted in 2001 and revised in 2014.
- An annular fissure (the term *annular tear* is considered nonstandard, so best to avoid it) is a separation between annular fibers, avulsion of fibers from their vertebral body insertions, or breaks through fibers that extend in a particular direction (Fig. 15.14).
  - There are three types of annular fissures: concentric, radial, and transverse, with the latter two being identifiable on MR. Transverse fissures are peripheral, disrupting Sharpey fibers. Radial fissures start from the nucleus and course through the annulus.
  - On MR, globular or linear high intensity can be observed on T2WI within the posterior annulus.

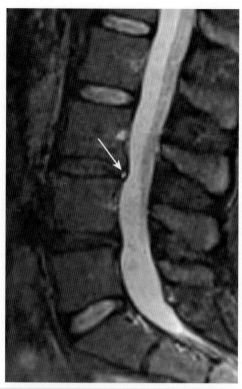

**Fig. 15.14 Annular fissure.** High signal intensity zone *(arrow)* at the margin of this disk represents an annular fissure. Signal intensity and associated enhancement do not imply acuity, etiology, symptomatology, or need for treatment.

Anterior radial annular fissures are rare but can be associated with back pain. Segmental instability may also be present. Annular fissures can enhance for years and show T2 hyperintensity for years; fissures do not imply acuity.

- A bulge is generalized displacement of disk material beyond the limits of the intervertebral disk space by greater than 25% of the disk circumference.
- A herniation is a *localized* displacement of disk material beyond the limits of the intervertebral disk space by less than 25% of the disk circumference (Fig. 15.15).
  - Herniations may be described as protrusions or extrusions.
  - Protrusions are defined as herniations that have a broader attachment at the junction with the parent disk than distally in any plane.
  - Extrusion is defined when the junction with the parent disk is narrower than its distal portion.
  - If there is separation of the herniated disk material from the parent disk, it is a sequestrated disk or free fragment, which is considered a type of disk extrusion.
  - If the herniated disk is displaced from the parent disk (regardless of whether it is sequestrated or not), it is termed a *migrated disk*. Disk migration occurs equally commonly up and down, right and left from the parent disk.
  - If the disk herniation is covered by the outer annulus and/or the posterior longitudinal ligament (defined as dark signal on MR pulse sequences), it is considered

contained or "subligamentous." If the disk herniation is uncovered, it is termed *uncontained* and/or *supraligamentous* (see Fig. 15.15D). This distinction aids the surgeon in knowing where to look for the disk fragment in the operating room. In extremely rare instances, disks have been reported to transgress the dura and lie intradurally.

- Further description should include the location of the herniation and the extent, if any, that a particular structure (nerve root, thecal sac, spinal cord) is compressed by the herniation.
  - The accepted terms to be used for describing disk position are (from the midline) *central, right/left central, subarticular, foraminal,* and *extraforaminal* (far lateral) (Fig. 15.16). Of course, there are anterior herniations in front of the vertebrae and intravertebral herniations, affectionately known as "Schmorl nodes." The disk may also, in a craniocaudal direction, be referred to as migrating to a *suprapedicular, pedicular,* or *infrapedicular* location.
- Another useful way of describing *herniations* or *osteophytes* is by their impact on the thecal sac or exiting nerve roots. The three terms that "tell it all" are *noncompressive, abutting,* and *compressing/displacing.* Thus, a herniation may:
  - be noncompressive without nerve contact and therefore unlikely to cause radiculopathy.
  - abut but not displace an exiting nerve root, implying that potentially, when weight-bearing or at stress it may displace and compress the nerve root (or not).
  - compress or displace the nerve root, even in nonweight-bearing positions. Compression of the nerve may occur with the nerve located within the thecal sac (central), as it leaves the thecal sac (right/left central), in the lateral recess (subarticular), in the neural foramen (foraminal), or exiting the foramen (extraforaminal).
- Disk fragments may have different intensities depending on their state of hydration and the particular pulse sequence used. Degenerated disks on MR generally have lower intensity on T2WI than normal disks, and disks containing gas (vacuum disks) or calcification have very low intensity on all pulse sequences.
  - Nitrogen gas from the vacuum disk that is within the spinal canal implies disk herniation (see Fig. 15.13). On CT and MR, air can be appreciated as linear low density and intensity. The presence of air in the disk space may indicate mobile spinal segment and should not be present in a fused spine.

## SCHMORL NODE

- Herniation of disk material through the endplate is termed a *Schmorl node* (intravertebral herniation), which usually has discrete margins and intensity similar to disk material and reveals rim enhancement. Schmorl nodes can be identified in patients with Scheuermann disease (wedge-shaped vertebrae leading to thoracic kyphosis in young adults) as well as asymptomatic patients and have been associated with infection, trauma, malignancy, osteopenia, and intervertebral osteochondrosis (Fig. 15.17).

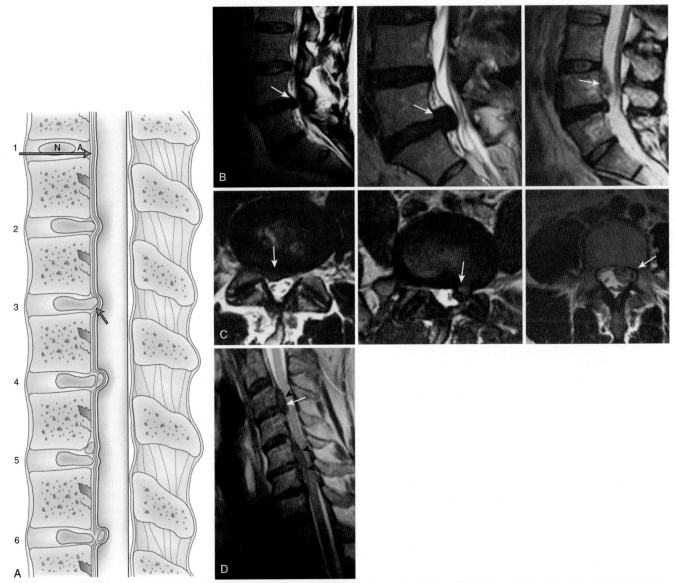

**Fig. 15.15 Disk nomenclature.** (A) Diagram of lateral spine demonstrating spectrum of disk lesions. 1. Normal configuration of nucleus pulposus (*N*), intact annulus fibrosis (*A*), posterior longitudinal ligament *(arrow)*, and dura. 2. Bulging disk with intact annulus fibrosus. 3. Subligamentous herniated disk with rupture of the annulus fibrosus *(arrow)*. 4. Herniated disk with a free fragment. 5. Herniated disk with a free fragment that has migrated superiorly. 6. Herniated disk that has ruptured through the posterior longitudinal ligament (PLL) and is against the thecal sac. In super rare instances, the disk can continue to head east and become intradural. (B) From left to right on sagittal scans, you have a protrusion, extrusion, and sequestrated disk herniation *(arrows)*. The base is wider in protrusion, narrower in extrusion, and detached in sequestration. (C) The same sequence on axial scans with wide base, narrow base, and no base *(arrows)* from left to right. (D) On this sagittal magnetic resonance image, we see disk herniations that are contained by the sharply defined PLL (subligamentous) denoted by *arrowheads*. However, at the *arrow*, you see the C3-C4 disk breaching the posterior longitudinal ligament (note blurred interface of the herniation and PLL). It is no longer "contained."

### TEACHING POINTS

Sure as Scheuermann

- This degenerative disease is noted in children, affecting males predominantly, with onset at puberty.
- It consists of vertebral wedging resulting in lower thoracic kyphosis.

■ Schmorl nodes are common.
■ The etiology is thought to be stress related through either congenitally or traumatically weakened portions of the cartilaginous endplates.

■ On MR, they appear as extensions of disk into the vertebral body surrounded by a rim of low intensity on T2WI representing reactive sclerosis. Occasionally, a Schmorl node may be associated with bone marrow edema (and pain, clinically), which can be confused with infection or metastatic lesion. Chronic Schmorl nodes may be associated with fatty endplate changes.
■ If the disk herniates into the anterior ring apophysis, it is termed a *limbus vertebra* (Fig. 15.18), and seen in children and associated with back pain.

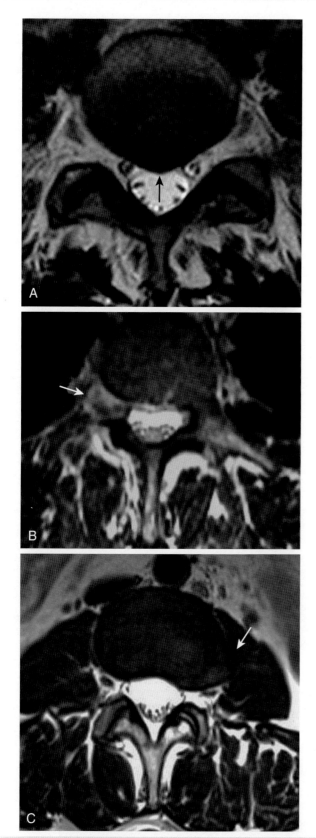

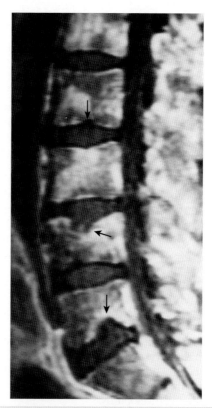

**Fig. 15.17** A Schmorl node causes the endplate to erode. Sagittal T1-weighted imaging demonstrates multiple intrabody disk herniations (Schmorl nodes) *(arrows)* in this patient who incidentally has acute myeloid leukemia (note generalized marrow heterogeneity).

**Fig. 15.16** Disk herniation descriptors: central (A, *arrow*), right central (see Fig. 15.15, C, left image, *arrow*), left subarticular (see Fig. 15.15, C, middle image, *arrow*), right foraminal (B, *arrow*), and left far lateral, also called extraforaminal (C, *arrow*).

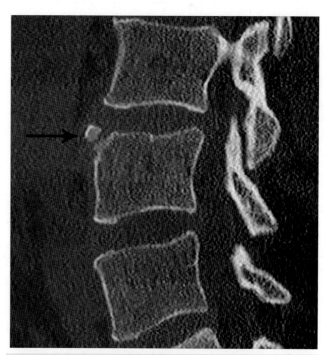

**Fig. 15.18 Limbus vertebra.** Well-corticated density *(arrow)* along the anterior aspect of the superior endplate of this lumbar occurs as a result of disk herniation into the anterior ring apophysis.

## OSTEOPHYTE FORMATION

- The combination of loss of disk height and disk shrinkage is associated with abnormal motion, particularly in the cervical region. Loss of height (but hopefully not of stature) and tissue shrinkage are what we have to look forward to with advancing age. Abnormal stress caused by the loss of disk height produces osteophyte formation and posterior displacement of the vertebral body. Because of the abnormal stress, subluxation of the facet joints may occur.
- Spur formation in the cervical spine takes place at the uncovertebral joints as the disks desiccate and get narrower leading to more grinding of the uncovertebral joint (UVJ) below and the vertebral body above (Fig. 15.19). Osteophyte formation at the UVJ produces foraminal stenoses, compression of the nerve root and clinical signs of cervical radiculopathy.
  - Note that while there are UVJs between C3-C4 and C6-C7, it is less common to have such a joint between C7-T1 and very rare at T1-T2. It can happen, but if you are apt to call UVJ-related stenosis of the neural foramen at C7-T1, it is probably a misnomer.
- At any spinal level, large osteophytes may form at the posterior edge of adjacent vertebral bodies, with narrowing of the subarachnoid space and spinal cord compression, producing myelopathy.
- Osteophyte formation also occurs at the facet joints; however, this is less significant in the cervical region than in the lumbar region. In the lumbar region, osteophytic compression occurs primarily in the lateral recess and at the neural foramen. Hypertrophy of the superior articular facets in the lumbar region is most important because it lies anterior to the inferior articular facet and closer to the nerve in the lateral recess and neural foramen (Fig. 15.20).

## ENDPLATE CHANGES

- In degenerative disease the signal intensity of the endplate vertebral marrow can be variable on conventional spin echo images, described as *Modic changes* (Fig. 15.21).

- Modic type 1 changes have been associated with acute low back pain and may be a marker of recent stress or spinal instability. Modic type 1 changes are more common in symptomatic low back pain patients than in asymptomatic

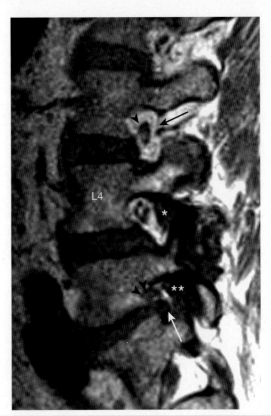

**Fig. 15.20 Foraminal stenosis.** Sagittal T1-weighted image shows varying degrees of foraminal patency. *L4* level is indicated. At L3-L4, the foramen is widely patent *(black arrow)*, with normal bright fat surrounding the exiting L3 nerve root *(black arrowhead)*. At L4-L5, ligamentum flavum infolding *(asterisk)* serves to narrow the posterior aspect of the foramen but the nerve root is just fine; we can call this mild foraminal narrowing. At L5-S1, there is pronounced ligamentum flavum infolding and facet hypertrophy *(double asterisks)* along with disk herniation *(white arrow)*, which serve to nearly completely efface the fat in the foramen, resulting in moderate to severe foraminal narrowing. Note the impact upon the exiting L5 nerve root *(double, black arrowheads)*, which is flattened and compressed.

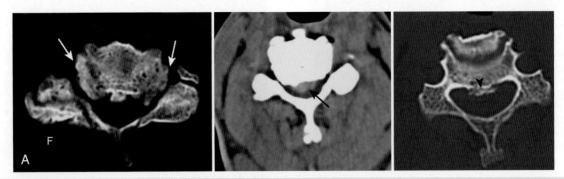

**Fig. 15.19 Cervical spine degenerative disease.** (A) Note the *white arrows* denoting uncovertebral joint osteophytes narrowing the neural foramina, accompanied by facet joint disease (F) on the right. A central disk protrusion is present *(black arrow)*, accompanied by ossification of the posterior longitudinal ligament *(black arrowhead)*. That'll give you a neck ache!

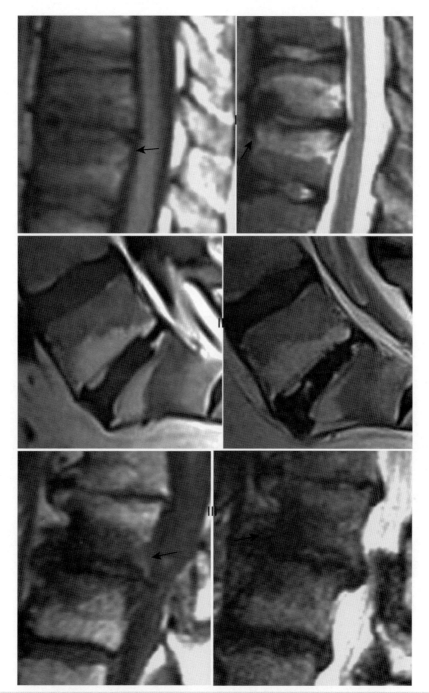

**Fig. 15.21 Modic endplate changes.** Modic type 1 at top with dark endplate on T1-weighted imaging (T1WI) on the left image and bright endplate on T2-weighted imaging (T2WI) on the right. In Modic type 2, middle set, endplates are bright on both T1WI and T2WI. Finally, the sclerotic Modic 3 form has dark intensity on both T1WI and T2WI (bottom set). Endplate changes are indicated by *arrows*.

**TEACHING POINTS**

Modic Changes

- Modic 1: Endplate vertebral marrow edema shows decreased intensity on T1-weighted imaging (T1WI) and increased intensity on T2-weighted imaging (T2WI).
- Modic 2: Endplate marrow signal can undergo subchondral fatty marrow conversion with increased intensity on T1WI and T2W1.
- Modic 3: Endplate marrow can undergo bony sclerosis, with hypointensity on T1WI and T2WI.

subjects. Some have suggested that there may actually be a low-grade infection occurring in patients with acute herniations and Modic type 1 changes, with studies showing clinical improvement after antibiotic therapy in patient with chronic low back pain. Unfortunately, Modic Type 1 degenerative changes look the same as early diskitis/vertebral osteomyelitis (DVO) and may show enhancement as well. Therefore, the high signal and enhancement of the disk and the endplate erosions and particularly perivertebral inflammatory soft tissue in DVO are critical adjunctive findings.

- Modic type 3 changes are static. Modic 1 and 2 may evolve or resolve.

## SYNOVIAL CYSTS

- Synovial cysts can present with pain, usually radicular, and neurologic deficits.
- They are associated with either side of the facet joint (medially or laterally) and appear as rounded postero-lateral extradural masses (medial cysts), but they may occur in the posterior paraspinal tissue (lateral cysts). They occur in the lumbar region, L4-L5 more commonly than L5-S1, although they have rarely been reported in other regions of the spine. Hemorrhage in these lesions, precipitating acute neurologic symptoms, has been reported, but often the hemosiderin seen in the wall of the cyst is not associated with acuity. This accounts for dark signal on T2WI surrounding fluid signal centrally.

- The diagnosis is made by the characteristic location and association with degenerative disease, including disk space narrowing, eburnation, and hypertrophic changes. Peripheral rim enhancement can be seen. There is an association with spondylolisthesis and abnormal movement of the facet joint.
- CT can rarely detect calcification in the cyst wall and gas in the cyst, but most often the periphery is just slightly hyperdense (Fig. 15.22). These lesions can display enhancement if associated with an inflammatory process.

## BAASTRUP DISEASE

- Baastrup disease represents inflammation of the interspinous ligaments usually found in the lumbar spine and isolated to one level. This may be because of excessive contact between the spinous processes resulting in their

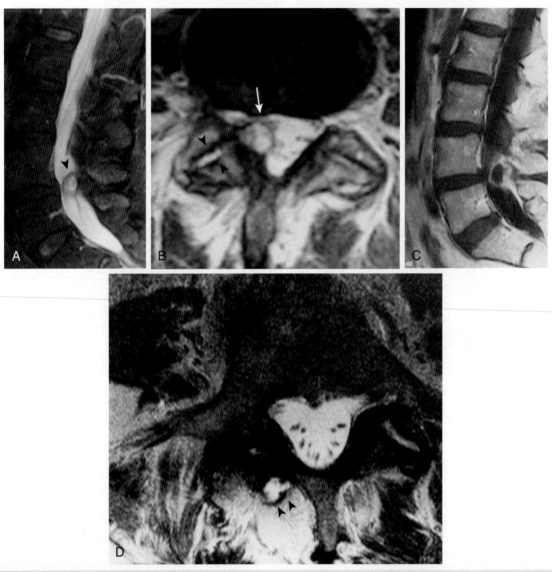

**Fig. 15.22 Synovial or juxta-articular cyst.** (A) Sagittal T2-weighted imaging (T2WI) shows a synovial cyst *(arrowhead)* that has a dark intensity rim and hyperintense center. (B) The origin from the facet joint *(arrowheads)* and the effect on the right-sided nerve roots *(arrow)* is demonstrated on the T2-weighted axial image. (C) After contrast, the wall of the cyst enhances. (D) Synovial cysts can also arise from the lateral aspect of the face joint and project into the paraspinal soft tissues as in this case *(black arrowheads).*

sclerosis, eburnation, and enlargement with pain maximal on extension. Many cases have associated cysts that may project in a number of directions, but they can project in the posterior epidural space in communication with the interspinous bursitis (Fig. 15.23). From there they may irritate the posteriorly located spinal nerve roots. Treatment is to remove the offending spinous processes.

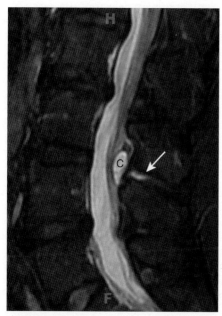

**Fig. 15.23 Baastrup disease.** Classic appearance on magnetic resonance (MR) imaging shows interspinous bursitis seen as high signal on short tau inversion recovery MR *(arrow)*, with a posterior epidural cyst *(C)*.

## OSSIFICATION OF THE POSTERIOR LONGITUDINAL LIGAMENT

■ As the name implies, ossification of the posterior longitudinal ligament (OPLL) is characterized by bone/marrow formation along the posterior longitudinal ligament. It is an inflammatory condition associated with degenerative disease and affects males and females typically in the fifth to seventh decades of life. OPLL occurs in 50% of patients with diffuse idiopathic skeletal hyperostosis (DISH; see following discussion). Although OPLL is a cervical spine entity, you often see coexisting thoracic spine ligamentum flavum infolding and calcification. It can produce compression of the spinal cord with myelopathic symptoms.

■ Thin ossifications on sagittal MR are difficult to detect and at times become apparent after identification of ventral compression of the cord. On T1WI, CSF and calcium have almost the same intensity. Axial T2WI aid in confirming extra-axial compression.

■ OPLL may be confused with osteophytic compression. Sometimes the ossification may truly have marrow fat and cortex in which case the bright signal marrow fat will be the giveaway on T1WI. Concurrent ligamentum flavum infolding is often present.

■ Remember that OPLL occurs along the full course of the posterior longitudinal ligament, whereas osteophytes are present only at the disk space. OPLL makes a strong case for CT and radiographs to establish the diagnosis (Fig. 15.24). OPLL is important to note in a report because it usually means that the surgeon must decompress via a posterior cervical laminectomy approach, not with anterior fusion.

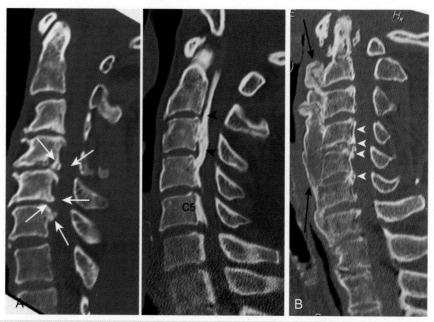

**Fig. 15.24** Ossification of the posterior longitudinal ligament (OPLL) versus osteophyte: Both can cause a canal that's too tight. (A) Contrast the osteophytes on the left-hand image *(white arrows)* with the OPLL on the middle image *(black arrowheads)*. OPLL is more likely to be flowing and continuous and may have breaks at the disk levels such as at C4-C5 and C5-C6. It may be just behind the vertebral body and not at the disk as at *C5*. (B) Diffuse idiopathic skeletal hyperostosis (DISH) causes enthesopathies of spinal aponeurosis. Note the appearance of osseous bridging *(black arrows)* at multiple contiguous levels. This is characteristic of DISH. OPLL coexists *(arrowheads)*.

## DIFFUSE IDIOPATHIC SKELETAL HYPEROSTOSIS

- DISH, or Forrestier disease, is characterized by ossification along the anterior and, to a lesser extent, lateral aspect of the spine (see Fig. 15.24). In addition, hyperostosis at the sites of tendon and ligamentous attachment to bone, ligamentous ossification (e.g., OPLL), and para-articular osteophytes in both the axial and appendicular skeleton are present. Findings of osseous bridging of at least four contiguous vertebral bodies, along with preservation of the intervertebral disk space and absence of apophyseal joints or sacroiliac inflammatory changes make the diagnosis. The entity is most commonly observed in the thoracic spine but can occur anywhere. Ossification of the ilio-lumbar and sacrotuberous ligaments with bony overgrowth of the inferior acetabular rim are findings in the pelvic region.
- DISH differs from spondylosis deformans in that calcification/ossification is present in the anterior longitudinal ligament with an associated proliferative enthesopathy at the site of attachment of the anterior longitudinal ligament to the anterior vertebral body surface.
- The differential diagnosis of DISH includes ankylosing spondylitis, which is not as florid as DISH and is associated with sacroiliitis (usually the first manifestation of the disease). You can observe erosion of the superior and inferior vertebral margins, producing squaring and bridging of the vertebral bodies (bamboo spine) in ankylosing spondylitis. The facet joints are involved in ankylosing spondylitis and not DISH, and the former is also associated with HLA-B27 and osteoporosis.

## SPONDYLOLYSIS AND SPONDYLOLISTHESIS

- The term *spondylolisthesis* is defined as slippage of one vertebra onto another whereas spondylolysis is a fracture through the pars interarticularis, which may or may not be associated with vertebral slippage (Fig. 15.25). A grading system is used to describe degree of slippage in the lumbar spine. Spondylolysis without spondylolisthesis is a cause of chronic low back pain, particularly in children and young adults. Effectively, this can present like a stress fracture in kids from repetitive injury, although the defect is also felt by some to arise on a developmental/congenital basis among other causes.

**TEACHING POINTS**

Grading Anterolisthesis in the Lumbar Spine

- A grading system is used on the basis of the position of the posterior margin of the subluxed vertebral body compared with the posterior margin of the inferior vertebral body.
- When the superior body is subluxed up to one fourth of a vertebral body width on the lateral film, it is termed grade I spondylolisthesis.
- Half a vertebral body is grade II.
- Three fourths a vertebral body is grade III.
- A whole width is grade IV.
- Spondyloptosis refers to a vertebral body plopping over the lower vertebral body (grade V).

**TEACHING POINTS**

Causes of Spondylolysis

- Congenital
  - Associated with dysplastic articular processes, abnormal orientation of articular processes, or kyphosis
- Acquired
  - Pars interarticularis lesions produced by stress fractures with persistent defects of the pars
  - The effects of degenerative facet disease associated with joint instability, most often occurring at L4-5, with a higher incidence in diabetics
  - Postsurgical lesions, which may be seen in the cervical or lumbar spine, resulting from altered stress on the joints after fusion surgery
  - Acute trauma with pedicle fractures
  - Pathologic conditions such as osteoporosis, metastasis, infection, osteopetrosis, or arthrogryposis

- Pars defects can be easily seen on plain spine films, particularly on oblique views and CT as a "break" in the neck of the Scottie dog, accompanied by anterior slippage of the affected body relative to the level below. The canal is generous, but neural foramina can be substantially narrowed, compromising the exiting nerve roots at the affected level. Findings on MRI, counterintuitively, are more challenging to appreciate.

**TEACHING POINTS**

Magnetic Resonance Imaging Findings of Spondylolysis

- Sagittal T1-weighted imaging (T1WI) and T2-weighted imaging (T2WI) can detect anterior slippage in association with break in the cortical margin of the pars and short tau inversion recovery (STIR) can see edema in the pars between the superior and inferior articular facets.
- Generous spinal canal.
- On sagittal images, altered shape of the neural foramina with a more horizontal configuration, loss of the foraminal fat, nerve root compression, and sharp angulation of the nerve root caused by slippage.
- "Continuous facet sign" on axial images, with pars defect mimicking appearance of facet joint, seemingly contiguous with the anatomic facet joint of the level above and below the defect.
- Disk herniation at the level of spondylolisthesis is unusual, but the more posterior disk is "uncovered" making it seem, to the "unrequisited" that the disk is herniated. It is really not, hence the term "pseudodisk/pseudoherniation"; it is just sticking with the appropriate more posterior endplate.

## SPINAL AND FORAMINAL STENOSIS

- Ultimately, the goal of imaging in the patient with spine pain is to characterize the impact of pathology on the patency of the canal and neural foramina to account for symptoms of radicular pain, claudication-like symptoms

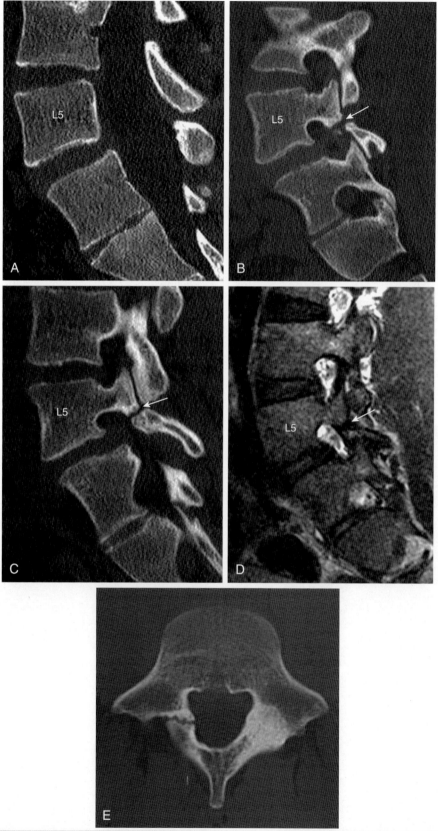

**Fig. 15.25 Spondylolysis of the spine with spondylolisthesis.** (A) Midline sagittal reconstruction from lumbar spine computed tomographic (CT) image shows a grade I anterolisthesis of L5 (indicated) on S1. (B) Right and (C) left parasagittal images from same exam show the bilateral *L5* pars defects *(arrows)*. (D) Sagittal T2-weighted image in the same patient shows the same defect on the left *(arrow)*. The defect is much harder to detect on magnetic resonance imaging (MRI) than CT, and sometimes you might think there is one on MRI only to find the pars intact on CT. So, make that MRI diagnosis with caution! (E) In another patient, a pars defect is well depicted on the axial CT. The horizontal orientation of the defect indicates that this is not a facet joint (a rookie mistake).

(which can be misdiagnosed as vascular disease), numbness, and tingling. With respect to degenerative pathology, the *bony* sagittal diameter may not be a sensitive indicator of stenosis because it does not take into account impact on canal or foraminal patency from soft tissues such as ligamentum flavum infolding, disk disease, epidural lipomatosis, and facet osteophytes. Spinal stenosis can occur in children and adolescents with achondroplasia (Fig. 15.26), mucopolysaccharidoses, congenital lipomas, and with acquired precipitating lesions such as an acute disk herniation in combination with preexisting idiopathic spinal stenosis.

- There are no specific measurement criteria in the diagnosis of canal or foraminal patency at any spinal level. In general, if the spinal canal has an AP diameter of greater than 10 mm, it is probably in good enough shape.

### PHYSICS PEARLS

- Magnetic resonance imaging tends to overestimate the degree of spinal stenosis compared with myelography and myelo-computed tomography.
- This is probably related to susceptibility effects, cerebrospinal fluid motion, and truncation artifact.

- For those less inclined to measure, the degree of canal or foraminal stenosis has been codified as mild if it narrows the thecal sac contents (with CSF effacement) or neural foramen (with fat effacement) by one third or less, moderate if narrowing one-third to two-thirds, and marked if more than two-thirds narrowed (see Fig 15.20).

## MYELOPATHY FROM DEGENERATIVE DISEASE

- Compressive cord myelopathy may result from either fixed stenosis, direct subclinical trauma, dynamic stretch injury with motion, arterial or venous ischemia, inflammation, or posttraumatic demyelination (Fig. 15.27). Myelopathy may be exacerbated if there is instability, which can be demonstrated on flexion extension radiographs.
- On MRI, myelopathy is best diagnosed on T2 images and may be seen as (1) edema within the cord (faint, indistinct high signal on T2WI); (2) gliosis (brighter, more well defined on T2WI); (3) demyelination; (4) cystic necrosis (bright, well defined on T2WI); and (5) myelomalacia (seen as elevated T2 signal with cord volume loss).
- After successful stabilization and decompression, the high intensity can resolve, suggesting an edematous etiology for the abnormality.

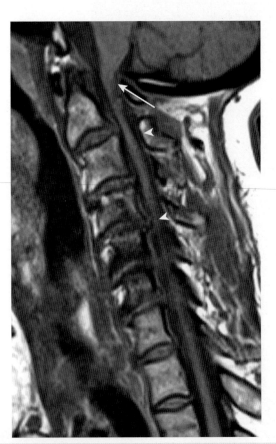

**Fig. 15.26 Achondroplastic dwarfism associated with tight foramen magnum.** Sagittal T1-weighted image shows spinal stenosis at the foramen magnum (*arrow*) as well as cervical spine stenosis (most severe level indicated by *arrowhead*). The anteroposterior and transverse diameter of the canal is often very stenotic throughout the spine.

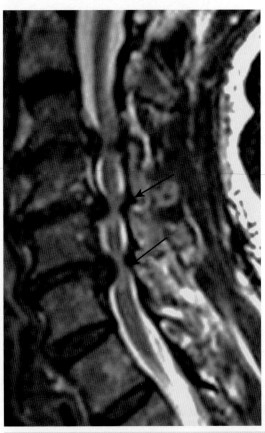

**Fig. 15.27 Spondylomyelopathy (a big word for cord injury because of degenerative disease).** Note the high signal intensity in the spinal cord on this T2-weighted image with multilevel degenerative disease and spinal stenosis (*arrows*).

## SURGICAL APPROACHES

- Spinal decompression from degenerative disease may be performed by anterior or posterior approach, often in concert with spinal fusion. The anterior approach is typically performed for disk removal and replacement often accompanied by anterior fusion hardware. Posterior approach most typically involves laminectomy with partial or complete removal of the lamina, the spinous process, and the ligamentum flavum. Posterior fusion hardware is often present to help promote spinal fusion for spine stability.
- In the lumbar and thoracic spine, posterior fusion is usually accomplished with pedicle screws transfixed with vertical and/or horizontal bars (the former particularly critical in scoliosis). In the cervical regions, except for C1, the posterior screws are usually placed in the laminae/ lateral mass. Anterior screws in the cervical region are usually attached to a plate but are located in the bodies.
- For functional fusion, the intended result calls for solid complete bridging bone across facet joints and/or intervertebral spaces around or through interbody spacer hardware. Keep in mind that although fusion surgery aids in spinal stability, the increased stresses can accelerate degenerative disease at adjacent nonfused levels, requiring revision fusion surgery—a real pain!

## POSTOPERATIVE IMAGING

- After the lengthy surgery for spinal stenosis, you will invariably receive the late-night CT scan for postoperative assessment that has become routine after hardware placement. Generally, this requires two parts to the report: one for hardware assessment and the other for immediate complications.
- Be on the lookout for lateral mass or pedicle screws that do not show adequate bony purchase. Errant screws may violate the medial pedicle margin and encroach on the thecal sac or lateral recess (Fig. 15.28). Screw tips that extend beyond the anterior cortex of a vertebral body can be ok, but if they abut critical structures (such as

the aorta, vertebral arteries in the foramen transversarium, esophagus, or nerves in the foramina) or violate the spinal canal, neural foramina, disk spaces, or facet joints, the surgeon should be notified with a courtesy call. Fractured or disengaged (i.e., screws not adequately transfixed by plate or rods) hardware should be reported.

- Intervertebral spacers of a variety of types may be placed for adding height between bodies and decompressing foramina. They should be symmetrically placed and should not overlap cortical edges on any plane.
- MRI might be performed in the immediate postoperative setting if there are new or concerning neurologic deficits that might suggest a postoperative complication.
  - On MRI, postoperatively, intermediate or high intensity on T2WI is observed in the region of the surgery. Mass effect (from the normal postoperative swelling, hemorrhage, and scar formation) can simulate preoperative disk herniation in size and signal intensity. This gradually resolves during a period of up to 6 months. Surgical disruption of the annulus appears as a line of high intensity on T2WI.
  - Immediately after surgery, mass effect on thecal sac may be present secondary to placement of absorbable surgical material for hemostasis, which appears like a folded sponge surrounded by fluid. Epidural hematomas may cause substantial mass effect on the thecal sac, requiring urgent surgical decompression in the setting of cord or thecal sac compression.
  - Extraspinal fluid collections reflecting hematomas or seromas can also be seen to compress the cord or cauda equina immediately postoperatively in the setting of a laminectomy procedure.
  - Scar tissue, evidenced by T1 and T2 hypointense, homogeneously enhancing tissue, can be seen in both asymptomatic and symptomatic patients and is dynamic over time. There is expected enhancement of the facet joint, paraspinal muscles, previously compressed nerve roots (which may enhance proximally up to the conus), the postdiskectomy disk space, and vertebral endplates. This enhancement is common and can persist for months or even longer.

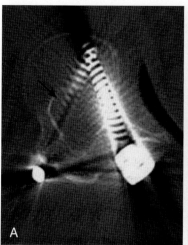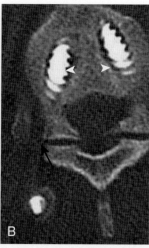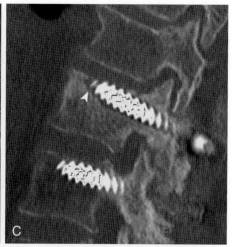

**Fig. 15.28 Pedicle screw misadventures.** (A) The tract of the right screw *(arrow)* can be seen to violate the spinal canal. Here it can irritate nerve roots or impact the thecal sac. (B) Not only does the right screw tract course lateral to the pedicle *(black arrow)*, both screws have lucency around them *(white arrowheads)* implying loosening (in a different patient). This is usually not an immediate postoperative finding but can be seen on follow-up. (C) If the screw violates the superior endplate *(arrowhead)* and enters the disk, it loses "purchase" and is unlikely to maintain stability.

## POSTOPERATIVE DISKITIS

■ The classic MR findings of postoperative diskitis are decreased signal intensity within the disk and adjacent vertebral body marrow on T1WI, increased signal on T2WI in the disk and adjacent marrow, and enhancement of the disk and endplate (Fig. 15.29). The trouble is asymptomatic patients after diskectomy may have some of these findings. Without perivertebral enhancing phlegmon or frank abscess formation, contrast enhancement of the residual disk material is not very specific in the postoperative patient to rule in or rule out diskitis. Suggest correlation with inflammatory markers like erythrocyte sedimentation rate or C-reactive protein and white blood cell (WBC) counts to help with the diagnosis.

## DURAL TEARS

■ Occasionally, the dura can be torn at the time of surgery or can occur after trauma or even spontaneously, with leakage of CSF from the wound (postoperatively) or with the formation of an organized CSF collection (pseudomeningocele), which can subsequently enlarge. This collection may need to be repaired if it is progressive and/or prone to infection and/or fistulizes to the skin. The differential diagnosis, particularly in the early postoperative period in the patient with pain and fever, is abscess, which might demonstrate significant peripheral enhancement. Seromas show minimal rim enhancement and are usually asymptomatic.

## FAILED BACK SURGERY SYNDROME (THE SURGEON'S WORST NIGHTMARE)

■ A large problem confronting the clinician (and secondarily the radiologist) is recurrent or residual low back pain in the patient after lumbar disk surgery. This condition has a reported incidence of 5% to 40%, and the syndrome has been termed the "failed back" or the "failed back surgery" syndrome (FBSS).

---

> **TEACHING POINTS**
>
> Causes of Failed Back Syndrome
>
> • Arachnoiditis
> • Epidural fibrosis/granulation tissue/scarring
> • Immediate postoperative complications including infection, hematoma, or surgical trauma to roots
> • Insufficient decompression of roots by residual soft tissue or bone
> • Mechanical instability
> • New disk disease at level adjacent to the surgery because of changes in stress
> • Pseudoarthrosis
> • Residual or recurrent disk
> • Spondylolisthesis
> • Surgery at wrong level

■ All patients have varying degrees of scar tissue at 4 months. However, scar tissue cannot necessarily be implicated as an etiology of postoperative back pain because everyone gets it and only some have chronic pain. In the failed back, it is critical to look carefully for other causes of pain including infection, residual or recurrent disk, or instability.

■ The diagnosis of scar versus residual/recurrent disk herniation is extremely important. Surgery is not indicated for scar (epidural fibrosis) but would be beneficial if disk can be diagnosed as the cause of the radiculopathy. Both may produce mass effect, although nerve root displacement is almost always associated with a recurrent herniated disk. IV contrast is key because immediate scanning of scar demonstrates diffuse enhancement on T1WI, whereas disk usually does not enhance or shows peripheral enhancement (Fig. 15.30). Fat saturation is really useful on postcontrast T1WI; without it, differentiation between scar (which shows T1 hyperintensity postcontrast) and fat (intrinsically T1 hyperintense) would be very difficult.

   ■ Scan immediately after contrast administration and with rapid sequences. If scanning is delayed more than 20 minutes, disk may imbibe the contrast and therefore enhance with an appearance identical to

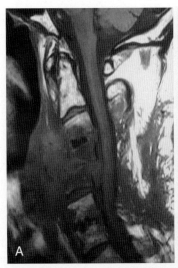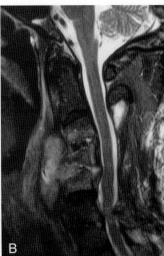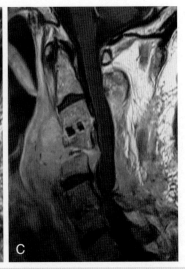

**Fig. 15.29 Postoperative diskitis.** (A) Sagittal T1-weighted imaging (T1WI) scan shows loss of disk space, hypointensity of the marrow, collapse, kyphosis, epidural compression, and an impressive prevertebral mass. (B) High signal in the disk and the adjacent marrow as well as the epidural and prevertebral mass is evident on this sagittal T2WI. (C) After contrast, one completes the picture with enhancing disk material, endplates, epidural phlegmon, and prevertebral abscess. Ouch!

scar. Enhancement also enables detection of the nerve root (not enhancing) surrounded by enhancing scar.

■ Nerve roots have been noted to enhance postoperatively. These roots are nearly always those compressed preoperatively, suggesting ongoing repair and regeneration associated with an impaired blood-nerve barrier. Relating clinical symptoms to root enhancement is controversial because this phenomenon occurs in 5% of symptomatic patients without surgery. An alternative explanation regarding lumbar root enhancement is that it results from obstruction of small radicular veins within the endoneurium of the nerve root related to nerve root compression. It may be the radicular veins (intravascular enhancement) and *not* roots that enhance.

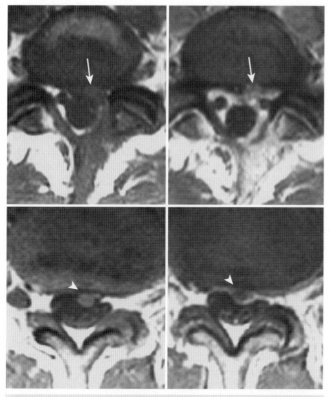

**Fig. 15.30 Scar versus residual disk.** Note that on the images above, the soft tissue in the left anterior epidural space after left hemilaminectomy shows enhancement on the top images *(arrows)*. Diagnosis: Scar! Contrast that (excuse the pun) with the images below where the soft tissue *(arrowheads)* does not enhance on the postcontrast scan. Diagnosis: Disk herniation.

## POSTOPERATIVE INSTABILITY

■ Instability has been defined as loss of motion segment stiffness as shown by an abnormal response to applied loads. An assessment of spinal stability after surgery begins with flexion and extension views to look for movement and change in angulation of the spine. If there is anterolisthesis or retrolisthesis with bending or if the width of the anterior intervertebral space changes significantly with position, it suggests the fusion is not solid. Vacuum phenomena in the disks implies movement is occurring and should not be seen at fused levels.

## ARACHNOIDITIS

■ Arachnoiditis, cited as a cause in up to 15% of cases of FBSS, is an inflammatory disorder of the spinal leptomeninges particularly affecting the nerve roots resulting in intradural adhesions. It can be responsible for the development of loculated arachnoid cysts particularly in the thoracic region.

   ■ Meningitis, subarachnoid hemorrhage, and contrast myelography using toxic dyes (Pantopaque is no longer on the market for this reason) can result in arachnoiditis.

   ■ Arachnoiditis can be diagnosed by MRI and CT myelography evidenced by (1) loss of the ability to distinguish the roots in the thecal sac and obliteration of the root sleeves (mild); (2) loss of the morphology of the thecal sac; (3) adhesion of the nerve roots to the dural tube ("empty sac"); or (4) clumping together of the nerve roots, leading to an appearance of a "pseudofilum" (Fig. 15.31). Arachnoiditis may or may not enhance.

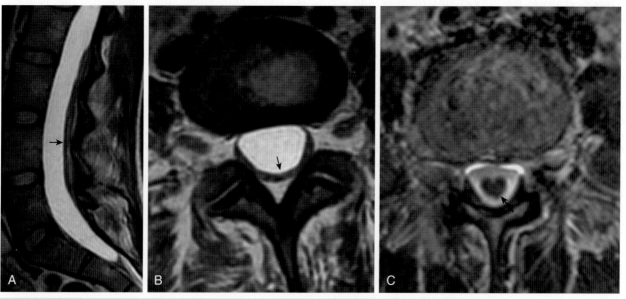

**Fig. 15.31 Empty thecal sac.** (A–B) These images show the nerve roots plastered along the posterior thecal sac such that the sac looks empty *(arrows)*. (C) Contrast that with this section through L4-L5 in a different patient where it looks like there is a spinal cord *(arrow)* present. Chiari with tethered cord? No, actually these are clumped nerve roots after surgery.

# Non-degenerative Disease of the Spine

MARGARET N. CHAPMAN

## Relevant Anatomy

- The following discussion focuses on the anatomy of the cord and spinal vasculature. Refer to Chapter 15 for a description of bone, disc, and neural anatomy.
- The spinal cord extends from the medulla oblongata, at the level of the upper border of the atlas, to about the T12-L2 spinal levels, where it terminates in the conus medullaris. At the apex of the conus, continuous with the pia mater, is the filum terminale, which initially descends in the thecal sac and then becomes covered with adherent dura as it leaves the thecal sac to insert in the coccyx. The cauda equina emanates from the conus medullaris and contains the nerve roots of the lumbar and sacral nerves.
- The spinal cord relays sensory and motor neural messages to and from the brain, along numerous white matter (peripheral) and gray matter (central) tracts (Fig. 16.1). The cord has two enlargements in its course, one in the cervical region from approximately C4 to approximately T1 and the other in the lower thoracic region from approximately T9 to T12. These enlargements correspond to the locations in the cord that supply the spinal nerves for the upper and lower extremities.
- The central canal (in the central spinal cord gray matter) extends from the obex of the fourth ventricle to the filum terminale, contains a small amount of cerebrospinal fluid (CSF), and is lined by ependymal cells. It can occasionally be seen on T2-weighted imaging (T2WI) but is usually less than 2 mm in diameter. In the region of the conus medullaris, the canal expands as a fusiform terminal ventricle, the ventriculus terminalis (fifth ventricle), which on MR imaging can be seen in children, very rarely in adults.
- In the cervical region, the anterior spinal artery is formed by branches that originate from the vertebral arteries just before joining the basilar artery (Fig. 16.2). The anterior spinal artery supplies the anterior two thirds/majority of the spinal cord, including the anterior column of the central gray matter, the corticospinal, the spinothalamic, and other tracts. The caliber of the anterior spinal artery at a particular spinal level is proportional to the metabolic demands of the spinal gray matter.
- In addition, paired posterior spinal arteries originate from the vertebral arteries and supply the dorsal portion of the cord (i.e., the posterior columns and the posterior horn of the central gray matter).
- The anterior spinal artery is in the midline, whereas the posterior spinal arteries lie off the midline. The anterior and posterior spinal arteries rarely originate at the same level. These two arterial systems do not usually have significant anastomoses between them and can lead to different ischemic myelopathic cord syndromes when compromised (Table 16.1).
- Radicular feeders from the vertebral, ascending cervical (anterior to the transverse process), and deep cervical (posterior to the transverse process) arteries anastomose with the spinal arteries. The radicular feeders enter the thecal sac through the intervertebral foramina and divide into the anterior and posterior branches coursing with the nerve roots. Because they follow the nerve root, the spinal arteries have a sharper angle in the lumbar region than in the cervical region.
- However, not all spinal nerves have radicular arteries. The cervical and upper two thoracic levels make up one vascular territory. The midthoracic region T3 to T7 is supplied by intercostal branches from the aorta, branches of the supreme intercostal arteries from the subclavians, and lumbar arteries. This region may have a tenuous blood supply.
- The lower thoracolumbar region to the filum terminale is supplied by the artery of Adamkiewicz. It is commonly located on the left side between T9 to L2 (85% of the time) and T5 to T8 (15% of the time). It enters the spinal canal with the nerve roots and makes a characteristic hairpin loop, giving off a small superior branch from the apex of the turn and a large descending branch, which supply the anterior spinal cord and anastomoses with the posterior spinal arteries in the region of the conus medullaris.
- The venous blood supply is comparable to the arterial blood supply with a variable amount of anterior and posterior spinal veins running with the spinal arteries.

## Imaging Techniques/Protocols

- Spinal imaging techniques are described in detail in Chapter 15. In terms of identifying nondegenerative pathologies in the spine, computed tomography (CT) and magnetic resonance imaging (MRI) are the main imaging modalities we have to work with.
- CT provides excellent bony detail and typically includes a smaller field of view centered on the spine and should be reviewed in axial, sagittal, and coronal planes. Typically, contrast is not necessary, unless there is clinical concern for paraspinal abscess. Intraspinal abscesses are difficult to perceive on CT even with contrast, and

MRI should be performed in those cases if there are no contraindications.

- Post-myelogram CT is an effective way to evaluate extra-medullary intradural pathology, including mass effect on cord and nerve roots in the event that MRI is contra-indicated. Similarly, nerve root avulsions after trauma can be elegantly demonstrated with post-myelogram CT studies.
- MRI provides excellent soft tissue detail and is very useful not only in identifying pathology but also in assessing extent and impact on cord and nerve roots with greater certainty than CT. For non-degenerative disease, intravenous (IV) contrast is usually very helpful in evaluation of cord and other intrathecal lesions.
- If vascular disease is suspected, magnetic resonance (MR) and CT angiographic techniques can be employed, but because we are talking about very tiny vessels, vascular stenosis–like occlusions and high-flow malformations are difficult to detect. In such cases, conventional angiography is the modality of choice.
- In the work-up for spinal CSF leak, high-resolution T2 images and pre- and postcontrast T1WI are needed to identify suspicious collections and meningoceles that might represent the culprit site of leakage. Post-myelogram high-resolution CT may also demonstrate subtle abnormalities and leaks.
- In cases of suspected cord infarct, cord abscess, and active demyelination, diffusion-weighted imaging of the cord can be enormously helpful.

---

**PHYSICS PEARLS**

- Diffusion-weighted imaging (DWI) of the cord is technically challenging because of its small size, physiologic motion artifacts from swallowing, cord motion from cerebrospinal fluid pulsations, and susceptibility artifacts from adjacent bones and lungs.
- Echo planar imaging (EPI) is the most commonly used technique, and image quality can be improved using reduced B values (400–500) and frequency encoding to shorten echo time, reduce tissue distortions, and improve signal to noise.
- Multishot EPI with smaller field of view can also help improve diagnostic quality.

## Pathology

### INFECTIOUS DISEASES OF THE SPINE AND SPINAL COVERINGS

#### Diskitis and Osteomyelitis

- Pyogenic disk space infections are usually the result of a blood-borne agent, often from the lung or urinary tract. *Staphylococcus* is the most commonly encountered pathogen.
- Clinical settings include a recent history of spine surgery, hematogenous dissemination from another infectious site, compromised immunity, infectious endocarditis, or IV drug use.
- Symptoms include focal back pain and can progress to radicular, meningeal, and spinal cord compressive symptoms if/as the disease advances.
- Vertebral osteomyelitis usually occurs in the setting of disk space infection; however, it can occur without disk space infection from hematogenous dissemination directly to the vertebral body.
- Vasculitis of the medullary arteries and/or veins may produce spinal cord symptoms/signs without epidural compression as one of the complications of pyogenic disk space infection or vertebral osteomyelitis.
- MRI is the most specific method for diagnosing infectious processes in the disk and/or vertebral body and can simultaneously provide information on involvement of the spinal canal and cord.
- Affected disks will demonstrate low signal intensity on T1-weighted imaging (T1WI) and higher than normal signal intensity on T2WI as a result of the associated edema (Fig. 16.3). If affected, the adjacent vertebral bodies (particularly the endplates) will also demonstrate similar signal abnormalities. The disk space, adjacent vertebral bodies, and the adjacent epidural and/or paravertebral soft tissues enhance if affected.
  - Modic type I degenerative marrow changes may appear similar to diskitis/osteomyelitis and may also enhance, making it difficult to distinguish between the two.
- Careful evaluation for epidural or paravertebral abscesses must also be performed because these may require surgical drainage.

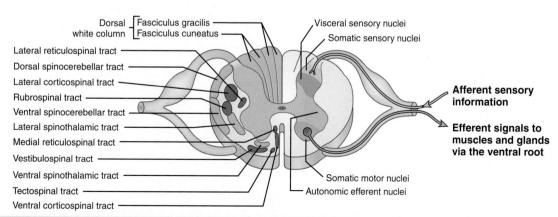

**Fig. 16.1 Schematic representation of spinal cord anatomy.** Grey matter visceral, somatic motor, somatic sensory and autonomic efferent nuclei are depicted along with white matter tracts, with ascending tracts depicted in *blue* and descending tracts depicted in *red*. Redrawn from https://www.chegg.com/flashcards/neurology-chapters-1-3-efb66f22-355f-45f6-b3ba-4be1cb1fa35e/deck and https://twitter.com/ptflashcards/status/1282933797470658560

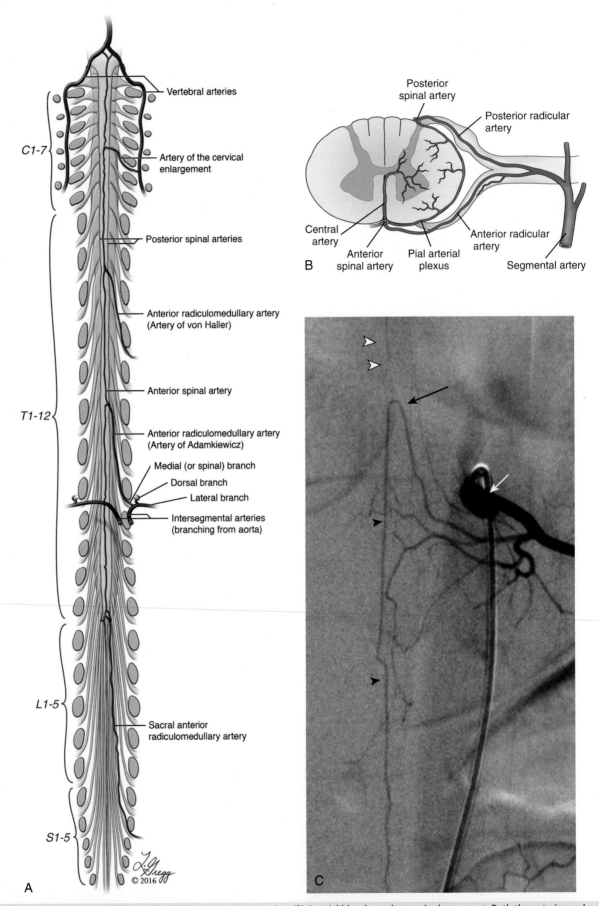

C1-7

Vertebral arteries

Artery of the cervical enlargement

Posterior spinal arteries

Anterior radiculomedullary artery (Artery of von Haller)

Anterior spinal artery

T1-12

Anterior radiculomedullary artery (Artery of Adamkiewicz)

Medial (or spinal) branch

Dorsal branch

Lateral branch

Intersegmental arteries (branching from aorta)

L1-5

Sacral anterior radiculomedullary artery

S1-5

© 2016

A

Posterior spinal artery

Posterior radicular artery

Central artery

Anterior spinal artery

Pial arterial plexus

Anterior radicular artery

Segmental artery

B

C

**Fig. 16.2 Arterial anatomy of the cord.** (A) Schematic representation. (B) Arterial blood supply at a single segment. Both the anterior and posterior medullary arteries are illustrated. This is not the typical arrangement. It is unusual for both anterior and posterior medullary arteries to enter at the same segment in any region of the cord. (C) Spinal arteriogram. Injection into the T9 left intercostal artery *(white arrow)* reveals filling of artery of Adamkiewicz with its characteristic hairpin turn *(black arrow)*. Anterior spinal artery is filling faintly above *(white arrowheads)* and more emphatically below *(black arrowheads)*. (A, Courtesy Lydia Gregg; B, From Krauss WE. Vascular anatomy of the spinal cord. *Neurosurg Clin North Am* 1999;10:10.)

**Table 16.1**  Cord Syndromes and Clinical Manifestations

| Syndrome | Part of Cord Affected | Manifestations | Less Common Manifestations | Typical Lesion |
|---|---|---|---|---|
| Anterior spinal artery syndrome | Anterior two thirds cord bilaterally | Bilateral motor loss and pain and temperature sensation loss | Hypotension, sexual dysfunction | Cord infarct (ASA) |
| Incomplete ASA syndrome | Just anterior horn cells | Paraplegia | Painful diplegia | Cord infarct (ASA) |
| Posterior spinal artery syndrome | Posterior column injury | Loss of proprioception, vibratory sense, total anesthesia at level of injury | Mild weakness, rarely bilateral | Cord infarct (PSA) |
| Brown-Sequard syndrome | Hemicord injury | Ipsilateral hemiparesis and loss of proprioception, contralateral loss of pain and temperature | — | Demyelinating diseases |
| Cauda equina syndrome | Conus, cauda equina injury | Back pain, saddle anesthesia, bowel and bladder dysfunction with incontinence, sexual dysfunction | Absent anal reflex, weakness in the legs, gait disturbance | Compression by bone/disk pathology |
| Central cord syndrome | Central cord | Bilateral loss of pain and temperature and motor control | Bladder dysfunction, urinary retention | Trauma, cervical spondylosis, cardiac arrest, hypotension |

*ASA,* Anterior spinal artery; *PSA,* posterior spinal artery.

■ Endplate destructive changes may be better appreciated by radiograph or CT. Nuclear medicine imaging may also provide information regarding adjacent osseous changes.

---

**TEACHING POINTS**

Nuclear Medicine Imaging of the Infected Spine

• A three-phase technetium bone scan can show increased blood flow and persistent osseous uptake on delayed images in osteomyelitis, although these findings are not specific.
• If there remains a question of degenerative disease versus infection, a gallium scan or indium-111–labeled leukocyte scan can help favor an infectious process by demonstrating increased uptake and correlating it with the positive bone scan.

---

## Granulomatous Infections

■ Tuberculosis, brucellosis, and fungal infections (blastomycosis, cryptococcus, and coccidiomycosis) are the most common granulomatous infections of the spine.
■ Spinal tuberculosis is an indolent process that most often affects the lower thoracic spine (Pott disease or tuberculous spondylitis). There is frequent associated epidural disease or adjacent paravertebral soft-tissue abscesses. The posterior elements may be involved, and the infection can spread along the anterior longitudinal ligament and involve multiple levels. Spinal deformity is common, including gibbus deformity.
■ Vertebral body destruction with relative sparing of the disk space occurs late in the disease. The disk can be of normal intensity on noncontrast MR but usually enhances.
■ Table 16.2 contrasts the features of bacterial infection, tuberculosis, and neoplasm.

## Intraspinal Infections

### Epidural Abscesses

■ Epidural abscesses result either from direct extension of vertebral osteomyelitis or hematogenous dissemination from an infectious source. *Staphylococcus aureus* is the most common pathogen.
■ Patients are often septic and may endorse a history of IV drug abuse, immunosuppression, urinary tract infections, recent surgery/trauma, and valvular infections.
■ Symptoms include tenderness over the spine, back pain, and progressive neurologic impairment.
■ MR is the modality of choice for imaging epidural abscesses (Fig. 16.4; see also Fig. 16.3). The epidural collection has low signal intensity on T1WI and has high signal on T2WI and can show diffusion restriction. There are three patterns of enhancement:
   ■ Homogeneous enhancement, representing diffuse inflamed tissue with microabscesses (phlegmonous granulation tissue), best seen with postcontrast fat-suppressed techniques
   ■ Peripheral enhancement consistent with frank abscess including a necrotic center
   ■ A combination of tissue enhancement and frank abscess
■ Precontrast T1WI images without fat suppression are helpful in detecting space-occupying processes in the epidural space because of effacement and/or replacement of the normal T1 bright epidural fat by abnormal tissue.
■ Epidural abscess produces symptoms by mass effect and/or septic thrombophlebitis with cord edema and infarction. Spinal cord infarction secondary to thrombophlebitis should be considered in the setting of epidural abscess and high signal on T2WI in the cord. Nowadays spinal diffusion-weighted imaging (DWI)/diffusion tensor imaging (DTI) sequences are available to readily diagnose spinal cord infarctions as intramedullary areas of apparent diffusion coefficient (ADC) restriction.

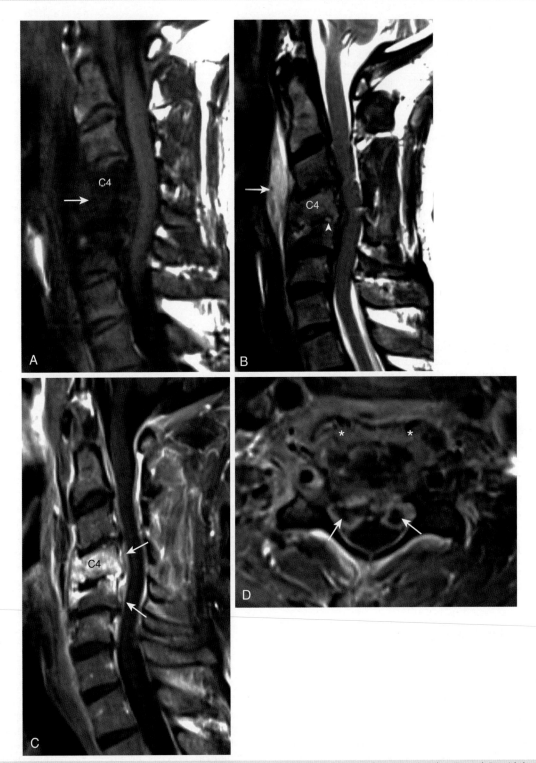

**Fig. 16.3 Cervical diskitis/osteomyelitis.** (A) Sagittal T1-weighted imaging (T1WI) shows abnormal marrow signal at C4 and C5 with loss of endplate definition *(arrow)*. There is a slight kyphotic angulation centered at this level. (B) Sagittal T2WI shows focal high signal within the C4 to C5 disk space *(arrow-head)*, although this alone is not sufficient to make a diagnosis of diskitis. It is the constellation of these and other findings, including prevertebral edema *(arrow)*, and (C) abnormal epidural enhancement *(arrows)* on postcontrast T1WI that support the diagnosis. (D) Note the presence of organized fluid collections within the ventral epidural space *(arrows)* resulting in canal compromise and thickening and enhancement of the longus colli musculature *(asterisks)*.

## Subdural Empyema

- Subdural empyema has a similar presentation to epidural abscess, although it is much rarer in occurrence and may occur after lumbar puncture, spinal anesthesia, and diskography. Discrimination between the subdural and epidural compartments is usually difficult on MR.

## Meningeal Inflammation

- Meningeal inflammation can occur either with or without the intraspinal infections previously described. Clinically, meningeal infection may lead to symptoms of myelopathy and/or radiculopathy, which can progress to paralysis.

**Table 16.2**   Salient Features of Nontuberculous Bacterial Infection, Tuberculosis, and Neoplasm

| Condition | Disk Space | Paraspinal Mass | Posterior Elements | Spread |
|---|---|---|---|---|
| Bacterial infection | Always involved early on | May or may not be present | Very uncommon | Contiguous |
| Tuberculosis | Occurs in the course of the disease | Usually large | Yes | May have skip areas |
| Neoplasm | Very rare | Yes | Yes | Noncontiguous |

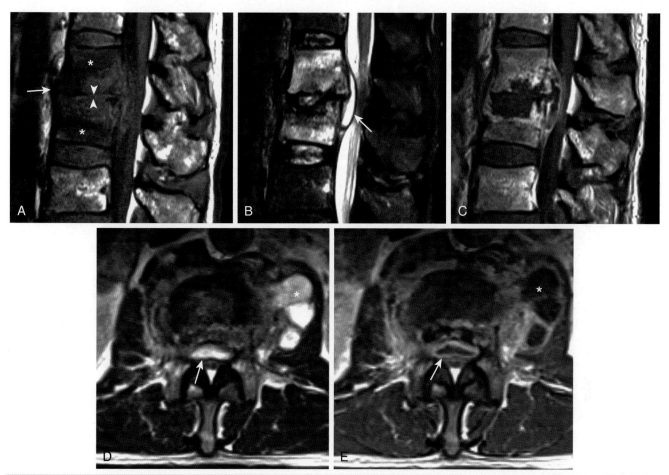

**Fig. 16.4  Tuberculous osteomyelitis.** (A) Sagittal T1-weighted imaging (T1WI) shows abnormal marrow signal involving two adjacent vertebral bodies *(asterisks)*, as well as loss of endplate cortical definition *(arrowheads)*. Note prevertebral component *(arrow)* along the anterior longitudinal ligament. (B) Sagittal short tau inversion recovery (STIR) image shows associated ventral epidural fluid collection compromising the spinal canal *(arrow)*. (C) On this sagittal postcontrast T1WI, the fluid collection shows peripheral enhancement, indicating organized abscess in communication with the intervertebral disk. (D) Axial T2-weighted imaging (T2WI) again shows the epidural fluid collection *(arrow)* and the extension of inflammation and fluid collection into the left psoas musculature *(asterisk)*. (E) Both fluid collections show peripheral rim enhancement on axial postcontrast T1WI indicating organized abscesses. Note perivertebral soft-tissue enhancement along the margins of the vertebral body.

- MR can show poor definition of the cord or subarachnoid space on T1WI and diffuse thick enhancement of the leptomeninges. This is often not readily discernible by CT, even with contrast administration.
- A normal MRI does not exclude meningeal inflammation, and if clinically suspected and no contraindications, lumbar puncture should be performed.
- Arachnoiditis may occur as a sequela of bacterial meningitis, which on MR or CT myelography is demonstrated by clumping of nerve roots within (pseudo cord sign) or around the periphery (empty sac sign) of the thecal sac (See Chapter 15). When acutely irritated, the nerve roots may enhance.

## Acquired Immunodeficiency Syndrome

- A variety of conditions affect the spinal canal and cord in patients with AIDS (Fig. 16.5).

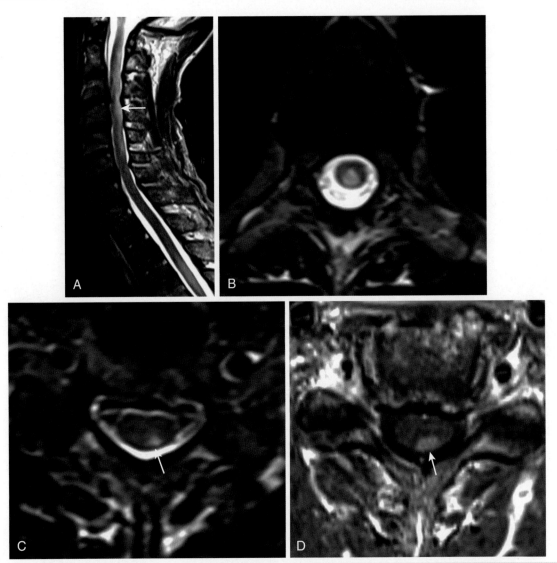

**Fig. 16.5 Acquired immunodeficiency syndrome–associated myelopathy.** (A) Long segment T2 hyperintensity predominantly affecting the dorsal cervical cord *(arrow)* is seen on this sagittal T2-weighted image (T2WI). Note additional multilevel signal abnormality at the upper thoracic cord. (B) Axial T2WI through the thoracic cord shows clear involvement of the dorsal cord. (C) More superiorly, this axial T2WI shows preferential involvement of the left dorsal cord *(arrow)*, and this lesion enhances on (D) postcontrast T1WI *(arrow)*.

**TEACHING POINTS**

Intramedullary Lesions in Acquired Immunodeficiency Syndrome

Viral (HIV, CMV, HSV, HZV) infection
Toxoplasmosis
Tuberculosis
Vacuolar myelopathy
Non Hodgkin lymphoma
Subacute necrotizing myelopathy
Syphilis

*CMV*, Cytomegalovirus; *HIV*, human immunodeficiency virus; *HSV*, herpes simplex virus; *HZV*, herpes zoster virus.

■ Unfortunately, nothing is specific about the MR appearance to separate AIDS from other non-AIDS intramedullary lesions. High intensity on T2WI is seen in a spinal cord that may be large, normal, or small in size.

# NON-INFECTIOUS INFLAMMATORY DISEASES OF THE SPINE AND SPINAL COVERINGS

## Renal Spondyloarthropathy

■ Patients undergoing dialysis can have changes in their spine (usually in the cervical region), which superficially may resemble infection (renal spondyloarthropathy).
■ There is destruction of the disk space and adjacent vertebral bodies; however, the signal intensity on T2WI is usually low rather than high as expected in infection. Paravertebral inflammatory tissue is absent.

## Sarcoidosis

■ Spinal neurosarcoidosis is rare, affecting only 6% to 8% of patients with neurosarcoidosis, most commonly in the cervical spine.
■ Intramedullary sarcoidosis may present as a diffuse inflammatory lesion or as a discrete mass with

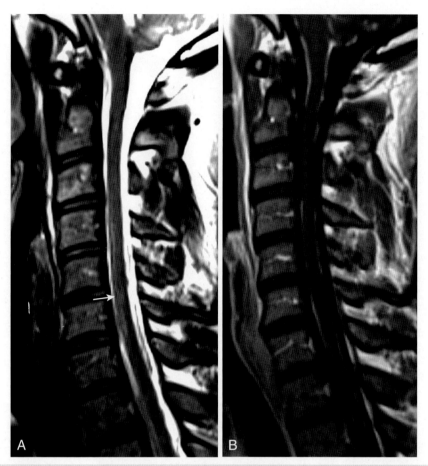

**Fig. 16.6 Sarcoidosis of cord.** (A) Sagittal T2-weighted imaging shows abnormal patchy intramedullary signal throughout the cervical spinal cord *(arrow)*. (B) On postcontrast T1-weighted imaging, there is striking enhancement of the leptomeninges.

intermediate to high signal intensity on T2WI (Fig. 16.6). Extramedullary manifestations include enhancing nodules on the surface of the cord or less commonly along individual nerve roots.

## Intramedullary Diseases

### Transverse Myelitis

- Transverse myelitis is a syndrome affecting the spinal cord associated with rapidly progressive neurologic dysfunction. Diseases causing this condition include acute disseminated encephalomyelitis, MS, and other demyelinating conditions such as neuromyelitis optica spectrum disorder and myelin oligodendrocyte glycoprotein (MOG)-associated disease, connective tissue diseases (lupus, rheumatoid arthritis, and Sjögren syndrome), sarcoidosis, vascular malformations, and vasculitides, or it may be idiopathic.
- The spinal cord is focally enlarged with high signal on T2WI and may show variable enhancement patterns including patchy, nodular, or meningeal enhancement (Fig. 16.7). The lesion extends over multiple spinal cord segments and involves the entire cross-section of the spinal cord.
- With idiopathic acute transverse myelitis, the clinical course occurs over days to weeks. In some cases, the

cauda equina enhances, suggesting a possible relationship with Guillain-Barré syndrome.

### Multiple Sclerosis

- Multiple sclerosis (MS) can affect the spinal cord and produce myelopathic signs and symptoms. It can be confined solely to the spinal cord (5%–24% of cases).
- MS lesions are isointense to cord or of low intensity on T1WI and high signal on T2WI. Sixty percent of the spinal cord lesions occur in the cervical region.
- The typical MS spinal cord lesion does not involve the entire cross-sectional area, is peripherally located, does not respect gray/white boundaries, and is less than two vertebral body segments in length (90% of the time) (see Fig. 16.8).
- The posterior columns are favored by MS. The cord is usually normal in size with enlargement seen in only 6% to 14% of cases and with possible atrophy detected over the course of the disease. The majority of lesions are patchy in configuration and rarely demonstrate enhancement unless the patient is referred for problems specific to new spinal cord signs/symptoms.
- MRI of the brain may be useful in distinguishing cord signal abnormalities related to transverse myelitis

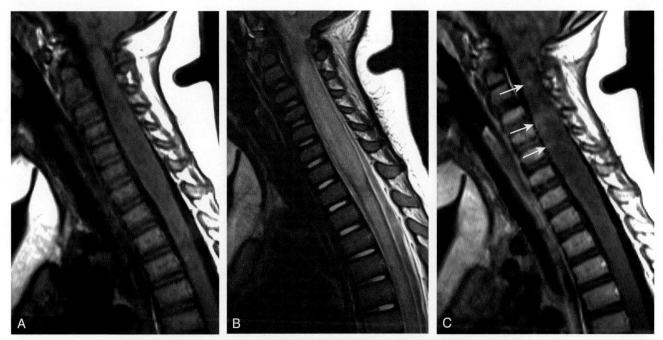

**Fig. 16.7  Transverse myelitis.** (A) Sagittal T1-weighted imaging (T1WI) shows marked enlargement of the imaged cord, particularly the cervical cord. (B) Sagittal T2-weighted imaging (T2WI) shows generalized increased T2 signal within the cord. (C) After contrast administration, patchy areas of subtle enhancement can be seen on this sagittal T1WI *(arrows).*

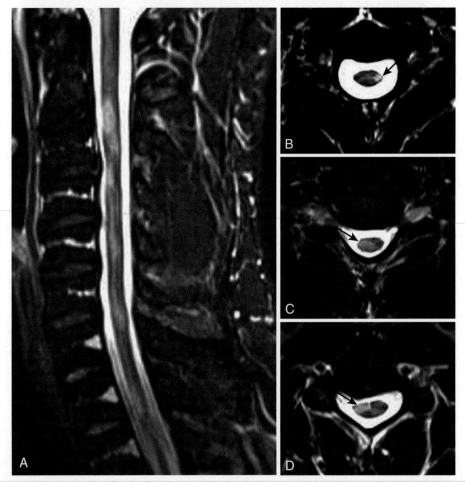

**Fig. 16.8  Multiple sclerosis.** (A) Multiple high signal intensity foci are depicted on this sagittal short tau inversion recovery (STIR) image through the cervical and upper thoracic cord. (B–D) Axial T2-weighted imaging through the cervical cord shows some of these lesions *(arrows).* Note that these typical lesions do not involve the entire cross-sectional area of the cord, are peripherally located, and do not respect great-white boundaries. Over time, cord volume loss may develop at these sites of disease.

or MS because asymptomatic high signal abnormalities in young adult brains help favor MS as the
cause.

■ Transverse myelitis and optic neuritis are seen with neuromyelitis optica spectrum disorder (NMOSD). NMOSD
shows long segment cord disease rather than short segment disease as in MS (which would more likely show
intracranial white matter disease than NMOSD). NMOSD
may be monophasic or polyphasic.

■ Anti-MOG (myelin oligodendrocyte glycoprotein)
myelitis falls within the demyelinating disease spectrum with MS and NMOSD, and longitudinal cord
lesions can be seen, usually in conjunction with optic
neuritis.

## Lupus Myelitis

■ Transverse myelitis presenting as back pain, paraparesis
or quadriparesis, and sensory loss may be a complication
of systemic lupus erythematosus. Etiology of the lesion
is vacuolar degeneration from an autoimmune process
or ischemia.

■ The spinal cord may be enlarged with high intensity
on T2WI involving four to five vertebral body segments
of the cord (Fig. 16.9). Contrast enhancement can be
detected in approximately 50% of cases.

## Radiation-Induced Changes

■ Spinal radiation converts normal bone marrow to fatty
marrow (Fig. 16.10) manifested on MR by diffuse high
signal on T1WI in the vertebral bodies and lower intensity on conventional T2WI.

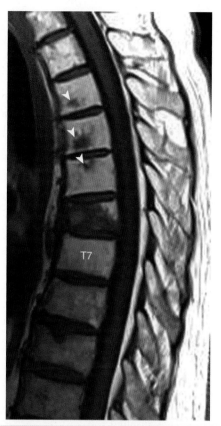

**Fig. 16.10 Radiation changes to spine.** In this patient with lung cancer treated with radiation, there is relatively bright T1 marrow signal
superiorly from T7. Compare with more normal heterogeneous marrow signal from T8 down. Unfortunately, this patient developed bone
metastases *(arrowheads)* with more confluent metastatic disease
nearly completely replacing the T6 marrow.

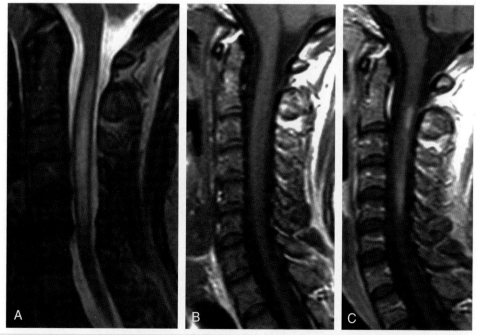

**Fig. 16.9 Lupus myelitis.** (A) Sagittal T2-weighted imaging (T2WI) shows diffusely increased T2 signal and mild enlargement of much of the
cervical cord. (B) When comparing precontrast sagittal T1-weighted imaging (T1WI) (C) with the postcontrast T1WI, note that there is patchy
enhancement present within this region of signal abnormality. It is difficult to know the diagnosis without the clinical history of systemic lupus
erythematosus.

Intensity Abnormalities of Vertebral Marrow on T1-Weighted Imaging

**Decreased Intensity**

> Any condition that produces edema, increased hematopoietic marrow, or fatty marrow replacement, such as infection, metastases, marrow packing disorders
> Any condition that produces sclerosis of the bone (e.g., metastases, osteopetrosis)
> Degenerative changes (Modic types I and III)
> Acquired Immune Deficiency Syndrome (AIDS)
> Anemia
> Paget disease (variable)
> Blood transfusions
> Hemochromatosis (iron overload)
> Chronic renal failure

**Increased Intensity**

> Any condition that produces fatty marrow, including normal aging
> Degenerative changes (Modic type II)
> Radiation
> Vertebral body hemangioma
> Hemorrhage
> Paget disease (variable)
> Fibrous dysplasia (variable)
> Steroid therapy/Cushing disease

- If the cord is high signal on T2WI, it may be the result of radiation myelitis or residual tumor if the reason for the initial therapy was a cord tumor. Cord atrophy is another manifestation of radiation therapy.

## Subacute Combined Degeneration

- Subacute combined degeneration, a complication of cobalamin (vitamin $B_{12}$) deficiency, causes a myelopathy affecting the cervical and upper thoracic spinal cord, but it can also produce lesions in the optic tracts, brain, and peripheral nerves. Folate deficiency and copper deficiency can lead to a similar spectrum of disease. This can be seen in patients with pernicious anemia, bariatric surgery, alcoholism, anorexia nervosa-bulimia syndromes, or other causes of nutritional imbalance.
- Clinical findings include paresthesias of the hands and feet, loss of position and vibratory sensation, sensory ataxia, spasticity, and lower extremity weakness.
- Pathologically, demyelination and axonal loss in the posterior and lateral spinal cord columns is seen.
- High intensity is observed longitudinally in the posterior columns on T2WI (Fig. 16.11). After treatment, this can regress and disappear; without treatment, permanent axonal loss and myelomalacia will be seen.
- There are several etiologies for posterior column disease.

Conditions Involving the Posterior Columns of the Spinal Cord

> Multiple sclerosis
> Cobalamin (vitamin $B_{12}$) deficiency
> Copper deficiency
> Folic acid deficiency
> Nitrous oxide toxicity
> Spinal trauma
> Tumor
> Tabes dorsalis (syphilis)
> Toxins
> Vacuolar myelopathy

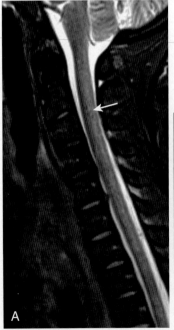
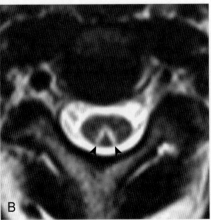

**Fig. 16.11 Subacute combined degeneration.** (A) Sagittal short tau inversion recovery (STIR) image shows subtle abnormal signal predominantly in the posterior spinal cord *(arrow)*. (B) On this axial T2-weighted image in a different patient, you can see the configuration of the posterior column disease *(arrowheads)*. Although vitamin $B_{12}$ and folate deficiency are the classic etiologies for this appearance, copper deficiency should also be on the differential diagnosis.

# CYSTIC LESIONS OF THE SPINAL CANAL

## Arachnoid Cyst

- Arachnoid cysts occur on a congenital basis or result from trauma, postoperative scarring, or inflammation. These cysts can be under pressure and produce symptoms by spinal cord compression as they enlarge.
- The cyst looks like CSF on MRI and CT; carefully scrutinize the cord margins for any suggestion of focal mass effect or cord displacement.
- On MRI, focal impression on the cord can be seen with intensity similar to that of CSF without enhancement (Fig. 16.12).
- On CT myelography, you will see an extramedullary mass, which may compress the cord. The cyst does not opacify at the time of initial intrathecal injection and may or may not fill with contrast on delayed imaging.
- A related entity is the spinal arachnoid web, which is a septation that can impress on the cord; some believe the web is caused by a disrupted or deflated arachnoid cyst.

The cord may be displaced, and the patient may develop pain and/or neurologic symptoms. A syringohydromyelia may result from abnormal CSF flow dynamics. The "scalpel sign" refers to the angulation of the cord appearing like a scalpel with its blade pointing posteriorly as a result of the web. These webs are most commonly thoracic and posterior in the intradural space.

- Cord herniation syndrome, a rare condition most commonly seen in the thoracic spine, mimics the imaging appearance of an arachnoid cyst. In this condition, a portion of the cord herniates through a dural defect, producing symptoms such as myelopathy, radiculopathy, sensory deficits, or Brown-Séquard syndrome. Dural defects may occur from prior surgery, trauma, a traumatic disk herniation, or a congenital dural defect.
  - MR demonstrates the cord to be small, rotated, and displaced with dilated CSF space opposite the herniation through the dura. As stated earlier, the appearance can mimic that of an arachnoid cyst displacing the cord, and a CT myelogram may need to be

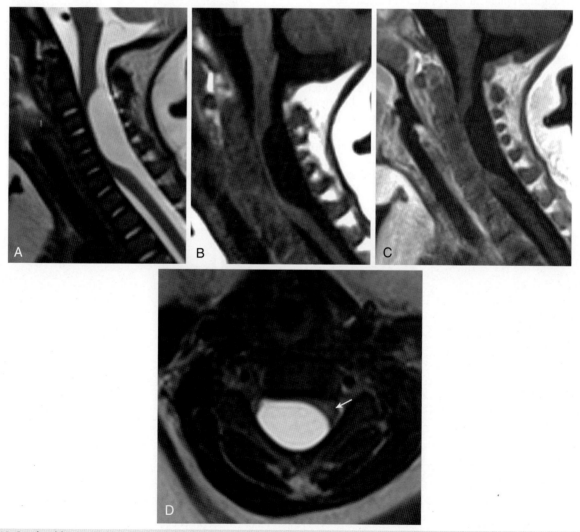

**Fig. 16.12 Arachnoid cyst.** (A) Sagittal T2-weighted imaging (T2WI) and (B) T1-weighted imaging (T1WI) show dramatic ventral displacement of the cervical cord by a space-occupying lesion within the posterior spinal canal, which is isointense to cerebrospinal fluid. (C) The lesion does not enhance after contrast administration on this axial T1WI. These findings indicate that this lesion is an arachnoid cyst. (D) Axial T2WI shows the marked displacement and compression of the cord *(arrow)* resulting from mass effect.

performed to distinguish between these two entities (Fig. 16.13). High signal intensity on T2WI may be seen in the cord if strangulated. Surgery is usually beneficial.

## Tarlov Cyst

- Cystic dilatation of the sacral root pouches can be large and may be associated with bone remodeling (Fig. 16.14). They occur in approximately 5% of individuals and vary in size from a few millimeters to several centimeters.
- There is a debate as to whether Tarlov cysts are symptomatic. When the nerve roots are compressed, one suspects that symptoms may occur but just foraminal expansion may be symptomatic.
- The differential diagnosis includes meningocele, arachnoid cyst, neurofibroma, and dural ectasia.

## Epidermoid Cyst

- Epidermoid cysts represent less than 1% of intraspinal tumors, with a higher incidence in children. They are usually extramedullary but rarely can be intramedullary. Congenital epidermoids result from displaced ectoderm inclusions occurring early in fetal life, usually in the lumbosacral region. The acquired cysts result from thecal sac instrumentation with inclusion of skin tissue in the spine.
- On MR, a discrete mass with variable signal intensity (depending on the cyst contents) is present. They often are bright on DWI, as elsewhere in the central nervous system (CNS). The lesion can calcify and rarely can be associated with peripheral enhancement.
- Other cysts include dermoid cysts (which contain fatty elements, bright on T1WI) and ependymal cysts (which follow CSF intensity) (Fig. 16.15).

## Syringohydromyelia

- States that alter the flow of CSF (Chiari malformations, arachnoid cysts, and adhesions) and/or produce abnormal CSF pressure may result in transmission of the fluid pressure into the central canal. This may result in syringohydromyelia. There are three types of syringohydromyelia:
- The first is a central canal dilatation that communicates with the fourth ventricle and is associated with

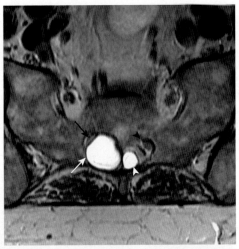

**Fig. 16.14 Tarlov cyst.** On this axial T2-weighted image, there is a lobulated sacral root cyst with large foraminal component on the right *(white arrow)* and smaller canal component *(white arrowhead)*. There is remodeling of the bony sacrum because of chronic cerebrospinal fluid pulsations. Note the displaced and compressed appearance of the exiting sacral nerve root on the right *(black arrow)*, compared with the more normal appearance on the left *(black arrowhead)*.

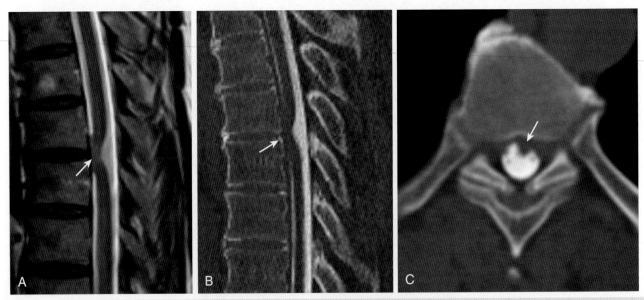

**Fig. 16.13 Thoracic cord herniation.** (A) Sagittal T2-weighted imaging shows ventral displacement of the spinal cord centered at a midthoracic disk level *(arrow)*. (B) Sagittal and (C) axial images from a computed tomography myelogram again shows the cord displacement centered at a midthoracic disk level with contrast opacification of the intraspinal cerebrospinal fluid space. The cord appears adherent to the disk *(arrow)* through a dural defect that cannot be appreciated on these images. An arachnoid cyst can fill with contrast on myelogram, but opacification would progress in a more delayed manner.

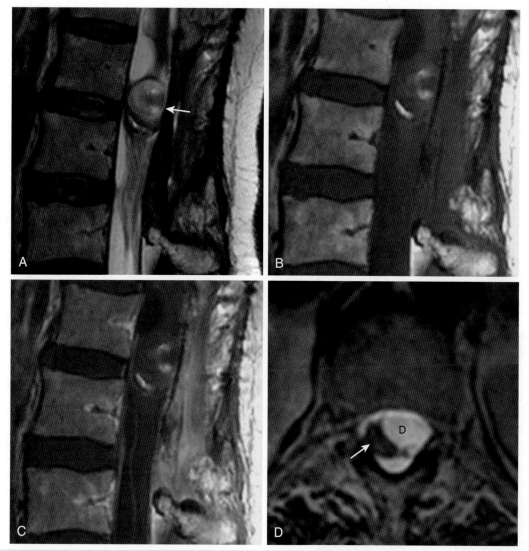

**Fig. 16.15 Lumbar dermoid.** (A) Sagittal T2-weighted imaging (T2WI) shows a heterogeneous intraspinal lesion at the L1 to L2 level *(arrow)*. Note the laminectomy defect at these levels. (B) On T1-weighted imaging (T1WI), high signal within the lesion indicates presence of fatty elements. (C) On this sagittal postcontrast T1WI, no enhancement is seen. Note the mass effect and displacement of the conus *(arrow)* by the extramedullary dermoid lesion (D).

hydrocephalus. These are produced by obstruction of CSF circulation distal to the outlets of the fourth ventricle.

■ The second occurs in a region of the central canal that is dilated but does not communicate with the fourth ventricle. These refer to Chiari I malformations, extramedullary intradural tumors, arachnoid cysts/arachnoiditis, cervical spinal stenosis, basilar invagination, and so forth (Fig. 16.16). These abnormalities have also been termed *hydromyelia*.

■ The third type of syringohydromyelia differs from the first two in that it is centered eccentrically in the spinal cord parenchyma rather than the canal (Box 16.7). These are found in watershed regions of the spinal cord and are associated with direct spinal cord injury such as trauma, infection, or infarction. This is usually termed a *syrinx*.

**TEACHING POINTS**

Lesions Associated with Hydromyelia

Basilar invagination
Chiari malformations
Diastematomyelia
Klippel-Feil syndrome
Paget disease
Spinal dysraphism
Tethered cord syndrome

**TEACHING POINTS**

Lesions Associated with Syringomyelia

Arachnoid cyst
Arachnoiditis
Cord infarction
Myelitis
Pott disease
Spondylotic compression
Trauma
Spinal cord neoplasm
Intradural extramedullary neoplasms
Vertebral body tumors

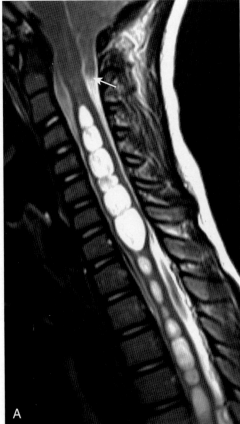

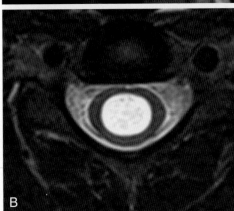

**Fig. 16.16 (A) Chiari I malformation with syringohydromyelia.** Sagittal T2-weighted imaging (T2WI) shows the cerebellar tonsils *(arrow)* extending well below the foramen magnum as well as a marked dilatation of the central canal throughout the imaged cord. (B) Axial T2WI shows the cyst is centrally based, indicating dilatation of the central canal within the cord. The lobulated appearance is because of glial adhesions and is classic in syringohydromyelia.

- Posttraumatic myelomalacia is a lesion with cord cavitation and volume loss, associated with significant spinal cord trauma, including hemorrhage or infarction. Altered CSF dynamics from adhesions may predispose to development of syrinx formation in this myelomalacic cavity.

### Cysts Associated With Neoplasia

- Neoplasms of the spinal cord commonly have cysts associated with them. These cysts have been termed tumoral (or intratumoral) and nontumoral (reactive) (Fig. 16.17).

Nontumoral Versus Tumoral Cysts

- Cysts rostral or caudal to the solid portion of the tumor (nontumoral) are secondary to dilatation of the central canal. They do not enhance, are not echogenic on intraoperative ultrasound, do not have septations, and usually disappear after resection of the solid lesion.
- Tumoral cysts (more common in astrocytoma) are part of the tumor itself and may show peripheral enhancement.

## NEOPLASTIC DISEASES INVOLVING THE SPINE AND CORD

### Intramedullary Tumors

- Spinal cord tumors represent approximately 5% of CNS neoplasms.
- Neoplasms have three general characteristics: (1) they tend to enlarge the cord either focally or diffusely, (2) on T2WI they produce high signal intensity, and (3) they frequently enhance.
- Neoplasm is not the only cause of cord enlargement; inflammatory and demyelinating diseases may also enlarge the spinal cord.

Causes of Spinal Cord Enlargement

**Demyelinating Diseases**
Acute disseminated encephalomyelitis
Multiple sclerosis
Transverse myelitis

**Intramedullary Infections**
**Tumor**
Metastases to cord
Primary spinal cord tumor

**Inflammation**
Sarcoid
Systemic lupus erythematosus

**Vascular Lesions**
Acute infarction
Arteriovenous malformation
Cavernous angioma
Hemorrhage
Venous hypertension (Foix-Alajouanine syndrome)

**Syringohydromyelia**

### Astrocytoma

- These make up approximately 40% of spinal tumors and usually occur in children (most common intramedullary tumor in children) and adults in their third to fifth decade of life. Males are affected more than females. Symptoms include pain and paresthesias followed by

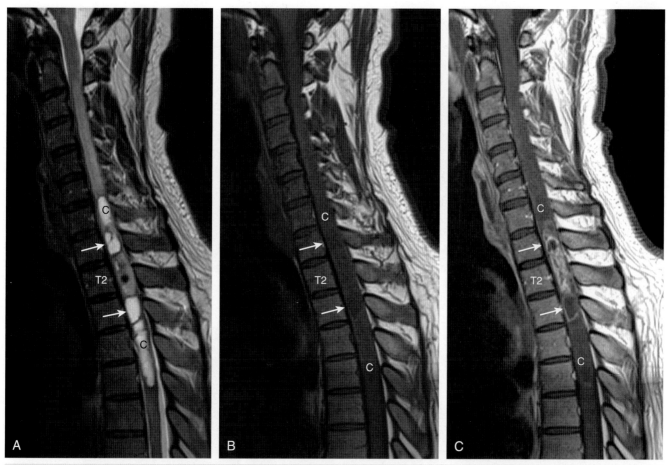

**Fig. 16.17 Neoplastic and nonneoplastic cysts in a patient with cord pilocytic astrocytoma.** (A) Sagittal T2, (B) sagittal T1, and (C) postcontrast sagittal T1-weighted imaging show a mass within the cord centered at the T2 level. Low signal within the segment of tumor at the T2 level on T2-weighted imaging (T2WI) indicates small focus of hemorrhage. There are cysts above and below the level of the T2 mass. Those labeled with *arrows* show rim enhancement, indicating they are part of the tumor proper. Those labeled with "C" at the extreme ends of the mass do not show rim enhancement and are therefore nontumoral cysts. Note edema within the cord extending to the C2 level on the T2WI.

motor signs. The cervicothoracic cord is most commonly involved.

- Astrocytomas are graded I to IV with grade I the pilocytic astrocytoma, II the low grade or fibrillary astrocytoma, III the anaplastic astrocytoma, and IV the glioblastoma. Most spinal cord astrocytomas are low grade (with grade I and grade II nearly equal in incidence), with less than 2% being glioblastomas.
- In children, these lesions behave as grade I pilocytic astrocytomas with a good prognosis. Adults have a worse outcome related to the infiltrative nature of the lesion and more cervical predominance.
- Cord astrocytomas are hypercellular, infiltrative, and often large without obvious margins and involve the full diameter of the cord but are more eccentric than ependymomas. The average length of involvement is seven body segments, although the size of the tumor does not necessarily reflect its malignant potential. These tumors are associated with neurofibroma type 1 (NF1) and generally not resectable.
- They are iso- to low intensity on T1WI and high intensity on T2WI and generally enhance, although the images may be uneven compared with the intense enhancement of ependymoma. They may have an associated

cystic component (usually tumoral, with small irregular or eccentric morphology) (see Fig. 16.17). Syrinx is more common in the pilocytic variety. Hemorrhage is uncommon. Exophytic components are sometimes present. Malignant potential is generally less than that of brain astrocytomas.

- These tumors may produce mild scoliosis, widened interpediculate distance, and vertebral scalloping but less than ependymomas.

**Ependymoma.**

- Ependymomas account for 50% to 60% of spinal cord tumors in the third to fifth decade of life (most common intramedullary neoplasm in adults) and may be sporadic or associated with neurofibromatosis type 2 (NF2).
- Ependymomas are generally more focal (involving an average of 3–4 vertebral body segments), although they can be extensive (reported to involve 15 vertebral body segments), and as they arise from ependymal cells from the central canal, they tend to occupy the central portion of the cord.
- Symptoms are generally mild, with back or neck pain being the most common complaint followed by sensory deficits and motor weakness, and bowel and bladder dysfunction.

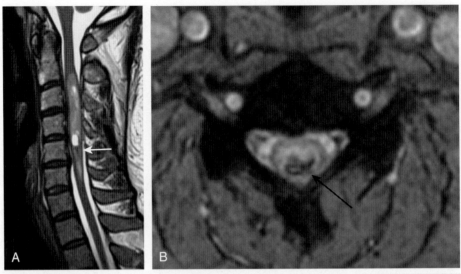

**Fig. 16.18 Ependymoma.** (A) Classic ependymoma in the cervical cord, with "cap sign" (low intensity inferiorly, *arrow*), which is more clearly demonstrated to be hemorrhage *(arrow)* on the axial gradient echo scan (B).

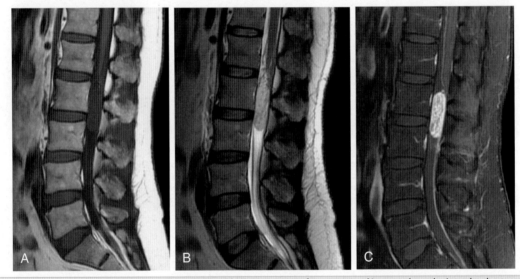

**Fig. 16.19 Myxopapillary ependymoma.** (A) Sagittal T1, (B) T2, and (C) postcontrast fat-suppressed images show the intradural extramedullary myxopapillary ependymoma, which is well defined and very bright on T2. The location is classic.

- They most commonly involve the cervical cord (32%), followed by the conus and cauda equina region (27%), cervicothoracic (16%), thoracic (16%), thoracolumbar (5%), and cervicomedullary (3%) locations.
- These neoplasms can be both intramedullary and extramedullary (affecting the filum). Ependymoma are well circumscribed, noninfiltrating, histologically benign with slow growth and, in certain circumstances, are totally resectable. The 5-year survival is greater than 80%. Metastatic spread to extraspinal sites is rare.
- Ependymomas appear isointense to hypointense with regard to the cord on T1WI and may have a multinodular high signal appearance on T2WI that occupies the whole width of the cord. Commonly there is edema surrounding the tumor. Ependymomas have a propensity to hemorrhage, with hypointense rims ("cap sign") on T2WI that histopathologically represent residual hemosiderin from hemorrhage (Fig. 16.18). Ependymomas may cause subarachnoid hemorrhage and associated hemosiderosis has been reported. Enhancement is common, and

the tumor may have sharply defined, intensely enhancing margins. They may be associated with extensive cyst formation (in up to 84% of ependymomas—mostly nontumoral cysts but tumoral cysts may also occur), which does not usually enhance.
- Other associated radiographic findings include scoliosis, canal widening with vertebral body scalloping, pedicle remodeling, or laminar thinning.
- Myxopapillary ependymoma (13% of all spinal ependymomas) may affect the filum with extension into the conus and the subcutaneous sacrococcygeal region. This lesion is most common in males with a mean age of diagnosis of 35 years. The presentation is of low back pain, leg pain, lower extremity weakness, and bladder dysfunction. These lesions are multilobulated, usually encapsulated, mucin-containing tumors that may hemorrhage and calcify. On MR, they are usually isointense on T1WI, high intensity on T2WI, and enhance (Fig. 16.19). However, as a result of calcification or hemorrhage, they may be high or low intensity on T1WI and T2WI.

### Hemangioblastoma.

- Hemangioblastomas are vascular tumors that may involve the cervical and thoracic spinal cord or appear on the surface of the cord and cauda equina nerve roots. They are the third most common primary intramedullary spinal neoplasm (1%–7% of all spinal cord neoplasms). The tumor is composed of a dense network of capillary and sinus channels. They diffusely widen the spinal cord and may have both a cystic and solid component, with the solid component enhancing intensely. These tumors are associated with considerable edema (Fig. 16.20). Hemangioblastoma may be solid in 25% of cases.
- Spinal cord hemangioblastomas may be an isolated lesion, but one third of cases are associated with von Hippel–Lindau disease and are multiple.
- Cord hemangioblastomas are more commonly thoracic than cervical, and 43% have associated cysts.
- On imaging, hemorrhagic components may be seen in the tumor nodule. There may be multiple lesions in the spine, and they may be eccentric, at times appearing extramedullary, or pial based, and they can occur on the nerve roots.
- On MR, intratumoral flow voids can be identified when the lesion is sizeable enough and prominent posterior draining veins can also be seen. They are variable intensity on T1WI and high intensity on T2WI. Edema can be noted surrounding the lesions. Avid homogeneous enhancement is visualized in the solid portion of the tumor.
- Spinal angiography shows dilated arteries, a tumor stain, and draining vein.

### Ganglioglioma/Gangliocytoma.

- The terms ganglioglioma and gangliocytoma are frequently used synonymously as the imaging features and treatment are similar. These rare lesions are more common in children and young adults, are slow growing, relatively benign neoplasms with the majority occurring in the cervical cord and less commonly the thoracic cord, conus, or entire spinal cord.
- Findings in this tumor include involvement consisting of long segments of tumor (commonly extending to over eight vertebral body segments) associated with scoliosis and bony remodeling, mixed signal on T1WI and high intensity on T2WI, prominent tumoral cysts, patchy enhancement that extends to the pial surface without central enhancement (15% of cases demonstrate no enhancement), lack of edema, hemosiderin, or calcification. Gross resection of the tumor is recommended.

### Paragangliomas.

- This is an avidly enhancing well-defined mass of neuroendocrine origin usually seen in adults in the conus and cauda equina region. A "salt-and-pepper" appearance with the lesion and/or flow voids within the tumor or along the cord surface aid in diagnosis.

### Intradural Intramedullary/Extramedullary Metastatic Disease

- Metastases can deposit on the dura, pia-arachnoid region, and rarely in the cord itself (Fig. 16.21). The incidence of leptomeningeal and intramedullary metastases (up to 3% of patients with metastatic disease) is increasing as patients with cancer live longer.
- Patients may have nonspecific symptoms (headache, back pain) or focal neurologic symptoms. Intramedullary lesions result from tumor growth along the Virchow-Robin spaces because of CSF spread or as a result of hematogenous dissemination.
- Intramedullary metastases enlarge the cord, are associated with cord edema, and enhance.

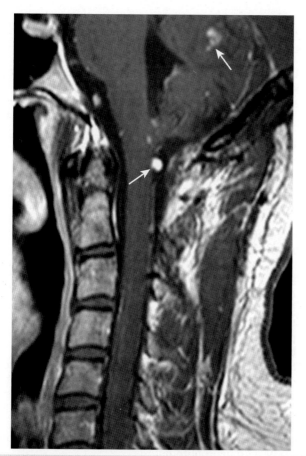

**Fig. 16.20 Hemangioblastoma.** The nature of these enhancing lesions in the cerebellum and along the dorsal surface of the cord *(arrows)* on this sagittal postcontrast T1-weighted imaging would be elusive without the known diagnosis of von Hippel–Lindau disease.

---

**TEACHING POINTS**

Tumors that Commonly Metastasize to the Spinal Cord or Leptomeninges

#### Children

Lymphoma, leukemia
Medulloblastoma
Pineal region tumors (e.g., germinoma, pineoblastoma)
Choroid plexus tumors
Ependymoma
Neuroblastoma
Retinoblastoma

(Continued)

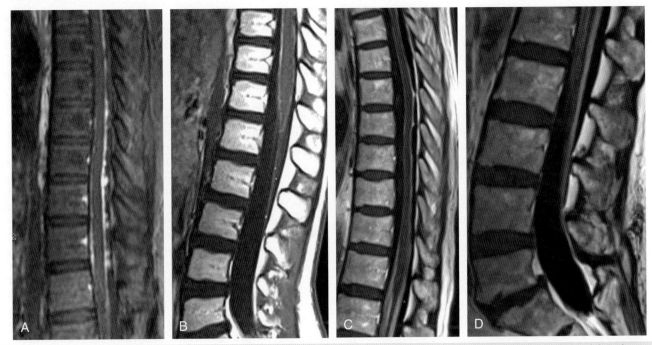

**Fig. 16.21 Leptomeningeal metastases.** (A) Enhanced fat-suppressed sagittal T1-weighted imaging (T1WI) shows diffuse linear and nodular enhancement on the posterior and anterior surface of the spinal cord in this patient with metastatic myxopapillary ependymoma. The appearance is likened to "sugar coating." (B) On this postcontrast T1WI, leptomeningeal spread along with dropped metastases along the cauda equina nerve roots are shown in this patient with metastatic medulloblastoma. (C–D) Smooth linear enhancement along the surface of the cord and cauda equina on this contrast-enhanced sagittal T1WI in this patient with breast cancer indicates metastatic leptomeningeal involvement.

**Adults**

Lymphoma, leukemia
Glioblastoma
Hemangioblastoma
Melanoma (primary or metastasis)
Metastases from lung > breast > melanoma > colorectal > renal > gastric carcinomas
Oligodendroglioma

## Intradural Extramedullary Lesions

### Meningioma

- Meningiomas are well-circumscribed lesions with a female predominance and constitute approximately 25% of spinal canal neoplasms. They are usually located in the thoracic region (approximately 80%) but can occur in any location throughout the spine. They favor the dorsal aspect of the meninges of the spine.
- They may coexist with schwannomas in patients with NF2. The vast majority are extramedullary intradural, but in rare cases, they can be both intradural and extradural or purely extradural (higher tendency to be malignant).
- These tumors are isointense to slightly hypointense on T1WI, isointense to slightly hyperintense relative to the spinal cord and are usually well demarcated by the brighter CSF on T2WI, enhance, and may show a dural tail. Most of the time these typical intradural extramedullary lesions are obvious on nonenhanced images (Fig. 16.22).
- Meningiomas are dural based in location, may compress the cord but do not invade it, may demonstrate calcification, and may widen the neural foramen but far less often than peripheral nerve sheath tumors.

Meningioma Versus Nerve Sheath Tumors

- It may be difficult to distinguish meningiomas from nerve sheath tumors. The following are clues that can help:
  - Meningiomas are more typically located posterolaterally, and nerve sheath tumors are anteriorly located within the canal
  - In general, multiplicity favors nerve sheath tumor over meningioma
  - Low-intensity central regions on postgadolinium T1-weighted imaging (T1WI) and T2-weighted imaging (T2WI) can be seen with nerve sheath tumors.

### Nerve Sheath Tumors: Schwannoma and Neurofibroma

- Two types of benign nerve sheath tumors can be distinguished histopathologically: the schwannoma and the neurofibroma.
- In patients with NF1, all spinal nerve root tumors are neurofibromas; however, neurofibromas can occur in patients without NF1. Very extensive plexiform neurofibromas can be seen in NF1.
- Schwannomas are the most common neurogenic tumors of the spine. In patients with neurofibromatosis type 2, almost all spinal nerve root tumors are schwannomas or mixed tumors rather than neurofibromas.
- Schwannomas are seen as solitary lesions (except in NF-2), whereas neurofibromas are often multiple and occur with neurofibromatosis.
- Schwannomas may occur in a purely intradural location (most common), be partially intradural and extradural, or purely extradural.

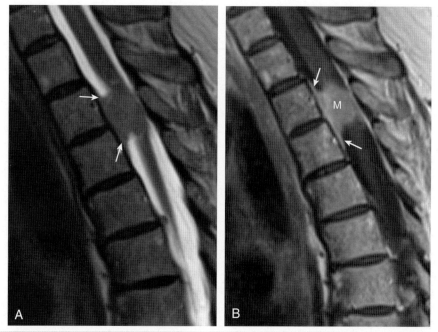

**Fig. 16.22 Meningioma.** (A) There is an intermediate intensity intradural extramedullary mass in the thoracic spinal canal on sagittal T2-weighted imaging (T2WI). Note the dural attachment *(arrows)*. Cord compression is present, and there is faint T2 high signal within the cord above and below the lesion indicating edema. (B) On contrast-enhanced sagittal T1-weighted imaging (T1WI), the mass *(M)* enhances as does the dural tail *(arrows)*.

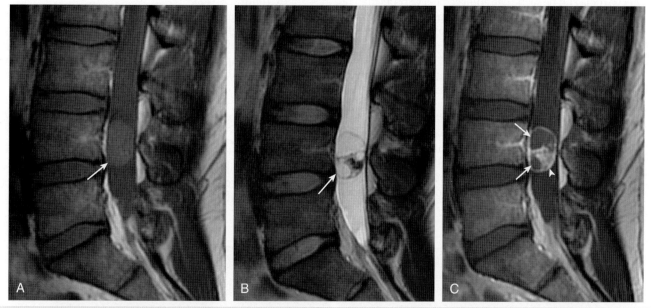

**Fig. 16.23 Schwannoma.** (A) Sagittal T1-weighted imaging (T1WI) shows an ovoid hypointense mass *(arrow)* at the L4 level. (B) Sagittal T2WI shows that the mass *(arrow)* has heterogeneous components, with areas of low T2 signal indicating hemorrhage. (C) After contrast administration, the lesion is shown to have solid *(arrowhead)* and cystic *(arrows)* components, a not uncommon feature of schwannomas.

■ It is difficult to distinguish schwannoma from neurofibroma by imaging, and thus they are clumped together. They are usually isointense on T1WI, hyperintense on T2WI, and enhance. If you're lucky, you may see central hypointensity on T2 (target sign), which is a feature of neurofibroma. Areas that are isointense or of high intensity on T1WI and low signal on PDWI and T2WI have been associated with hemorrhage (Fig. 16.23). Calcification is rare.

■ Other findings that are associated with neurofibromatosis include enlarged neural foramina and vertebral scalloping secondary to dural ectasia, lateral meningocele, or an arachnoid cyst.

### Hereditary Motor and Sensory Neuropathies

■ Hereditary motor and sensory neuropathies (HMSN) make up a group of diseases that are, in some cases, associated with hypertrophic peripheral and/or cranial nerves (Fig. 16.24). These diseases are characterized by concentric proliferation of Schwann cells, interspersed with collagen, in response to multiple episodes of demyelination and remyelination. This process results in an "onion bulb" appearance to the nerve.

Types of Hereditary Neuropathies

- Charcot-Marie-Tooth disease (CMT or HMSN 1) is usually an autosomal dominant disease that presents with slowly progressive distal atrophy (common peroneal muscular atrophy) and weakness in conjunction with pes cavus and scoliosis. The posterior columns, optic nerve, and acoustic nerve may be involved. Enlarged peripheral nerve roots can be seen on magnetic resonance imaging (MRI). There may be minimal or no abnormal enhancement seen.
- Dejerine-Sottas disease (HMSN 3) is an autosomal recessive condition with slowly progressive motor and sensory loss and ataxia. Scoliosis and pes cavus are frequent. There are enlarged peripheral and cranial nerves with hypomyelination. Imaging findings included enlarged nerves best demarcated on T2-weighted imaging (T2WI) with variable enhancement.
- HMSN 2 and 4 have no associated imaging features.

- On MR, enlargement and, at times, enhancement of the nerve roots can be seen. The enlarged nerve roots may be seen in the cervical or lumbar regions and may extend beyond the neural foramina into the extradural space.

## Inflammatory Neuropathies

- Chronic inflammatory demyelinating polyradiculoneuropathy (CIDP) is an acquired demyelinating condition of peripheral nerves characterized by the slow onset of proximal weakness, paresthesias, and numbness.
  - On MRI, cranial and peripheral nerves may be enlarged and can enhance (Fig. 16.25). Imaging findings are often bilateral and symmetric. CIDP is often associated with lesions in the brain that appear similar to those of MS. CIDP is considered to be a chronic version of Guillain-Barré syndrome (GBS).

- GBS is an autoimmune disorder that can occur after viral or bacterial infection. Patients typically present with symptoms ranging from ascending weakness to flaccid paralysis. Several subtypes exist, including acute inflammatory demyelinating polyradiculopathy, axonal subtypes, and regional syndromes (including the Miller-Fisher variant in which ataxia and areflexia are the dominant features).
  - In patients with GBS, MRI may reveal enlarged and enhancing nerve roots (preferentially ventral nerve roots but dorsal nerve roots can also enhance), usually at the cauda equina level (Fig. 16.26).
  - Most cases of GBS follow a gastrointestinal (campylobacter) or respiratory viral infection. Occasionally surgery will trigger the syndrome. In rare cases, vaccinations and infections by flu, cytomegalovirus, Epstein Barr virus, and Zika virus may increase the risk of GBS.

## Lipoma

- Lipomas (Fig. 16.27) are usually seen in the first three decades of life and are most common in the thoracic region. In the lumbar region, they are associated with myelodysplasia or tethered cord (see Chapter 8). They are commonly identified in the filum terminale (1.5%–5% prevalence). Lipomas may be intradural (60% of cases) or extradural (40%).
- Imaging characteristics of lipomas include low density on CT or high signal on T1WI and T2WI. With fat suppression, they appear dark. These lesions can be extensive and compress the spinal cord. Chemical shift artifact can be identified along the frequency encoding axis.

Chemical Shift Artifact

- A type of artifact seen in the frequency-encoding direction because of the differences in resonance frequencies of fat and water.

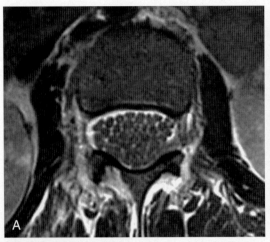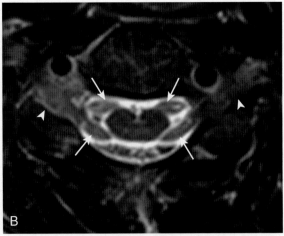

**Fig. 16.24 Charcot-Marie-Tooth disease.** (A) Markedly thickened lumbar nerve roots are present in this patient with Charcot-Marie-Tooth disease. (B) In this same patient, even the ventral and dorsal nerve roots arising from the cervical cord are massively enlarged *(arrows)* as are the exiting nerve roots within the neural foramina *(arrowheads)*.

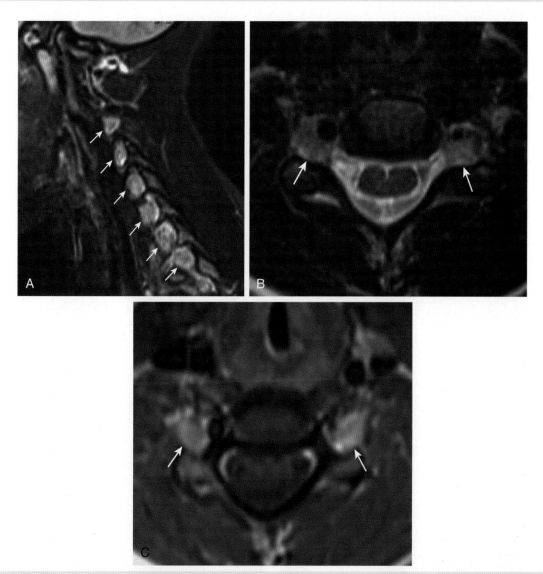

**Fig. 16.25 Chronic inflammatory demyelinating polyradiculoneuropathy (CIDP).** (A) Far lateral image from sagittal short tau inversion recovery (STIR) sequence shows marked enlargement of the cervical nerve roots as they exit the neural foramina *(arrows)*. (B) Axial T2-weighted imaging (T2WI) again shows the marked enlargement of the exiting cervical nerve roots *(arrows)*, and (C) postcontrast axial T1WI shows these nerve roots to enhance avidly *(arrows)* in this patient with CIDP.

Teratoma can be considered if a fat-containing sacrococcygeal mass is seen. Lesions present as a large expansile mass with fatty, cystic, and solid components and may even be hemorrhagic. There is a female predominance and a high incidence (as high as 60%) of malignant transformation, especially in male patients.

### Tethered Cord
- Symptoms of adult tethered cord/tight filum terminale syndrome include diffuse back and perianal pain, leg weakness, and urinary tract dysfunction.
- Imaging reveals the neural placode to be below L2, which is considered the lower limit of normal, and a thickened filum (>2 mm). It is sometimes difficult to distinguish between a thickened filum and a low-lying conus.

### Metastases
- Intraspinal metastases are usually low intensity on T1WI and high intensity on T2WI (prominent edema surrounding the tumor nodule) with avid homogeneous enhancement of the tumor nodule. Cerebral MR is necessary in this situation because leptomeningeal metastases may be the result of CSF seeding from brain parenchymal metastases. Non-CNS primary tumors from the breast, lung, and kidney may also lead to leptomeningeal seeding.

**TEACHING POINTS**

Imaging Features of Intraspinal Metastases

- The entire subarachnoid space can enhance (sugar-coated appearance), and tumor nodules can be seen on nerve roots or in the cauda equina.
- Pial metastases reveal linear enhancement on the surface of the cord.
- The CSF on T1WI can be more intense than normal and the conspicuity between CSF and cord may be diminished.

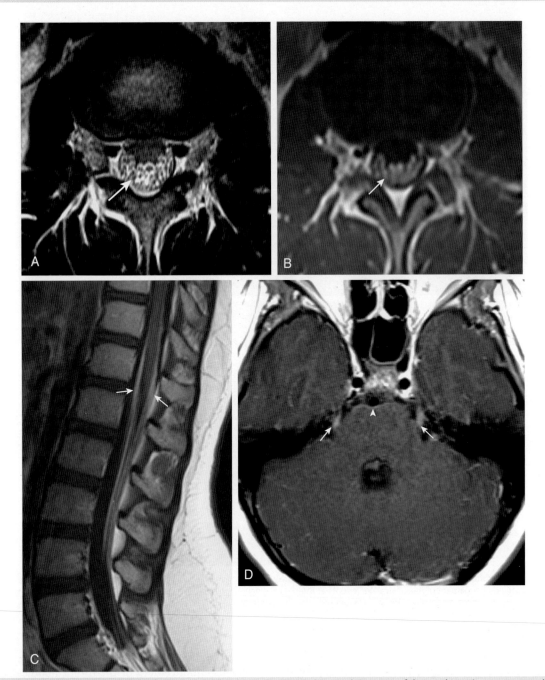

**Fig. 16.26  Guillain-Barré syndrome (GBS).** (A) Axial T2-weighted imaging (T2WI) shows enlargement of the cauda equine nerve roots *(arrow)*. (The dark signal in the ventral aspect of the thecal sac is because of cerebrospinal fluid pulsation artifact.) (B) Axial and (C) sagittal postcontrast T1-weighted imaging (T1WI) show marked enhancement of the cauda equine nerve roots *(arrows)*. (D) Intracranially, abnormal enhancement of the prepontine segment of the trigeminal nerves *(arrows)* and leptomeninges *(arrowhead)* is also seen in this patient with GBS.

- Parameningeal masses are a preferred presentation for leukemia (termed chloromas), which can grow through the intervertebral foramina, a mode of spread also noted in both Hodgkin disease, non-Hodgkin lymphoma, and neuroblastoma. CNS lymphoma rarely occurs as an intramedullary lesion (3%). Leukemic cell spread to the CSF may be invisible on MR and better diagnosed by lumbar puncture.

### Extradural Lesions

- The vertebral bodies are the most frequent site of metastatic disease to the spine. Lesions may be osteolytic or

a combination of osteolytic and osteoblastic. Multiplicity of lesions in the vertebral column should raise suspicion for metastatic disease.
- On MRI, usual fatty marrow is replaced with associated hypointense signal on T1WI and high signal on short tau inversion recovery (STIR) (Fig. 16.28). On conventional T2WI, the tumor-replaced marrow may appear as high signal intensity compared with the normal fatty marrow with lytic lesions or may appear as lower signal intensity with sclerotic lesions.
- Metastatic disease is therefore most conspicuous on unenhanced T1WI and may be difficult to perceive on

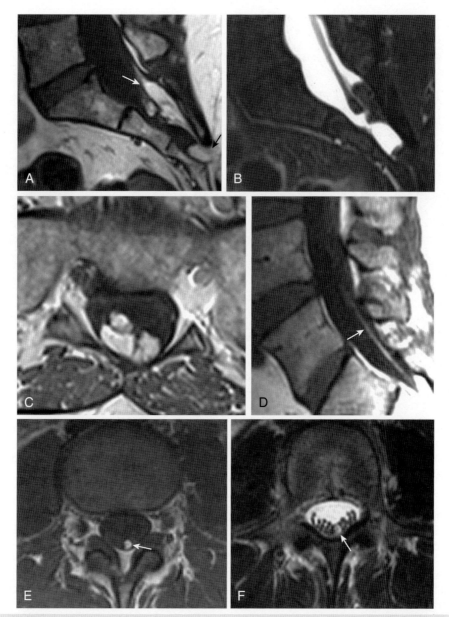

**Fig. 16.27 Fatty intraspinal masses.** (A) Extramedullary lipoma *(white arrow)* is seen on this sagittal T1-weighted image (T1WI) with inferior extent of the lipoma extending through a bony defect in the dorsal sacrum *(black arrow)*. (B) The lipoma signal suppresses completely on short tau inversion recovery (STIR) image. (C) The lipoma is again shown on axial T1WI. (D) This sagittal T1WI in a different patient shows incidental asymptomatic fatty filum *(arrow)*. Fatty filum in a different patient seen as (E) T1 hyperintensity and (F) T2 hyperintensity, paralleling the course of the cauda equina *(arrows)*.

T2 or fat-suppressed T2 images. In and out of phase imaging may help identify bone marrow–replacing lesions.

- Common cancers associated with spinal metastasis include breast, prostate, lung, and kidney. Lymphoma rarely can present as an epidural mass without bone involvement.
- Carefully evaluate for pathologic fracture, extraosseous soft-tissue extension into the perivertebral and intraspinal spaces, cord compression, and cord signal changes.

## Osteoporotic Compression Fractures

- Osteoporosis is characterized by decreased bone mass. It is associated with compression fractures that are spontaneous or associated with minimal trauma, usually located in the midthoracic region and thoracolumbar junction. Osteoporosis is the most common cause of

compression fractures and is particularly observed in elderly females.

- It may be difficult to distinguish between acute osteoporotic vertebral collapse and acute collapse from metastatic disease (Fig. 16.29).

**TEACHING POINTS**

Computed Tomography Features of Benign and Malignant Compression Fractures

**Benign**

Cortical fractures of the vertebral body without cortical bone destruction (puzzle sign)

Retropulsion of a bone fragment of the posterior cortex of the vertebral body into the spinal canal

*(Continued)*

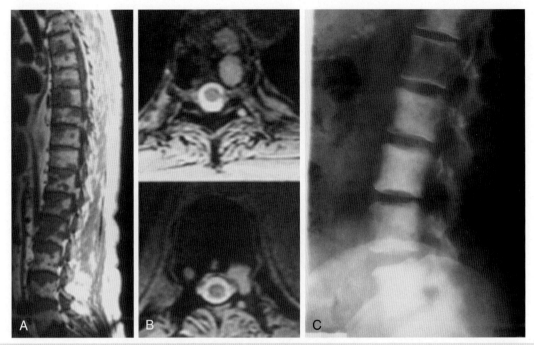

**Fig. 16.28 Metastatic lesions.** (A) Note the low-intensity lesions outlined by residual fat in the vertebral bodies on this sagittal T1-weighted imaging (T1WI) scan in a patient with breast metastases. (B) Same patient as A; axial T2-weighted imaging (T2WI) scan of one vertebra reveals multiple high-intensity metastases in the vertebral body and pedicles. (C) Lateral spine radiograph in a different patient with metastatic breast cancer shows extensive osteoblastic metastases.

Fracture lines within the cancellous bone of the
   vertebral body
Thin diffuse paraspinal soft-tissue mass (the hematoma)
Intravertebral vacuum phenomenon

**Malignant**
   Destruction of the anterolateral or posterior cortical
      bone of the vertebral body
   Destruction of the cancellous bone of the vertebral
      body
   Destruction of the vertebral pedicle
   Focal paraspinal soft-tissue mass (extraosseous tumor)
   Epidural mass (extraosseous tumor)

- On MR, both nonpathologic and pathologic compression fractures may have low signal on T1WI and high signal on T2WI and enhance. Both could involve multiple vertebral bodies and be associated with soft-tissue masses. Features that might help distinguish nonpathologic and pathologic compression fractures on MRI are summarized below.

Magnetic Resonance Features of Benign and Malignant Spine Fractures

**Benign**
   Low-intensity T1 acutely but returns to normal signal
      over 4 to 6 weeks
   High intensity T1 chronically
   Stripes of dark and bright on T1-weighted imaging
   Smaller paraspinal soft-tissue mass (perivertebral
      hematoma)

Posterior elements less commonly affected
Higher ADC values
Usually not associated with an epidural mass

**Malignant**
   Low-intensity T1; only returns to normal signal after
      radiation
   Complete replacement of vertebral body with low intensity on T1-weighted imaging
   Larger paraspinal soft-tissue mass (extraosseous tumor)
   Posterior elements more commonly involved
   Lower ADC values when there is cellular packing of the
      marrow
   Epidural mass (extraosseous tumor)

*ADC,* Apparent diffusion coefficient.

- In the case of a single collapsed vertebral body, a repeat examination in 4 to 6 weeks is recommended because often it is not possible to distinguish between acute, nontraumatic benign, and metastatic vertebral body collapse. In this interval, benign collapse progresses to isointensity on T1WI and T2WI, with decreased enhancement, whereas metastatic disease remains stable or progresses without a change in intensity. A full workup for occult malignancy, including bone scan to determine whether there are other lesions, is recommended. If waiting is not an option, bone biopsy is the only definitive test for distinguishing benign versus malignant disease.

**Neural Crest Tumors**
- Tumors of neural crest origin occur in infancy and arise from the sympathetic plexus. These include neuroblastoma (patients <5 years old), ganglioneuroblastoma

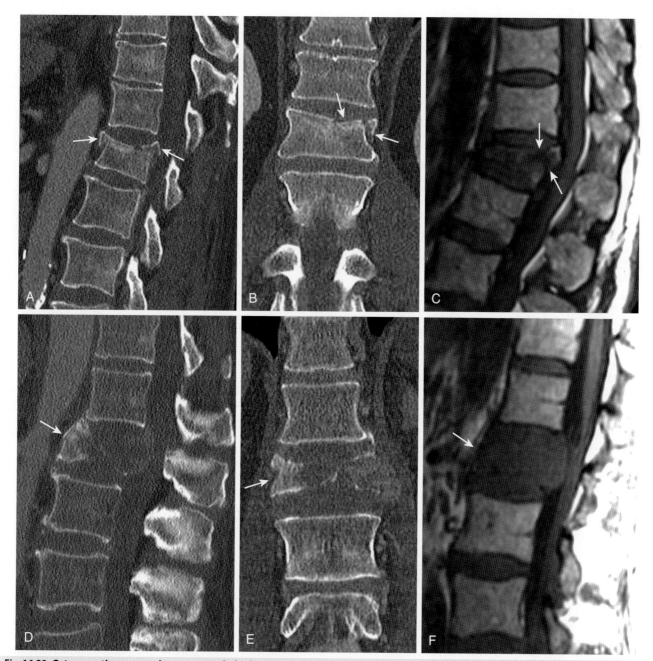

**Fig. 16.29 Osteoporotic compression versus pathologic compression fractures.** (A) Sagittal and (B) coronal reconstructions from noncontrast computed tomography (CT) show acute compression deformity with multiple superior endplate fracture fragments that can be pieced together like a puzzle *(arrows)*, a very good indicator of benign fracture. (C) Sagittal T1-weighted imaging (T1WI) in a different patient with benign fracture also shows compression deformity with fragments that could conceivably be pieced together *(arrows)*. Compare that case to this one in which (D) sagittal and (E) coronal reconstructions from noncontrast CT show extensive disruption and compression deformity of a single vertebral body *(arrows)*, but the margins of the fracture fragments are not clearly seen and lack the "puzzle" configuration of a benign fracture. (F) Sagittal T1WI in this same patient shows that the marrow space at this level is completely replaced by soft-tissue tumor *(arrow)*, without discernible fracture plane. This is a pathologic compression fracture resulting from metastatic disease.

(5–8 years old), and ganglioneuroma (>8 years old) (Fig. 16.30). Calcification occurs in 30% of cases, and hemorrhage has been reported. These enhancing paravertebral masses, which usually occur in the thoracic region, can extend through the neural foramina to compress the thecal sac. Fifty percent of paraspinal neuroblastomas enter the spinal canal.

■ Extramedullary hematopoiesis, a process of red cell production outside the marrow compartment that occurs

when normal erythropoiesis in the marrow fails because of disorders in hemoglobin production (e.g., sickle cell disease) and myeloproliferation (e.g., myelofibrosis or chronic myelogenous leukemia), may also produce a paraspinal mass. Hepatosplenomegaly is more commonly seen, but more rarely, extramedullary hematopoiesis can be seen in the chest as well defined, lobulated, unilateral, or bilateral paraspinal soft tissue masses (see Fig. 16.30).

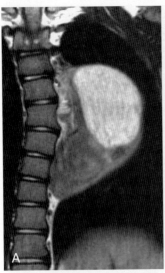
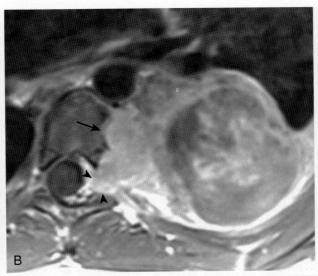
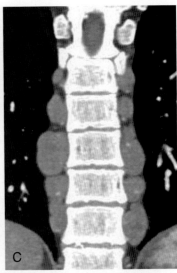

**Fig. 16.30 Paraspinal masses.** (A) Coronal T2-weighted image (T2WI) on an 8-year-old child shows a bulky mixed intensity left paraspinal mass with associated scoliosis of the adjacent thoracic spine. (B) Axial postcontrast T1-weighted imaging (T1WI) shows the same bulky mass scalloping the adjacent thoracic vertebral body *(arrow)* and sneaking its way into the spinal canal (between *arrowheads*) through an expanded neural foramen. This turned out to be a ganglioglioma. (C) Contrast with this case of extramedullary hematopoiesis, where there are multiple bilateral paraspinal masses in an adult patient with thalassemia.

## Hemangioma

- Hemangiomas are common benign neoplasms of the vertebral body and are most often incidental findings. They are composed of fully developed adult blood vessels. More than 50% of solitary hemangiomas occur in the vertebral bodies. Multiple hemangiomas can occur in approximately one third of cases.
- These lesions most often present in the vertebral bodies as round geographic lesions but rarely can be extensive, replacing the entire vertebral body with involvement of the pedicles, arches, and spinous processes. The cortical margins are usually distinct.
- On CT and plain films, thick trabeculae with a striated appearance are seen. The vertical striations represent vascular channels interspersed with thickened trabeculae. MR reveals high signal intensity on T1WI and (fast spin echo) T2WI because of their fat and water content (Fig. 16.31). On nuclear scintigraphy, tagged red blood cell scan, these lesions show metabolic activity and on spinal angiography, these lesions are vascular.
- Although benign, vertebral bodies with hemangiomas can have compression fractures. Rarely, these may be aggressive with epidural extension resulting in compromise of the spinal canal or neural foramen. With extraosseous extension, the signal intensity of the exophytic portion of the lesion may be dark on T1WI and high on T2WI.
- The differential diagnosis is focal fatty marrow replacement. Atypical hemangiomas may simulate bone metastases by having low signal on T1WI and brightness on T2WI. Even with these unusual signal intensity combinations, the CT appearance still is classic for hemangiomas, and the diagnosis can be made with greater confidence when CT is performed in conjunction with MRI. Otherwise, patients may need to go to biopsy (which could get messy) or undergo follow-up imaging to assess for interval change.

## Chordoma

- Chordomas are slow growing, locally invasive neoplasms derived from remnants of the notochord, with approximately 50% originating in the sacral region, 15% affecting the spine (particularly the cervical region), and the rest affecting the clivus.
- In the spine, the tumor mass is associated with lytic lesions of the bone, at times with a sclerotic rim and calcification. MR imaging features are variable with most lesions demonstrating very high signal on T2WI. These lesions may involve the disk space and multiple vertebral bodies. In the differential diagnosis, think about chordoma in bizarre spinal lesions that resemble large, herniated disks, schwannoma, or unusual osteomyelitis (Fig. 16.32).

## Chondrosarcoma

- Chondrosarcoma may also occur in the spine and is associated with destruction of bone in the body or posterior elements. The hallmark of this lesion is chondroid calcification, which is much better detected on CT or plain film and T2 hyperintensity on MRI.

## Aneurysmal Bone Cyst, Giant Cell Tumor, Osteoblastoma, and Osteoid Osteoma

- Benign bony tumors of the spine include aneurysmal bone cyst, giant cell tumor, osteoblastoma, and osteoid osteoma and are best imaged on CT and radiographs.
- Osteoblastoma (>1.5 cm) is larger than osteoid osteoma (<1.5 cm) and is much more common in the spine. Both have a propensity for the posterior elements or transverse process, have a lytic and/or calcific nidus surrounded by a sclerotic rim, and are associated with pain, which in the case of osteoid osteoma is classically described as nocturnal and relievable by aspirin (Fig. 16.33).
- Giant cell tumors are lytic lesions found commonly in the sacrum and vertebral bodies; tumor margins can be thin

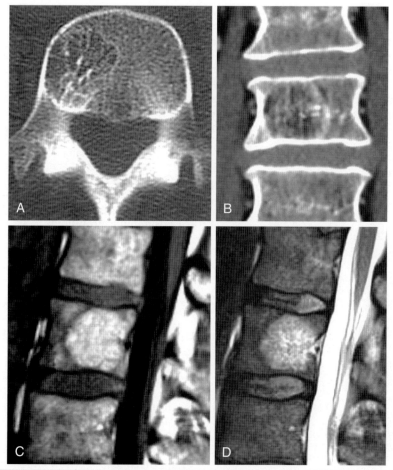

**Fig. 16.31 Hemangioma.** (A) Unenhanced computed tomography (CT) shows the characteristic speckled appearance because of vertical trabecular striations, with low-density areas and high-density spicules in this hemangioma in the right aspect of this vertebral body. (B) Coronal CT reconstruction in a different patient shows the vertical trabeculated striations, which accounts for the "corduroy" appearance initially described on plain radiograph. (C) Sagittal T1-weighted imaging (T1WI) in another patient shows a high-intensity bony mass in the vertebral body. (D) The lesion is also bright on T2-weighted imaging (T2WI).

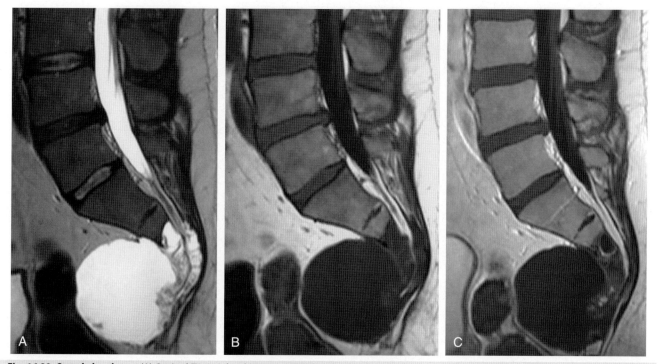

**Fig. 16.32 Sacral chordoma.** (A) Sagittal T2-weighted imaging (T2WI) shows a very hyperintense mass arising from the lower sacral elements and bulging into the presacral space. The T2 hyperintensity is characteristic for chordoma. (B) Sagittal T1 and (C) postcontrast sagittal T1-weighted imaging (T1WI) show little to no enhancement within the lesion. Histopathology confirmed chordoma.

or dehiscent and soft-tissue component of the mass may be present.

■ Aneurysmal bone cysts are usually circumscribed multiloculated lytic lesions, occasionally containing hemorrhage (with fluid levels) and involving the posterior elements, particularly the lamina (Fig. 16.34). Some of these entities (i.e., giant cell lesion and aneurysmal bone cyst and osteoblastoma) coexist within the same lesion or evolve into each. Aneurysmal bone cysts can also coexist with osteosarcomas.

## Eosinophilic Granuloma

■ Eosinophilic granuloma (part of the Langerhans cell histiocytosis spectrum) affects children and when seen

in the spine predominantly involves the vertebral body. It is a rapidly growing tumor, producing bone loss and vertebral collapse associated with normal vertebral disk spaces (vertebra plana) (Fig. 16.35). There may be associated soft-tissue extension from the vertebral body posteriorly into the vertebral canal or anteriorly into the prevertebral tissues.

---

### TEACHING POINTS

Causes of Vertebral Plana

Osteoporosis
Steroids
Tumors (leukemia, myeloma)
Eosinophilic granuloma
Fracture
Mucopolysaccharidoses

---

## Osteochondroma

■ These lesions usually arise from the posterior elements and commonly involve the thoracic or lumbar vertebrae. They are commonly found in teenagers where they grow and occasionally cause neurologic symptoms. On MR, these lesions are heterogeneous showing high intensity on T2WI (from the cartilaginous portion of the lesion) and low intensity on all pulse sequences from the ossified part of the tumor. Ollier's syndrome and Mafucci's syndrome are associated with multiple osteochondromas.

## Paget Disease

■ Paget disease commonly involves the spine and produces enlargement of all the vertebral elements. It usually demonstrates thickened bone cortex with disorganized

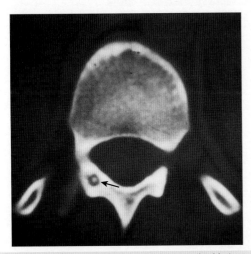

**Fig. 16.33 Osteoid osteoma.** There is a circumscribed lytic region in the right lamina on this computed tomography (CT) scan with bone windows. In the central portion of the hypodense region *(arrow)* is a punctate area of high density.

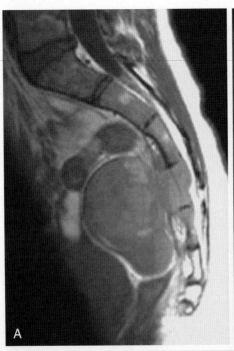 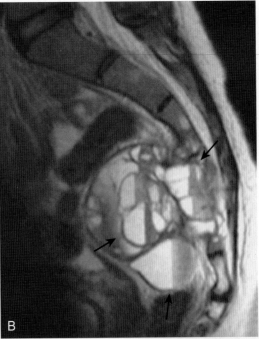

**Fig. 16.34 Aneurysmal bone cyst.** (A) T1-weighted imaging (T1WI) and (B) T2-weighted imaging (T2WI) in the sagittal plane shows blood-fluid levels *(arrows)* in a bone lesion projecting from the lower sacrum into the anterior pelvis. The fluid levels are characteristic of aneurysmal bone cysts.

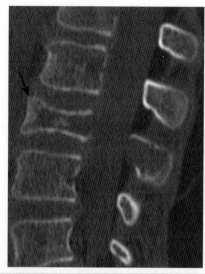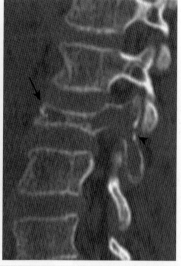

**Fig. 16.35 Eosinophilic granuloma of the spine.** Sagittal reconstructions from computed tomography (CT) lumbar spine shows loss of height at L3 *(arrows)* with lytic appearance within the medullary compartment including posterior elements *(arrowhead)*. This loss of height, *vertebra plana*, is characteristic of eosinophilic granuloma involving the spine.

trabecular pattern (distinguishing it from fibrous dysplasia), and sclerosis (late phase), with low intensity on T1WI and T2WI. An early lytic phase has also been described.

- Involvement is associated with back and neck pain and neurologic dysfunction associated with facet arthropathy, lateral recess syndrome, and stenosis of the spinal canal.

- It is difficult at times to distinguish from osteoblastic metastatic disease because Paget disease is polyostotic in more than two thirds of cases. There is the possibility of malignant transformation to osteogenic sarcoma in approximately 10% of cases: the rate of malignancy is 20 times greater in pagetoid bone than in nonpagetoid bones. The appearance of osteogenic sarcoma is variable, depending on whether the lesion is lytic, blastic, or mixed. Osteoid matrix or calcification appears as a signal void on all MR pulse sequences.

### Multiple Myeloma

- In multiple myeloma, three patterns of marrow involvement have been observed on sagittal MR.
  - The most common type reveals focal lesions with low intensity on T1WI and high intensity on T2WI (Fig. 16.36). Rarely, lesions may be hyperintense on T1WI, probably because of hemorrhage within the myeloma foci.
  - A second pattern consists of a variegated (inhomogeneous) appearance with tiny foci of hypointensity on T1WI and hyperintensity on T2WI.
  - The third diffuse pattern represents total marrow involvement so that on T1WI the replaced fatty marrow is hypointense to disk. The diffuse and variegated appearance on T1WI can be difficult to distinguish from inhomogeneous distribution of fat in older patients.

- Vertebral compression may occur without the marrow being diffusely abnormal on MR and have a vertebra plana pattern. Vertebral compression fractures occur in

50% to 70% of patients and spinal cord compression in 10% to 15% of these cases.

- Radiographs and CT demonstrate purely lytic lesions or diffuse osteopenia. It is unusual for myeloma to involve the pedicles. On CT, destruction of cortical bone is much less common in myeloma than metastatic disease, whereas cancellous vertebral body destruction occurs in both metastatic and myelomatous lesions.

- Myeloma may be difficult to detect with bone scans. A solitary plasmacytoma may be indistinguishable from a lytic metastasis and is a harbinger of multiple myeloma.

### Epidural Lipomatosis

- Epidural lipomatosis can occur from a number of different causes including obesity, steroid use (usually after prolonged use of oral steroids), and Cushing syndrome. The fatty tissue is seen most often in the posterior epidural space and can contribute to spinal stenosis and can produce significant cord or cauda equina compression.

- On MRI, prominent epidural fat is demonstrated to distort the normal round or oval-shaped configuration of the thecal sac, resulting in crowding and compression of thecal sac contents. Treatment involves weight loss and cessation of steroid use, depending on the cause.

## VASCULAR LESIONS

### Infarction

- Spinal cord ischemia and infarction can occur at any location in the cord but has a propensity for the upper thoracic or thoracolumbar regions, particularly the ventral cord because of the tenuous blood supply. Infarction can result from problems associated with the descending aorta, such as atheroma, aortic surgery, and dissecting aneurysm, or from vertebral artery occlusion/dissection, vascular or vasculitic processes, or infectious etiologies, to name a few.

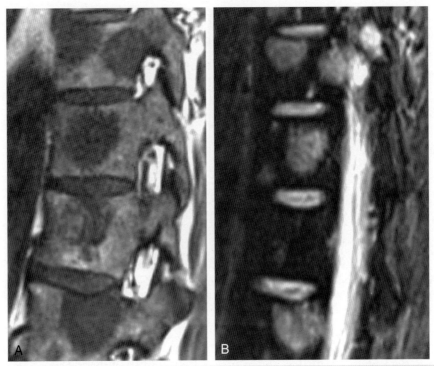

**Fig. 16.36 Multiple myeloma.** (A) Sagittal T1 and (B) sagittal short tau inversion recovery (STIR) images through the midthoracic spine show multiple discrete T1 hypointense and STIR hyperintense marrow lesions in this patient with known multiple myeloma.

- The clinical presentation includes impairment of bowel and bladder function, loss of perineal sensation, and moderate impairment of sensory and motor function of the lower extremities. Ischemia to the conus may result from poor collateral supply after occlusion of the dominant blood supply (artery of Adamkiewicz). Rarely, posterior spinal artery infarcts can be seen.
- On MR, high signal on T2WI is noted in the cord, most commonly the ventral cord, which is usually enlarged, and enhancement may or may not be present (Fig. 16.37). Diffusion restriction in the cord will be seen in the acute setting. Occasionally, vertebral body high signal intensity on T2WI can be identified and is most likely the result of concomitant infarction. Careful attention should be paid to the aorta for aortic dissection or aneurysms as a cause.

## Vascular Malformations

- Spinal vascular malformations are separated into spinal dural arteriovenous fistula (SDAVF), spinal cord arteriovenous malformation (SCAVM), and spinal cord (or perimedullary) arteriovenous fistula (SCAVF) (Fig. 16.38). Treatment of spinal vascular malformations is dependent on many factors, including age, malformation type, and neurologic condition, and consists of embolization, surgery, or a combination of the two. Blood supply to the malformation is very important in determining whether to proceed with embolization or to perform surgery.
- When malformations produce increased venous pressure, they can produce cord edema (Foix Alajouanine syndrome) or subarachnoid hemorrhage. If the venous drainage is intracranial (particularly with SCAVF), patients may present with intracranial subarachnoid hemorrhage. Therefore, the workup for subarachnoid

hemorrhage without clear etiology should include imaging of the spine. There is a differential diagnosis of subarachnoid hemorrhage and hematomyelia.

**TEACHING POINTS**

Spinal Subarachnoid Hemorrhage and Hematomyelia Differential Diagnosis

Trauma
Iatrogenic/postoperative
Coagulation disorders/anticoagulation
Dissections
High-flow vascular malformation
Cavernous angioma
Spinal cord tumor
Spinal artery aneurysm
Spinal venous aneurysm
Vasculitis

## Spinal Dural Arteriovenous Fistula

- SDAVF is the most common spinal vascular malformation having a nidus at or near the nerve root sleeve. This malformation, whose draining veins are most frequently found on the dorsal aspect of the lower thoracic cord or conus medullaris, sometimes has the eponym Foix-Alajouanine syndrome attached to it, to describe the myelopathy secondary to venous hypertension in the cord.
- In approximately 85% of cases, a single radicular artery with systemic pressure is identified draining directly into spinal pial vein(s). However, there are cases with many

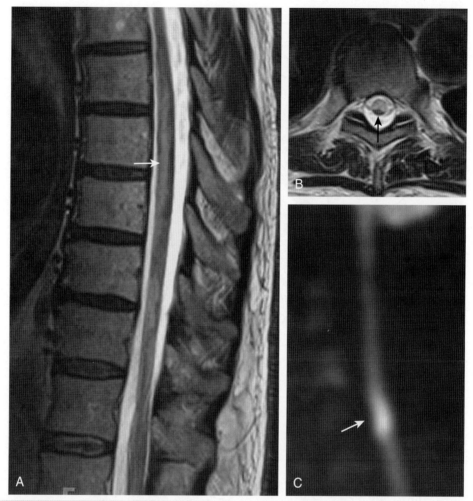

**Fig. 16.37 Cord infarct.** (A) Sagittal T2-weighted imaging (T2WI) shows a long segment abnormal high signal intensity and swelling within the ventral cord at the mid to lower thoracic spine levels *(arrow)*. (B) Axial T2WI confirms involvement of the ventral cord, with preserved normal signal only within the dorsal aspect of the spinal cord *(arrow)*. Although the imaging findings carry a differential diagnosis, the clinical context of abrupt loss of sensation and weakness abruptly after aortic aneurysm repair should make the diagnosis of cord infarct a no-brainer. (C) Diffusion-weighted imaging from another patient shows high signal at the level of cord infarct *(arrow)* relative to the normal cord.

arterial feeders originating from either single or multiple levels that may be either unilateral or bilateral. The systemic pressure in the spinal veins initially dilates these vessels with subsequent kinking and poor venous drainage. This results in venous hypertension defined histopathologically by stasis, edema, ischemia, and leading to swelling and subsequent infarction of the spinal cord. The veins may also appear serpentine.

- Symptoms begin with an insidious onset of lower extremity weakness or sensory changes, associated with nonradiating pain starting in the caudal spinal segments and progressing superiorly. There is a propensity for these to occur in males in their fifth or sixth decade of life or older. This clinical presentation can sometimes be mistaken for degenerative disk disease. CSF protein can be increased mistakenly leading to the thought of a spinal cord tumor.
- The MR findings are key (Fig. 16.39). The spinal cord may be of normal size or enlarged with intramedullary high intensity seen on T2WI, reflecting swelling from venous congestion. T2 hypointense hemorrhage may be seen within the cord or along the leptomeninges. Prominent

vessels on the posterior aspect of the spinal cord are often seen. These vessels enhance and the spinal cord itself, in addition to the veins, may or may not enhance slightly. Spinal MR angiography, when performed appropriately, can be used to localize the arteriovenous fistula and even the feeding vessels.

- Conventional spinal angiography should be performed in equivocal cases, in cases where no clear abnormality is seen on MRI/MR angiography (MRA) but clinical suspicion for high flow vascular malformation remains and for treatment planning purposes.
- Usually, the anterior spinal artery does not arise at the same level as the SDAVF. If it does, then an endovascular approach is contraindicated, and surgical treatment is required. If the malformation is supplied by other vessels, embolization with permanent occlusive agents would be the procedure of choice.
- Occasionally, intracranial dural arteriovenous fistulas may have intraspinal drainage (<5%) via meningeal branches of the external carotid artery or the vertebral artery. These usually involve the medulla or cervical spine and may present acutely with hemorrhage,

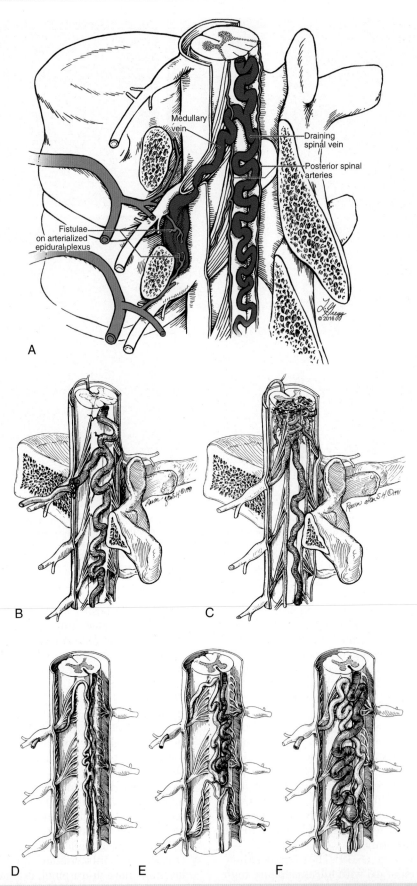

**Fig. 16.38 Schematic representations of vascular malformations of the spinal canal with part of lamina and dura removed.** The more common sites of spinal arteriovenous fistulas include the epidural compartment near the nerve root sleeve (A) and in the proximal nerve root sleeve (B). (C) An intramedullary spinal arteriovenous malformation can have multiple arterial feeders from both the anterior and posterior spinal arteries. The nidus is located within the spinal cord and drains into a dilated venous plexus. (D–F) Variations of perimedullary arteriovenous fistulas: in all three types, the fistulous connection is intradural. These can range from small fistula to large arterial feeder and a massively dilated venous system. Venous aneurysms are often associated with these lesions. (A, Courtesy Lydia Gregg; B–F, Courtesy Barrow Neurological Institute.)

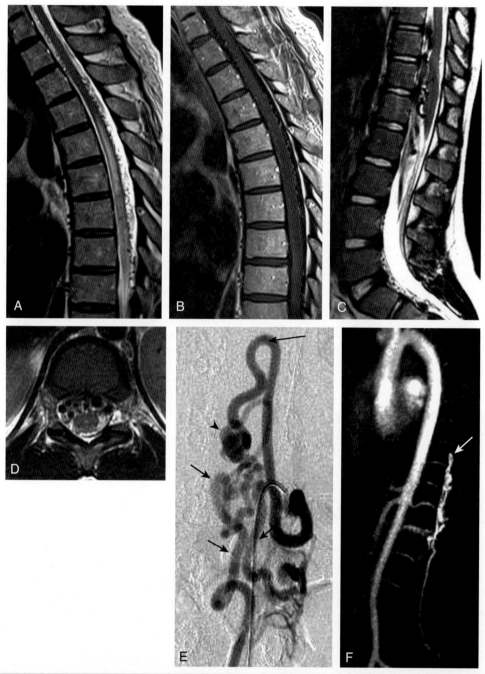

**Fig. 16.39 Arteriovenous malformation.** (A) Sagittal T2-weighted image (T2WI) in a patient with progressive lower extremity weakness shows innumerable flow voids along the surface of the cord, predominantly along the dorsal surface. There is increased T2 signal and expansion of the lower thoracic cord because of venous congestion. (B) Postcontrast sagittal T1-weighted imaging (T1WI) shows some enhancement within these prominent flow voids. Spinal angiogram confirmed presence of a dural arteriovenous fistula, which was successfully embolized. (C) Sagittal and (D) axial T2WI show enlarged serpentine flow voids along the ventral aspect of the lower spinal cord without associated cord signal change. This 6-year-old patient was asymptomatic, and the abnormality was picked up incidentally on another imaging study performed for a different reason, prompting this magnetic resonance imaging (MRI). (E) Conventional spinal angiogram followed, showing a markedly enlarged and tortuous artery of Adamkiewicz *(large arrow)* with a direct fistulous connection to a dilated venous pouch *(arrowhead)* with multiple enlarged draining veins coursing caudally from the fistula *(small arrows)*. (F) Follow-up contrast-enhanced spinal MRA after partial embolization of the fistula shows the fistula and artery of Adamkiewicz *(arrow)* to be much smaller in caliber.

quadriparesis, or medullary dysfunction. High intensity on T2WI in the medulla and/or cervical cord associated with peripheral cord hypointensity should suggest this possible diagnosis.

## Spinal Cord Arteriovenous Malformation

- SCAVMs are intramedullary lesions with a well-defined nidus fed by branches of the anterior or posterior spinal arteries and draining into spinal veins.

- Acute symptoms are caused by intramedullary hemorrhage. Unlike SDAVF, there is no sex predilection, and progressive myelopathy is less common.

## Spinal Cord Arteriovenous Fistula

- SCAVF are intradural extramedullary ("perimedullary") arteriovenous fistulas (without an intervening capillary network) located on the pial surface. They involve the anterior or posterior spinal arteries with a single arteriovenous communication.
- Clinical presentations can vary from progressive myelopathy to hemorrhage, including subarachnoid hemorrhage (up to 30%). Venous aneurysm can be seen with this malformation.

## Cavernous Malformation

- Cavernous malformations of the spinal cord are uncommon intramedullary vascular lesions. They appear similar to those in the brain, which are common.
- The clinical presentation includes pain, weakness, and paresthesias, which may be progressive or episodic and progressive.
- MR is the imaging study of choice, with the malformation appearing round with regions of high signal intensity (methemoglobin) on T1WI and T2WI surrounded by low signal intensity on T2WI (hemosiderin) (Fig. 16.40). There is minimal mass effect or edema unless there has been recent hemorrhage. These lesions may show minimal contrast enhancement. Myelography may be normal or may reveal atrophy or cord expansion. Calcification has been reported. Angiography is usually negative in these cases, although late venous pooling or abnormal draining veins may be found.

## (Hemo)Siderosis

- Recurrent hemorrhage from spinal vascular malformations or hemorrhagic tumors such as an ependymoma or hemangioblastoma is associated with hemosiderin deposition throughout the leptomeninges and intracranially.

## SPINAL TRAUMA/INJURY

- Imaging is required to assess integrity of the spine in the circumstance of severe pain, distracting injuries, and altered awareness. In acute spinal injury, CT is the best method for detecting fractures and dislocations of the bony spine and has replaced radiograph examination at many trauma centers (Fig. 16.41).
- It is very important that thin section axial CT images be reviewed in conjunction with coronal and sagittal

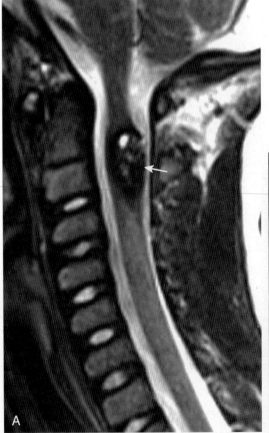
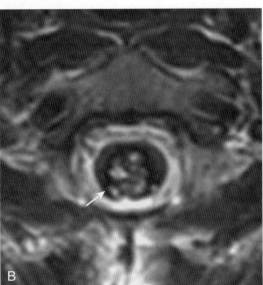

**Fig. 16.40 Cord cavernous malformation.** (A–B) Just like in the brain, a popcorn-shaped lesion with high signal intensity centrally (extracellular methemoglobin) and dark signal peripherally (hemosiderin) in the cord on T2-weighted imaging (T2WI) is characteristic of a cavernoma *(arrows)*. Note absence of high signal within the cervical cord despite the size of the lesion.

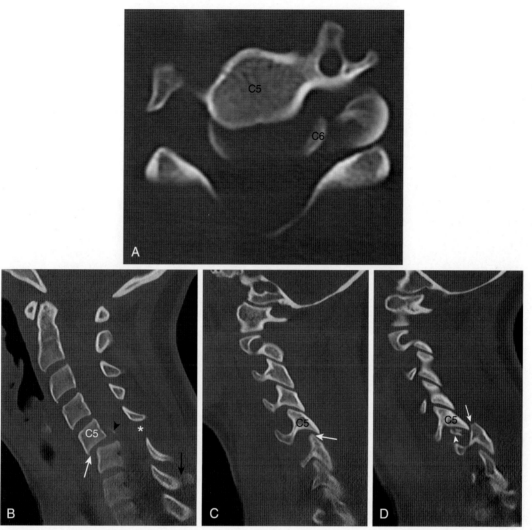

**Fig. 16.41 Cervical spine trauma on computed tomography.** (A) Axial computed tomography (CT) image of the cervical spine at the C5 to C6 level shows both C5 and C6 vertebral bodies present on the same slice. (B) Sagittal CT reconstruction helps us understand what is going on, showing traumatic anterolisthesis of C5 on C6 *(white arrow)* and widening of the interspinous interval *(asterisk)*. A small chip fragment from C5 was left behind *(arrowhead)* during the migration of C5 anteriorly. Note nondisplaced fracture of the C7 spinous process *(black arrow)*. (C) More laterally on the same reconstructed series, there is abnormal widening of the C5 to C6 facet articulation with partial "uncovering" of the facet joint *(arrow)*, disrupting the normal "shingled" appearance of the fact joints. (D) On the other side, the inferior articulating facet of C5 has "jumped" over the superior articulating facet of C6 *(arrow)*, which is fragmented *(arrowhead)*. Three-column injury is *definitely* unstable. A magnetic resonance (MR) image is warranted (barring any contraindications) to assess for potential cord and/or ligamentous injuries and/or intraspinal hemorrhages before urgent spine surgery for stabilization.

reconstructions and that areas of suspicion be confirmed in multiple planes.

■ Angiography by CT, MR, or conventional techniques can assess the integrity of the carotid and vertebral arteries, which can be traumatized in certain types of spine injuries.

■ MR is the only technique that can reliably reveal intrinsic injury to the cord and ligaments (Fig. 16.42). The fibrous nature of the spinal ligaments results in their normal hypointensity on all MR pulse sequences. They should have well-demarcated margins throughout their course. Tears or partial tears resulting in edema are best visualized on STIR images (and almost as well on fat-suppressed T2WI) as high intensity.

■ The sagittal plane depicts injury to the anterior and posterior longitudinal ligaments, the ligamentum flavum, and the interspinous ligaments. High signal within and surrounding facet joints at levels of injury can indicate facet capsular rupture. High T2 signal and ligamentous discontinuity at the tectorial membrane, transverse, and alar ligaments indicate craniocervical ligamentous injury.

■ Injury to these structures may be present even if no fractures are evident by CT. The presence of prevertebral swelling on radiograph or CT should raise suspicion for soft-tissue injury involving the anterior column.

■ In acute spinal cord injury, abnormalities include intramedullary hemorrhage, which may be petechial or diffuse, and swelling, both of which can be appreciated on MR. In severe spinal cord trauma, lacerations and spinal cord transections can be appreciated by MR. Hemorrhage in the cord, hematomyelia, is associated with a poor prognosis.

■ MR can also visualize subluxations and vertebral body fractures, hematomas around ligamentous tears, cord

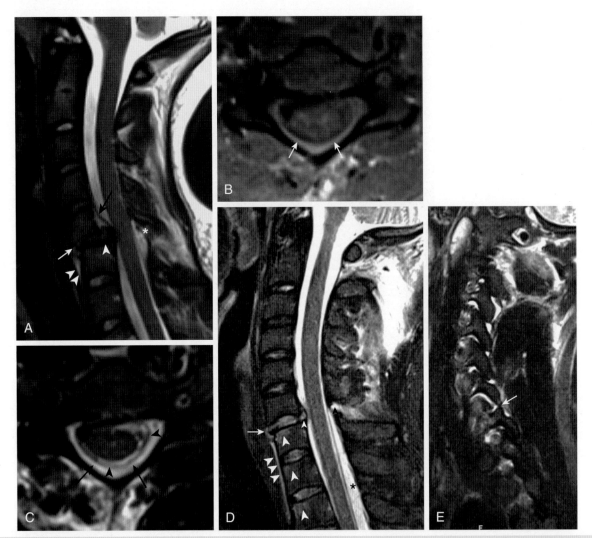

**Fig. 16.42  Magnetic resonance imaging and ligamentous injury.** (A) Sagittal T2-weighted (T2WI) imaging on the same patient as in Fig. 16.41 shows the same traumatic anterolisthesis of C5 on C6 *(white arrow)*. Now we can see the injuries to the soft tissues. There is edema within the prevertebral soft tissues *(double arrowheads)*. There is laxity and disruption of the posterior longitudinal ligament *(black arrow)*. There is elevated T2 signal within the disk, indicating acute disk rupture *(single arrowhead)*. There is disruption of the ligamentum flavum *(asterisk)*, normally seen as dark signal at this level. Note associated widening of the interspinous interval here. The cord looks tight within the canal, but at least the cord signal looks good. (B) Axial gradient echo, and (C) axial T2 images show epidural hematoma surrounding the thecal sac *(arrows)* contributing to the crowding of the cord within the thecal sac. In the cervical spine, the dural margins should approximate the bony canal margins, but in this case, they are lifted off as a result of the epidural hematoma (see C, *arrowheads*). (D) In a different patient with similar injury, sagittal short tau inversion recovery (STIR) shows anterior longitudinal ligament disruption *(arrow)* and associated edema in the prevertebral tissues *(triple arrowheads)*, acute disk rupture *(small arrowhead)*, ligamentum flavum disruption *(black arrowhead)*, and abnormal T2 high signal within the interspinous ligament (at and posterior to the *black arrowhead*), as well as marked edema within the soft tissues of the upper neck. Note the elevation of the dura posteriorly, resulting from epidural fluid collection *(black asterisk)*. Bone contusions along the superior endplates of C7, T1, and T2 *(large single arrowheads)* were not appreciable by computed tomography (CT) but are clearly present on STIR. (E) In this same patient, the inferior articulating facet of C6 is "perched" on the superior articulating facet of C7, and edema around the facet joint *(arrow)* indicates facet capsular rupture.

compression, and traumatic disk herniations. Sometimes the linear areas of high signal on STIR images may indicate a fracture/bone edema that is not evident (initially) on the multiplanar high resolution CT scan.

- Patients with acute spinal cord injury without radiographic abnormalities (SCIWORA) and normal MR findings have the best prognosis, whereas patients with hemorrhage and/or low or high signal intensity on T1WI and high signal on T2WI within the cord have the poorest prognosis.
- The pathologic consequences of significant spinal cord trauma include (1) atrophy, (2) myelomalacia,

(3) posttraumatic syrinx, (4) arachnoid cyst, and (5) arachnoiditis.

- Radiographs can also play an important role in assessing cervical spine instability in both the acute and nonacute settings. Changes in alignment of the spine on radiographs obtained in flexed, neutral, and extended positions can indicate ligamentous laxity. These patients can benefit from spine-stabilizing surgery. In the acute setting, these examinations should be performed under the direct supervision of a clinician who knows and has examined the patient before acquiring images. The patient's neck should not be directly manipulated by the technologist or any physician who has not performed a thorough clinical assessment of the patient.

- In the lumbar spine, transverse process fractures outnumber vertebral body compression fractures as most common. They are often seen in association with motor vehicle collisions (MVCs). There is a high rate of concomitant abdominopelvic visceral injury.
- Beware the transverse process fracture of the cervical spine. These may be subtle, may involve the foramen transversarium, and may lead to vertebral artery injury.

## Cervical Nerve Root Avulsions

- These are the result of traction injuries on the upper extremities that tear the roots from the spinal cord (Fig. 16.43). The roots are absent on one side, and the cord is consequently pulled to the contralateral side. Thin section MR or CT myelographic images can show the nerve root disruption. Pseudomeningoceles are associated with this injury. They result from tears of the arachnoid and dura, which can be identified on MR or CT myelography.

## Spine Fractures and Dislocations

- Spinal stability has been defined as the capacity of the spine under physiologic loads to limit displacement so as not to compromise or damage the spinal cord and nerve roots. Stability also denotes prevention of deformity or pain secondary to anatomic changes. Conversely, clinical

instability may be defined as greater than normal range of motion within a spinal segment so as to assume a risk of neurologic injury. Bones and ligaments are responsible for spinal cord stability.

- The implication of clinical instability is that surgical intervention is necessary to stabilize the spine and protect the cord. Although certain fracture types can be characterized as stable or unstable based on radiographic appearance, not all can, and very often the clinical evaluation also plays a crucial role in determining spine stability in conjunction with imaging findings.

**TEACHING POINTS**

Stability of Cervical Spine Fractures

**Typically Considered Stable**

Pillar fracture
Posterior neural arch fracture, atlas
Unilateral facet dislocation
Spinous process fracture
Clay-shoveler fracture
Transverse process fracture
Compression fracture of <25% of vertebral body height
Anterior wedge fracture
Isolated avulsion without ligamentous tear
Type I odontoid fracture
Type III odontoid fracture (usually)

(Continued)

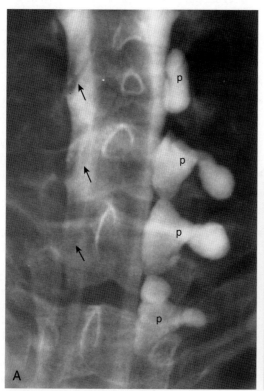

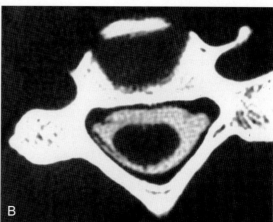

**Fig. 16.43 Cervical root avulsion.** (A) Myelogram illustrates multiple cervical nerve root avulsions manifested by multiple pseudomeningoceles (*p*) from the torn arachnoid and dura. Ipsilateral nerve roots are not seen, having been torn and retracted. Contralateral nerve roots (*arrows*) can be identified. (B) Note the absence of anterior and posterior roots on the *left* side with an incipient pseudomeningocele from the empty root sleeve on this computed tomography (CT) myelogram.

Endplate fracture
Osteophyte fracture (not including corner or teardrop fracture)
Trabecular bone injury

**Typically Considered Unstable**

Atlantooccipital subluxation/dislocation
Bilateral C1-C2 dislocation
Bilateral facet, laminae, or pedicle fractures and/or dislocation
Chance fractures
Extension teardrop fracture
Flexion teardrop fracture
Hangman fracture
Hyperextension fracture-dislocation
Type II odontoid fracture
Jefferson fracture

- The spinal column can be divided into three columns. The anterior column is composed of the anterior longitudinal ligament, the anterior annulus, and the anterior portion of the vertebral body. The middle column is delineated by the posterior longitudinal ligament, the posterior portion of the annulus, and the posterior aspect of the vertebral body and disk. The posterior column contains the neural arch, facet joints and capsules, ligamentum flavum, and all other posterior spinal ligaments.
- The middle column is critical because instability occurs when two of the three columns are injured (Fig. 16.44). Compression fractures result in anterior column injury (usually stable), whereas burst fractures affect the anterior and middle columns (unstable). Flexion-distraction injuries affect the middle and posterior columns, and

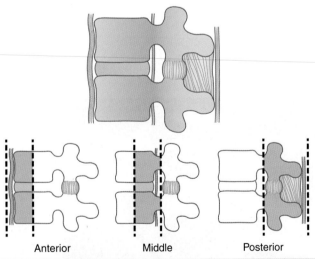

**Fig. 16.44** The three-column classification model of the spine proposed by Denis represented an advance in thinking about spinal injuries over the previous two-column model. The concept of the middle column, composed of the posterior longitudinal ligament, the posterior aspect of the annulus fibrosus, and the posterior portion of the vertebral body and disk were added. *(From Garfin SR, Blair B, Eismont FJ, Abitbol JJ. Thoracic and upper lumbar spine injuries. In: Browner BD, Jupiter JB, Levine AM, et al., eds. Skeletal Trauma: Fracture, Dislocations, Ligamentous Injuries. 2nd ed. Philadelphia: Saunders; 1998:967; Vol 1.)*

Anterior          Middle          Posterior

fracture-dislocation injuries result in a three-column injury.
- Hyperflexion is a forward rotation and/or translation of a vertebra with both distraction of the posterior column and compression of the anterior column.
- Hyperextension injuries involve posterior rotation/translation. Here the anterior and middle columns bear the brunt of the injury (anterior longitudinal ligament, disk, and posterior longitudinal ligament).
- "Sprains" are minor tears of the supraspinous, interspinous, and facet capsules from flexion-distraction injuries, which can result in anterior subluxation.
- Anterior subluxation is seen as a hyperkyphotic angulation of the cervical spine with widening of the distance between the spinous processes and interlaminar space compared with other levels (fanning). Other findings include narrowing of the anterior disk space with widening of its posterior aspect with or without anterior translation of the involved vertebral body, widening of the space between the subluxed vertebral body and the superior articular facet of the lower vertebral body, and subluxation of the facet joints. Flexion-extension radiographs can best demonstrate this injury.
- There are a range of facet-related injuries from fractures to facet subluxations to perched facets to facet dislocations (jumped facets) that can be unilateral or bilateral (see Figs. 16.41 and 16.42).
- Rotational facet injury is a generic term used to describe unilateral facet dislocation/subluxation and unilateral facet fractures with malalignment.
- Facet subluxations without fractures occur in only 25% of cases but have a higher rate of cord injury and therefore should be stabilized. It is usually the inferior articulating facet of the vertebral body above that fractures. Facet fractures with vertebral injury lead to rotational instability and require surgical fixation.

## Atlanto-occipital Dislocation

- Atlantooccipital dislocation (otherwise known as craniocervical dissociation) occurs as a result of injury to the stabilizing ligaments at the craniocervical junction (Fig. 16.45). This is typically considered a fatal injury, although there are many case reports of survival.
- Severe injuries include pontomedullary junction laceration, contusion or laceration of the inferior medulla and spinal cord, injury to the midbrain, subarachnoid hemorrhage, subdural hemorrhage, and vascular dissection.
- The incidence is increased in children, predominantly because of their small occipital condyles and horizontal plane of the atlantooccipital joints.
- Atlantooccipital dislocation can be associated with severe hyperextension, type I odontoid fracture (see Odontoid Fracture subsection), loss of the normal relationship of the occipital condyles to C1, and prevertebral swelling. Longitudinal distraction and anterior or posterior dislocation of the occiput relative to the atlas is observed as a result of tearing of the tectorial membrane and alar ligaments (Fig. 16.46) and is seen as increased distance between the basion and dens (greater than 12 mm on lateral radiograph).
- CT can detect basion and condylar fractures; however, if there is no associated bony fracture, this severe injury

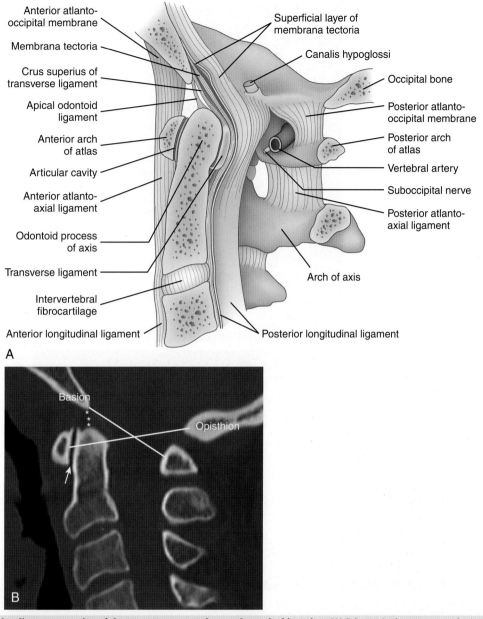

Anterior atlanto-occipital membrane
Membrana tectoria
Crus superius of transverse ligament
Apical odontoid ligament
Anterior arch of atlas
Articular cavity
Anterior atlanto-axial ligament
Odontoid process of axis
Transverse ligament
Intervertebral fibrocartilage
Anterior longitudinal ligament

Superficial layer of membrana tectoria
Canalis hypoglossi
Occipital bone
Posterior atlanto-occipital membrane
Posterior arch of atlas
Vertebral artery
Suboccipital nerve
Posterior atlanto-axial ligament
Arch of axis
Posterior longitudinal ligament

A

Basion
Opisthion

B

**Fig. 16.45 Stabilizing ligaments and useful measurements at the craniocervical junction.** (A) Schematic demonstrates the important stabilizing ligaments at the craniocervical junction. (B) Useful measurements at the craniocervical junction to keep in mind include the anterior atlantodental interval *(arrow)*, which should measure no greater than 3 mm in an adult, and should not change in flexed and extended positions as well as the basion-axial interval *(asterisks)*, which should measure less than 12 mm. Powers ratio is calculated as the distance between the basion and spinolaminar line of C1 divided by the distance between the anterior arch of C1 and the opisthion. A ratio greater than 1 implies occipitoatlantal dislocation.

can be altogether missed when reviewing axial CT images alone. Review of multiplanar images is critical, and in this type of injury, coronal and sagittal reformatted images will demonstrate widening between the lateral masses of C1 and the occipital condyles. MR with T2WI and STIR images reveal prevertebral soft-tissue injury, ligamentous tears, epidural hematoma, spinal cord injury, and brainstem injury. Occipital condyle fractures may appear as avulsion type injuries.

■ In children, this diagnosis can be problematic because of variable bone ossification in the craniocervical junction, especially in the dens where the basion-dens interval is reported to be unreliable in patients younger than 13 years of age.

■ Fig. 16.47 shows the three types of occipital condyle fractures.

## Atlantoaxial Distraction

■ This injury occurs as a result of severe extension. There is disruption of the articular capsules, alar ligaments, transverse ligament, and tectorial membrane between C1 and C2. Occasionally, there is a type I dens fracture. There is obvious widening of the space between C1 and C2. Look for prevertebral swelling on plain films and CT. On MR, edema can be identified on STIR or T2WI in the prevertebral, interspinous, and nuchal ligaments. Other reported findings may be facet widening, epidural hematoma, and focal increased T2 signal intensity in the spinal cord.

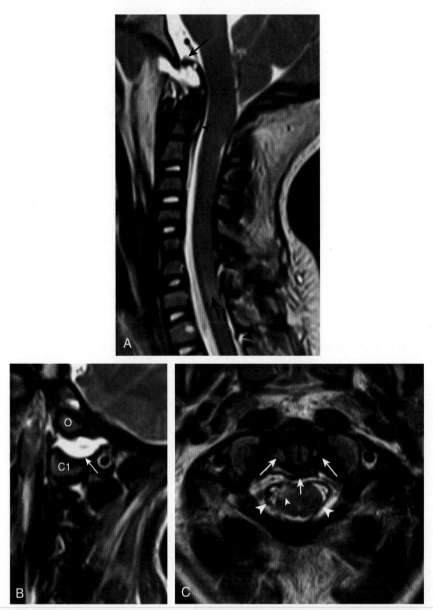

**Fig. 16.46 Craniocervical dissociation.** (A) Sagittal T2-weighted imaging (T2WI) shows disruption and redundancy of the tectorial membrane *(small arrow)*. There is widening of the space between the tip of the clivus and the dens with absence of the apical ligament usually seen connecting the tip of clivus to the dens, also disrupted. The transverse ligament *(small arrowhead)* is elevated off of the posterior aspect of the dens. Despite the severe injury at the craniocervical level, the atlantodental interval is preserved so the C1 to C2 relationship is maintained appropriately anteriorly. Multiple foci of ligamentum flavum disruption are present at other cervical levels *(large arrowheads)* and there is T2 high signal indicating edema within the cord at the C7 level *(large arrow)*. (B) Far lateral image from the same series shows abnormal widening and fluid *(arrows)* between the occipital condyle (O) and C1 lateral mass *(CI)*, which was present bilaterally (only one side shown here). Also note that the occipital condyle is ever so slightly anteriorly displaced relative to the lateral mass of C1. (C) Axial T2 image shows high signal at the attachment of the bilateral alar ligaments at the dens *(large arrows)* and elevation and laxity of the transverse ligament *(small arrow)*. There is elevation of the dura within the spinal canal *(large arrowheads)* as a result of epidural hematoma and there is another contusion within the cord *(small arrowhead)*.

## Atlantoaxial Rotatory Subluxation

■ Atlantoaxial rotatory subluxation results in torticollis, so that the atlas is rotated and dislocated from the articular processes of the axis. Head rotation does not correct what appears to be an asymmetric widening of the space between the odontoid with respect to the lateral masses of C1, nor does the spinous process of C1 move. CT or plain radiography performed with the head turned to the left, right, and in the neutral position can reveal the lack of correction.

## Atlantoaxial Instability

■ Atlantoaxial dislocation can be caused by trauma with associated fractures and rupture of the transverse ligament or may be seen in nontraumatic situations associated with transverse ligament laxity or odontoid process malformations (os odontoideum, ossiculum terminale, or agenesis of the odontoid base, apical segment, or the entire base). This injury can be fatal, yet patients can be completely asymptomatic.

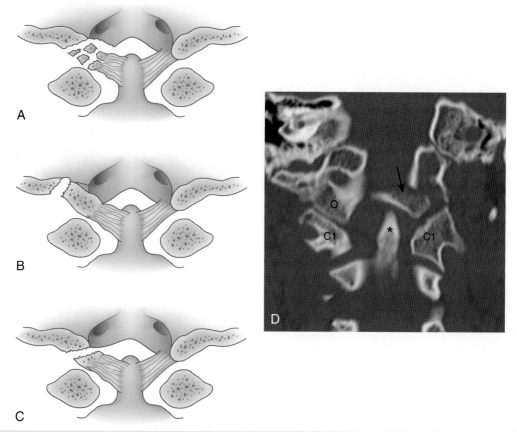

**Fig. 16.47** The classification of Anderson and Montesano describes three basic types of occipital condyle fractures. The first (A) is an impaction-type fracture, which is usually the result of an asymmetric axial load to the head; it may be associated with other lateral mass fractures in the upper cervical spine. (B) The next type is a basilar skull-type occipital condyle fracture, which may be the result of a distraction force applied through the alar and apical ligament complex. (C) Type III avulsion-type occipital condyle fracture. (D) Coronal computed tomography (CT) reconstruction shows the normal relationship between the occipital condyle (O) and C1 lateral mass (C1) on the *right*. The dens of C2 is indicated by an *asterisk*. On the *left*, there is an occipital condyle fracture with displacement and angulation of the occipital condyle fracture fragment *(arrow)*. Disruption of the apical and alar ligaments was demonstrated on subsequent magnetic resonance imaging (MRI) (not shown). (B, Redrawn from Anderson P, Montesano P. Morphology and treatment of occipital condyle fractures. *Spine*. 1988;13:731.)

---

**TEACHING POINTS**

Nontraumatic Causes of Atlantoaxial Instability

- Odontoid process malformations
- Infections such as tonsillitis and pharyngitis (Grisel syndrome)
- Down syndrome (trisomy 21)
- Marfan syndrome
- Neurofibromatosis
- Ankylosing spondylitis
- Rheumatoid arthritis
- Calcium pyrophosphate deposition disease
- Bone tumors

---

- The anterior atlantodental interval can be abnormally widened as a result of ligamentous laxity and can vary in width on patient positioning (Fig. 16.48).

## Basilar Invagination/Basilar Impression

- These are descriptions for congenital or acquired upward migration of the dens above the level of the foramen magnum. The term *impression* is reserved for cases where the underlying bone is abnormal, whereas invagination implies no intrinsic bone pathology (Fig. 16.49).

**TEACHING POINTS**

Causes of Basilar Impression/Invagination

Congenital causes:
- Osteogenesis imperfecta
- Klippel-Feil syndrome
- Achondroplasia
- Chiari malformations

Acquired causes:
- Pannus formation from rheumatoid arthritis
- Paget disease
- Metastatic disease
- Metabolic derangements such as hyperparathyroidism and rickets

---

- The displaced dens can impress upon the brainstem and can cause neurologic compromise, hydrocephalus, syrinx, and can even be fatal.
- On imaging, if the dens extends greater than 3 mm above a line drawn from the hard palate to the opisthion (Chamberlain line), or greater than 5 mm above a line drawn from hard palate to the inferior-most margin of the occipital bone (McGregor line), then basilar invagination is present. Surgical stabilization is typically required in these cases.

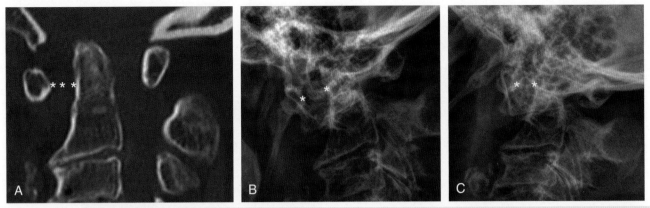

**Fig. 16.48  Atlantoaxial instability.** (A) Sagittal computed tomography (CT) image shows abnormal widening of the anterior atlantodental interval (demarcated by *asterisks*). This should be no wider than 3 mm in an adult and is enlarged in this case as a result of degenerative pannus (not shown). (B) Flexion and (C) extension radiographs of the cervical spine show that despite this patient's limited excursion, this interval is wider in the flexed position than the extended position, indicating ligamentous laxity and instability.

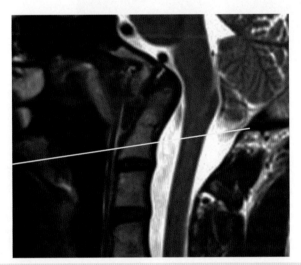

**Fig. 16.49  Basilar invagination.** Sagittal T2-weighted imaging (T2WI) scan from a patient with Klippel-Feil syndrome shows superior migration of the dens relative to the McGregor line (*white line* depicted), indicating basilar invagination. The marrow is normal, hence the term *invagination*, rather than impression. There is mild mass effect on the ventral medulla as a consequence, although (good news!) there is no abnormal signal in the brain stem. Note the flattened appearance of the clivus: the basal angle measured 150 degrees, indicating platybasia.

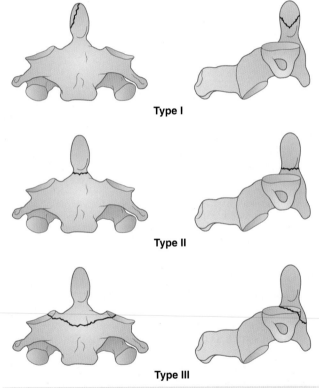

**Type I**

**Type II**

**Type III**

**Fig. 16.50  Types of odontoid fractures.** This diagram illustrates the configuration of the three types of odontoid fractures from frontal (*left-sided* images) and lateral (*right-sided* images) perspectives. (From Modic M, Masaryk T, Ross J. *Magnetic Resonance Imaging of the Spine*. 1st ed. Mosby; 1989.)

## Odontoid Fracture

■ Odontoid fractures have been divided into oblique fractures through the upper portion of the dens (type I), transverse fractures through the junction of the dens with the body of the axis (type II) (unstable), and fractures extending into the cancellous portion of the body of the axis (type III) (Fig. 16.50).

## Os Odontoideum

■ Os odontoideum is a round smooth bony ossicle that is seen superior to the base of the dens. Its position is variable either in the position of the odontoid process (orthotopic) or at the foramen magnum near the base of the occiput (dystopic). Originally thought to be a congenital or developmental anomaly, it is now thought to be the result of an acquired or posttraumatic cause. There is

an association, albeit infrequent, with Klippel-Feil syndrome, myelodysplasia, Morquio syndrome, Down syndrome, and spondyloepiphyseal dysplasia.

■ On lateral radiographs, there is commonly a smoothly marginated bone ossicle, separated by a zone of radiolucency, above the superior facets of axis (Fig. 16.51).

■ The os is embedded within the transverse atlantoaxial ligament and is associated with atlantoaxial instability, translating over the axis and at times producing spinal

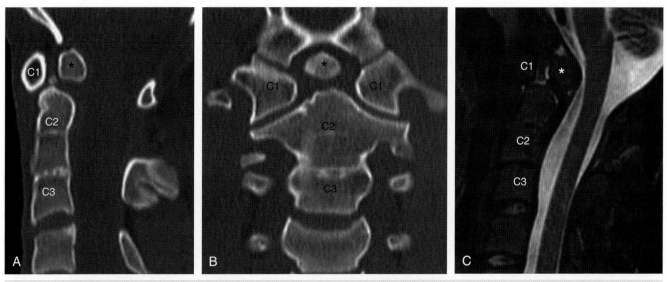

**Fig. 16.51 Os odontoideum.** (A) Sagittal and (B) coronal computed tomography (CT) reconstructions along with (C) sagittal short tau inversion recovery (STIR) image show well-corticated ossific density *(asterisk)* above the dens of C2, representing the os. There is a calcific density between the anterior arch of C1 and the os on the sagittal CT image, suggesting possible previous trauma. There is incomplete segmentation of the C2 and C3 vertebral bodies.

cord compression. This usually requires surgical correction by posterior atlantoaxial fusion.

■ The issue for radiologists is the differentiation of the os from a type I or type II odontoid fracture. Acute fractures do not have smoothly corticated margins as seen with os odontoideum; rather they have sharp radiolucent margins.

## Jefferson Fracture

■ Jefferson fractures are breaks in the ring of the atlas that were classically described as having four sites (junctions of the anterior and posterior arches with the lateral masses, which are where the bone is thinnest), although there are many variations in the number of fractures (Fig. 16.52). They are caused by compressive forces. Tears of the transverse ligament are associated with Jefferson fracture.

## Hangman Fracture

■ Hangman fractures result from hyperextension of the neck and are fracture dislocations of C2. The spectrum of traumatic spondylolisthesis is seen in Fig. 16.53. When both pedicles are fractured, there is anterior subluxation of the body of C2 on C3, whereas the posterior ring does not move, being fixed by the inferior articular processes.

## Thoracolumbar Spine Fractures

■ Numerous classification schemes for categorizing thoracolumbar spine fractures have been proposed to guide clinical management, with the thoracolumbar injury classification and severity score (TLICS) most recently introduced to provide a clearer basis for the need for urgent surgical intervention by including both imaging and clinical parameters in the decision process. This classification scheme takes into account and applies a numerical scoring system (1–10) to injury morphology, integrity of the posterior ligament complex, and the patient's clinical symptomatology in determining the need for urgent surgical spine stabilization (score >5).

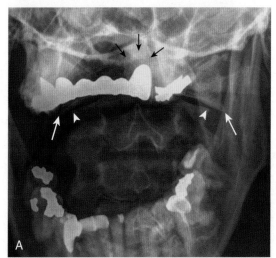

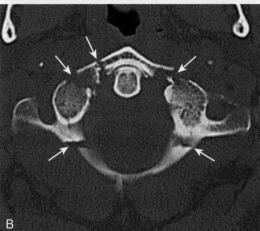

**Fig. 16.52 Jefferson fracture.** (A) Open mouth odontoid view radiograph shows lateral subluxation bilaterally of the lateral masses of C1 *(white arrows)* with regard to the lateral margins of the lateral masses of C2 *(arrowheads)*. Normally, these structures should line up with each other. The tip of the dens in indicated by *black arrows*. (B) Axial computed tomography (CT) image from the same patient shows multiple fractures *(arrows)* through the anterior and posterior arches of C1. The anterior atlantodental interval is not widened in this case.

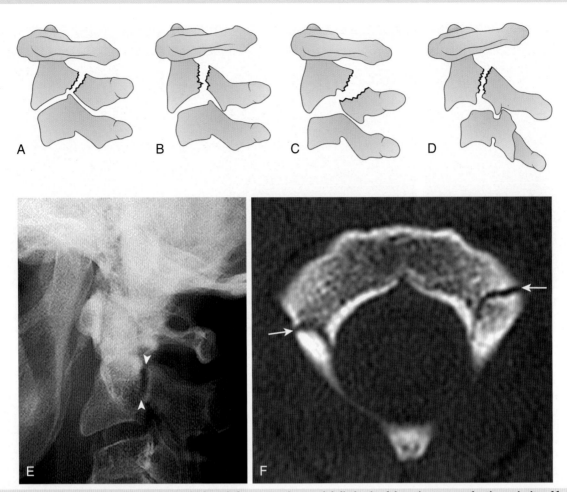

**Fig. 16.53   The classification devised by Levine and Edwards for traumatic spondylolisthesis of the axis accounts for the majority of fractures of this type.** (A) The most common pattern is type I, which is characterized radiographically by a fracture through the neural arch with minimal translation (<3 mm) and minimal angulation. Not pictured in the classification is the later addition of type IA, which has also been called *atypical hangman fracture*. (B) Type II fractures have significant angulation (>3 degrees) and translation (>3 mm) and are much more unstable than type I fractures. (C) Type IIA fractures are identified radiographically by an oblique fracture line with minimal translation but significant angulation. (D) Type III axial fractures combine bilateral facet dislocation between C2 and C3 with a fracture of the neural arch of the axis. (E) Lateral radiograph shows acute fracture through the pars interarticularis of C2 *(arrowheads)*. Note slight anterolisthesis of C2 with regard to C3. (F) Axial computed tomography (CT) image shows a fracture defect extending through the pars interarticularis of C2 bilaterally *(arrows)*. (A-C, From Levine AM, Edwards CC. The management of traumatic spondylolisthesis of the axis. *J Bone Joint Surg Am*. 1985;67:217–226; D, From Levine AM, Edwards CC. Treatment of injuries in the C1-C2 complex. *Orthop Clin North Am*. 1986;17:42.)

- Several observations should be recorded in the report that can aid the spine surgeon to decide as to whether or not urgent intervention is required (Fig. 16.54). This includes a description of the fracture pattern (compression, burst, translation/rotation, distraction).
  - Compression fractures are those that involve endplate injuries with or without anterior cortex injuries but with preservation of the posterior vertebral body wall.
  - Burst fractures are comminuted fractures that involve the posterior vertebral body with displacement of superior endplate fragments into the spinal canal and are a result of axial loading injury.
  - Translational injuries result in lateral displacement of one vertebral body with respect to another.
  - Distraction injuries result in widening of bony relationships in vertical plane.
- For all injury types, percent vertebral body height loss; presence of retropulsion and impact on spinal canal diameter; kyphosis; and the presence of intraspinal hemorrhage should be described in the radiology report.

- Additionally, presence of posterior ligament complex injury should be assessed, evidenced by facet joint or interspinous distance widening, spinous process avulsion injury, or vertebral body dislocations on radiograph or CT. On MRI, injury to the supraspinous and interspinous ligaments, ligamentum flavum, facet capsules, imply injury to the posterior ligament complex. Increased T2 signal within these structures and focal discontinuity of the T2 dark stabilizing ligaments can suggest the diagnosis of posterior ligament complex injury.
- Presence of intraspinal hemorrhage and cord/nerve root injury should also be reported.
- Chance fractures are flexion/distraction injuries that occur at the thoracolumbar junction and are typically seen as a result of lap seat belt injury in an MVC or fall from an axial loading injury. The vertebral body, including anterior and posterior aspects as well as the posterior elements, are fractured. All three columns are involved, and there is a high probability of concomitant abdominal injury.

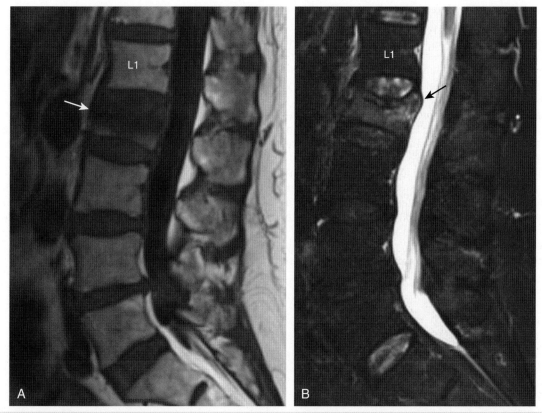

**Fig. 16.54 Acute compression fracture.** (A) Sagittal T1-weighted imaging (T1WI) and (B) short tau inversion recovery scans show abnormal signal intensity indicating edema at the L2 vertebral body *(arrows)*. Specifically, there is disruption along the superior endplate, resulting in at the most 25% loss of height of L2. There is minimal posterior bulging of the superior L2 endplate into the spinal canal, without frank disruption of the posterior ligament complex and without significant canal compromise. There is no cord signal abnormality, and no intraspinal hemorrhage is present.

- The most common fractures seen in MVCs involving the lumbar spine are transverse process avulsion fractures. These are often at multiple levels and bilateral and occur as a result of psoas muscle contractions leading to avulsions or from extreme rotation or sideways bending from MVC impact. These are stable fractures, although when seen, you should look carefully for other potentially unstable fractures elsewhere in the spine.
- Vertebral compression fractures are next most common.

## Insufficiency Fractures of the Sacrum

- These pathologic injuries result from the inability of abnormal bone to withstand normal stress and are seen after radiation therapy or secondary to postmenopausal or steroid-induced osteoporosis.
- The major finding is linear defect running vertically (parallel to the sacroiliac joints) in the sacral alae, usually at the first through third sacral segments. The underlying marrow disease can make the fractures difficult to appreciate on CT.
- On MRI, T1 and T2 hypointense signal reflecting the fracture defect, with or without edema in the adjacent marrow is seen.
- Radionuclide bone scans reveal increased uptake ("Honda" sign).

## Spinal Cord Injury Without Radiologic Abnormality

- Spinal cord injury without radiologic abnormality (SCIWORA) presents as myelopathy after a traumatic

event, but the imaging of the cord is normal. This is more commonly seen in children with cervical spine injuries. It is presumed that the ligamentous laxity that children have can lead to injuries not apparent on plain film or CT. The cause is usually a hyperextension injury and patients may present with central cord symptoms. MRI may show ligamentous injuries and/or cartilaginous fractures. Treatment is immobilization.

## AO Spine Classification System

- You have already seen a number of fracture classification systems discussed in this chapter, which are used heterogeneously among imagers and spine surgeons. Well here comes another!
- The AO spine classification system aims to unify fracture descriptions so that we are all speaking the same language. As such, it is gaining in favor as a means of incorporating fracture morphology with clinical factors to aid in clinical decision-making.
- In addition to morphologic descriptors, each classification system considers neurological signs (N0–N4, neurologically intact to complete spinal cord injury). This part is for our clinical colleagues examining the patient.
- Each of the classification systems also has its own specific variables (modifiers) that may affect clinical outcome (e.g., underlying clinical conditions like ankylosing spondylitis or osteoporosis) and can be optionally added to the classification to inform management.

- *The Upper Cervical Injury Classification System* categorizes injury by site including occipital condyle and craniocervical junction (I), C1 ring or C1 to C2 joint (II), and C2 and C2 to C3 joint (III). These site-specific injuries are then further classified by type: bony injury (A), tension band/ligamentous injury (B), or translation injuries (C). The injury in Fig. 16.46 would be considered IC, for example.

- *The Subaxial Injury Classification System* categorizes injuries into compression (A), tension band (B), translation (C), and facet related injuries (F). Types A, B, and F are further subclassified numerically by morphology (A0-A4, from no morphologic injury to burst fracture), location (B1-B3, anterior and/or posterior tension band) or both (F1-F4, from nondisplaced to subluxation) with a higher number signifying a higher level of injury. The injuries in Fig 16.42 would be classified as type C.

- *The Thoracolumbar Injury Classification System* similarly classifies injury by morphology and includes compression (A), distraction (B), and displacement/translational injuries (C). Types A and B are also further subclassified with a numerical descriptor of morphology (A0-A4, from no morphologic injury to burst fracture) and pattern (B1-B3, transosseous tension band, posterior tension band, hyperextension injuries). The injury in Fig 16.54 would be classified as A3.

- *The Sacral Injury Classification System* also categorizes injuries by type including lower sacrococcygeal (A), posterior pelvic (B), and spinopelvic (C) injuries. A numerical subclassification further characterizes each type by morphology.

- Whether or not you choose to use this classification system or another, the most important take home point is the need for clear and concise communication with the clinical team. So pick up that phone or reach out on your secure chat platform and let them know what you see!

# Index

Page numbers followed by *b* indicate boxes; *f,* figures; and *t,* tables.

## A

# O